Sleep and Breathing in Children

LUNG BIOLOGY IN HEALTH AND DISEASE

Executive Editor

Claude Lenfant

Former Director, National Heart, Lung, and Blood Institute
National Institutes of Health
Bethesda, Maryland

The opinions expressed in these volumes do not necessarily represent the views of the National Institutes of Health.

Sleep and Breathing in Children

Second Edition

Developmental Changes in Breathing During Sleep

Edited by

Carole L. Marcus
University of Pennsylvania School of Medicine
Philadelphia, Pennsylvania, USA

John L. Carroll
University of Arkansas for Medical Sciences
Little Rock, Arkansas, USA

David F. Donnelly
Yale University School of Medicine
New Haven, Connecticut, USA

Gerald M. Loughlin
Weill Medical College of Cornell University
New York, New York, USA

informa
healthcare

New York London

Informa Healthcare USA, Inc.
52 Vanderbilt Avenue
New York, NY 10017

© 2008 by Informa Healthcare USA, Inc.
Informa Healthcare is an Informa business

No claim to original U.S. Government works
Printed in the United States of America on acid-free paper
10 9 8 7 6 5 4 3 2 1

International Standard Book Number-10: 1-4200-6082-1 (Hardcover)
International Standard Book Number-13: 978-1-4200-6082-9 (Hardcover)

For Corporate Sales and Reprint Permissions call 212-520-2700 or write to: Sales Department, 52 Vanderbilt Avenue, 16th floor, New York, NY 10017.

Visit the Informa Web site at
www.informa.com

and the Informa Healthcare Web site at
www.informahealthcare.com

Introduction

> Sleep is the only medicine that gives me ease.
>
> Sophocles (496–406 BC), *Philoctetes*

Philoctetes, a play written and presented by Sophocles in 409 BC, is based on the adventures, or rather misadventures, of the hero Philoctetes, who was the son of the mythological king of Thessaly. He had been deported by the Greeks on an island where he suffered physically and psychologically. It is while commenting on his fate that he stated, "Sleep is the only medicine that gives me ease."

Of course, at that time, no one knew much about the biology of sleep, but it appears that it was already recognized that (good) sleep is an effective regulator of many biological and mental functions. Today, sleep research and sleep medicine have clearly demonstrated that sleep is a determinant of good health. Impaired or disordered sleep is associated with numerous conditions, some quite serious like sleep apnea and/or hypertension, among others.

We have learned that infants, children, and adolescents are, as adults, affected by sleep disorders; this is a critical problem because physiological and mental functions develop during the early years of life. The younger the age, the more the sleep required. We also have learned that adolescents of school age will be at risk of learning, health, behavioral, and mood impairments if they do not have enough sleep (8 to 9.5 hours) or if their sleep is disordered. At the same time, we have also learned through extensive research that sleep is a complex process and that sleep patterns evolve during the years of physical growth and maturation. In addition, during these years, many physiological functions develop—respiratory, circulatory, and endocrine.

In 2000, the series of monographs *Lung Biology in Health and Disease* introduced a volume titled *Sleep and Breathing in Children* The editors, Drs. Gerald M. Loughlin, John L. Carroll, and Carole L. Marcus, aimed to emphasize the importance of the interactions of sleep and breathing during the developmental journey from infancy to adolescence. The authors and editors underscored the need for further research to understand and hopefully to eventually correct the disordered patterns of sleep and breathing in early life so that these disorders would not spill into, and worsen, during adult life.

Since then, a considerable amount of research has been done and our knowledge on the development of sleep and breathing and the relationship—perhaps interdependency—between these two functions has markedly increased. Thus, it is with thanks and gratitude that the series of monographs Lung Biology in Health and Disease welcomes the publication of this new volume, *Sleep and Breathing in Children: Developmental Changes in Breathing During Sleep*. Although the title is partly similar to that of the Loughlin et al. volume, the scope of the two volumes is very different. This current edition is in two volumes; one focuses on developmental changes in sleep patterns and the other on developmental changes in breathing during sleep.

The editors of this new monograph, Drs. Carole L. Marcus, John Carroll, David Donnelly, and Gerald Loughlin, have reached out to experts from several countries and institutions to present a complete state of our current knowledge. The readership of these volumes will undoubtedly be stimulated by the new developments presented by the authors and will appreciate that it brings us closer to helping infants and children suffering from disordered sleep and breathing. As the executive editor of this series of monographs, I am thankful for their valuable contribution.

Claude Lenfant, M.D.
Gaithersburg, Maryland, U.S.A.

Foreword

Human infants at birth spend more time asleep than awake, but for a long time limited attention was given to the sleep of children. Interestingly, it was while observing sleeping infants that Aserinski and Kleitman (1) noticed periods of sleep characterized by bursts of eye movements with seemingly half-opened eyes. These researchers decided to place electrodes and monitor eye movements. This experiment lead to the discovery of two types of eye movements during sleep, one fast and the other slow, with the fast eye movements occurring episodically several times during sleep. William C. Dement (2), a student in the Kleitman laboratory, continued the work started by Aserinski and placed EEG electrodes alongside the eye electrodes to investigate infant sleep, thus discovering REM sleep in humans. During such monitoring, it was noted that bursts of rapid eye movements were associated with irregular breathing and short respiratory pauses. The question arose: why? Was control of vital functions different during periods of wake and sleep?

Much work has been done since these discoveries in the mid-1950s. We have a better understanding of the physiology of sleep and the mechanisms that underlie the two different sleep states. We have also integrated sleep and wake within the 24-hour cycle, which led, for example, to distinguishing hormones whose secretory patterns are circadian dependent from those that are sleep dependent, such as growth hormone. We have deciphered differences in the control of some vital functions, such as the dependence of respiratory rhythm on central chemosensitivity during slow wave sleep (the "quiet sleep" of infants). We have begun to understand the mechanism behind congenital central hypoventilation syndrome. Our progress in understanding the mechanisms underlying sleep and wakefulness and in understanding the progressive "buildup" of sleep during the nocturnal period has led to better approaches to sleep-related disorders, as well as better diagnostics and treatment options. I recall an occasion in 1972 (3) when I had to tell the mother of a 12-year-old girl who had failed to improve following adenotonsillectomy that the only treatment available for her newly diagnosed obstructive sleep apnea syndrome (OSAS) was a tracheostomy. I also recall the joy of mother and daughter in the fall of 1981 when I contacted them to indicate that there was a potential new treatment, developed in Australia, called "nasal continuous positive airway pressure" (CPAP)(4). Colin Sullivan sent one of his technicians to show us how to make a mask by hand, but it was a young craniofacial otolaryngologist, Nelson Powell, who helped us pull things together. We used a homemade CPAP device made by a small firm in South San Francisco that could probably have powered a small motorcycle. Carleen, since my encounter with her in 1972, underwent every treatment advance for OSAS and finally became free of medical care after a maxillomandibular advancement. Another patient, a three-year-old boy, at first misdiagnosed with atonic seizures due to his "drop attacks," still requires one or two short naps daily despite modafinil and sodium oxybate. Despite his narcolepsy-cataplexy syndrome, he completed his Ph.D. this year, but vigilantly watches his food intake to avoid losing the battle of inappropriate weight gain. The discovery that narcolepsy-cataplexy was related to the destruction of hypocretin/orexin neurons located in the lateral hypothalamus, as predicted by Von Economo (5) in the mid-1920s, has allowed both a better understanding of the different clinical features of the syndrome and better treatment of symptoms.

Pediatric sleep medicine is an integral part of pediatrics. All children sleep, and sleep mechanisms may trigger or worsen many disorders seen in daily pediatric practice. Difficulty falling asleep, sleep terrors, sleepwalking, and enuresis are common complaints, but so are problems associated with sleep disorders such as nasal allergies, enlarged adenoids and tonsils, difficulties in school, attention deficit hyperactivity disorder, and even orthodontic treatment. When to recommend adenotonsillectomy or to avoid nocturnal headgear as an orthodontic treatment?

Sleep medicine is young, and we do not necessarily have all the answers, but we have much to contribute. We can respond better to the needs of children with a better understanding of issues and problems associated with pediatric sleep medicine. Medical students rotating through pediatric departments should be exposed to the basics of sleep medicine, and all pediatricians should be exposed to it during their residency.

This book has many chapters authored by experts on the subject, and it contains important information for all health professionals dealing with children. The different chapters with their many vignettes and well-constructed bibliographies will help in responding to questions from parents and their children. It will be helpful to many in their regular practice, and not simply to those interested in pediatric sleep medicine.

Christian Guilleminault, M.D., D.M., Biol.D.
Stanford University
Palo Alto, California, U.S.A.

References

1. Aserinsky E, Kleitman N. Regularly occurring periods of eye motility, and concomitant phenomena, during sleep. Science 1953; 118:273–274.
2. Dement WC, Kleitman N. Cyclic variations in EEG during sleep and their relation to eye movements, body motility, and dreaming. Electroencephalogr Clin Neurophysiol 1957; 9:673–690.
3. Guilleminault C, Dement WC, Monod N. Mort Subite du Nourrisson, apnée lors du sommeil: nouvelle hypothèse. Nouv Presse Med 1973; 2:1355–1358.
4. Sullivan CE, Issa FG, Berthon-Jones M, et al. Reversal of obstructive sleep apnoea by continuous positive airway pressure applied through the nares. Lancet 1981; 1:862–865.
5. Von Economo C. Sleep as a problem of localization. J Nerv Men Dis 1930; 71: 249–259.

Preface

Depending on age, infants and children spend one- to two-thirds of their life asleep. Despite this, very little attention was paid until recently to understanding both normal sleep and sleep-related abnormalities during development. However, the last few years have seen burgeoning research and publications in this area. Important developments have occurred in the field since the publication of the first edition of this book in 2000. Thus, the book has been totally revised. The basis of the book remains rigorously conducted scientific research. The chapters have been authored by an international group of outstanding scientists. As several clinical pediatric sleep books have been published since the first edition of this book, we have shifted the focus of the book away from some of the more clinically oriented chapters toward developmental physiology. In addition, we have divided the book into two volumes to accommodate the increased amount of literature that is now available. One volume concentrates on sleep alone, and the other on breathing during sleep. It should be noted, however, that not all chapters could be so neatly categorized, and thus the two volumes are synergistic.

This volume is devoted to breathing during sleep, its changes with development (from the fetus onward), and the pathophysiology of sleep-related breathing disorders. The concluding chapter reviews the history of our young field and outlines future directions.

Breathing influences sleep, and sleep influences breathing. During sleep, there is a change in upper airway resistance, ventilatory drive, and respiratory muscle tone, all of which will affect breathing. Conversely, respiratory abnormalities such as upper airway occlusion and hypercapnia can result in arousal from sleep. Normal changes in breathing during sleep are magnified in patients with respiratory disease. Thus, in addition to sleep-specific respiratory disorders (such as obstructive sleep apnea and congenital central hypoventilation syndrome), breathing during sleep is worse than breathing during wakefulness in virtually any child with lung disease. There are profound changes in breathing, and sleep, during growth and maturation. An example of this interaction is seen in the young child with obstructive sleep apnea, compared with an adult. The child may have marked paradoxical inward rib cage motion due to the compliant rib cage, resulting in a low functional residual capacity and desaturation. In conjunction with this, the young child has a high arousal threshold, allowing the apnea to be prolonged.

The success of the book depends, of course, on the quality of the individual contributors. We therefore want to thank the many authors who have contributed to the book. They are all leaders in the field and, as such, have many demands on their time. Nevertheless, as the reader will appreciate, they have devoted time and energy into writing outstanding chapters.

We would like to dedicate this book to the children and families who have willingly participated in sleep research experiments. Without them, this book would not exist.

We thank Mary Anne Cornaglia for her invaluable assistance with the book preparation.

Carole L. Marcus
John L. Carroll
David F. Donnelly
Gerald M. Loughlin

Contributors

Michael J. Ackerman Mayo Clinic College of Medicine, Rochester, Minnesota, U.S.A.

Ruben Alvaro University of Manitoba, Winnipeg, Manitoba, Canada

Raouf Amin University of Cincinnati, Cincinnati, Ohio, U.S.A.

Raanan Arens Albert Einstein College of Medicine, Bronx, New York, U.S.A.

Elizabeth M. Berry-Kravis Rush University, Chicago, Illinois, U.S.A.

Peter S. Blair University of Bristol, Bristol, U.K.

Lee J. Brooks University of Pennsylvania, Philadelphia, Pennsylvania, U.S.A.

Robert T. Brouillette McGill University, Montreal, Quebec, Canada

John L. Carroll University of Arkansas for Medical Sciences, Little Rock, Arkansas, U.S.A.

Ronald D. Chervin University of Michigan, Ann Arbor, Michigan, U.S.A.

Sally L. Davidson Ward University of Southern California, Los Angeles, California, U.S.A.

David F. Donnelly Yale University School of Medicine, New Haven, Connecticut, U.S.A.

Nalton F. Ferraro Children's Hospital, Boston, Massachusetts, U.S.A.

Peter Fleming University of Bristol, Bristol, U.K.

Ralph F. Fregosi The University of Arizona, Tucson, Arizona, U.S.A.

Claude Gaultier Hospital Robert Debré and University Paris 7 Denis Diderot, Paris, France

David Gozal University of Louisville School of Medicine, Louisville, Kentucky, U.S.A.

Ronald M. Harper University of California, Los Angeles, Los Angeles, California, U.S.A.

Shiroh Isono Graduate School of Medicine, Chiba University, Chiba, Japan

Athanasios G. Kaditis University of Thessaly School of Medicine and Larissa University Hospital, Larissa, Greece

Thomas G. Keens University of Southern California, Los Angeles, California, U.S.A.

Brian J. Koos University of California, Los Angeles, Los Angeles, California, U.S.A.

Mary L. Marazita University of Pittsburgh, Pittsburgh, Pennsylvania, U.S.A.

Carole L. Marcus University of Pennsylvania School of Medicine, Philadelphia, Pennsylvania, U.S.A.

Louise M. O'Brien University of Michigan, Ann Arbor, Michigan, U.S.A.

Aloka L. Patel Rush University Medical Center, Chicago, Illinois, U.S.A.

Jean-Paul Praud Université de Sherbrooke, Sherbrooke, Canada

Susan Redline Case Western Reserve University, Cleveland, Ohio, U.S.A.

Henrique Rigatto University of Manitoba, Winnipeg, Manitoba, Canada

Carol L. Rosen Case Western Reserve University School of Medicine, Cleveland, Ohio, U.S.A.

Nathalie Samson Université de Sherbrooke, Sherbrooke, Canada

Martin P. Samuels Keele University and University Hospital of North Staffordshire, Staffordshire, U.K.

Jean M. Silvestri Rush University Medical Center, Chicago, Illinois, U.S.A.

James C. Spilsbury Case Western Reserve University, Cleveland, Ohio, U.S.A.

Riva Tauman Tel Aviv University, Tel Aviv, Israel

Bradley T. Thach Washington University, St. Louis, Missouri, U.S.A.

Karen A. Waters University of Sydney and The Children's Hospital at Westmead, Sydney, Australia

Debra E. Weese-Mayer Northwestern University Feinberg School of Medicine, Chicago, Illinois, U.S.A.

Contents

1

Breathing and Sleep States in the Fetus and at Birth

BRIAN J. KOOS
University of California, Los Angeles, Los Angeles, California, U.S.A.

I. Introduction

The fetus has a number of distinctive features that include a low arterial PO_2 (~30 Torr), parallel ventricular function with increased combined cardiac output, umbilical circulation, and the placenta, which is the organ of exchange for respiratory gases, nutrients, and waste products. The pulmonary vascular resistance is very high, which necessitates a direct conduit (i.e., ductus arteriosus) from the right ventricular outflow tract to the aorta. Fetal breathing movements, which start long before birth, contribute to normal lung growth and differentiation, respiratory muscle development, and establishment of neural pathways controlling respiration (1–4). Fetal breathing has unique features that include the requirement for a physiological environment (intrauterine or exteriorized in a warm saline bath) and the dominating control by sleep and behavioral states.

II. Animal Studies

Developmental studies on sleep and breathing have been performed primarily in chronically catheterized fetal sheep, which have a gestational length of 147 days.

The brain of the sheep fetus is largely developed in utero, like that of the human, although the fetal sheep brain is functionally more mature at birth.

A. Electrocortical Activity

In fetal sheep, the electrocorticogram (ECoG) differentiates at 110 to 115 days of gestation, with clearly distinguishable low-voltage fast activity (45–50% of the time), high-voltage slow activity (35–45% of the time), and transitional states after 120 days of gestation (1,5).

B. Eye Movements

Virtually continuous eye activity changes to episodic rapid eye movements (REM) after 107 days of gestation, with coincidence of REM with low-voltage activity after 120 days' gestation (1).

C. Behavioral States

Fetal behavioral states (>120 days' gestation) have been identified that are similar to REM sleep (low-voltage ECoG, REM, and absent nuchal muscle activity) and quiet sleep (high-voltage ECoG, absent REM, and nuchal muscle tone), which reflects the development of thalamocortical and intracortical innervation patterns (1,2,5,6). An aroused state (low-voltage ECoG, REM, and sustained activity of the dorsal neck muscles) occurs ∼5% of the time (4,5), but wakefulness, as defined by open eyes and purposeful movements of the fetal head, has not been detected (6).

D. Breathing

Fetal breathing (>120 days' gestation) primarily involves contractions of the diaphragm that reduce intratracheal pressure by 3 to 4 mmHg. Caudal displacement of the diaphragm with inspiration coupled with minimal change in intrathoracic volume (<1.0 mL) results in paradoxical or rocking motion due to inward movement of the anterior chest and outward protrusion of the abdomen. Very little amniotic fluid is inspired because of the high viscosity of tracheal fluid relative to that of air and the resistance of the upper respiratory tract (1,2).

    The posterior cricoarytenoid muscles (dilators of the larynx) phasically contract with inspiration. Laryngeal dilatation in expiration allows egress of tracheal fluid, which reduces lung volume over a breathing episode (2). In apnea, secretion of lung fluid along with a high resistance of the upper respiratory tract due to contraction of laryngeal constrictor muscles establishes a small positive tracheal pressure gradient relative to that of amniotic fluid that maintains fluid lung volume (∼40 mL/kg body weight), which approximates the functional residual capacity. Electromyographic (EMG) recordings indicate that diaphragmatic activity is present as early as 40 to 50 days of gestation (fetal period in

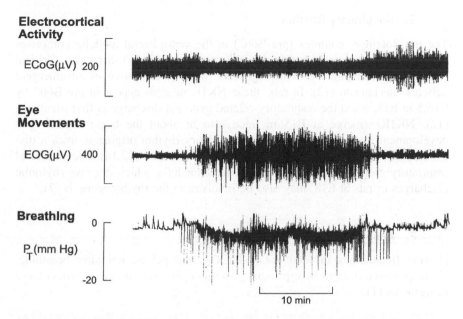

Figure 1 The ECoG, EOG, and P_T recordings from a near-term sheep fetus. Breathing is depicted by negative deflections in P_T. *Abbreviations*: ECoG, electrocorticogram; EOG, electrooculogram; P_T, tracheal pressure.

sheep begins at 34 days), although it lacks significant brainstem control. Later in gestation, breathing occurs almost continuously with apneic episodes usually lasting <2 minutes. After 107 days, breathing evolves into an episodic pattern of rapid (≤ 4 Hz), irregular (in rate and amplitude) movements that are coincident with REM. With ECoG differentiation, both REM and breathing are virtually confined to low-voltage states (Fig. 1), along with variable occurrence of phasic intercostal activity and infrequent contractions of the dorsal neck muscles. The emergence of episodic, behavior-related breathing reflects the maturation of the rostral brain (1).

In rats, low-frequency (~8 breaths/hr) respiratory-like activity develops by embryonic day (E) 16.5 to 17 (fetal period starts ~E14–15), with an increase in rate to ~300/hr by E20. Breathing becomes episodic by ~E18, but this pattern is not observed in isolated medullary preparations, which confirms the modulatory role of rostral brain sectors on breathing pattern (7).

In sheep, the incidence and amplitude of breathing vary over the day, with peak values at 1900 to 2100 hours and a nadir at 0400 to 0900 hours. This circadian variation, which follows changes in the incidence of low-voltage ECoG (8,9), appears to be entrained by the maternal melatonin rhythm that is regulated by the light-dark cycle (10,11).

E. Respiratory Rhythm

The pre-Bötzinger complex (pre-BötC) in the ventrolateral medulla comprises glutamatergic neurons with neurokinin-I receptors (NK1Rs) that have a critical role in rodent respiratory rhythmogenesis, which likely involves an emergent network mechanism (12). In rats, these NK1R neurons appear in pre-BötC by E16.5 to E18, when the respiratory-related neuronal discharge is first identified (12). NK1Rs emerge at E15 in mice also at about the beginning of fetal development in this species, but the respiratory rhythm originates from a distributed neuronal network rather than a single pacemaker (13,14). The parafacial respiratory group in the rostral ventrolateral medulla, which displays rhythmic discharges in rats at E18, may also be involved in the rhythmogenesis (7).

F. Respiratory Modulators

Normal fluctuations in fetal PaO_2, $PaCO_2$, and pH do not alter breathing, although larger changes in respiratory gases and pH can significantly affect these movements (1).

Carbon Dioxide

Hypercapnia increases the incidence of low-voltage ECoG, REM, and breathing as well as the amplitude and regularity of breathing (1,15). However, it does not induce breathing in high-voltage states, except in fetuses with lateral pontine lesions (1,16). Conversely, lowering fetal $PaCO_2$ will virtually arrest breathing without altering the normal cycling of REM or ECoG (17).

Oxygen

Isocapnic hypoxia inhibits breathing but does not alter the amplitude or respiratory period. Hypoxic inhibition is dose dependent once the end-capillary PO_2 of the fetal brain falls below 13 Torr, as shown in Figure 2 (18). The parallel depressant effects of hypoxia on REM (>0.8 term) suggest that hypoxia inhibits breathing indirectly by reducing REM, although the mechanism is developmentally regulated because hypoxia blunts diaphragmatic activity before the emergence of REM (1,15).

Hypoxic inhibition is mediated through effects of low O_2 tensions on the supramedullary brain, and thus it does not involve direct hypoxic depression of respiratory motoneurons (1,19–21). More recent work has shown that bilateral neuronal lesions that encompass the parafascicular nuclear complex (Pf) of the posteromedial thalamus abolish the depressant effects of hypoxia on breathing (22) and that electrical stimulation of this locus inhibits breathing in normoxic fetuses (23). Pf participates in tonic cortical activation associated with increased discharge rates in desynchronized states of wakefulness and REM. The involvement of Pf in sleep and breathing is consistent with the hypothesis that

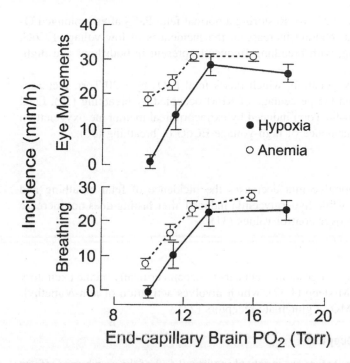

Figure 2 Incidence of breathing and eye movements in fetal sheep (>0.8 term) during
one hour of graded hypoxia or anemia. Incidence is depicted as a function of the effective
PO_2 at the end of an average brain capillary, which was calculated from jugular venous
PO_2 and the average distance between red cells. Low-voltage ECoG was not significantly
reduced at this level of O_2 deprivation. Vertical bars represent SE. *Abbreviation*: ECoG,
electrocorticogram. *Source*: From Ref. 18.

changes in sleep and behavioral state underlie respiratory depression of acute,
moderately severe hypoxia.

Hypoxia-induced degradation of extracellular adenine nucleotides appears
to be the primary source of the neuromodulator adenosine that is critically
involved in the inhibition of REM and breathing (24). Activation of adenosine
A_{2A} receptors coupled with G-protein (G_s) triggers the depression (25). A_{2A}
receptors in Pf are a potential locus of adenosine action relative to hypoxic
inhibition of REM and breathing (26). Hypoxic inhibition of fetal breathing may
also involve α_2-adrenergic depression of noradrenergic facilitatory tone that
involves activation of K^+ currents (27).

The brain PO_2 set point for hypoxic inhibition rapidly adapts to reductions
in PaO_2 (hypoxia) and O_2 carrying capacity (anemia). The decline in breathing
elicited by moderate O_2 deprivation is followed by a return to normal levels,
although this recovery does not occur in severe hypoxia with a progressive

metabolic acidemia (2,27,28). Restoring a normal fetal PaO_2 after prolonged O_2 deficiency creates a rebound increase in the incidences of low-voltage ECoG, REM, and breathing, with breathing frequently present in both low- and high-voltage ECoG (28).

Hyperbaric oxygenation, which raises fetal PaO_2 by ~20 Torr, increases the aroused state and the percentage of REM occupied by breathing (29). Fetal hyperoxia (PaO_2 50–90 Torr) induced by extracorporeal membrane oxygenation does not alter the incidence of high-voltage ECoG or breathing (30).

Glucose

Fasting-induced hypoglycemia decreases the incidence of fetal breathing and low-voltage ECoG, while hyperglycemia induced after fasting does not increase breathing incidence over control values (31).

REM Sleep

Breathing (>115 days of gestation) appears to depend critically on the excitatory drive of phasic REM sleep (1,32), which involves activation of non-N-methyl-D-aspartate (non-NMDA) glutamate receptors (27).

G. Chemoreceptors

Central H^+ chemoreceptors are involved in virtually all of the respiratory effects of systemic hypercapnia (1,15,20). In vitro studies have shown pH-sensitive, respiratory-like activity in the brainstem of mice ($\geq$E13) and rats ($\geq$E20) (33).

The peripheral arterial chemoreceptors have little involvement in hypoxic inhibition of breathing. Eliminating hypoxic inhibition by disrupting neurons and fiber tracts of the rostral brainstem results in hypoxic stimulation of breathing (1), an excitation that is abolished by sino-aortic denervation (34). Thus, in hypoxic fetuses, supramedullary sectors appear to be involved in blocking stimulatory input from the carotid sinus nerves to respiratory motoneurons.

H. Pulmonary Reflexes

Hering-Breuer inflation and deflation reflexes can be demonstrated experimentally in fetal sheep; however, the normal changes in lung volume per breath (<1 mL) are insufficient to activate the pulmonary stretch receptors (1).

I. Neurotransmitters and Neuromodulators

The expression and function of neurotransmitters and neuromodulators and their receptors depend on the stage of development (35). In fetal sheep (>0.8 term), the neurotransmitters and neuromodulators involved in central respiratory regulation generally have qualitatively similar effects to those observed postnatally (1,27,35). However, a major difference in central regulation of fetal breathing is the state-dependent episodic pattern, which is of particular interest because of the necessary transition to continuous breathing at birth.

Cerebroventricular infusion of muscarinic cholinergic agonists increases the amplitude of breathing as well as the incidence of low-voltage ECoG, REM, and breathing activity; breathing in high-voltage ECoG via activation of M_1 receptors has also been reported (1,36,37). Muscarinic cholinergic antagonists promote high-voltage ECoG states (37). These effects on behavioral state are presumably mediated through cholinergic pathways in the medial pontine reticular formation, as postulated for adults.

Systemic administration of 5-hydroxytryptamine, which induces quiet sleep in adult mammals by elevating brain serotonin levels, dissociates breathing from sleep state by eliciting prolonged high-voltage ECoG activity accompanied by cessation of REM but with vigorous breathing (1).

Intracisternal injection of norepinephrine or dopamine increases the amplitude of breathing (38), which likely involves activation of α_1-adrenoreceptors (39). Catecholamine-stimulated breathing continues through both low- and high-voltage ECoG activity (38). By reducing medullary prostaglandin E_2 (PGE$_2$) concentrations, cyclooxygenase inhibitors induce a similar pattern of prolonged breathing, which is also independent of the ECoG and may involve increased central 3,4-dihydroxyphenylacetic acid concentrations (1,40).

In fetal sheep, adenosine, via A_{2A} receptors, tonically suppresses low-voltage ECoG, REM, and breathing. Thus, higher extracellular adenosine levels in REM compared with high-voltage states would provide a negative feedback loop that would promote quiet (NREM) sleep; however, fetal brain adenosine levels are yet to be measured with respect to ECoG (41). Adenosine acting on A_1 receptors likely enhances high-voltage ECoG activity in hypoxic conditions that increase brain adenosine levels (41). Plasma concentrations (and presumably brain levels) of adenosine (42,43) are elevated in the fetus compared with those in the newborn, which suggests a more prominent role in modulating breathing and sleep state in utero.

PGE$_2$ inhibits fetal breathing without altering REM or ECoG, and the high fetal levels of PGE$_2$ may be involved in the modulating fetal behavior and breathing (1,44,45). Allopregnanolone may contribute to fetal sleep-like behavior through activation of central GABA$_A$ receptors (46), while GABA-induced stimulation of GABA$_A$ receptors may be involved in the inhibition of breathing in high-voltage ECoG (45). Endogenous opiates dampen breath amplitude (47), while corticotrophin-releasing factor may tonically facilitate breathing (48).

J. Pharmacologic Agents

Activators of GABA$_A$ receptors (e.g., pentobarbital, diazepam, alcohol) or selective opiate receptors abolish fetal breathing at doses that do not significantly depress maternal respiration, although low doses of morphine stimulate breathing via activation of central μ_1 receptors (1,49). Respiratory stimulants such as caffeine or doxapram increase the incidence of REM as well as the frequency and depth of breathing, but they do not induce breathing in high-voltage ECoG (50).

K. Parturition

Breathing incidence declines within two days prior to the onset of parturition and falls further with the onset of spontaneous labor in normoxic fetal sheep, which is often associated with increased incidence of high-voltage ECoG (51–53).

III. Human Studies

The inability to record ECoG and EMG and to determine purposeful activity limits sleep analysis in human fetuses. However, behavioral states can be identified through ultrasound detection of movements involving the eyes, limbs, and trunk.

A. Activity Cycles

Frequent, virtually random movements are initially detected in the late embryogenesis (5–6 weeks postconception), which become clustered by 14 weeks' gestation with ~5-minute activity-free epochs separating episodes of movement (54). Between 24 and 28 weeks' gestation, sporadic, short-duration movements average about 13% of the time (55). Quiet-active cycles become clearly developed after 24 to 28 weeks of gestation, with quiescence occurring about 20–26% of the time and activity about 70–80% (56–59). The mean incidence and number of movements vary in a circadian manner with peak values at 2100 to 0100 hours (60,61).

REM can be detected by ~20 weeks of gestation with the emergence of NREM episodes from 28 to 31 weeks of gestation. Distinct cycling of REM and NREM phases becomes evident after 32 weeks of gestation (62,63). At 36 to 40 weeks of gestation, REM occupies about 60% of the time, with a mean duration of REM episodes of ~29 minutes; NREM states occur about 24% of the time, with an average length of ~21 minutes (63). After 36 weeks, REM is almost exclusively associated with states that are suggestive of REM sleep (58,64).

B. Behavioral States

Behavioral states in the human fetus have been defined as recurrent, nonrandom coincidence of behavior in which the defining components change virtually simultaneously at transitions from one state to another (65). Four behavioral states (states 1F–4F) have been identified on the basis of the linkage of fetal body movements (absent, incidental, periodic, continuous) with eye activity (absent, present) (Table 1). Although coordination of movements starts earlier (66,67),

Table 1 Behavioral States in the Human Fetus

State	1F	2F	3F	4F
Eye movements	absent	present	present	present
Gross body movements	incidental	periodic	absent	continuous
Breathing[a]	regular	irregular	regular	irregular
Heart rate accelerations	incidental	present	absent	present

[a]If present.
Source: From Ref. 65.

the critical gestational age for the emergence of synchronized behavioral patterns is ~36 weeks, when coherent behavioral states that are comparable to those in the newborn are established in about 80% of fetuses (58,65). Of the four states, 1F (~30% time, analogous to quiet sleep) and 2F (~58% time, similar to REM sleep) are the most frequently observed (67). Fetal movements are usually associated with accelerations of the fetal heart rate (FHR), and thus FHR can be used to detect active and quiet states after 27 weeks of gestation (68).

On the basis of heart rate and eye and somatic movements, fetal states 3F and 4F have been considered virtually identical to awake states 3 (S3, quiet awake) and 4 (S4, active awake) in the newborn (65), although this conclusion is disputed (67). Open eyelids have been detected in the fetus (28–39 weeks of gestation) for only very brief (<30 seconds), infrequent periods (69), but whether purposeful gaze or activity occurs is unknown.

C. Breathing

Ultrasound imaging techniques can be used to detect fetal breathing, which involves paradoxical motion of the sternum and abdominal wall and caudal excursions of the diaphragm and liver. Breathing can also be detected from Doppler velocimetry of umbilical venous blood and of nasal and tracheal fluid.

The incidence of breathing increases from ~2% at 10 weeks of gestation to ~6% at 19 weeks (54,70). At 20 to 22 weeks of gestation (71), median values are greater in the afternoon and evening (~12%) than in the morning (2%). Breathing incidence increases to 24–35% by 30 to 32 weeks' gestation (57,67). Mean breath interval (cycle time) increases from ~0.64 seconds at 22 to 25 weeks' gestation to ~1.00 second at ≥30 weeks' gestation, which is accompanied by a reduction in inspiratory time and a rise in breath amplitude (72–74).

D. Relation to Behavioral State

Breathing increasingly correlates with REM after 20 weeks' gestation, with a high coincidence after 27 weeks' gestation (58,63). Between 28 and 36 weeks of gestation, fetal breathing is more associated with active states than quiet phases

(58,75,76). The rate and amplitude of breathing is more irregular in active than in quiet states. After 36 weeks, breathing occurs more in the active 2F state than in the quiet 1F state (58,76) (Fig. 3).

E. Glucose and Ultradian Rhythm

The incidence of breathing, with no body movements, increases significantly postprandially after 22 to 30 weeks' gestation as a result of a rise in fetal glucose concentrations (71,77–80), which significantly shortens the maximum apneic periods to <0.75 hours (79). No postprandial changes occur in breath interval or amplitude (81), which argues against a direct effect on respiration. A glucose-independent rise in breathing incidence is present in the early morning (0400–0700 hours) over the last 10 weeks of pregnancy (78).

F. Respiratory Gases

Maternal hypercapnia significantly increases the incidence of fetal breathing, particularly after 28 weeks' gestation, while hypocapnia induced by hyper-ventilation reduces breathing activity (82,83). Changes in $PaCO_2$ do not affect somatic activity. Clinical studies indicate that breathing is more sensitive than limb or body movements to the depressant effects of hypoxia (84). Increasing the maternal inspired O_2 fraction to 0.5, which increases fetal PaO_2 by ~6 Torr, does not normally alter breathing activity, although it can increase breathing in growth-restricted fetuses that are presumably O_2 deficient (85,86).

G. Parturition

In human fetuses, breathing incidence declines within three days of the onset of parturition (87). Breathing is generally reduced in labor, although states 1F and 2F continue to cycle normally (88).

IV. Transition to Postnatal Respiration

Heightened sensation and asphyxia traditionally have been considered to play critical roles in the transition from intrauterine to extrauterine respiration, which involves circulatory changes, absorption of lung fluid, gaseous expansion of the lungs, and the onset of continuous breathing (89,90). Rhythmic breathing can commence directly in noncyanotic human infants or after a prolonged single inspiration or asphyxial gasping (89). Effective pulmonary ventilation is nor-mally achieved in infants with an intact umbilical circulation by about the fifth breath, which occurs within 30 seconds of delivery (91).

A single trigger for the onset of continuous breathing has not been iden-tified. Factors that may be involved include asphyxia, vagal afferent traffic related to respiratory and/or circulatory transitions, umbilical cord occlusion, and cutaneous cooling (92–94). The rise in PaO_2 associated with established

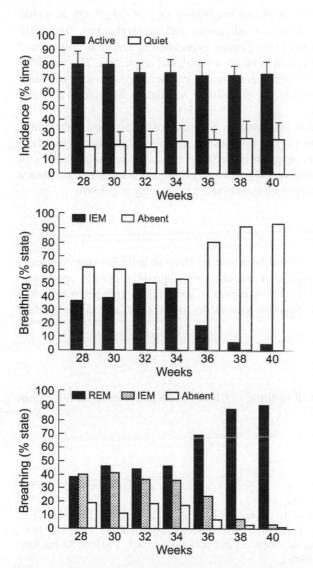

Figure 3 Fetal behavioral states and breathing in the third trimester of human pregnancy determined by ultrasound and FHR variability. (*Top*) Incidence of active and quiet states. Transition states accounted for <3% of time across gestational age. Vertical bars represent mean ± SD. (*Middle*) Distribution of fetal breathing in quiet phases according to the presence or absence of IEM. (*Bottom*) Distribution of breathing in active epochs coincident with REM, IEM, or absent eye movements. *Abbreviations*: FHR, fetal heart rate; IEM, intermittent eye movement; REM, rapid eye movement. *Source*: From Ref. 58.

respiration probably provides additional respiratory support (28,29,95), as would the fall in the newborn's levels of adenosine and prostaglandins. The birth process likely triggers changes in the genetic expression of neurotransmitters and neuromodulators that are involved in sleep, arousal, and respiration. The threshold and sensitivity of central and peripheral arterial chemoreceptors undergo adjustment over time in the newborn, as established ventilation increases PaO_2 and decreases $PaCO_2$.

The placenta has been proposed as a source of respiratory depressants, such as PGE_2 and adenosine (45), but it does not appears to be critically involved in the onset of continuous respiration because episodic breathing persists in sheep fetuses in which normal blood gases and pH are maintained in the absence of a placenta by an extracorporeal membrane gas exchanger (93,96).

V. Summary

Fetal breathing is episodic, primarily driven by sleep or behavior-related stimuli rather than metabolic signals, and inhibited by hypoxia. Episodic apnea and hypoxic depression in the fetus likely persist to a variable degree postnatally and contribute to sleep apnea, hypoxic ventilatory depression, and sudden infant death syndrome (97).

Acknowledgment

Supported in part by National Institute of Child Health and Human Development Grant HD-18478.

References

1. Dawes GS. The central control of fetal breathing and skeletal muscle movements. J Physiol (Lond). 1984; 346:1–18.
2. Harding R. Development of the respiratory system. In: Thorburn GD, Harding R, eds. Textbook of Fetal Physiology. New York: Oxford University Press, 1994:140–167.
3. Copland I, Post M. Lung development and fetal lung growth. Paediatr Respir Rev. 2004; 5(suppl A):S259–S264.
4. Inanlou MR, Kablar B. Contractile activity of skeletal musculature involved in breathing is essential for normal lung cell differentiation, as revealed in *Myf-/-:myoD-/-*embryos. Dev Dynamics. 2005; 233(3):772–782.
5. Szeto HH, Hinman DJ. Prenatal development of sleep-wake patterns in sheep. Sleep. 1985; 8(4):347–355.
6. Rigatto H, Moore M, Cates D. Fetal breathing and behavior measured through a double-wall plexiglass window in sheep. J Appl Physiol. 1986; 61:160–164.
7. Greer JJ, Funk GD, Ballanyi K. Preparing for the first breath: prenatal maturation of respiratory neural control. J Physiol. 2006; 570(3):437–444.

8. Boddy K, Dawes GS, Robinson JS. A 24-hour rhythm in the fetus. In: Comline KS, Cross KW, Dawes GS, et al., eds. Foetal and Neonatal Physiology. Proceedings of the Sir Joseph Barcroft Centenary Symposium Held at the Physiological Laboratory, Cambridge 25–27 July 1972. Cambridge, UK: Cambridge University Press, 1972: 63–66.

9. Callea J, McMillen IC, Walker DW. Effect of feeding regimen on diurnal variation of breathing movements in late-gestation fetal sheep. J Appl Physiol. 1990; 68(5): 1786–1792.

10. McMillen IC, Nowak R, Walker DW et al. Maternal pinealectomy alters the daily pattern of fetal breathing in sheep. Am J Physiol. 1990; 258(1 pt 2):R284–R287.

11. Houghton DC, Walker DW, Young IR, et al. Melatonin and the light-dark cycle separately influence daily behavioral and hormonal rhythms in the pregnant ewe and sheep fetus. Endocrinology. 1993; 133(1):90–98.

12. Del Negro CA, Morgado-Valle C, Hayes JA, et al. Sodium and calcium current-mediated pacemaker neurons and respiratory rhythm generation. J Neurosci. 2005; 25(2):446–453.

13. Thoby-Brisson M, Trinh JB, Champagnat J, et al. Emergence of the pre-Bötzinger respiratory rhythm generator in the mouse embryo. J Neurosci. 2005; 25(17):4307–4318.

14. Eugenin J, Nicholls JG, Cohen LD, et al. Optical recording from respiratory pattern generator of fetal mouse brainstem reveals a distributed network. Neuroscience. 2006; 137:1221–1227.

15. Jansen AH, Chernick V. Fetal breathing and development of control of breathing. J Appl Physiol. 1991; 70(4):1431–1446.

16. Johnston BM, Gluckman PD. Lateral pontine lesions affect central chemosensitivity in unanesthetized fetal lambs. J Appl Physiol. 1989; 67(3):1113–1118.

17. Kuipers IM, Maertzdorf WJ, De Jong DS, et al. Effect of mild hypocapnia on fetal breathing and behavior in unanesthetized normoxic fetal lambs. J Appl Physiol. 1994; 76(4):1476–1480.

18. Koos BJ, Matsuda K, Power GG. Fetal breathing and cardiovascular responses to graded methemoglobinemia in sheep. J Appl Physiol. 1990; 69(1):136–140.

19. Gluckman PD, Johnston BM. Lesions in the upper lateral pons abolish the hypoxic depression of breathing in unanaesthetized fetal lambs in utero. J Physiol (Lond). 1987; 382:373–383.

20. Koos BJ, Sameshima H. Effects of hypoxaemia and hypercapnia on breathing movements and sleep state in sinoaortic-denervated fetal sheep. J Dev Physiol. 1988; 10(2):131–144.

21. Walker DW, Lee B, Nitsos I. Effect of hypoxia on respiratory activity in the foetus. Clin Exp Pharmacol Physiol. 2000; 27:110–113.

22. Koos BJ, Chau A, Matsuura M, et al. A thalamic locus mediates hypoxic inhibition of breathing in fetal sheep. J Neurophysiol. 1998; 79(5):2383–2393.

23. Koos BJ, Kawasaki Y, Hari A, et al. Electrical stimulation of the posteromedial thalamus modulates breathing in unanesthetized fetal sheep. J Appl Physiol. 2004; 96(1):115–123.

24. Koos BJ, Kruger L, Murray TF. Source of extracellular brain adenosine during hypoxia in fetal sheep. Brain Res. 1997; 778(2):439–442.

25. Koos BJ, Maeda T, Jan C, et al. Adenosine A$_{2A}$ receptors mediate hypoxic inhibition of fetal breathing in sheep. Am J Obstet Gynecol. 2002; 186(4):663–668.

26. Yan X, Koos BJ, Kruger L, et al. Characterization of [125I]ZM241385 binding to adenosine A_{2A} receptors in pineal gland of sheep brain. Brain Res. 2006;1096.

27. Bissonnette JM. Mechanisms regulating hypoxic respiratory depression during fetal and postnatal life. Am J Physiol. 2000; 278(6):R1391–R1400.

28. Matsuda K, Ducsay C, Koos BJ. Fetal breathing, sleep state, and cardiovascular adaptations to anaemia in sheep. J Physiol. 1992; 445:713–723.

29. Tiktinsky-Rupp MH, Hasan SU, Bishop B, et al. Hyperbaric oxygenation increases arousal and breathing movements in fetal lambs. J Appl Physiol. 1994; 77(2): 902–911.

30. Blanco CE, Chen V, Maertzdorf W, et al. Effect of hyperoxia (PaO_2 50–90 mmHg) on fetal breathing movements in the unanesthetized fetal sheep. J Dev Physiol. 1990; 14(4):235–241.

31. Richardson B, Hohimer AR, Mueggler P, et al. Effects of glucose concentration on fetal breathing movements and electrocortical activity in fetal lambs. Am J Obstet Gynecol. 1982; 142:678–683.

32. Ioffe S, Jansen AH, Chernick V. Fetal respiratory neuronal activity during REM and NREM sleep. J Appl Physiol. 1993; 75:191–197.

33. Eugenín J, von Bernhardi R, Muller KJ, et al. Development and pH sensitivity of the respiratory rhythm of fetal mice in vitro. Neuroscience. 2006; 141:223–231.

34. Koos BJ, Chao A, Doany W. Adenosine stimulates breathing in fetal sheep with brain stem section. J Appl Physiol. 1992; 72(1):94–99.

35. Hilaire G, Duron B. Maturation of the mammalian respiratory system. Physiol Rev. 1999; 79(2):325–360.

36. Bissonnette JM, Hohimer AR, Knopp SJ. A cholinergic mechanism involved in fetal breathing during the high voltage ECoG state. Respir Physiol. 1994; 96(2–3):151–162.

37. Morrison JL, Carmichael L, Homan J, et al. The effects of "sleep promoting agents" on behavioural state in the ovine fetus. Dev Brain Res. 1997; 103(1):1–8.

38. Joseph SA, Walker . Effects of intracisternal monoamines on breathing movements in fetal sheep. Am J Physiol. 1993; 264(6):R1139–R1149.

39. Giussani DA, Moore PJ, Bennet L, et al. α_1- and α_2-adrenoreceptor actions of phentolamine and prazosin on breathing movements in fetal sheep in utero. J Physiol (Lond). 1995; 486:249–255.

40. Joseph SA, Walker DW. Monoamine concentrations in cerebrospinal fluid of fetal and newborn sheep. Am J Physiol. 1994; 266(2):R472–R480.

41. Koos BJ, Takatsugu M, Calvin J. Adenosine A_1 and A_{2A} receptors modulate sleep state and breathing in fetal sheep. J Appl Physiol. 2001; 91(1):343–350.

42. Koos BJ, Doany W. Role of plasma adenosine in breathing responses to hypoxia in fetal sheep. J Dev Physiol. 1991; 16(2):81–85.

43. Sawa R, Asakura H, Power GG. Changes in plasma adenosine during simulated birth of fetal sheep. J Appl Physiol. 1991; 70:1524–1528.

44. Adamson SL, Kuipers IM, Olson DM. Umbilical cord occlusion stimulates breathing independent of blood gases and pH. J Appl Physiol. 1991; 70(4):1796–1809.

45. Thorburn GD. The placenta and the control of fetal breathing movements. Reprod Fertil Dev. 1995; 7:577–594.

46. Crossley KJ, Nitsos I, Walker DW, et al. Steroid-sensitive $GABA_A$ receptors in the fetal sheep brain. Neuropharmacol. 2003; 45(4):461–472.

47. Adamson SL, Patrick JE, Challis JR. Effects of naloxone on the breathing, electrocortical, heart rate, glucose and cortisol responses to hypoxia in the sheep fetus. J Dev Physiol. 1984; 6(6):495–507.
48. Bennet L, Johnston BM, Vale WW, et al. The effects of corticotrophin-releasing factor and two antagonists on breathing movements in fetal sheep. J Physiol (Lond). 1990; 421:1–11.
49. Szeto HH, Cheng PY, Dwyer G, et al. Morphine-induced stimulation of fetal breathing: role of μ1-receptors and central muscarinic pathways. Am J Physiol. 1991; 261:R344–R350.
50. Jansen AH, Ioffe S, Chernick V. Drug-induced changes in fetal breathing activity and sleep state. Can J Physiol Pharmacol. 1983; 61(4):315–324.
51. Berger PJ, Walker AM, Horne R, et al. Phasic respiratory activity in the fetal lamb during late gestation and labour. Respir Physiol. 1986; 65(1):55–68.
52. Wallen LD, Murai DT, Clyman RI, et al. Effects of meclofenamate on breathing movements in fetal sheep before delivery. J Appl Physiol. 1988; 64(2):759–766.
53. Schinozuka N, Nathanielsz PW. Electrocortical activity in fetal sheep in the last seven days of gestation. J Physiol. 1998; 513(1):273–281.
54. de Vries JI, Visser GH, Mulder EJH. The emergence of fetal behaviour. I. Qualitative aspects. Early Hum Dev. 1982; 7:301–322.
55. Natsello-Paterson C, Natale R, Connors G. Ultrasonic evaluation of fetal body movements over twenty-four to twenty-eight weeks' gestation. Am J Obstet Gynecol. 1988; 158:312–316.
56. Dierkei LJ, Pillay SK, Sorokin Y, et al. Active and quiet periods in the preterm and term fetus. Obstet Gynecol. 1982; 60:65–70.
57. Natale R, Nasello-Paterson C, Turliuk R. Longitudinal measurement of fetal breathing, body movements, heart rate, and heart rate accelerations and decelerations at 24-32 weeks of gestation. Am J Obstet Gynecol. 1985; 151:256–263.
58. Arduini D, Rizzo G, Giorlandino C, et al. The development of fetal behavioural states: a longitudinal study. Prenat Diagn. 1986; 6(2):117–124.
59. Pilli M, James DK, Parker M. The development of ultradian rhythms in the human fetus. Am J Obstet Gynecol. 1992; 167:172–177.
60. Roberts AB, Little D, Cooper D. Normal patterns of fetal activity in the third trimester. Br J Obstet Gynecol. 1979; 86:4–9.
61. Patrick J, Campbell K, Carmichael L, et al. Patterns of gross fetal body movements over 24-hour observation intervals during the last 10 weeks of pregnancy. Am J Obstet Gynecol. 1982; 142:363–371.
62. Inoue M, Koyanagi T, Nakahara H, et al. Functional development of human eye movement in utero assessed quantitatively with real-time ultrasound. Am J Obstet Gynecol. 1986; 115(1):170–174.
63. Okai T, Kozuma S, Shinozuka N, et al. A study on the development of sleep-wakefulness cycle in the human fetus. Early Hum Dev. 1992; 29:391–396.
64. Koyanagi T, Horimoto N, Nakano H. REM sleep determined using in utero penile tumescence in the human fetus at term. Biol Neonate. 1991; 60(suppl 1):30–35.
65. Nijhuis JG, Prechtl HFR, Martin CB Jr., et al. Are there behavioural states in the human fetus? Early Hum Dev. 1982; 6:177–195.
66. Visser GHA, Poelmann-Weesjes G, Cohen TMN, et al. Fetal behavior at 30–32 weeks of gestation. Pediatr Res. 1987; 22(6):655–658.

67. Pillai M, James D. Behavioral states in normal mature human fetuses. Arch Dis Child. 1990; 65:39–43.
68. Visser GH, Dawes GS, Redman CW. Numerical analysis of the normal human antepartum fetal heart rate. Br J Obstet Gynecol. 1981; 88(8):792–802.
69. Kozuma S, Okai T, Ryo E, et al. Differential development process of respective behavioral states in human fetuses. Am J Perinatol. 1998; 15(3):203–208.
70. de Vries JIP, Visser GHA, Prechtl HFR. The emergence of fetal behavior. II. Quantitative aspects. Early Hum Dev. 1985; 12:99–120.
71. de Vries JI, Visser GH, Mulder EJH, et al. Diurnal and other variations in fetal movement and heart rate patterns at 20-22 weeks. Early Hum Dev. 1987; 15:333–348.
72. Dornan JC, Ritchie JWK, Ruff S. The rate and regularity of breathing movements in the normal and growth retarded fetus. Br J Obstet Gynaecol. 1984; 91:31–36.
73. Andrews J, Shime J, Gare D, et al. The variability of fetal breathing movements in normal human fetuses at term. Am J Obstet Gynecol. 1985; 151(2):280–282.
74. Trudinger BJ, Cook CM. The fetal breath cycle. Early Hum Dev. 1990; 21:181–191.
75. Timor-Tritsch IE, Dierker LJ Jr., Hertz RH, et al. Regular and irregular human fetal respiratory movement. Early Hum Dev. 1980; 4(3):315–324.
76. van Vliet MA, Martin CB, Nijhuis JG, et al. The relationship between fetal activity and behavioral states and fetal breathing movements in normal and growth-retarded fetuses. Am J Obstet Gynecol. 1985; 53(5):582–588.
77. Lewis PJ, Trudinger BJ. Effect of maternal glucose ingestion on fetal breathing and body movements in late pregnancy. Br J Obstet Gynecol. 1978; 85(2):86–89.
78. Patrick J, Campbell K, Carmichael L, et al. Patterns of human fetal breathing during the last 10 weeks of pregnancy. Obstet Gynecol. 1980; 56:24–30.
79. Patrick J, Campbell K, Carmichael L, et al. A definition of human apnea and the distribution of fetal apneic intervals during the last 10 weeks of pregnancy. Am J Obstet Gynecol. 1980; 136:471–477.
80. Harper MA, Meis PJ, Rose JC, et al. Human fetal breathing response to intravenous glucose is directly related to gestational age. Am J Obstet Gynecol. 1987; 157(6): 1403–1405.
81. Adamson SL, Bocking A, Cousin AJ, et al. Ultrasonic measurement of rate and depth of human fetal breathing: effect of glucose. Am J Obstet Gynecol. 1983; 147 (3):288–295.
82. Ritchie JWK, Lakhani K. Fetal breathing movements in response to maternal inhalation of 5% carbon dioxide. Am J Obstet Gynecol. 1980; 136:386–388.
83. Connors G, Hunse C, Carmichael L, et al. The role of carbon dioxide in the generation of human fetal breathing movements. Am J Obstet Gynecol. 1988; 158: 322–327.
84. Platt LD, Manning FA, Lemay M, et al. Human fetal breathing: relationship to fetal condition. Am J Obstet Gynecol. 1978; 132:514–518.
85. Ritchie JWK, Lakhani K. Fetal breathing movements and maternal hyperoxia. Br J Obstet Gynaecol. 1980; 87:1084–1086.
86. Dornan JC, Richie JWK. Fetal breathing movements and maternal hyperoxia in the growth retarded fetus. Br J Obstet Gynecol. 1983; 90:210–213.
87. Carmichael L, Campbell K, Patrick J. Fetal breathing, gross fetal body movements, and maternal and fetal heart rates before spontaneous labor at term. Am J Obstet Gynecol. 1984; 148:675–679.

88. Griffen RL, Caron FJM, van Geijn HP. Behavioral states in the human fetus during labor. Am J Obstet Gynecol. 1985; 152(7 pt 1):828–833.
89. Barcroft J. Researches on Pre-Natal Life, vol. 1. Oxford: Blackwell Scientific, 1946:267–276.
90. Pagtakhan RD, Faridy EE, Chernick V. Interaction between arterial PO_2 and PCO_2 in the initiation of respiration of fetal sheep. J Appl Physiol. 1971; 30(3):382–387.
91. Chou PJ, Ullrich JR, Ackerman BD. Time of onset of effective ventilation at birth. Biol Neonate. 1974; 24:74–81.
92. Dawes GS. Foetal and Neonatal Physiology. Chicago: Year Book Medical Publishers, 1968:131.
93. Kuipers IM, Maertzdorf WJ, Keunen H, et al. Fetal breathing is not initiated after cord occlusion in the unanesthetized fetal lamb in utero. J Dev Physiol. 1992; 17 (5):233–240.
94. Wong KA, Bano A, Rigaux A, et al. Pulmonary vagal innervation is required to establish adequate alveolar ventilation in the newborn lamb. J Appl Physiol. 1998; 85:849–859.
95. Baier RJ, Hasan SU, Cates DB, et al. Effects of various concentrations of O_2 and umbilical cord occlusion on fetal breathing and behavior. J Appl Physiol. 1990; 68 (4):1597–1604.
96. Kozuma S, Nishina H, Unno N, et al. Goat fetuses disconnected from the placenta, but reconnected to an artificial placenta, display intermittent breathing movements. Biol Neonate. 1999; 75(6):388–397.
97. Koos BJ, Kawasaki Y, Kim YH, et al. Adenosine A_{2A} receptor blockade abolishes the roll-off respiratory response to hypoxia in awake lambs. Am J Physiol Regul Integr Comp Physiol. 2005; 288(5):R1185–R1194.

2

Laryngeal Function and Neonatal Respiration

JEAN-PAUL PRAUD and NATHALIE SAMSON
Université de Sherbrooke, Sherbrooke, Canada

I. Introduction

The upper airways, especially the larynx, exert an important influence on breathing from the fetal period onward. In addition to participating in fetal lung growth, in the successful transition toward air breathing at birth and in the maintenance of optimal lung ventilation thereafter, the larynx of the newborn is also involved in reflexes such as nutritive and nonnutritive swallowing (NNS) and protection of the lower airways. Furthermore, neural immaturity in the newborn is often responsible for reflexes originating from the laryngeal region, the laryngeal chemoreflexes (LCR), which are inhibitory to cardiorespiratory function.

This review will focus on recent findings on laryngeal function in relation to neonatal apneas, LCR, breathing and NNS coordination, and the laryngeal responses to nasal application of positive pressure. The clinical importance of these findings is ultimately linked to their application in the understanding and treatment of severe pathological respiratory conditions of the newborn. While not reviewed herein, the other components of the upper airways are also of vital importance for neonatal respiration, and the reader is referred to a recent review on the subject (1).

19

II. Overview of Laryngeal Function

A detailed account of laryngeal development and anatomy is beyond the scope of the present review and can be found elsewhere (2). We will limit our focus herein to a few key points that are important for the understanding of respiratory functions of the neonatal larynx.

The first lungfish acquired the ability to use environmental air to fulfill its metabolic requirements more than 370 million years ago. For the first time, a vertebrate was able to ventilate a primitive lung intermittently. The simultaneous appearance of a closing valve, the primitive larynx, was critical to this evolutionary step to protect the lungs from flooding during water diving. Though lower airway protection is still one of the most important functions of the larynx in mammals, this rudimentary valve has evolved into a sophisticated organ involved in various important functions such as pulmonary ventilation, phonation, defecation, and parturition.

From a respiratory standpoint, the mammalian larynx is a "tuning organ" with two components. First, it is a sensory organ generating abundant afferent input arising from the highest concentration of sensory receptors within the airways. Aside from flow (cold temperature), pressure, and movement mechanoreceptors, the laryngeal mucosa contains chemoreceptors, which are sensitive to CO_2, water, H^+ ions, low chloride ion content, etc. Second, it is a motor organ harboring a rich set of constrictor and dilator glottal muscles, which are highly coordinated both with each other and with the thoracic respiratory muscles. Available studies on glottal muscles most frequently focus on the thyroarytenoid muscle as representative of a glottal constrictor and on the posterior cricoarytenoid muscle as the main glottal dilator muscle. In addition, the cricothyroid muscle also behaves as a glottal dilator, including in the neonatal period (3). With this entire sensory and motor armamentarium, the larynx can generate a wide range of responses, from gross modifications of lung ventilation to very fine modulation of inspiratory and expiratory airflow patterns and respiratory phase length. Current knowledge ascribes an essential role of the larynx during the perinatal period, in conjunction with the establishment of successful lung ventilation for the newborn in its transition from the intra- to the extrauterine environment.

III. Perinatal "Respiratory" Function of the Larynx

A. Respiratory Function of the Larynx in Fetal Life

Part of laryngeal functioning in the fetus is aimed at ensuring successful pulmonary ventilation at birth. In addition, knowledge of laryngeal functions in fetal life offers important clues for understanding laryngeal function in the first postnatal weeks, especially after preterm birth. Fetal lung growth relies heavily on the increase in pressure of liquid-filled airways generated during NREM (non–rapid eye movement) sleep-like state by active glottal closure, which opposes the efflux of lung liquid continuously secreted by the future airways (4,5). It is also suggested that the larynx defends the entrance of the trachea against influx of amniotic fluid via reflex glottal closure, due to laryngeal receptors sensitive to the lower chloride concentration of the amniotic fluid, as opposed to lung liquid. This theory would explain the LCR in response to low chloride content fluids in postnatal life (6). Interestingly, coordination between glottal muscles and the diaphragm is already present prenatally. This has been observed in the fetal lamb for both the glottal dilators, i.e., the posterior cricoarytenoid and the cricothyroid muscle (7), and the glottal constrictor muscle, i.e., the thyroarytenoid muscle (5), during REM sleep-like epochs with fetal breathing movements. Finally, breathing-swallowing coordination will allow oral feeding around 35 weeks of gestation, as seen in the newborn infant after premature birth (8).

B. Respiratory Function of the Larynx at Birth and in the Early Postnatal Period

At birth, complete, active glottal closure throughout the very first expirations allows the vital establishment of an end-expiratory lung volume of air, the initial functional residual capacity (7). In the first hours after birth, an active laryngeal airflow braking, sometimes heard as an expiratory grunting, is frequently observed in early expiration. Increased pulmonary water is one of the factors that enhance this post-inspiratory glottal constrictor contraction via stimulation of capsaicin-sensitive pulmonary fibers (9), especially in pathological conditions such as hyaline membrane disease. By decreasing lung emptying, laryngeal airflow braking also represents a crucial energy cost–efficient mechanism for defending an optimal end-expiratory lung volume against low lung compliance present in the newborn and young infant (10). Normally, activity of the glottal muscles is precisely coordinated from birth thereafter, in order to optimize lung ventilation. Hence, phasic inspiratory electrical activity (EMG) of the glottal dilator muscles occurs with or just before diaphragm EMG (3,11) to decrease the inspiratory work of breathing. The importance of this inspiratory coordination, which is less consistent in the preterm infant (11), is particularly due to the bulky arytenoids in the newborn, which tend to increase laryngeal inspiratory resistance. In addition, while glottal constrictor EMG is typically observed in only the first part of expiration, leading to an active, post-inspiratory laryngeal airflow braking, glottal dilator EMG is observed in the second part of expiration, presumably to decrease expiratory resistance to lung deflation at that time and to allow a sufficient tidal volume (3) (Fig. 1). Of note, glottal muscle EMGs are markedly influenced by REM sleep, which is characterized by the disappearance of post-inspiratory glottal constrictor EMG and a marked increase in inspiratory and expiratory cricothyroid EMG, consequently participating in the well-known decrease in functional residual capacity in REM sleep (Fig. 2).

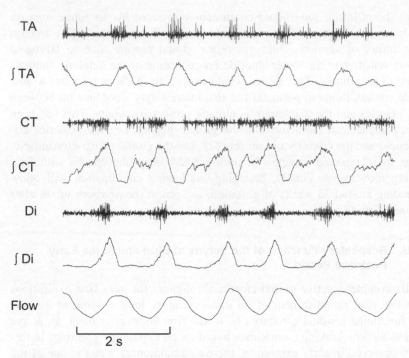

Figure 1 Respiratory phasic activity of glottal constrictor and dilator muscles. Note that while phasic expiratory TA EMG occurs during early expiration, phasic expiratory CT EMG occurs during the second part of expiration. *Abbreviations*: TA, raw thyroarytenoid muscle (a glottal constrictor muscle) electrical activity (EMG); ∫TA, moving time averaged TA EMG (time constant: 100 ms); CT, cricothyroid muscle (a glottal dilator muscle) EMG; ∫CT, moving time averaged CT EMG; Di, diaphragmatic muscle EMG; ∫Di, moving time averaged Di EMG; Flow: nasal airflow (inspiration upward).

In summary, precise control of the glottis aperture throughout the respiratory cycle is an essential mechanism in the newborn aimed at optimizing pulmonary ventilation in normal and pathological conditions. Central coordination of glottal muscles between each other, with the pharyngeal muscles, and with the thoracic respiratory muscles is of great importance and is normally initiated in fetal life. This central coordination involves numerous afferent messages originating in part from upper airway receptors (especially in the larynx) and bronchopulmonary receptors. The majority of these influences on laryngeal function are still poorly understood (12), especially in the newborn. Inability of the central "respiratory centers" to integrate their rich array of inputs and/or generate the "ideal" central respiratory output, e.g., due to neural immaturity, can translate in a suboptimal or even inadequate laryngeal functioning with regard to respiration.

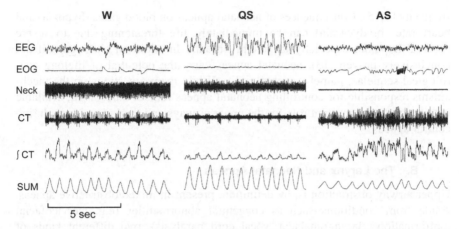

Figure 2 Effect of active sleep on inspiratory and expiratory CT EMG. From left to right: W, wakefulness; QS, quiet sleep; AS, active sleep. Note the increase in both the phasic inspiratory and expiratory CT EMG in AS, whereas tonic neck muscle EMG virtually disappears. *Abbreviations*: EEG, electroencephalogram; EOG, electrooculogram; Neck, neck muscle EMG; CT, cricothyroid muscle (a glottal dilator muscle) EMG; ∫CT, moving time averaged CT EMG; Sum, variations of lung volume, assessed from respiratory inductance plethysmography.

IV. The Larynx and Apneas in the Newborn

A. Neonatal Apneas

Apneas, which are basically defined as breathing cessation corresponding to at least "two missed breaths," are very frequent in the neonatal period, especially in the preterm newborn. Short isolated apneas without bradycardia or decline in oxygenation are especially frequent following sighs and with body movements or arousals, and are most often of no clinical concern. While apneas accompanied by bradycardia or a significant decline in oxygenation, regardless of apnea duration, are basically the only apneas of real importance for the clinician, there is no consensus on what constitutes a significant bradycardia or decline in oxygenation (13). The frequency of such apneas is directly proportional to gestational age at birth, so that preterm infants born before 27 weeks of gestation or with a birth weight less than 1000 g are virtually all affected by significant apneas of prematurity. As a whole, neonatal apneas are more frequent, longer, and more frequently associated with severe hypoxemia and bradycardia during REM sleep. Three types of apneas have been reported in newborn humans: central, obstructive, and mixed. Central apneas occur with greater frequency in non-REM sleep, often as periodic breathing, which is defined as the alternation of central apneas and regular breathing. Apneas become predominantly mixed when they are longer than 10 seconds. Purely obstructive apneas are much less frequent (14,15). Consequences of neonatal apneas on blood gases (hypoxia) and heart rate (bradycardia) can be immediately life threatening due to severe cerebral hypoxia, especially in preterm infants. In addition, although still not conclusively proven (13), neonatal apneas carry the potential of lifelong neurological sequelae, namely cerebral palsy. While many questions on the mechanisms responsible for controlling neonatal apneas remain unresolved, available data suggest an important role for the upper airways and the larynx, even during central apneas.

B. The Larynx and Neonatal Apneas

Upper airway obstruction is, by definition, present in mixed/obstructive apneas. Aside from conditions such as congenital abnormalities (e.g., cervicofacial malformations, laryngomalacia, vocal cord paralysis), two different kinds of upper airway obstruction can be involved in mixed/obstructive apneas in the newborn. The most frequently recognized mechanism is passive pharyngeal collapse during inspiration (15), which is favored by conditions such as cervical flexion, nose obstruction, or pharyngeal muscle-diaphragm discoordination due to central neural immaturity or abnormalities. In addition, it is well accepted that active glottal closure can occur as part of the LCR, which are triggered by stimulation of laryngeal mucosal receptors by liquids.

Although less often recognized, upper airway closure during central apneas now appears to be frequent in the newborn mammal. Again, passive pharyngeal collapse has been observed during central apneas, both isolated and during periodic breathing epochs (15). Mounting evidences also support the presence of frequent active glottal closure during central apneas in the human newborn. Indeed, endoscopic observation of sustained glottal closure during central apneas has been shown during apneas of prematurity, both isolated and during periodic breathing (15), a fact reported for years by clinicians during attempts at endotracheal intubation. Several animal studies in the 1980s reported rare observations of active glottal closure during central apneas in the newborn mammal, including lambs (7), dog pups (16), and newborn opossums (17). However, given the paucity of spontaneous apneas observed in newborn mammals born at term and the difficulty of documenting glottal closure in human infants, these observations were largely ignored.

Data from our laboratory, obtained over the last 15 years in nonsedated lambs, have further underlined the importance of active glottal closure during central apneas in the neonatal period. First, in full-term lambs, we were able to show that a complete active glottal closure was consistently observed throughout artificially induced central apneas, while the pharynx was not closed (18) (Fig. 3). An identical observation of a complete, active glottal closure with maintenance of a high apneic lung volume throughout apneas was consistently noted during spontaneous epochs of periodic breathing in our unique model of

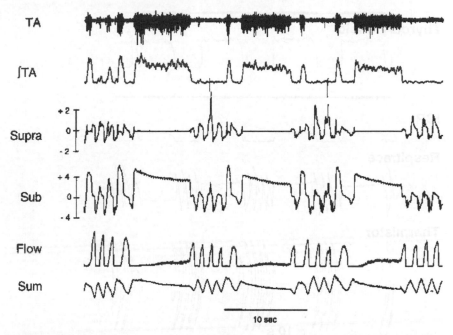

TA

∫TA

Supra

Sub

Flow

Sum

10 sec

Figure 3 Active glottal closure during artificially-induced central apneas in a full-term lamb. Complete glottal closure during central apneas is indicated by maintenance of positive subglottal pressure throughout the apnea, while supra-glottal pressure is atmospheric. The latter indicates further that the pharynx is open during central apneas. *Abbreviations*: TA, raw thyroarytenoid muscle (a glottal constrictor muscle) electrical activity (EMG); ∫TA, moving time averaged TA EMG (time constant: 100 ms); Supra, supra-glottal (hypopharyngeal) pressure; Sub, sub-glottal pressure; Flow, nasal airflow (inspiration upward); Sum, variations of lung volume, assessed from respiratory inductance plethysmography.

preterm lambs (Fig. 4) (19,20). In addition, the vast majority of spontaneous post-sigh apneas were characterized by continuous active glottal closure during the initial two thirds of the apneas, in both preterm and full-term lambs. Simultaneously, active glottal opening was consistently absent during periodic breathing apneas. It was also absent during post-sigh apneas, apart from the last third of post-sigh apneas in less than 10% of cases, where it was accompanied with a decrease in apneic lung volume (Fig. 5) (3). Finally, this precise coordination between glottal constrictor and dilator muscles during central apneas was lost on rare occasions, when glottal constrictor and dilator EMGs overlapped during isolated spontaneous apneas in preterm lambs, either after arousal, or with sneezing and movements during wakefulness (3).

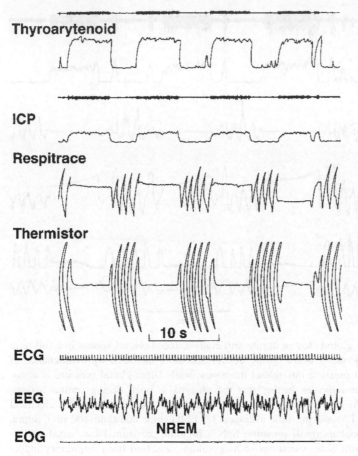

Figure 4 Active glottal closure throughout central apneas during a spontaneous epoch of periodic breathing in a preterm lamb. Continuous TA EMG without CT EMG is characteristic of periodic breathing apneas during NREM sleep. Note that the apneic volume is maintained in an inspiratory position during central apneas (central apnea = inspiratory breath-holding). *Abbreviations*: Thyroarytenoid, Thyroarytenoid muscle EMG, raw and moving time averaged signals; ICP, Inferior constrictor of the pharynx (synergistic to the glottal constrictor muscles), raw and moving time averaged signals; Respitrace, sum signal of the respiratory inductance plethysmograph; Thermistor, nasal airflow (inspiration upwards); ECG, electrocardiogram; EEG, electroencephalogram; EOG, electrooculogram.

C.   Consequences of Glottal Closure During Neonatal Central Apneas

Consequences of active glottal closure throughout central apneas can theoretically be either beneficial or deleterious and are not fully determined as of yet. Benefits are related to consequences of inspiratory breath-holding, i.e., maintenance

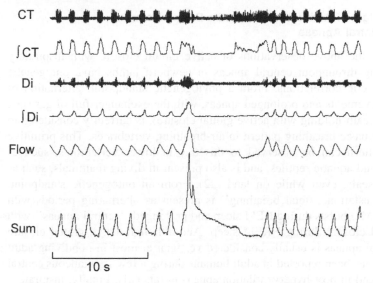

CT

∫CT

Di

∫Di

Flow

Sum

|_____|
10 s

Figure 5 Active glottal opening at the end of a post-sigh central apnea in a full-term lamb. Note the simultaneous presence of CT EMG and decrease in lung volume in the last portion of a central post-sigh apnea, indicating active glottal opening. *Abbreviations*: CT, cricothyroid muscle (a glottal dilator muscle) EMG; ∫CT, moving time averaged CT EMG; Di, diaphragmatic muscle EMG; ∫Di, moving time averaged Di EMG; Flow: nasal airflow (inspiration upward); Sum, variations of lung volume, assessed from respiratory inductance plethysmography.

of a high lung volume, maintenance of positive subglottal pressure, and resumption of breathing with expiration. We have shown that maintenance of a high pulmonary volume during central apneas increases alveolar O_2 stores and limits post-apneic arterial O_2 desaturation (19). In addition, maintenance of positive subglottal pressure likely increases lower airway stability and lung compliance, hence decreasing the tendency for atelectasis and further hypoxemic apnea. Finally, resumption of breathing with expiration from a higher apneic lung volume could conceivably minimize aspiration of secretions, which may have accumulated in the hypopharynx during apnea. Conversely, while one can speculate on the deleterious effects of inspiratory breath-holding in newborns, the importance of such effects remains to be demonstrated. Despite the fact that breathing cessation in an inspiratory position could theoretically inhibit the next inspiration through the Hering-Breuer inhibitory reflex and thereby prolong apnea duration, this has not been supported by our findings in preterm lambs (19). Finally, while the return of inspiratory efforts despite ongoing laryngeal closure (mixed apnea) is indeed possible (21), it has been rarely observed in our preterm ovine model (3,19,20).

D. Origin of Active Glottal Closure During Neonatal Central Apneas

Interestingly, the above observations of active glottal closure with inspiratory breath-holding throughout central apneas in newborn lambs have ontogenetic and phylogenetic correlations. From a phylogenetic standpoint, alternation of breathing movements and prolonged apneas, with the exchanger full of gas (i.e., inspiratory breath-holding with active glottal closure), is currently considered to represent the basic breathing pattern in air-breathing vertebrates. This primitive breathing pattern can be observed to this day in lower vertebrates, such as amphibians and aquatic reptiles, and is also present in diving mammals, such as whales and seals, even while on land (22). From an ontogenetic standpoint, during late gestation, "fetal breathing" is present as alternating periods with diaphragm EMG bursts during REM sleep and prolonged "central apneas" with active glottal closure during NREM sleep. And although active glottal closure during central apneas is usually considered vestigial at most in nondiving adult mammals, it has been reported in adult humans during a few spontaneous central apneas (23) and in post-hyperventilation apneas in rats (21). Finally, inspiratory breath-holding with active glottal closure is commonly observed throughout life with Valsalva maneuvers in conditions such as defecation, micturition, parturition, and heavy load carrying. However, contrary to induced apneas in full-term lambs (24), Valsalva maneuvers are associated with forceful tonic abdominal muscle contraction throughout inspiratory breath-holding.

Data in the literature on laryngeal control during apnea are scarce and unclear. Insofar as central mechanisms are concerned, the demonstration that stimulation of α_2 adrenergic agonists induces tonic glottal constrictor EMG during central apneas in awake goats has led to speculation on the direct involvement of brainstem α_2 adrenergic receptors in active glottal closure during apneas (25). More recently, the involvement of serotonin and its 5HT1 receptor have been proposed from data obtained in a transgenic mouse model of neonatal ventilatory instability displaying numerous central apneas with post-inspiratory vagal activity (surrogate for glottal constrictor EMG) (26). These hypotheses remain to be confirmed, however. As for the effect of peripheral input, investigators have previously speculated that increased vagal afferent activity related to decreased lung volume is responsible for continuous glottal constrictor EMG during central apneas in full-term lambs (7). However, glottal constrictor EMG is still observed throughout induced central apneas in full-term lambs, despite thoracic vagotomy (27) or maintenance of a high lung volume (28). These observations are also independent of the presence of laryngeal afferent activity, as shown after severing of both superior laryngeal nerves (18). Glottal constrictor EMG is not modified either by various conditions of arterial PO_2 or PCO_2 (18,27,28). This observation demonstrates that neither central nor peripheral chemoreceptor activity is the primary factor responsible for active glottal closure throughout central apneas in full-term lambs.

Of interest, active glottal closure is also present throughout inspiratory breath-holding, alternating with gasps during anoxic gasping in lambs (29). Since gasping respiration is speculated to originate from brainstem centers other than those implicating eupnea, such observations suggest that reciprocal inhibition between motoneurons driving glottal constrictor muscles and inspiratory bulbospinal neurons is a consistent feature despite varying respiratory control circumstances, including eupnea, apnea, and gasping respiration.

In summary, upper airway closure appears to be an important feature of neonatal apneas, including not only during obstructive/mixed apneas, but also during central apneas. Current evidence supports the view that both passive pharyngeal collapse and active glottal closure are involved in neonatal apneas. Interestingly, this active closure, which seems particularly well suited to the newborn with numerous apneas, is increasingly recognized. This includes spontaneous as well as artificially induced central apneas, in both newborn (dog, sheep, opossum, mouse) and adult mammals (human, goat, rat, diving mammals) of various species.

V. Laryngeal Chemoreflexes

The LCR are triggered by the contact between liquids—especially acid or with low chloride content—and receptors of the laryngeal mucosa in mammals. For several decades now, it has been known that LCR are lung protective reflexes in mature mammals beyond infancy, consisting primarily of swallowing, coughing, and arousal, aimed at limiting contact duration with the laryngeal mucosa and at preventing subglottal aspiration (6). Since the initial observations of Johnson et al. (30) in anesthetized lambs, over fifty studies have reported that inhibitory cardiorespiratory responses to application of distilled water on the larynx are characteristic of the immature, newborn mammal. Classically, in the latter, LCR are composed of a vagal efferent component, which includes laryngospasm, central or mixed/obstructive apnea, oxygen desaturation and bradycardia, and a sympathetic efferent component, which includes systemic hypertension and redistribution of blood flow to vital organs, such as the brain and heart (6). Clinical relevance of LCR stems from the common observation that LCR can be triggered by gastropharyngeal reflux, bottle-feeding, or oral intake of medications (e.g., vitamins or iron) in preterm neonates. In addition, LCR can be responsible, in a few infants, even when born after full term gestation, for apparent life-threatening events and probably some cases of sudden infant death syndrome (SIDS) (6,31). While numerous studies have assessed LCR in response to various liquids in newborn mammals, most were of disputed clinical relevance, due to inherent experimental conditions (use of anesthesia or sedation, instillation of liquids on the tracheal side of the larynx, use of distilled water, etc.). In particular, the effects of acid solutions (as a surrogate for gastric liquid) have been much less studied than that of water. This recognition provided us the impetus to engage in a research program on LCR using full-term and preterm newborn lamb models, while focusing on experiments relevant to clinical conditions.

A. LCR in Preterm vs. Full-Term Lambs

Findings from a study conducted on LCR in nonsedated, full-term lambs during NREM sleep reveal that instillation of both distilled water and acid solutions elicit very mild cardiorespiratory responses. However, lower airway protective reflexes, including swallowing, cough and arousal, are prominent, especially following acid solutions, suggesting that the latter are more potent stimuli than distilled water for these reflexes (32). Accordingly, results in nonsedated piglets using distilled water similarly yielded mild cardiorespiratory responses, while eliciting both swallowing and arousal (33). Conversely, recent findings in preterm lambs have shown much more potent cardiorespiratory responses to both distilled water and hydrochloric acid, including prolonged and, at times, life-threatening apneas with oxyhemoglobin desaturation and bradycardia (34) (Fig. 6). Our findings in lambs of a relationship between gestational age and the degree of cardiorespiratory responses mimic clinical observations in human preterm infants, in whom immature LCR, characterized by prominent cardiorespiratory responses, are primarily observed (35). However, unusual neural immaturity or abnormal conditions in full-term newborn infants, such as respiratory syncytial virus infection (36), likely exacerbates the potentially dangerous (immature-type) cardiorespiratory components of the LCR.

LCR elicited by acid solutions (e.g., gastric liquid) warrant further scrutiny because of their clinical relevance (gastropharyngeal reflux). Differences between LCR triggered by acids and water are likely related to stimulation of different laryngeal receptors. Two types of water receptors have been described in the laryngeal mucosa, responding either to low chloride concentrations or to hypo-osmolality (37). By comparison, extracellular acidification can alter the activity of several ionic channels, including the vanilloid receptor TRPV1, the acid-sensitive Na^+ channels ASIC, and the acid-sensitive K^+ channels TASK. TRPV1 receptors have previously been shown to be present in the laryngeal mucosa in adult rats (38), and preliminary personal observations suggest the presence of ASIC1 and TASK1 channels in the laryngeal mucosa of full-term lambs in the first postnatal week (unpublished observations). Capsaicin-sensitive laryngeal fiber endings (with TRPV1 receptors) have been shown to be sensitive to citric acid but insensitive to water in adult guinea pigs (39). Similarly, our previous results in lambs suggest that while capsaicin-sensitive laryngeal fibers are functional in the neonatal period, they are insensitive to water (40). Further experiments are needed to assess the possibility of inhibiting acid-triggered LCR by specific blockade of the acid-sensing receptors.

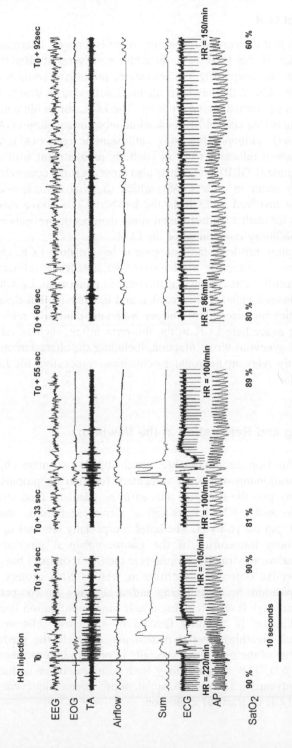

Figure 6 Laryngeal chemoreflexes triggered by injection of 0.5 mL hydrochloric acid on the larynx in a preterm lamb (gestational age 132 days) during quiet sleep at postnatal day 7. Note the potentially life-threatening cardiorespiratory responses with prolonged, repetitive central apneas, marked bradycardia, and desaturation. *Abbreviations:* EEG, electroencephalogram; EOG, electrooculogram; TA, raw thyroarytenoid muscle (a glottal constrictor muscle) electrical activity (EMG); Airflow, nasal airflow; Sum, variations of lung volume, assessed from respiratory inductance plethysmography; ECG, electrocardiogram; AP, arterial pressure; SatO$_2$, arterial hemoglobin saturation (pulsed oximetry).

B. Modulation of LCR

Previous results suggest that the central respiratory drive is a major determinant of the apnea component of the LCR (41). In addition, several studies have examined the possibility of decreasing the immature, prominent cardiorespiratory component of the LCR in the newborn mammal with various drugs. The more notable results can be summarized as follows. The LCR can be blunted by various interventions, including central M_3 muscarinic receptor antagonists (42), β-adrenergic agonists (43), aminophylline (44), antihistamine agents (45), acetazolamide (46), and topical lidocaine (47). In addition, pretreatment with calcitonin gene-related peptide (CGRP) antagonists also prevents some components of the LCR elicited by water in piglets (48), which suggests that capsaicin-sensitive fibers may be involved in LCR in the newborn. The above results certainly form the basis for further studies aimed at the therapeutic prevention of the cardiorespiratory inhibitory component of the LCR.

In conclusion, healthy full-term lambs appear to have mature LCR, characterized by lower airway protective mechanisms and absence of clinically significant apnea-bradycardia. The converse is also true in preterm lambs, which exhibit severe and prolonged apneas, bradycardia, and oxyhemoglobin desaturation. Additional studies are needed to further ascertain clinically relevant conditions presumed to exacerbate LCR in the full-term infant, such as reflux laryngitis or respiratory syncytial virus infection, including the characterization of the likewise clinically relevant neuronal mechanisms responsible for LCR triggered by acid solutions.

VI. Swallowing and Respiration in the Newborn

Swallowing is a vital function throughout life, which fulfills two main objectives. First, nutritive swallowing serves an alimentary function by propulsing food from the oral cavity into the stomach, thus ensuring adequate food intake and normal growth. Secondly, NNS clears saliva, airway secretions, and/or gastric content refluxed into the pharynx. The latter is especially relevant in the newborn infant, in whom immaturity of the gastroesophageal junction is responsible for regurgitations in virtually all infants in the first months of life. By carrying out their respective objectives, nutritive as well as NNS protect the lower airways from aspiration. Since breathing and swallowing are competing functions at the upper airways level, breathing-swallowing coordination is crucial. While this coordination is certainly favored by the close relationship between swallowing and breathing central pattern generators in the medulla (49,50), neural immaturity of the newborn, especially in preterm infants, impairs that coordination (8,51,52). This situation may lead to apneas of prematurity, with hypoxemia and bradycardia, as well as to apparent life-threatening events of infancy and SIDS, via LCR or tracheal aspiration.

This section will primarily focus on recent data on NNS and its coordination with breathing in newborns. The reader interested in a more detailed review on nutritive swallowing in the newborn is referred to recent reviews on the subject (52,53).

A. Swallowing in the Neonatal Period

The precise neurophysiology of swallowing has been summarized in recent reviews (49,50). Briefly, nutritive swallowing is comprised of three phases: oral (nutritive sucking in the newborn), pharyngeal, and esophageal. Efficient nutritive sucking is lacking prior to 32 weeks' postconceptional age (PCA) and reaches a mature pattern at about 36 weeks' PCA (8,51,52). The pharyngeal phase associates closure of both the velopharyngeal sphincter and the larynx, relaxation of the crico-esophageal sphincter, and contraction of the pharynx in order to propel the bolus into the esophagus. Finely coordinated contraction of a number of pharyngeal and laryngeal muscles (~ 20 pairs of muscles) is crucial during this phase, in order to ensure perfect breathing-swallowing coordination. A short obligatory respiratory pause is present with laryngeal closure. Breathing-swallowing coordination undergoes maturation between 32 and 36 weeks' PCA, and rhythmic (mature) breathing during nutritive swallowing is usually established at 36 weeks' PCA (8). Finally, the third swallowing phase, namely the esophageal phase, ensures progression of the bolus toward the stomach.

As opposed to nutritive swallowing, NNS begins with the pharyngeal phase and is triggered by afferent messages in the pharyngeal and the superior laryngeal nerves. Relevance for addressing NNS and its coordination with breathing stems from the fact that NNS is a major component of the mature LCR and from the temporal coincidence reported between apneas of prematurity and NNS, which has led to suggest that NNS may cause neonatal apneas (see below). We will review some factors impacting first on the frequency of NNS in the neonatal period, then on breathing-swallowing coordination.

B. Factors Influencing the Frequency of NNS

States of Alertness

In the neonatal period, all studies but one (54) have reported that NNS frequency is at its highest in REM sleep and at its lowest in NREM sleep (33,55–57). In addition, NNS bursts are much more frequent in REM sleep (55–57). The reason why NNS frequency is higher in REM sleep is unclear and might simply be related to a higher production of saliva during REM sleep. However, it is well documented that REM sleep also triggers irregular and higher respiratory and heart rates. Given the close localization and organization of the central pattern generators driving NNS, respiration, and heart rate, it may not be surprising that REM sleep exerts a similar influence on all of these functions. As for the higher NNS frequency in wakefulness than in NREM sleep, the wakefulness stimulus may influence the swallowing central pattern generator, as it does for the respiratory central pattern generator (58).

Pre- and Postnatal Development

While gestational age does not seem to have an impact on the frequency of isolated NNS, the frequency of NNS bursts is higher in preterm than in full-term lambs, regardless of the state of alertness (55–57). Similar results have been reported in preterm infants (59), leading to the speculation that preterm birth leads to an increase in pharyngolaryngeal sensitivity. The physiological consequences of these repeated swallows still remain to be proven, some authors considering them as ineffectual (59).

In adult humans (60) and adult sheep (61), NNS frequency is higher in REM sleep than in NREM sleep and NNS burst frequency is at its highest during REM sleep in adult sheep (61). Hence, regardless of the cause for higher NNS and NNS burst frequency during REM sleep, the relationship between NNS frequency and states of alertness seem to be similar among humans and animals, irrespective of the maturation process of the organism.

Nasal Application of Positive Pressure

Nasal application of positive pressure, either intermittently (nasal intermittent positive pressure ventilation, or nIPPV) or continuously (nasal continuous positive airway pressure, or nCPAP), is increasingly used in the neonatal period as a treatment for mild respiratory distress syndrome (62), apneas of prematurity (63) and as a means of reducing the rate of extubation failure following endotracheal mechanical ventilation (64,65). However, a few results suggest that nCPAP or nIPPV can influence swallowing function. Indeed, nCPAP has been shown to inhibit swallowing in awake human adults (66) and to decrease isolated NNS in NREM sleep and bursts of NNS in REM sleep in the newborn lamb. In comparison, the effects of nIPPV on NNS frequency were more variable (67). Studies are currently ongoing to understand the mechanisms responsible for decreasing NNS frequency in NREM sleep in the lamb. Our preliminary results suggest that stimulation of slow adapting bronchopulmonary receptors are involved in the decrease in NNS frequency observed with nCPAP (68). Accordingly, two separate studies have implied that stimulation of slow adapting bronchopulmonary receptors inhibits water-induced swallowing in awake adult humans (69,70). Regardless of the mechanism(s) involved, awareness of the decreasing effect of nCPAP on NNS is potentially of high clinical relevance. Indeed, in addition to the important role of NNS in clearing the upper airways from secretions and frequent gastric regurgitations, prolonged application of nCPAP in the immature newborn with high neural plasticity might lead to a further delay in swallowing maturation or even long lasting disturbance in swallowing function. This however remains to be tested.

Hypoxia and Hypercapnia

While hypoxic and/or hypercapnic conditions are very frequent in the neonatal period, at times for several weeks, consequences of these respiratory challenges on NNS are totally unknown. Current knowledge on the effects of hypoxia on swallowing is restricted to one report concluding that acute hypoxia inhibits swallowing induced by stimulation of the superior laryngeal nerve in decerebrate adult cats (71). However, our recent results revealed that moderate hypoxia induced by breathing 10% O_2 during a four-hour period ($PaO_2 = 45$ to 50 mmHg) does not modify NNS frequency in nonsedated newborn lambs, regardless of the state of alertness (72). With regards to hypercapnia, available data are also restricted to acute hypercapnia and have yielded contradictory results. While a first study reported that hypercapnia had no effect on swallowing activity in anaesthetized cats (71), more recent studies showed that hypercapnia decreased water-induced swallowing in adult humans (73,74) and decreased nutritive swallowing frequency in newborns (75). However, our recent results suggest that a moderate hypercapnia induced by breathing 5% CO_2 during a four-hour period ($PaCO_2 = 50$ mmHg) increases NNS frequency in all states of alertness in the nonsedated newborn lamb (72). The mechanisms involved are still under study and may involve stimulation of upper airway receptors by hypercapnia (76) or the consequent hyperventilation, stimulation of saliva production (77), or direct hypercapnic stimulation of neurons of the swallowing centers, which share common medullary locations with the respiratory centers (49,50). Potential consequences of such observations on aspirations, apneas, and swallowing maturation ultimately need to be addressed in future studies.

C. Factors Influencing Breathing-Swallowing Coordination

Breathing and swallowing share common structures in the oropharyngeal cavity and are therefore competing functions of the upper airways (52). Breathing and NNS cannot be performed simultaneously and must be perfectly coordinated. A short obligatory respiratory pause is present with laryngeal closure during NNS. Interestingly, swallowing and respiratory central pattern generators are also located in the neighboring regions in the brainstem, mainly in the regions of the nucleus tractus solitarius and the nucleus ambiguus (49). This anatomical proximity thereby facilitates both reciprocal inhibition and coordination (53).

Four types of NNS can be described in relationship with its occurrence within the respiratory cycle (Fig. 7). They include the e-type NNS, followed and preceded by expiration, the i-type NNS, followed and preceded by inspiration, the ie-type NNS, occurring at the transition between inspiration and expiration, and finally the ei-type NNS, occurring at the transition between expiration and inspiration. Relevance for studying the precise NNS-breathing coordination arises from the premise that NNS occurring during inspiration carries a higher risk of aspiration (51) and NNS occurring during expiration may carry a higher risk of apnea.

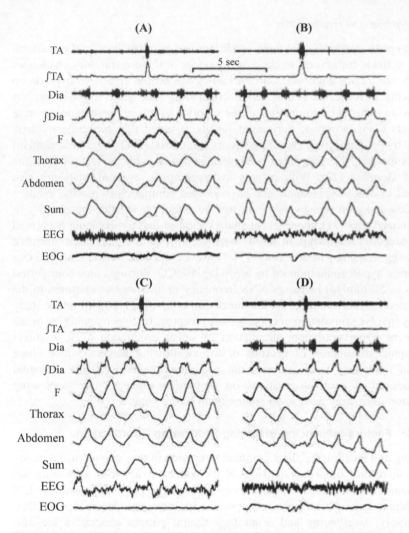

Figure 7 Various types of NNS-breathing coordination. (**A**) i-type NNS (preceded by and followed by inspiration). (**B**) e-type NNS (preceded by and followed by expiration). (**C**) ie-type NNS (at the phase transition between inspiration and expiration). (**D**) ei-type NNS (at the phase transition between expiration and inspiration). *Abbreviations*: NNS, nonnutritive swallowing; TA, raw thyroarytenoid muscle (a glottal constrictor muscle) electrical activity (EMG); ∫TA, moving time averaged TA EMG (time constant: 100 ms); Di, diaphragmatic muscle EMG; ∫Di, moving time averaged Di EMG; F, nasal airflow (inspiration upward); Thorax, variations of thoracic volume, assessed from respiratory inductance plethysmography; Abdomen, variations of abdominal volume, assessed from respiratory inductance plethysmography; Sum, variations of lung volume, assessed from respiratory inductance plethysmography; EEG, electroencephalogram; EOG, electrooculogram.

Influence of the States of Alertness and Age

To our knowledge, the only data available on the influence of the states of alertness on breathing-swallowing coordination and respiration were obtained in sheep. In the neonatal period, in both full-term and preterm lambs and in the adult sheep, results reveal the same pattern of NNS distribution during quiet wakefulness, NREM sleep, and REM sleep (56,57,61). While the i-type represents the most frequent NNS type (roughly 40%), the e-type is the least frequent (less than 10%). Hence, NNS-respiration coordination in sheep seems to be established early in life, even prenatally. Previous results in humans suggest however the presence of a more complex postnatal maturation. Indeed, while NNS occurred throughout the respiratory cycle in preterm infants (78), most NNS were of the e-type in young (18–34 years old) adult humans during wakefulness. In addition, prevalence of NNS occurring during inspiration was increased in older adult humans (63–83 years old) (79). Of note, a similar postnatal maturation was observed for nutritive swallowing in humans, with up to 50% of nutritive swallowing being preceded by an inspiration in the preterm infant (8,51), and the majority of induced water or nutritive swallows in adult humans being consistently of the e-type (73,79,80).

Influence of Species and Experimental Conditions

While data on breathing-swallowing coordination in adult humans reported mostly e-type NNS (73,79–81), observations in adult goats (82), dogs (83), and rabbits (84) during wakefulness, and in adult sheep during all states of alertness (61) reported a predominance of NNS occurring during inspiration. Discrepancies between results obtained in adult animals and humans may be related to (1) experimental conditions, such as the technique used to induce swallowing, i.e., NNS induced by a bolus of water in adult humans vs. spontaneous NNS in goats, sheep, dogs, vs. nutritive swallows in rabbits; (2) species differences, including the fact that goats and sheep are ruminants with different body positions (biped vs. quadruped). Regarding the latter, available data suggest that while breathing-swallowing coordination is identical in the supine and upright position in adult humans (e-type NNS, either spontaneous or water-induced) (79,85), occurrence of nutritive swallows is altered from late- to early-expiration from the hand and knees to the upright position (86).

External Influences on Breathing-Swallowing Coordination

Numerous external influences can probably impact on breathing-swallowing coordination in the neonatal period. Preliminary results in newborn lambs suggest that the increase in NNS during hypercapnia is entirely due to an increase in ie-type NNS; in comparison, the small decrease in ei-type NNS observed in hypoxia, though statistically significant, is of doubtful physiological significance (72). Studies are currently ongoing to assess the influence of secondary tobacco smoke in the first postnatal weeks on NNS frequency and breathing-swallowing coordination in relation with the suggested relationship between tobacco smoke exposure and SIDS (87,88). Finally, we are currently studying the impact of respiratory syncytial virus infection in relation with the reported abnormalities in swallowing reflex and a higher risk of aspiration in previously healthy infants (89).

D. Apnea and NNS

Breathing in human infants (90,91) and adults (92) is suspended for a short period during swallowing. Duration of this breathing pause has recently been estimated to be 0.5 seconds for nutritive swallows and 0.8 seconds for NNS in the human infant (91). In addition, as opposed to adult humans, up to 55% of nutritive swallows in the newborn are preceded and followed by a breathing pause (8,51). While NNS have been reported with isolated central, obstructive, or mixed apneas in the human newborn (54,78,93), the majority of these NNS-associated apneas were either obstructive or mixed. In the preterm lamb, NNS are absent during central apneas observed with periodic breathing and, overall, only 10% of apneas are associated with NNS, mostly during REM sleep (Fig. 8) (57). The mechanisms involved in the temporal association between apneas and

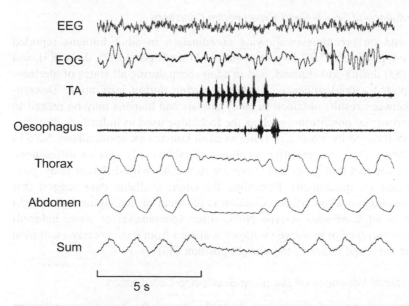

Figure 8 Spontaneous central apnea associated with NNS burst in a full-term lamb during active sleep. *Abbreviations*: EEG, electroencephalogram; EOG, electrooculogram; TA, raw thyroarytenoid muscle (a glottal constrictor muscle) electrical activity (EMG); Oesophagus, oesophageal muscle EMG; Thorax, variations of thoracic volume, assessed from respiratory inductance plethysmography; Abdomen, variations of abdominal volume, assessed from respiratory inductance plethysmography; Sum, variations of lung volume, assessed from respiratory inductance plethysmography.

NNS remain controversial. While virtually all spontaneous NNS (either isolated or in bursts) associated with apneas in preterm lambs occur after onset of the apnea (57), data in infants before six months of age suggest that NNS could trigger up to 25% of apneas (54). Some arguments support the hypothesis of a peripheral origin to this association, while others are supportive of a central origin (57). In the peripheral hypothesis, stimulation of chemo- and/or mechanoreceptors at the laryngeal or pharyngeal levels would produce both apneas and swallowing. Alternatively, the development of negative pressure during obstructive apneas could trigger NNS via stimulation of upper airway receptors. In the central hypothesis, NNS occurrence during apneas is likely related to the disinhibition of the swallowing central pattern generator during central inspiratory drive arrest. However, this is inconsistent with the higher incidence of NNS during obstructive/ mixed apneas, when central inspiratory drive is present.

In summary, NNS, and its relationship with breathing, is an important consideration in understanding respiration in normal and pathological conditions of the newborn. Many factors can influence the frequency of NNS, such as states of alertness, nasal ventilatory support, and hypercapnia. Limited available data suggest the establishment of a precise coordination between NNS and phases of the breathing cycle at birth, even before term, at least in the ovine model. However, differences were observed in regards to this coordination between humans and animal models and may be related to the posture during feeding or experimental conditions. As in the case of apneas, NNS—especially, when occurring in bursts—is associated with some obstructive/mixed spontaneous apneas in REM sleep but absent with central apneas of periodic breathing in NREM sleep.

VII. Laryngeal Function and Nasal Ventilatory Support

Nasal positive pressure ventilation (nIPPV) is increasingly used in the neonatal period and somewhat preferred to endotracheal tube ventilation as a means to prevent the various complications associated with the latter. An important difference, however, in using a nasal interface as opposed to an endotracheal tube for ventilatory support is the interposition of the larynx. Indeed, previous endoscopic observations in adult humans reported a glottal narrowing during nIPPV (94), thus suggesting that the larynx can act as a closing valve and prevent transmission of positive pressure from a mechanical ventilator to the lungs. Further, personal recent observations in newborn lambs have yielded striking changes in glottal muscle electrical activity (EMG) in nIPPV. Indeed, we demonstrated that nIPPV, either in the pressure support or volume control mode, induced both a decrease in phasic laryngeal dilator EMG and the onset of phasic laryngeal constrictor EMG simultaneously to ventilator insufflations (Fig. 9) (95). Simultaneously, a significant relationship was shown between the increase in glottal constrictor EMG and the increase in trans–upper airway pressure, strongly suggesting the development of an active glottal narrowing

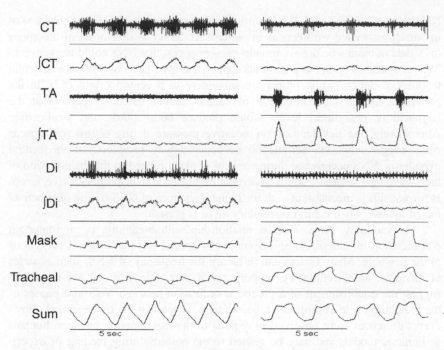

Figure 9 Active glottal closure developing with nasal intermittent positive ventilation (pressure support mode) in one full-term lamb during wakefulness. Left: CPAP = 4 cmH$_2$O; Right: 10/4 cmH$_2$O. Note the disappearance of inspiratory CT and diaphragm EMG, and the appearance of TA EMG, simultaneously with the increase in mask pressure (ventilator strokes). *Abbreviations*: CT, cricothyroid muscle (a glottal dilator muscle) electrical activity (EMG); ∫CT, moving time averaged CT EMG; TA, raw thyroarytenoid muscle (a glottal constrictor muscle) EMG; ∫TA, moving time averaged TA EMG (time constant: 100 ms); Di, diaphragmatic muscle EMG; ∫Di, moving time averaged Di EMG; Mask, mask pressure; Tracheal, tracheal pressure; Sum, variations of lung volume, assessed from respiratory inductance plethysmographie.

against ventilator insufflations, which increasingly limited lung ventilation, in parallel with augmentation in ventilatory support (95). This limitation was more marked in volume control than in pressure support mode of ventilation. Results were identical in wakefulness and quiet sleep. The mechanisms responsible for enhancing active glottal closure in inspiration during nIPPV are currently under investigation. Since results obtained to date do not favor the involvement of hypocapnia, reflex activity originating from various upper and/or lower airway receptors is likely involved. Such laryngeal behavior during nIPPV is of high clinical importance and has been linked to lung hypoventilation during sleep in adult humans (96). In addition, diversion of positive pressure from the airways can lead to increased gastric distension (97) as well as the risk of vomiting and even gastric perforation in neonates.

VIII. Conclusion

Consideration of laryngeal function is imperative for understanding neonatal respiration in normal and pathological conditions. Available data on neonatal apneas suggest that active laryngeal closure can occur and be beneficial in the newborn, especially by limiting hypoxemia following repetitive central apneas during periodic breathing epochs. In addition, we believe that immaturity of the reflexes originating from the laryngeal chemoreceptors, including LCR and NNS, contributes to the occurrence of apneas, bradycardia, and oxyhemoglobin desaturation in early life, with at times potentially dramatic consequences. This finding indubitably underscores the need for additional research in the area of laryngeal function and respiration in the postnatal period.

Acknowledgments

Jean-Paul Praud is a "national researcher scholar" of the *Fonds de la recherche en santé du Québec*. Nathalie Samson holds a Canada graduate scholarship award. This work was supported by the Canadian Institutes of Health Research (NRF 15558) and the Quebec Foundation for Research into Children's Diseases. Studies in preterm lambs were made possible thanks to a gracious donation of BLES surfactant by BLES Inc, London, Ontario, Canada.

References

1. Gauda SB. Upper-airway muscle control during development-application to clinical disorders that occur in preterm infants. In: Mathew OP, ed. Respiratory Control and Disorders in the Newborn. New York: Marcel Dekker, Inc., 2003:115–137.
2. Henick DH, Holinger LD. Laryngeal development. In: Holinger LD, Lusk RP, Green CG, eds. Pediatric Laryngology and Bronchoesophagology. Philadelphia: Lippincot-Raven, 1997:1–17.
3. Samson N, Lafond JR, Moreau-Bussiere F, et al. Cricothyroid muscle electrical activity during respiration and apneas in lambs. Respir Physiol Neurobiol 2007; 155 (2):147–155.
4. Harding R, Hooper SB. Regulation of lung expansion and lung growth before birth. J Appl Physiol 1996; 81:209–224.
5. Kianicka I, Diaz V, Dorion D, et al. Coordination between glottic adductor muscle and diaphragm EMG activity in fetal lambs in utero. J Appl Physiol 1998; 84:1560–1565.
6. Thach BT. Maturation and transformation of reflexes that protect the laryngeal airway from liquid aspiration from fetal to adult life. Am J Med 2001; 111:69S–77S.
7. Harding R. The upper respiratory tract in perinatal life. In: Johnston BM, Gluckman PD, eds. Respiratory Control and Lung Development in the Fetus and Newborn. Ithaca, NY: Perinatology Press, 1986:332–376.
8. Mizuno K, Ueda A. The maturation and coordination of sucking, swallowing, and respiration in preterm infants. J Pediatr 2003; 142:36–40.

9. Diaz V, Dorion D, Renolleau S, et al. Effects of capsaicin pretreatment on expiratory laryngeal closure during pulmonary edema in lambs. J Appl Physiol 1999; 86: 1570–1577.

10. Mortola JP. Dynamics of breathing in newborn mammals. Physiol Rev 1987; 67: 187–243.

11. Eichenwald EC, Howell RG III, Kosch PC, et al. Developmental changes in sequential activation of laryngeal abductor muscle and diaphragm in infants. J Appl Physiol 1992; 73:1425–1431.

12. Bailey EF, Fregosi RF. Modulation of upper airway muscle activities by bronchopulmonary afferents. J Appl Physiol 2006; 101:609–617.

13. Finer NN, Higgins R, Kattwinkel J, et al. Summary Proceedings from the apnea-of-prematurity group. Pediatrics 2006; 117:S47–S51.

14. Baird TM. Clinical correlates, natural history and outcome of neonatal apnoea. Semin Neonatol 2004; 9:205–211.

15. Milner AD, Greenough A. The role of the upper airway in neonatal apnea. Semin Neonatol 2004; 9:213–219.

16. England SJ. Laryngeal muscle and diaphragmatic activities in conscious dog pups. Respir Physiol 1985; 60:95–108.

17. Farber J. Development of pulmonary reflexes and pattern of breathing in the Virginia opossum. Respir Physiol 1972; 14:278–286.

18. Fortier P-H, Reix P, Arsenault J, et al. Active upper airway closure during induced central apneas in lambs is complete at the laryngeal level only. J Appl Physiol 2003; 95:97–103.

19. Reix P, Arsenault J, Dome V, et al. Active glottal closure during central apneas limits oxygen desaturation in premature lambs. J Appl Physiol 2003; 94:1949–1954.

20. Renolleau S, Létourneau P, Niyonsenga T, et al. Thyroarytenoid muscle electrical activity during spontaneous apneas in preterm lambs. Am J Respir Crit Care Med 1999; 159:1396–1404.

21. Sun QJ, Berkowitz RG, Pilowsky PM. Response of laryngeal motoneurons to hyperventilation induced apnea in the rat. Respir Physiol Neurobiol 2005; 146: 155–163.

22. Mortola JP, Limoges M-J. Resting breathing frequency in aquatic mammals: A comparative analysis with terrestrial species. Respir Physiol Neurobiol 2006; 154:500–514.

23. Insalaco G, Kuna ST, Catania G, et al. Thyroarytenoid muscle activity in sleep apneas. J Appl Physiol 1993; 74:704–709.

24. Kianicka I, Diaz V, Canet E, et al. Laryngeal and abdominal muscle electrical activity during periodic breathing in non sedated lambs. J Appl Physiol 1998; 84:669–675.

25. Hedrick MS, Dwinell MR, Janssen PL, et al. Differential respiratory muscle recruitment induced by clonidine in awake goats. J Appl Physiol 1998; 84: 1198–1207.

26. Stettner GM, Huppke P, Dutschmann M. The C57BL/6J mouse strain: an animal model to study spontaneous obstructive apnoea? Experimental Biology meeting abstracts [CD-ROM]. FASEB J 2006; 20:231.8.

27. Praud J-P, Canet E, Bureau MA. Chemoreceptor and vagal influences on thyroarytenoid muscle activity in awake lambs during hypoxia. J Appl Physiol 1992; 72: 962–969.

28. Praud J-P, Kianicka I, Leroux J-F, et al. Prolonged active glottis closure after barbiturate-induced respiratory arrest in lambs. Respir Physiol 1996; 104: 221–229.

29. Thuot F, Lemaire D, Dorion D, et al. Active glottal closure during anoxic gasping in lambs. Respir Physiol 2001; 128:205–218.

30. Johnson P, Dawes DS, Robinson JS. Maintenance of breathing in newborn lamb. Arch Dis Child 1972; 47:151.

31. Page M, Jeffery H. The role of gastro-oesophageal reflux in the aetiology of SIDS. Early Hum Dev 2000; 59:127–149.

32. St-Hilaire M, Nsegbe E, Gagnon-Gervais K, et al. Laryngeal chemoreflexes induced by acid, water and saline in nonsedated newborn lambs during quiet sleep. J Appl Physiol 2005; 98:2197–2203.

33. Page M, Jeffery HE, Marks V, et al. Mechanisms of airway protection after pharyngeal fluid infusion in healthy sleeping piglets. J Appl Physiol 1995; 78: 1942–1949.

34. St-Hilaire M, Samson N, Nsegbe E, et al. Postnatal maturation of laryngeal chemoreflexes in the preterm lamb. J Appl Physiol, 2007; 102:1429–1438.

35. Thach BT. The role of respiratory control disorders in SIDS. Respir Physiol Neurobiol 2005; 149:343–353.

36. Lindgren C, Jing L, Graham B, et al. Respiratory syncytial virus infection reinforces reflex apnea in young lambs. Pediatr Res 1992; 31:381–385.

37. Anderson JW, Sant'Ambrogio FB, Mathew OP, et al. Water-responsive laryngeal receptors in the dog are not specialized endings. Respir Physiol 1990; 79:33–43.

38. Yamamoto Y, Taniguchi K. Immunolocalization of VR1 and VRL1 in rat larynx. Auton Neurosci 2005; 117:62–65.

39. Forsberg K, Karlsson JA, Theodorsson E, et al. Cough and bronchoconstriction mediated by capsaicin-sensitive sensory neurons in the guinea-pig. Pulm Pharmacol 1988; 1:33–39.

40. Roulier S, Arsenault J, Reix P, et al. Effects of C fiber blockage on cardiorespiratory responses to laryngeal stimulation in conscious lambs. Respir Physiol Neurobiol 2003; 136:13–23.

41. Van Der Velde L, Curran AK, Filiano JJ, et al. Prolongation of the laryngeal chemoreflex after inhibition of the rostral ventral medulla in piglets: a role in SIDS? J Appl Physiol 2003; 94:1883–1895.

42. Richardson BE, Pernell KJ, Goding GS, Jr. Effect of antagonism at central nervous system M3 muscarinic receptors on laryngeal chemoresponse. Ann Otol Rhinol Laryngol 1997; 106:920–926.

43. Grogaard J, Kreuger E, Lindstrom D, et al. Effects of carotid body maturation and terbutaline on the laryngeal chemoreflex in newborn lambs. Pediatr Res 1986; 20: 724–729.

44. Lee JC, Stoll BJ, Downing SE. Properties of the laryngeal chemoreflex in neonatal piglets. Am J Physiol 1977; 233:R30–R36.

45. Downs DH, Johnson K, Goding GS Jr. The effect of antihistamines on the laryngeal chemoreflex. Laryngoscope 1995; 105:857–861.

46. Heman-Ackah YD, Goding GS Jr. Effects of intralaryngeal carbon dioxide and acetazolamide on the laryngeal chemoreflex. Ann Otol Rhinol Laryngol 2000; 109: 921–928.

47. McCulloch TM, Flint PW, Richardson MA, et al. Lidocaine effects on the laryngeal chemoreflex, mechanoreflex, and afferent electrical stimulation reflex. Ann Otol Rhinol Laryngol 1992; 101:583–589.
48. Bauman NM, Wang D, Jaffe DA, et al. Effect of intravenous calcitonin gene–related peptide antagonist on the laryngeal chemoreflex in piglets. Otolaryngol Head Neck Surg 1999; 121:1–6.
49. Ertekin C, Aydogdu I. Neurophysiology of swallowing. Clin Neurophysiol 2003; 114:2226–2244.
50. Jean A. Brain stem control of swallowing: neuronal network and cellular mechanisms. Physiol Rev 2001; 81:929–969.
51. Lau C, Smith EO, Schanler RJ. Coordination of suck-swallow and swallow respiration in preterm infants. Acta Paediatr 2003; 92:721–727.
52. Oommen MP. Respiratory control during oral feeding. In: Oommen MP, ed. Respiratory Control and Disorders in the Newborn. Lung Biology in Health and Disease. Vol. 173. New York: Marcel Dekker, 2004:373–393.
53. Miller MJ, Kiatchoosakun P. Relationship between respiratory control and feeding in the developing infant. Semin Neonatol 2004; 9:221–227.
54. Don GW, Waters KA. Influence of sleep state on frequency of swallowing, apnea, and arousal in human infants. J Appl Physiol 2003; 94:2456–2464.
55. Jeffery HE, Ius D, Page M. The role of swallowing during active sleep in the clearance of reflux in term and preterm infants. J Pediatr 2000; 137:545–548.
56. Reix P, Fortier P-H, Niyonsenga T, et al. Non-nutritive swallowing and respiration coordination in full-term newborn lambs. Respir Physiol Neurobiol 2003; 134:209–218.
57. Reix P, Arsenault J, Langlois C, et al. Nonnutritive swallowing and respiration relationships in preterm lambs. J Appl Physiol 2004; 97:1283–1290.
58. Longobardo G, Evangelisti CJ, Cherniack NS. Effects of neural drives on breathing in the awake state in humans. Respir Physiol 2002; 129:317–333.
59. Pickens DL, Schefft GL, Thach BT. Pharyngeal fluid clearance and aspiration preventive mechanisms in sleeping infants. J Appl Physiol 1989; 66:1164–1171.
60. Lichter I, Muir RC. The pattern of swallowing during sleep. Electroencephalogr Clin Neurophysiol 1975; 38:427–432.
61. Roberge S, Samson N, Dorion S, et al. Non-nutritive swallowing and respiration coordination among states of alertness in the adult sheep. J Otolaryngol 2007; 36:140–147.
62. Tooley J, Dyke M. Randomized study of nasal continuous positive airway pressure in the preterm infant with respiratory distress syndrome. Acta Paediatr 2003; 92:1170–1174.
63. Davis P, Henderson-Smart DJ. Nasal continuous positive airways pressure immediately after extubation for preventing morbidity in preterm infants. Cochrane Database Syst Rev 2003; 3:CD000143.
64. De Paoli AG, Davis PG, Lemyre B. Nasal continuous positive airway pressure versus nasal intermittent positive pressure ventilation for preterm neonates, a systematic review and meta-analysis. Acta Paediatr 2003; 92:70–75.
65. Espagne S, Hascoet JM. Noninvasive ventilation of premature infants. Arch Pediatr 2002; 9:1100–1103.
66. Nishino T, Sugimori K, Kohchi A, et al. Nasal constant positive airway pressure inhibits the swallowing reflex. Am Rev Respir Dis 1989; 140:1290–1293.

67. Samson N, St-Hilaire M, Nsegbe E, et al. Effect of nasal continuous or intermittent positive pressure on non-nutritive swallowing in the newborn lamb. J Appl Physiol 2005; 99:1636–1642.
68. Samson N, Duvareille C, Clapperton V, et al. CPAP inhibits non-nutritive swallowing through stimulation of bronchopulmonary receptors. Paediatr Respir Rev 2006; 7:S267.
69. Kijima M, Isono S, Nishino T. Modulation of swallowing reflex by lung volume changes. Am J Respir Crit Care Med 2000; 162:1855–1858.
70. Yamamoto F, Nishino T. Phasic vagal influence on the rate and timing of reflex swallowing. Am J Respir Crit Care Med 2002; 165:1400–1403.
71. Nishino T, Kohchi T, Honda Y, et al. Differences in the effects of hypercapnia and hypoxia on the swallowing reflex in cats. Br J Anaesth 1986; 58:903–908.
72. Duvareille C, Lafrance M, Samson N, et al. Effects of hypoxia and hypercapnia on non nutritive swallowing in newborn lambs. J Appl Physiol 2007; 103:1180–1188.
73. Nishino T, Hasegawa R, Ide T, Isono S. Hypercapnia enhances the development of coughing during continuous infusion of water into the pharynx. Am J Respir Crit Care Med 1998; 157:815–821.
74. Sai T, Isono S, Nishino T. Effects of withdrawal of phasic lung inflation during normocapnia and hypercapnia on the swallowing reflex in humans. J Anesth 2004; 18:82–88.
75. Timms BJM, DiFiore JM, Martin RJ, et al. Increased respiratory drive as an inhibitor of oral feeding of preterm infants. J Pediatr 1993; 123:127–131.
76. Nishijima K, Tsubone H, Atoji Y. Contribution of free nerve endings in the laryngeal epithelium to CO2 reception in rats. Auton Neurosci 2004; 110:81–88.
77. Hoover WH, Sawyer MS, Apgar WP. Ovine nutritional responses to elevated ambient carbon dioxide. J Nutr 1971; 101:1595–1600.
78. Wilson SL, Thach BT, Brouillette RT, et al. Coordination of breathing and swallowing in human infants. J Appl Physiol 1981; 50:851–858.
79. Shaker R, Li Q, Ren J, et al. Coordination of deglutition and phases of respiration: effect of aging, tachypnea, bolus volume, and chronic obstructive pulmonary disease. Am J Physiol 1992; 263:G750–G755.
80. Smith J, Wolkove N, Colacone A, et al. Coordination of eating, drinking and breathing in adults. Chest 1989; 96:578–582.
81. Hiss SG, Treole K, Stuart A. Effects of age, gender, bolus volume, and trial on swallowing apnea duration and swallow/respiratory phase relationships of normal adults. Dysphagia 2001; 16:128–135.
82. Feroah TR, Forster HV, Fuentes CG, et al. Effects of spontaneous swallows on breathing in awake goats. J Appl Physiol 2002; 92:1923–1935.
83. Kawasaki M, Ogura J.H, Takenouchi S. Neurophysiologic observations of normal deglutition. I. Its relationship to the respiratory cycle. Laryngoscope 1964; 74: 1747–1765.
84. McFarland DH, Lund JP. An investigation of the coupling between respiration, mastication, and swallowing in the awake rabbit. J Neurophysiol 1993; 69:95–18.
85. Barkmeier JM, Bielamowicz S, Takeda N, et al. Laryngeal activity during upright vs. supine swallowing. J Appl Physiol 2002; 93:740–745.
86. McFarland DH, Lund JP, Gagner M. Effects of posture on the coordination of respiration and swallowing. J Neurophysiol 1994; 72:2431–2437.

87. McDonnell M, Mehanni M, Mc Garvey C, et al. Smoking: the major risk factor for SIDS in Irish infants. Ir Med J 2002, 95:111–113.

88. McMartin KI, Platt MS, Hackman R, et al. Lung tissue concentrations of nicotine in sudden infant death syndrome (SIDS). J Pediatr 2002; 140:205–209.

89. Khoshoo V, Edell D. Previously healthy infants may have increased risk of aspiration during respiratory syncytial viral bronchiolitis. Pediatrics 1999; 104: 1389–1390.

90. Hanlon MB, Tripp JH, Ellis RE, et al. Deglutition apnoea as indicator of maturation of suckle feeding in bottle-fed preterm infants. Dev Med Child Neuro 1997; 39:534–542.

91. Kelly BN, Huckabee M-L, Jones RD, et al. Nutritive and non-nutritive swallowing apnea duration in term infants: Implications for neural control mechanisms. Respir Physiol Neurobiol 2006; 154:372–378.

92. Issa FG, Porostocky S. Effect of continuous swallowing on respiration. Respir Physiol 1994; 95:181–193.

93. Miller MJ, DiFiore JM. A comparison of swallowing during apnea and periodic breathing in premature infants. Pediatr Res 1995; 37:796–799.

94. Rodenstein DO. The upper airway in noninvasive ventilation. In: Hill NS, ed. Long-term Mechanical Ventilation Lung Biology in Health and Disease, Vol. 152. New York: Marcel Dekker, 2001:87–103.

95. Moreau-Bussière F, Samson N, St-Hilaire M, et al. Laryngeal response to nasal ventilation in non-sedated lambs. J Appl Physiol 2007; 102:2149–2157.

96. Delguste P, Aubert-Tulkens G, Rodenstein DO. Upper airway obstruction during nasal intermittent positive-pressure hyperventilation in sleep. Lancet 1991; 338 (8778):1295–1297.

97. Garland JS, Nelson DB, Rice T, et al. Increased risk of gastrointestinal perforations in neonates mechanically ventilated with either face mask or nasal prongs. Pediatrics 1985; 76:406–410.

3

Postnatal Development of Carotid Chemoreceptor Function

JOHN L. CARROLL
University of Arkansas for Medical Sciences, Little Rock, Arkansas, U.S.A.

DAVID F. DONNELLY
Yale University School of Medicine, New Haven, Connecticut, U.S.A.

I. Overview

Regulation of arterial oxygen levels is critically important in mammals, particularly during early life. Peri- and postnatal hypoxia may lead to death, impaired cognitive development, and abnormalities in cardiovascular function, breathing control maturation, and lung function (1–5).

The main sensors of arterial O_2 tension are the carotid body chemoreceptors, which are located bilaterally at the bifurcations of the common carotid arteries. Carotid chemoreceptor sensory afferents, via the carotid sinus nerves (CSN), project to the nucleus tractus solitarius and other brain stem nuclei, providing the major source of O_2-mediated ventilatory drive. Neural signals from the carotid chemoreceptors to the brain stem cardiorespiratory control nuclei also mediate critically important respiratory reflexes, such as arousal from sleep during hypoxia, and cardiovascular reflexes that modulate heart rate and blood pressure (6).

Perhaps surprisingly, given their importance, the carotid chemoreceptors have a low sensitivity to hypoxia at the time of birth and become more sensitive to hypoxia over the first few days of life. In some species a slower phase of carotid chemoreceptor maturation has been described, with O_2 sensitivity increasing slowly over weeks or months (7). This enhanced hypoxia sensitivity of the arterial chemoreceptors (rightward shifting of the O_2 response curve) after birth is termed "resetting," and it occurs in both carotid and aortic chemoreceptors (8). Although it is clear that the increase in oxygen tension at birth is a major factor initiating carotid chemoreceptor resetting (9), the exact mechanism and sites of maturation are unknown.

The critical importance of carotid chemoreceptor function during infancy has been demonstrated by experiments in which the CSN are severed just after birth. Adults survive bilateral carotid denervation (CD) (10). In sharp contrast, bilateral CD in newborns leads to hypoventilation, increased frequency of central apnea, prolonged duration of apnea, abnormal breathing pattern development, and mortality rates as high as 66% during the neonatal period (11–15).

Taken together, available data suggest that a "vulnerable period" exists in mammalian postnatal development, during which functioning carotid chemoreceptors are crucial for maintaining normal respiration. Abnormalities in respiration or the respiratory pattern may be especially critical in neonates because of their low pulmonary O_2 stores and higher O_2 consumption/body surface area ratio. This leads to rapid oxyhemoglobin desaturation (rapidly developing hypoxemia) during periods of hypoventilation due to apnea, upper airway obstruction, rebreathing (e.g., bedding material covering face), or illness.

In addition to hypoxia, the carotid chemoreceptors also respond to changes in CO_2, pH, temperature, osmolarity, elevated K^+, glucose, and several pharmacological stimuli (16). Lowering Po_2 increases carotid chemoreceptor sensitivity to CO_2 and raising CO_2 increases sensitivity to hypoxia, a phenomenon known as O_2-CO_2 interaction. A detailed description of the response to all of these stimuli as well as maturational changes in the responses is beyond the scope of this chapter. Instead, we will focus on (1) the role of the carotid chemoreceptors in normal breathing control during development, (2) maturation of the response to hypoxia, (3) developmental changes in carotid chemoreceptor neural responses to natural stimuli, (4) mechanisms of carotid body development, and (5) the carotid chemoreceptors in selected states of abnormal cardiorespiratory control.

II. The Carotid Chemoreceptors in Normal Breathing Control in Childhood

As noted above, the function of carotid chemoreceptors may be grossly assessed by comparing subjects whose chemoreceptors have been resected with normal subjects. This is more readily undertaken in animal studies; therefore, much of the information on the carotid chemoreceptors in maturation of breathing control derives from studies in rats, rabbits, cats, goats, ponies, dogs, and pigs. In the past, a population of human patients underwent carotid body resection for the treatment of intractable asthma and thus became a useful study population (17). Today, studies of human subjects necessarily employ indirect techniques, such as the Dejours transient O_2 test, that measure complex integrated responses (18). Although a great deal has been learned from the denervation approach, it is worth noting that the extent to which these studies can be extrapolated to human respiratory control maturation remains unclear.

A. Onset of Breathing at Birth

Studies in lambs show that the carotid chemoreceptors are not necessary for the onset of normal breathing at birth (19,20). However, they play important roles in a variety of other respiratory responses during development and in the mature mammal. Several studies using the CD approach have revealed striking effects on cardiorespiratory control during postnatal development. It should be noted that the neural output from carotid sinus baroreceptors also runs in the CSN; therefore, cutting the CSN also results in denervation of carotid sinus baroreceptors in addition to chemoreceptors. Clearly, this complicates interpretation of studies using this approach.

B. Breathing Control Development

Denervation of carotid chemoreceptors in the newborn has been shown to cause severe respiratory abnormalities in piglets, rats, and sheep. For instance, Donnelly and Haddad compared piglets undergoing CD and, in some cases, carotid and aortic denervation (CAD) at less than nine days of age with piglets undergoing denervation at about 30 days of age (13). Studies on the days following denervation showed particular abnormalities in breathing control in the young piglets characterized by prolonged apneas and O_2 desaturation. Of particular note, $\sim 60\%$ of the young CD piglets died after three to seven days following surgery, while none in the older denervated or sham operated groups died (13). Coté et al. subsequently performed a more extensive study of denervated piglets with surgery performed at ~ 5, 10, 15, and 21 days of age. CD again resulted in prolonged apnea, severe hypoxemia, and flattening of the electroencephalogram (EEG), but the effect was confined to the 15-day group and only during quiet sleep (21). Prolonged apnea and hypoxemia were not observed at other ages or during active sleep at any age. Although the reasons for the difference in mortality rates between the studies are unclear, it is clear that the effect of CD in the first weeks of life can have major effects on respiratory rhythm generation (21).

As in piglets, denervation in other species results in breathing abnormalities and increased mortality. Newborn lambs with CD at one to two days of age died suddenly and unexpectedly in 43% of the cases. They died between 4-5 weeks of age, suggesting that the carotid chemoreceptors become important for survival within a particular age range during development (11). These investigators also reported that minute ventilation (V_E) in intact lambs, adjusted for body weight, decreased with age between 7 and 70 days, accompanied by characteristic changes in breathing pattern. In contrast, lambs that underwent CD just after birth exhibited hypoventilation and little change in V_E or breathing pattern during the same time frame (12). Similarly, CD in immature rats resulted in hypoventilation, especially during rapid eye movement (REM) sleep and mortality rates of ∼50% (14,15). Sectioning of the aortic depressor nerves alone did not have this effect.

Thus, it is clear that CD is associated with cardiorespiratory control abnormalities and an increased probability of mortality in immature mammals across species. However, caution must be exercised in the interpretation of survival data. The reasons for increased mortality in these studies are unknown. In addition, the extent to which the increased mortality was related to chemo-versus baro-denervation or to other factors is unclear. Nevertheless, it seems clear that neural input from the carotid chemoreceptors, baroreceptors, or both is critically important for ensuring survival during a vulnerable period of postnatal development.

C. Central Apnea Termination

Central apnea is common in infants but is usually not prolonged beyond ∼20 to 25 seconds. It is not associated with bradycardia and is generally not accompanied by severe or prolonged hypoxemia (22). In general, these normal apneas terminate spontaneously. However, considering the vulnerability of the newborn to rapid O_2 desaturation, termination of spontaneous apnea must be considered of vital importance. Therefore, the mechanisms responsible for the termination of central apnea and resumption of normal breathing are of particular interest and here the carotid body appears to play a vital role.

Studies on the unanesthetized, awake lamb indicated that carotid chemoreceptors have a major influence on the blood-gas threshold for the resumption of breathing following apnea (23). Apnea was induced by passive hyperventilation in lambs aged between 1 day and 15 days under normoxic, hyperoxic, and hypoxic conditions. The apnea termination threshold (ATT) was determined by measuring the Pao_2 and $Paco_2$ at which breathing resumed. The effect of CD was also examined in lambs younger than two days old. The results were striking. Figure 1 shows the apnea termination threshold for Pao_2 ($PATT_{O2}$) plotted against the apnea termination threshold for $Paco_2$ ($PATT_{CO2}$). In 14-day-old lambs, as Pao_2 was lowered from ∼150 to ∼40 mmHg, the CO_2 threshold for resumption of breathing became progressively lower, from ∼50 to ∼30 mmHg (Fig.1, open circles). A similar relationship, although not as steep, was observed for lambs younger than two days (Fig. 1, filled circles). In sharp contrast, in the CD group (open triangles) across the full range of Pao_2 from ∼400 to 30 mmHg, $PATT_{CO2}$ remained elevated at ∼50 to 55 mmHg (Fig. 1, triangles). Thus, in the absence of functioning carotid chemoreceptors, the $Paco_2$ threshold for resumption of breathing during central apnea is abnormally high and independent of Pao_2. In other words, input from the carotid chemoreceptors

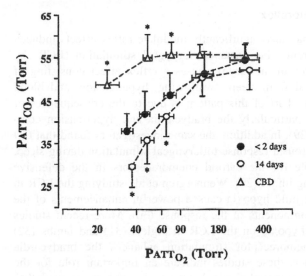

Figure 1 Mean $PATT_{CO_2}$ values calculated for each $PATT_{O_2}$ range (severe hypoxia, moderate hypoxia, normoxia, moderate hyperoxia, hyperoxia) in each group of lambs [the groups were (●) <2 days CB intact, (○) 14 days CB intact, (△) <2 days CB denervated). $PATT_{O_2}$ is plotted on a logarithmic scale. Values are mean ± SD. *Significant difference from the lamb group less than 2 days old, $P < 0.05$. *Abbreviation*: CB, carotid body. *Source*: From Ref. 23.

appears to modulate the level of $PaCO_2$ at which breathing resumes after central apnea. Another important finding of this study was that hypoxia consistently failed to promote the occurrence of apnea; instead, it lowered the $PaCO_2$ apnea threshold even in CD lambs. Therefore, although it appears that the input from carotid chemoreceptors modulates the $PaCO_2$ apnea threshold, the carotid chemoreceptors are not required for reinitiation of breathing.

D. Bradycardia

In mammals, stimulation of the carotid chemoreceptors may lead to profound vagally mediated bradycardia and negative inotropic effects (24,25). However, the situation is complex as input from the carotid chemoreceptors to the brain stem cardiovascular control areas is gated by respiratory phase, modulated by the level of $PaCO_2$, and also modulated by the level of input from pulmonary stretch receptors (25). Nevertheless, prolonged expiratory apnea is a particularly dangerous condition for developing infants, because rapidly developing hypoxemia is likely and the resulting powerful, hypoxia-driven cardioinhibitory reflexes are unopposed by cardiostimulatory input from pulmonary stretch receptors (24). Although in the term-fetal sheep hypoxia induces profound bradycardia via reflex mechanisms driven by the carotid chemoreceptors (26), little is known about the same reflex during postnatal life.

E. Laryngeal Chemoreflex

Carotid chemoreceptors may also significantly modulate reflex effects induced by other respiratory afferents. For instance, laryngeal stimulation (LCR) by water or foreign substances in the larynx causes a reflex effect consisting of apnea, bradycardia, arousal from sleep, swallowing, hypertension, and blood flow redistribution (27,28). Part of this pattern is due to the consequences of carotid body stimulation, particularly the bradycardia and hypertension components of this reflex (27,29). In addition, the same investigators found that CD markedly attenuated the arousal response to laryngeal stimulation during sleep, indicating yet another role for the carotid chemoreceptors in the defensive responses of the developing infant (29). Wennergren et al., studying the LCR in human infants, found that mild hypoxia caused powerful enhancements of the bradycardic and apneic components of the response (30). More recent studies examining the effects of hypoxia on the LCR in piglets (31) and lambs (32) report that peripheral chemoreceptor stimulation enhances the bradycardia component. Taken together, these studies indicate an important role for the carotid chemoreceptors in the modulation of heart rate during hypoxia as well as significant interactions with other reflexes, such as the LCR.

F. Respiratory Control Stability

The breathing pattern of the newborn and developing neonate is characterized by instability and exaggerated responses to perturbations, such as sigh, movement, or apnea (33). Studies in adult mammals indicate a significant role for the carotid chemoreceptors in maintaining respiratory stability (34). Indirect evidence and theoretical modeling suggest that the carotid chemoreceptors play a role in newborn respiratory pattern instability, such as postsigh apnea or oscillation (33,35,36). Although it is plausible that postnatal maturation of carotid chemoreceptor sensitivity plays a role in the development of respiratory system stability, and modeling approaches support this, direct evidence is lacking.

G. Arousal from Sleep

Arousal from sleep in response to hypoxic or hypercapnic challenge is a critically important defense mechanism. A recent study of full-term infants during the first six months of life suggests that arousal from sleep in response to acute hypoxia, especially during active sleep, is a vital survival mechanism (37).

Fewell and Baker studied the arousal from sleep in response to rapidly developing hypoxemia by challenging lambs with mild, moderate, or severe hypoxia during sleep (38). More severe levels of hypoxia resulted in a markedly faster rate of arterial desaturation. Arousal from sleep in response to hypoxia occurred in $\sim 94\%$ of the challenges, and during quiet sleep the lambs aroused at oxygen saturation (Sao_2) of about 80%, no matter how rapidly Sao_2 fell. However, during active sleep, more rapidly developing hypoxemia correlated with arousal occurring at progressively lower Sao_2 levels. Interestingly, repeated exposure to rapidly developing hypoxemia further impaired the arousal response (39). The same authors later showed that CD markedly blunted arousal from sleep in response to rapidly developing hypoxemia, with only 28% of challenges resulting in arousal before Sao_2 reached 30% (40). Because CD also denervates the carotid sinus baroreceptors, these authors could not determine the relative contribution of the chemo- versus baroreceptors in their findings. However, it was clear that the carotid chemo- and/or baroreceptors play a major role in arousal from sleep in response to rapidly developing hypoxemia.

Arousal from sleep in response to upper airway obstruction or hypercapnia is another crucial defense mechanism in the developing infant. Igras and Fewell showed that in three- to four-week-old lambs, nasal or tracheal airway occlusion usually results in arousal from sleep, although the arousal response is significantly delayed in active compared to quiet sleep (41). Repeated airway obstruction further delayed the arousal response in active sleep (42). CD markedly impaired the arousal response to airway obstruction. Following CD, although airway obstruction still produced arousal from sleep, the response was markedly delayed and occurred at lower Sao_2 levels (43). In addition to mediating arousal responses to hypoxia and airway obstruction, Fewell et al. also reported that the carotid chemoreceptors play a major role in the arousal response to alveolar hypercapnia (44). Taken together, these studies indicate that the carotid chemoreceptors play a significant role in modulating arousal responses to hypoxemia, hypercapnia, and airway obstruction and that active sleep is a condition during which infants are likely to be particularly vulnerable to these stressors.

H. Ventilatory Response to Hypoxia—Selected Aspects

The neonatal ventilatory response to hypoxia is complex, reflecting a balance between increased neural input from the carotid chemoreceptors, central nervous system (CNS) inhibition (45,46), and hypoxic hypometabolism (47,48). The carotid chemoreceptors provide nearly all of the stimulatory input driving the ventilatory response to hypoxia (49). Nearly four decades ago, Schwieler reported that CD in kittens eliminates the ventilatory response to hypoxia (50), and numerous studies have confirmed the key role of the carotid chemoreceptors in driving the V_E response to hypoxia in developing mammals.

In all mammalian species studied to date, the increase in V_E during hypoxia is relatively small in the newborn and increases with age (51–55). Furthermore, at all ages, the increased V_E in response to a constant level of hypoxia is not sustained. Initially, upon exposure to hypoxia, V_E rises, reaching maximum within several minutes and thereafter slowly declines (termed the "late decline in ventilation," "biphasic response," or "V_E rolloff") (Fig. 2). The major differences between mature and immature responses to hypoxia are that in mature mammals the V_E response declines more slowly and is ultimately

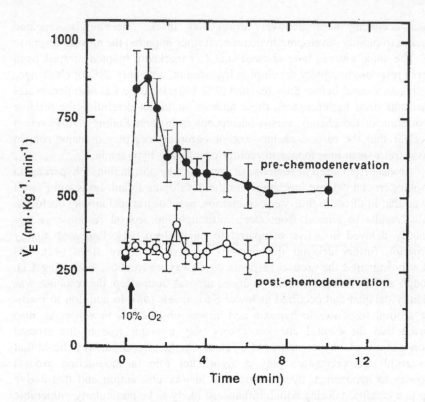

Figure 2 Time course of ventilatory responses to acute hypoxia in five rabbits before (*filled circles*) and after (*open circles*) peripheral chemodenervation. Data represent mean ± SE of minute ventilation adjusted for body weight. Note that after CD, there is no V_E response to hypoxia but also no ventilatory depression. *Abbreviations*: CD, carotid denervation; V_E, minute ventilation. *Source*: From Ref. 57.

sustained at a higher level compared to neonates. The late decline in V_E during hypoxia is particularly pronounced in neonates, especially in premature infants, and nonhuman species that are relatively immature at birth.

A recent study of the hypoxic ventilatory response in full-term human infants during sleep showed that the immature biphasic response persists until five to six months of age, which is substantially longer than previously reported (37). In addition, between birth and six months of age in human infants, arousal was shown to be the predominant response to hypoxia during active sleep, and maturation of the hypoxic ventilatory response only occurred during quiet sleep (37). Postnatal development of V_E and arousal responses to hypoxia in human infants has recently been reviewed (56).

There is strong evidence that the late V_E decline during hypoxia is mediated by inhibitory mechanisms operating at the level of the central nervous system

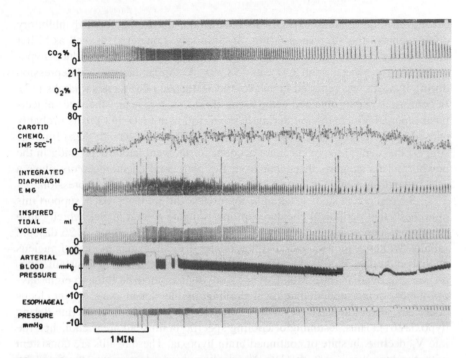

Figure 3 Anesthetized kitten 17 days old. Effect on breathing of abruptly reducing inspired O_2 to 6% for 4.5 minutes. There are breaks in the blood pressure tracing where blood samples were taken. After the initial increase, breathing frequency and tidal volume fell below control by the end of the hypoxia period. Note that carotid chemoreceptor spiking frequency is maintained throughout the hypoxia period. *Source*: From Ref. 75.

(CNS). Possible mechanisms underlying the late V_E decline are discussed further in the chapter by Alvaro and Rigatto and will not be repeated here. However, intriguing results from recent studies raise interesting questions about a possible role for the carotid chemoreceptors in the late-phase V_E decline during hypoxia.

Figure 3 shows the effect of breathing 6% O_2 on a 17-day-old anesthetized kitten. After an initial rise in breathing frequency and tidal volume, both fell progressively during the 4.5 min challenge. Blood pressure declined as well. However, throughout this classical example of the biphasic V_E response, neural output from the carotid chemoreceptors was sustained. This would appear to be consistent with the mechanism outlined above; stimulation from the carotid chemoreceptors is counteracted or "gated out" by depression at the CNS level. However, several lines of evidence suggest that it is not that simple and, to the contrary, suggest that the carotid chemoreceptors may mediate both the excitatory and significant proportions of the inhibitory components.

Schramm and Grunstein in 1987 reported that ventilatory depression occurred during hypoxia in 1- to 33-day-old rabbits, but that it required intact carotid chemoreceptors (57). CD abolished both the excitatory and inhibitory components of the VE response (Fig. 2). Similarly, Long et al. as well as Miller and Tenney reported that mild to moderate hypoxia failed to induce hypoventilation in awake, adult CD cats (58,59). A similar lack of V_E depression during hypoxia was reported in awake, unanesthetized CD neonatal lambs (12). In contrast to results obtained without anesthesia, studies in anesthetized subjects have reported V_E depression during hypoxia following CD, but this is probably caused by the effects of anesthesia (58). Although controversial, these findings suggest that central hypoxia cannot account for the ventilatory depression in the newborn. This suggests that input from the peripheral chemoreceptors plays a role in both the ventilatory excitation as well as the subsequent depression.

Several recent studies, taking a completely different approach, support this hypothesis that peripheral chemoreceptors stimulate central nuclei, which cause ventilatory depression. In vagotomized, paralyzed, decerebrate ~ 26-day-old rabbits, Waites et al. demonstrated that bilateral small lesions in the red nucleus abolished the late V_E (phrenic nerve output) decline, resulting in a sustained V_E response to hypoxia (60). Moore et al., studying anesthetized three to eight day-old-lambs, demonstrated that focal cooling in the dorsal pons, at the locus coeruleus, also eliminated (reversibly) the late respiratory output decline during hypoxia (61). Thus, lesioning or cooling specific brain stem areas abolished the late V_E decline, in spite of continued brain hypoxia. These results are consistent with the hypothesis that the late V_E decline during hypoxia is mediated by stimulation of brain stem neurons that are inhibitory to respiratory output (61). Combined with the observation that the late V_E in hypoxia decline (at least in unanesthetized subjects) depends on having intact carotid chemoreceptors, these data suggest that the neurons inhibiting the V_E response to hypoxia are stimulated by neural input from the carotid chemoreceptors.

The studies described above raise some intriguing possibilities. If the degree of cardiorespiratory depression during hypoxia depends on a complex balance between chemoreceptor-driven excitatory versus inhibitory neuron pools, then differences in rates of maturation of the neurons involved in the V_E response to hypoxia could result in imbalances and vulnerability during particular periods of development. Little is known about potential sources of developmental vulnerability to hypoxic stress and more work is needed in this critically important area.

III. Developmental Changes in O_2 Chemoreflexes

Numerous studies have attempted to assess the role of the carotid chemoreceptors in the maturation of breathing control using the transient O_2 test developed by Dejours (18). In this test, the inspired gas is suddenly switched from room air to 100% O_2 for a few breaths, causing Pa_{O_2} to suddenly rise and peripheral chemoreceptors to abruptly reduce their spiking rates. As a result, V_E

falls, and the drop in V_E is proportional to the amount of V_E drive arising from the carotid chemoreceptors at the moment of the test (18). Using this approach, it was shown that in human infants transient exposure to 100% O_2 had no effect on two- to six-hour-old newborns but caused an $\sim 10\%$ fall in V_E in two- to six-day-old infants (62). Comparable results were obtained in other species (53,63). Because hyperoxia is applied systemically, the response includes contributions by the entire peripheral and CSN neural pathway, and it does not assess peripheral chemoreceptor output per se. Maturational changes in the relative contribution of the peripheral chemoreceptors to overall V_E drive may be entirely due to changes in central gating or processing of chemoreceptor inputs. In addition, the magnitude and time profile of the stimulus may be affected by lung function.

There are several alternative methods of assessing peripheral chemo-receptor function in developing intact animals. In the opposite sense to the Dejours test, peripheral chemoreceptor may be selectively stimulated by switching to a few breaths of N_2 or brief injection of a low dose of cyanide. When a subject is suddenly exposed to two to three breaths of pure N_2, there is a sudden large drop in Pao_2 and corresponding transient increase in V_E. Theoretically, this should allow measurement of the immediate, dynamic V_E response to hypoxia, without the confounding effects of hypocapnia, blood pH shifts, and brain hypoxia that occur with more prolonged challenges. Using this test in lambs, Canet et al. reported that the V_E response to three breaths of N_2 nearly doubled between ~ 24 hours of age versus 12 days (64). As with the transient O_2 test, this one also uses V_E as an output measure and is therefore not a direct test of peripheral chemoreceptor output. A variation of this approach involves administration of intravenous NaCN to stimulate the peripheral chemoreceptors in developing animals. With this method it was demonstrated in lambs that the V_E response to 0.1 mg/kg intravenous NaCN increased nearly fourfold between 2 and 10 days of age, with no further increase at 21 days (53). However, this test also uses V_E as the outcome measure and suffers from the limitations described above.

Still another method of assessing O_2 chemoreflex maturation is the alternating breath technique, which alternates the fraction of inspired oxygen (Fio_2) between normoxia and hypoxia in every other breath. This oscillating input function, sensed by the peripheral chemoreceptors, generates an alternating output function in the form of breath-to-breath alternation of instantaneous V_E. The degree of V_E alternation produced by the alternating Fio_2 is taken as measure of peripheral chemoreceptor sensitivity. With this method it was demonstrated, in unanesthetized kittens, that the alternation response was absent on day 1 and increased after day 4 of age, again indicating a developmental increase in the O_2 chemoreflex response (65). This test, which shares the limitations discussed in the preceding paragraphs, has also been used in human infants. Calder et al. used this method on human infants, reporting that the alternation response was present by ~ 43 hours and was not increased further at 47 days (66). They concluded that, in humans, the "resetting" of peripheral chemoreceptor responses to hypoxia was ~ complete by 24 to 48 hours of age. However, they did not study older infants or intermediate ages, leaving open the possibility for a missed peak (at an intermediate age between 2 and 47 days) or a slower rate of maturation over many months. In any case, by any method of testing, it is clear that developmental changes in O_2 chemoreflex strength occur in all species studied to date.

IV. Developmental Changes in Afferent Chemoreceptor Nerve Activity

As discussed above, the carotid chemoreceptors modulate resting respiratory control as well as driving ventilatory arousal and other critically important defensive responses to environmental stressors such as hypoxia. Therefore, it is noteworthy that important developmental changes also occur at the level of the peripheral chemoreceptors (9). In the newborn, the sensitivity of the neural response to hypoxia and hypercapnia is less than in the adult and, in some studies, the neural response is not as well-sustained compared to the adult.

The concept of hypoxia sensitivity may be viewed from two perspectives. Firstly, it may be viewed from the viewpoint of a relative change in nerve activity, which is usually assessed by recording from many nerve fibers simultaneously and normalizing all measurements to baseline activity or to peak activity. Alternatively, chemoreceptor activity may be considered an absolute, that is, in terms of spiking activity of individual axons. This type of recording represents the minimal unit of chemoreceptor activity, since no further subdivision of a functioning chemoreceptor unit is possible. When viewed from both perspectives, significant developmental changes occur in peripheral chemoreceptor function.

A. Hypoxia Sensitivity and Response

On both absolute and relative scales, the level of spiking activity for a given level of hypoxia is less in the newborn than in the adult, and maturation appears to occur in the weeks after birth. This observation was first unequivocally demonstrated by Mulligan in piglets in which she employed single-axon recordings, in vivo, from cell bodies of chemoreceptor neurons in the petrosal ganglion (Fig. 4) (67). Based on recordings from a population of single axons, the increase in spiking activity in response to graded hypoxia was approximately twofold greater in 12- to 20-day-old piglets compared with one- to five-day-old piglets.

Not only was the peak frequency of discharge greater in the older piglets but the response curve was shifted to the right (sensitivity increased). Similar rightward shifts in the response curves were also found in kittens (68,69) and lambs (9). This developmental increase in hypoxia sensitivity is not limited to

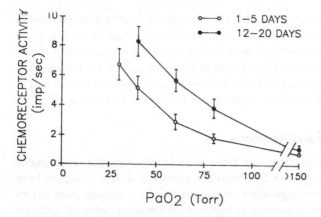

Figure 4 Single-cell carotid chemoreceptor afferent responses to isocapnic hypoxia in young (1- to 5-day-old) and older (12- to 20-day-old) piglets. (Mean ± SEM, n = 10 for each age group). Chemoreceptor activity was significantly greater in the older age group at all Po_2 levels except hyperoxia. *Source*: From Ref. 74.

the carotid chemoreceptors since a 50% increase in the response to hypoxia was also observed in recordings from aortic chemoreceptors, in vivo (8). This increased responsiveness is of some import because the chemoreceptor response curve is not linear, but approximates the hyperbolic dissociation curve of hemoglobin (70). The rightward shift of the chemoreceptor response curve with development would, thus, provide a greater safety margin in avoiding significant oxygen desaturation.

Before birth, chemoreceptor activity is even more reduced as compared to the newborn. Some studies indicate that fetal chemoreceptor activity is low or absent and, when present, fails to respond to hypoxia, at least in the presence of normal sympathetic activity (71,72). Results of other studies indicate that fetal chemoreceptor activity is present but the response curve is far leftward shifted compared with the newborn and adult response curves. For instance, it was necessary to reduce fetal Pao_2 to below 20 mmHg in order to increase chemoreceptor nerve activity two- to fourfold (9). In comparison, a Pao_2 of 60 to 70 mmHg would be expected to increase chemoreceptor activity threefold in the adult (73).

In addition to a reduced sensitivity to hypoxia, the newborn may also be less able to sustain a neural carotid chemoreceptor response to hypoxia. Mulligan noted this in her piglets in which a strong hypoxic stimulus (below 30 mmHg) resulted in a decrease, rather than an increase in spiking activity (74). Several of the axons, in fact, ceased to continue spiking and required reoxygenation to resume spiking. This observation was confirmed and extended by Marchal et al. and Carroll et al. who observed significant accommodation to a hypoxic stimulus. Using single-fiber recording of kitten chemoreceptors, Marchal observed that 46% of one- to three-day-old kitten, chemoreceptor fibers accommodated to a hypoxic stimulus, but this was not observed in fibers recorded from 15-day-old kittens (69). Similar results were obtained using whole-nerve recordings in kittens (68). However another study, using whole-nerve recordings from the carotid chemoreceptors in 5- to 34-day-old anesthetized kittens, found that CSN output was sustained during a five-minute exposure to 6–12% acute hypoxia (75).

B. CO_2 Sensitivity and Response

Compared with experiments addressing hypoxia sensitivity, less data are available on the developmental changes in CO_2 sensitivity, and some of these data have been inconsistent. Recordings of single-fiber chemoreceptor nerve activity from kittens indicate some developmental increase in hypercapnia sensitivity over the first two weeks of life (69). Calder and colleagues reported a similar developmental increase in single-fiber nerve activity in lambs (76). Other data suggest that the developmental increase continues over a much longer period. In studies of kitten chemoreceptor, there was no significant change in the whole-nerve response to hypercapnia between one week and eight weeks of age, but there was a significant increase to adulthood, suggesting that maturation of the CO_2 response is quite slow in this species (68). On the other hand, some studies indicate that the response to hypercapnia is unchanged after birth (77) or that, while the steady-state response to CO_2 may increase after birth, the dynamic response to CO_2 is unchanged (76). Finally, Bamford et al., using multifiber CSN recording in excised superfused carotid bodies from rats aged term-fetal to 21 days, found no significant maturational increase in the carotid chemoreceptor response to 15% CO_2 (78).

Confounding a clear interpretation to these (sometimes) conflicting data are uncertainties introduced by normalization parameters. For instance, one study calculated the percentage increase in nerve RMS voltage during application of a 6% inspired CO_2 stimulus and determined that this increased with age (68). However, normalization to whole-nerve baseline spiking activity may have introduced an age bias if the newborn had a greater level of non-chemoreceptor activity or higher baseline spiking rates than the adult. In another study, nerve activities were normalized to that obtained during superfusion of a chemoreceptor, in vitro, with saline equilibrated to 70 mmHg Po_2. In this case, it was claimed that hypercapnia sensitivity did not change with age (77). However, since spiking rates during hypoxia are higher in older animals (67,79), normalization to the higher spiking rates may have obscured a developmental increase in hypercapnic responsiveness. A recent study of Bamford et al., also using an in vitro superfusion approach, found no developmental increase in the CO_2 response during the first three weeks of life in rats (78). This study did not employ normalization. It is clearly difficult or even impossible to fully appreciate the biases introduced by normalization procedures applied to multifiber nerve activities, but it is worthwhile to keep in mind that they may introduce a variable which may have a significant effect on the conclusions.

Despite some evidence that the CSN response to CO_2 increases with age, the increased responsiveness does not appear to be reflected in the ventilatory output. Analysis of the ventilatory response to a transient hypercapnia stimulus (which is assumed to specifically stimulate the peripheral chemoreceptors) showed no developmental change in lambs over the course of 1 to 12 days of age in response to 13% CO_2 in the air (64). Similar results were obtained in maturing piglets using a sophisticated systems analysis to isolate the fast (peripheral) chemoreceptor part of the ventilatory response to CO_2 (80). Taken together these observations suggest that there may be a developmental increase in CO_2 sensitivity in some species but that the magnitude is smaller and the time course is slower than maturation of the hypoxia response.

C. Interactions in CO_2 and O_2

Not only do hypoxia and acidity stimulate chemoreceptor activity, but they interact together, enhancing activity beyond that expected for a simple summation of stimuli. This is perhaps best observed in the family of CO_2 response curves as developed against several different Po_2 backgrounds. The slope of the CO_2 response line is steeper as the level of oxygen is decreased (68). In contrast, the same experiment in the newborn yields CO_2 response curves that show little interaction between CO_2 and hypoxia (68).

This observation was placed on a more quantitative basis by Kumar and colleagues who deconvolved the response of rat chemoreceptors recorded in vitro into three components: (1) a response to hypoxia alone, (2) response to CO_2 alone, and (3) a term $CO_2 \times$ hypoxia (77). In this case, all chemoreceptor activities were normalized to 100% (defined as the spiking activity observed during superfusion with 70 mmHg O_2). Using this normalization scheme, there was no change with age in the sensitivity to CO_2 alone or to hypoxia alone, but age significantly enhanced the stimulus interaction between CO_2 and hypoxia. The effect of the combined stimuli was super-additive in the adult but not in the newborn. These findings are consistent with a recent study from Bamford et al., which used multifiber CSN recording in excised superfused carotid bodies from rats aged term-fetal to 21 days (78). Although they found no developmental increase in the carotid body response to CO_2, O_2-CO_2 interaction was absent in carotid bodies from rats near-term fetal to 11 days, but increased fivefold by 16 to 21 days of age (78). Thus, it appears that development specifically targets O_2-CO_2 interaction and not the response to hypercapnia per se.

V. Mechanisms of Developmental Changes

A greatly simplified overview of the carotid chemoreceptor is shown in Figure 5. The chemoreceptor complex consists of the afferent nerve fibers whose cell bodies are in the petrosal ganglia. The axons enter the carotid body, bifurcate and terminate on O_2-sensitive secretory cells (glomus cells). The terminations may

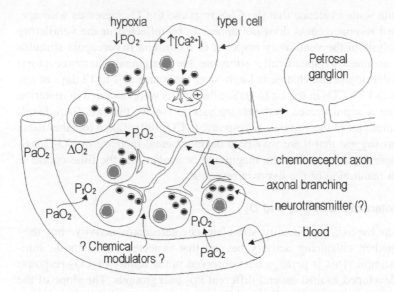

hypoxia   type I cell
↓PO₂ → ↑[Ca²⁺]ᵢ

Petrosal
ganglion

P₁O₂

PaO₂   ΔO₂

chemoreceptor axon

P₁O₂   axonal branching

PaO₂   neurotransmitter (?)

P₁O₂

blood

? Chemical   PaO₂
modulators ?

Figure 5 Schematic drawing of mammalian carotid body. See text for explanation.

be quite extensive. A cat carotid body contains approximately 10,000 glomus cells each of which averages a single nerve terminal. The sinus nerve contains about 500 axons, resulting in an estimated 20 glomus cells/single chemoreceptor axon (81). Because of the synaptic arrangement, it is universally speculated that glomus cells transduce hypoxia and acidity, resulting in the release of an excitatory transmitter(s). The purported excitatory transmitter causes nerve depolarization and enhanced spiking activity on the afferent nerve.

Although this transduction path is reasonably based on some biophysical responses of glomus cells (described below), it is hardly established. What is most lacking is the identification of an excitatory transmitter since pharmacological blockade of many candidate neurotransmitters yields no change in afferent nerve activity or increased, not decreased, afferent nerve activity. For instance, the application of an antagonist to dopamine D2 receptors, which should block the effects of released catecholamine (a major transmitter released by glomus cells), causes an enhancement of the nerve response to hypoxia, especially in rats exposed to chronic hypoxia (82). Recently, adenosine triphosphate (ATP) was proposed as a strong candidate for the excitatory transmitter released from glomus cells during hypoxia (83), and acetylcholine (ACh) has long been promoted as a putative excitatory transmitter (84). However, recent studies in cat carotid bodies indicate that the CSN response to hypoxia persists even in the presence of pharmacological antagonists that completely block CSN responses to cholinergic and ATP stimulation (85,86). These results strongly suggest that release of ATP or ACh, singly or in combination, cannot account entirely for hypoxia-induced excitation of the CSN. In addition, there is a body of evidence suggesting that the afferent nerve terminals may possess an endogenous sensitivity to hypoxia, thus obviating the necessity to postulate the existence of an excitatory neurotransmitter (87). Data are currently lacking to reach a definite conclusion regarding the mechanism of afferent nerve excitation, but for the purposes of this chapter we will stay with the conventional model in which the glomus cell is the transducing element and releases a neurotransmitter that excites the afferent nerve endings. On occasion, we will speculate on alternate models.

A. Changes in Organ Anatomy

Despite the high level of blood flow to the carotid body, the tissue O_2 tension is considerably lower than in arterial blood, and the level of tissue O_2 pressure undergoes a developmental change. Measurements of carotid body tissue Po_2 indicate that in fetal sheep, the arterial-to-tissue O_2 difference is negligible. Birth and transition to pulmonary ventilation lead to a rise in Pao_2 and the arterial-to-tissue O_2 difference rises to adult levels (88). This observation likely reflects changes in blood vessel control, since no anatomical vascular changes occur over this time period (89–91), which strengthens the case for the importance of local neural control of the circulation. This is further supported by the observations that sympathetic stimulation causes afferent activity to increase (92) and that parasympathetic stimulation causes nerve activity to decrease (93), apparently related to local blood flow changes. This modulation may be particularly potent around the time of birth because chemoreceptor activity may be switched from absent to present, in part, by sympathetic stimulation in the fetus (72).

B. Changes in Humoral Factors

In addition to local flow changes, factors in the blood may modulate chemoreceptor activity, such as changes in serum K^+, Na^+, or osmolarity. For instance, the slight increase in K^+, which occurs with exercise, causes a 20–30% increase in the sensitivity to hypoxia (94). In addition, an isotonic decrease in sodium by 20% may reduce chemoreceptor-spiking rates by over 50% (95), and a small increase in serum osmolarity also decreases afferent nerve activity (96). Whether these circulatory factors contribute to the postnatal changes in chemosensitivity in the newborn period remains unexplored.

Circulatory neurochemicals may also potentially modulate carotid chemoreceptor activity in the newborn period. Endorphin levels decrease in the newborn period and application of exogenous endorphins cause an inhibition of hypoxia sensitivity (97). Thus, the postnatal enhancement of chemoreceptor activity may, in part, be due to a reduction in endorphin-based inhibition. An additional, but unidentified, neurochemical is also implicated based on the work of Joels and Neil in 1968. These investigators noted that chemoreceptors perfused with artificial plasma became unresponsive over time, but could be functionally restored by the addition of as little as 5% blood to the perfusate, suggesting the presence of a vital factor in blood which is not present in artificial plasma (98). On the other hand, fetal blood may contain an inhibitory modulator on the basis of the observation that chemoreceptor nerve activity is difficult to record in situ, but may be readily recorded from the same chemoreceptor after removal and perfusion with saline (72).

C. Morphologic Changes in Synapses and Nerve Terminals

In addition to developmental changes in vascular control or hormonal factors, there is strong evidence that developmental changes occur within the chemoreceptor complex itself. Removal and superfusion of the organ with oxygenated saline would be expected to eliminate all circulatory factors. Under these conditions, the level of spiking activity recorded on individual axons during severe hypoxia clearly increases with age (79). This correlates well with results of an anatomical study, which demonstrated that the number of synapses between afferent nerve endings and glomus cells increase four to five times between birth and 20 days of age (99).

What is less clear is whether there is an actual increase in hypoxia sensitivity as compared to an increase in spike generation sites. While it is well established that the nerve activity at a given Po_2 is less in the newborn (Fig. 4), there are two ways to interpret this difference. The newborn response may be "left-shifted" from the adult such that one may overlay the response lines by shifting the adult curve to the left by approximately 30 mmHg, suggesting a change in the sensitivity of the oxygen sensor. On the other hand, the lines may be superimposed by multiplying the newborn response by a constant without changing the apparent sensitivity to hypoxia, suggesting no change in sensitivity but an increase in spike generating sites. There is insufficient data to discriminate between these possibilities based on published studies or from recordings, in vivo. However, from rat chemoreceptors, in vitro, the apparent sensitivity to hypoxia (expressed as a rate constant for a decrease in activity with an increase in superfusate Po_2) was unchanged with development, suggesting no change in the sensor's sensitivity to hypoxia (77).

D. Glomus Cell Anatomy and Physiology Responses

A general schema for the release of an excitatory transmitter from glomus cells may involve three steps: (1) glomus cell depolarization and activation of voltage-dependent calcium currents, (2) a rise in intracellular calcium, and (3) enhanced neurotransmitter secretion due to the rise in intracellular calcium. None of these steps are unequivocally established as essential for carotid body O_2 sensing, but, nevertheless, provide a framework for addressing some developmental changes in glomus cell properties.

Glomus Cell Membrane Depolarization with Hypoxia

Depolarization of the glomus cell by hypoxia is likely the first critical step in the transduction cascade, but the mechanism for the depolarization is far from resolved. Several investigators have proposed that hypoxia inhibits a K^+ current that leads to cell depolarization. Several different types of K^+ currents which are inhibited by hypoxia have been described in glomus cells and can be broadly categorized as (*i*) transient (100), (*ii*) calcium dependent (101), and (*iii*) background or "leak" (102). Of all these O_2-sensitive K^+ currents, the Po_2-current inhibition relationship of the background K^+ current (102) most closely matches the Po_2-$[Ca^{2+}]_i$ relationship of dissociated glomus cells (103–105) and the tissue Po_2-nerve activity relationship of the carotid body (106). In the case of the transient K^+ current, the sensitivity to hypoxia appears to be abnormally high with complete inhibition at Po_2 levels considerably higher than that for the $[Ca^{2+}]_i$ response or organ response to hypoxia (107). The O_2-response curve for the calcium-dependent current has not been elucidated, to date. Whether or not a hypoxia-sensitive background K^+ conductance is responsible for depolarizing glomus cells in response to hypoxia remains to be demonstrated.

To date, formal developmental studies have been undertaken for the calcium-dependent current and the background K^+ current. Both currents are found to mature in the newborn period. The magnitude of the calcium-dependent current increases with age over the first one to two weeks of life (Fig. 6) (108), and this current is reduced by raising the animals in chronically hypoxic conditions (109). This experimental maneuver appears to eliminate the physiologic signal for chemoreceptor maturation, and it is established that animals so treated maintain an immature response to hypoxia (65). Similarly, a recent study from one of our laboratories demonstrated that the O_2 sensitivity of the background or "leak" K^+ conductance (102) is small in glomus cells from newborn rats and increases over the first two weeks of life (7). Although the maturational time course for both currents matches the known time course of glomus cell $[Ca^{2+}]_i$ response maturation (104) and nerve activity hypoxia response maturation (79), a causal nature to the relationship has not been unequivocally established for either O_2-sensitive current.

Calcium Responses of Glomus Cells

Depolarization of the glomus cell leads to activation of voltage-dependent calcium currents and a rise in intracellular calcium. Based on recording from a large number of glomus cells, the magnitude of the calcium response is significantly greater in the glomus cells harvested from older animals compared with younger animals (104). Wasicko et al. characterized the $[Ca^{2+}]_i$ response to graded hypoxia in glomus cells isolated from term-fetal rats that were 1, 3, 7, 11, 14, and 21 days old (104). The response was hyperbolic at all ages. Two major developmental changes were noted, an increase in the maximal $[Ca^{2+}]_i$ response to anoxia, and an apparent rightward shift in the response curve with age (Fig. 7).

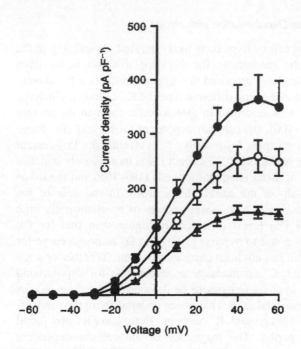

Figure 6 Current density-voltage plots of glomus cell K^+ currents from 4-day-old (▲, n = 40 cells), 10-day-old (○, n = 47 cells), and adult rats (●, n = 46 cells). Currents were evoked by step depolarizations from −70 mV to between −30 and +50 mV in 20-mV increments. *Source*: From Ref. 108.

The developmental increase in the glomus cell $[Ca^{2+}]_i$ response to graded hypoxia occurred between 3 days and 11 to 14 days of age, which agrees well with the reported time course for maturation of carotid body nerve responses to anoxia (79).

    The lower calcium response of the immature cell does not appear to be due to a lack of voltage-gated calcium channels, since the calcium channel density is similar in four- and 10-day-old rats (108). In addition, Wasicko et al. found no change in the glomus cell $[Ca^{2+}]_i$ response to elevated extracellular K^+ between 3 and 14 days of age, the same time frame during which all of the developmental increase in the $[Ca^{2+}]_i$ response to hypoxia occurred (104). If elevated K^+ is taken to be a nonspecific depolarization stimulus, these results indicate that the immature glomus cell is capable of mobilizing large amounts of $[Ca^{2+}]_i$ with depolarization, suggesting that maturation of the $[Ca^{2+}]_i$ response is not due to changes in voltage-gated calcium channels. Furthermore, chronic hypoxia after birth increases, not decreases, the magnitude of the whole-cell calcium current in response to a depolarization (110), although this may largely be caused by the hypertrophy associated with chronic hypoxia (111). In addition, a recent study

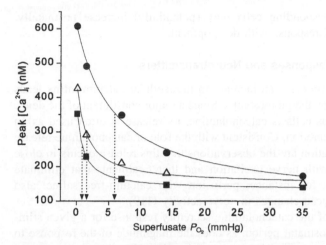

Figure 7 Rightward/upward shift in glomus cell $[Ca^{2+}]_i$ response to hypoxia with age. Mean peak $[Ca^{2+}]_i$ responses of dissociated carotid chemoreceptor cells from three age groups plotted against superfusate P_{O_2} [the age groups were as follows: ■, fetal 1 day (n = 28 glomus cell clusters); △, 3–7 days (n = 15 clusters); ●, 11–21 days (n = 34 clusters)]. Arrows indicate superfusate P_{O_2} at half-maximal $[Ca^{2+}]_i$ response. *Source*: From Ref. 104.

reported that glomus cells harvested from 11-day-old rats reared in chronic hypoxia had minimal or no $[Ca^{2+}]_i$ response to hypoxia, while $[Ca^{2+}]_i$ responses to elevated extracellular K^+ and CO_2 were unaffected (112). Taken together, these results suggest that the postnatal development of glomus cell $[Ca^{2+}]_i$ response to hypoxia depends on maturation of an O_2 sensor or its ability to depolarize the cell.

A second possible area of maturation is in the number of responding cells. Several studies conclude that a significant number of glomus cells fail to depolarize with hypoxia (113) and many glomus cells fail to increase their intracellular calcium levels with hypoxia (114–117). Why many cells fail to respond is presently unclear, although methods of cell preparation and stimulus strength may be important. For example, Bright et al. used 35 mmHg superfusate P_{O_2} as the "hypoxia" challenge and found that only 20% of isolated glomus cells responded with an increase in $[Ca^{2+}]_i$ (114). However, 35 mmHg P_{O_2} is in the normoxic range of carotid body microvascular (tissue) P_{O_2} (106), which may explain the low proportion of glomus cell $[Ca^{2+}]_i$ responses reported by these authors. In a study using superfusate P_{O_2} values of 0, 2, 7, and 14 mmHg, the great majority of glomus cells significantly raised $[Ca^{2+}]_i$ in response to hypoxia (104). Nevertheless, patch clamp recordings of intact glomus cells demonstrate a suppression of calcium-dependent K^+ current in many cells under normoxic conditions (118), suggesting that calcium currents may be inhibited, in situ. If so, then the number of responding cells may (potentially) increase postnatally, providing an enhanced response with development.

E. Secretory Responses and Neurotransmitters

As in adrenal chromaffin cells, an increase in intracellular calcium influx leads to enhanced secretion by the glomus cells. Since a major constituent of the dense core vesicles in glomus cells is catecholamine, its release is often used as an index of glomus cell secretion. Consistent with the role of catecholamine release in afferent nerve excitation are the observations that this release occurs in close temporal association with nerve excitation and that treatments that eliminate catecholamine release, for instance, perfusion with calcium-free saline, also eliminate hypoxia-induced changes in nerve activity (119).

The magnitude of the catecholamine secretory response for a given stimulus increases in the postnatal period, as does the magnitude of the response to hypoxia. This concept was first demonstrated by observing the response to an anoxic stimulus that rapidly increases both nerve activity and free tissue catecholamine (Fig. 8) (120,121). A similar increase in the total release of catecholamine following a 1-hour incubation in solution equilibrated with 8% O_2 was recently described for isolated rabbit carotid bodies in which release as a proportion of total dopamine was larger in 25 days old and adult rabbits than in rabbit pups (122).

The increased secretion of catecholamine is paralleled by an increased expression of D2 receptors in the petrosal ganglia (location of the cells bodies whose axons innervate the carotid body) and in the carotid body itself. D2 receptor mRNA in both the ganglia and carotid body increases fivefold between day 1 and day 25 of life in developing rabbits (123). However, in the opposite sense, pharmacological antagonism of D2 receptors with domperidone has a greater effect on the hypoxia sensitivity in the newborn than in the older cat (124). Although the role of dopamine receptors in organ function is presently unresolved, it is clear that catecholamine secretion as well as catecholamine receptors undergo changes in the postnatal period.

Most studies show that stimulation of catecholamine receptors inhibits carotid body activity. Application of dopamine antagonists generally excite chemoreceptor activity in both the newborn and adult (70,124). This demonstrated inhibitory effect gave rise to an alternate theory of the lower sensitivity in the newborn period. Instead of a lack of excitation, it was proposed that excessive secretion of catecholamines may lead to an active inhibition in the newborn period (63,125). This is supported by data showing a higher turnover rate for catecholamine in rat carotid body immediately after birth, and decreasing over the first 12 to 18 hours after birth (63). Furthermore, postnatal hypoxia, which appears to impair maturation of the normal adult pattern, perpetuates the high turnover of catecholamine (125). While this alternative model offers some explanation for the postnatal maturation, it appears that the maturation of the

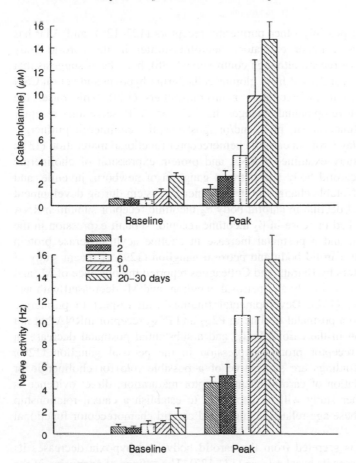

Figure 8 Baseline and peak values for rat carotid sinus nerve activity and carotid body catecholamines. Mean ± SEM for carotid bodies harvested from rats aged 1 (n = 6), 2 (n = 6), 6 (n = 5), 10 (n = 7), and 20 to 30 days (n = 11). Note age-dependent increase in both tissue catecholamines and CSN response to anoxia. *Source*: From Ref. 120.

turnover rate occurs too rapidly. The period of high catecholamine turnover occurs only within the first six hours after birth, while the developmental changes in nerve and calcium responses appear to occur over the first two weeks (78,79,104,112).

Recent studies have explored developmental changes in other carotid body neurotransmitters, most notably ACh, adenosine, and ATP. As noted above, cholinergic receptors are located on glomus cells and on CSN nerve terminals, and ACh has been proposed as an excitatory neurotransmitter and modulator of glomus cell function (84,126). Purinergic receptors (e.g., $P2_{X2}$ and $P2_{X3}$) are located in the petrosal ganglion and on CSN nerve terminals, glomus cells express $P2_{Y2}$ and possibly other purinergic receptors (127–129), and ATP has been proposed as a major excitatory neurotransmitter in the carotid body (83,130). A popular recent, although controversial (86), hypothesis suggests that ATP and ACh are coreleased from glomus cells during hypoxia and act on CSN nerve terminals as major excitatory neurotransmitters (130). This raises the possibility that developmental changes in ACh or ATP secretion, receptor expression, or function of pre- and/or postsynaptic cholinergic/purinergic receptors could play a role in carotid chemoreceptor functional maturation (131).

A recent study examined mRNA and protein expression of cholinergic receptors in the carotid body and petrosal ganglion of newborn, juvenile, and adult cats (129). Notable changes in the cholinergic system during development included a marked decline in carotid body α_3 nicotinic receptor subunit mRNA expression, a marked increase in β_2 nicotinic receptor subunit expression in the petrosal ganglion, and a postnatal increase in choline acyltransferase protein expression in both carotid body and petrosal ganglion (129). A recent study of muscarinic receptors by Bairam and Colleagues reported the presence of M_1 and M_2 receptors in carotid body and petrosal ganglion, and M_1 decreased with age while M_2 did not (132). Developmental findings with respect to purinergic receptors included a postnatal decline in $P2_{X2}$ and $P2_{X3}$ receptor mRNA but not protein expression in the carotid body, and a substantial postnatal decrease in $P2_{X2}$ and $P2_{X3}$ receptor protein expression in the petrosal ganglion (129). Although these findings are suggestive of a possible role for cholinergic or purinergic modulation of carotid chemoreceptor maturation, direct evidence is lacking and further study will be necessary to establish a causal relationship between any of these age-related changes and carotid chemoreceptor functional maturation.

Adenosine is secreted from the carotid body, and hypoxia decreases its content and increases its basal release (131,133). The actions of adenosine in the carotid body are complex; exogenous adenosine appears to stimulate CSN activity via an A2a receptor–mediated mechanism (134), while adenosine inhibits the hypoxia-induced rise in intracellular calcium via an A2a receptor mechanism (135). Although postnatal decline in carotid body A2a receptor mRNA expression has been reported (136), little is known about the potential functional role of adenosine in carotid body maturation. Recently, complex interactions between the adenosine and ACh roles in carotid body O_2 sensing have been proposed, but their functional roles remain speculative and beyond the scope of this chapter.

Given the many neurotransmitters, neurotransmitter receptors, and their subtypes in the carotid body and petrosal ganglion, the multiple actions of these neurochemicals at different sites and the complexity of interactions between neurotransmitters, both pre- and postsynaptically, elucidation of specific roles of neurotransmitters in carotid body maturation remains a major challenge. Carotid chemoreceptor glomus cell maturation (137) and developmental changes in neurotransmitter secretion (84,131) were reviewed recently.

F. Carotid Body Maturation in Altered O_2 Environments

As noted above, chronic hypoxia in the perinatal period blunts maturation of carotid body O_2 sensing at the whole carotid body, glomus cell $[Ca^{2+}]_i$, and depolarization levels (109,112,138,139). On the opposite end of the O_2 spectrum, multiple studies show that chronic hyperoxia during the perinatal period blunts ventilatory and carotid body responses to acute hypoxia challenge (140–142). Chronic intermittent hypoxia (CIH), which more closely mimics hypoxia patterns seen in sleep apnea and other clinical conditions, causes sensitization of the carotid body hypoxia response and long-term sensory facilitation in adults (143). However, in neonates, CIH induces sensitization of the carotid body hypoxia response but not long-term sensory facilitation, indicating potentially important development-related differences in the effects on CIH on carotid body function (144). This is an important area of carotid chemoreceptor development with substantial translational potential, which clearly deserves further study.

VI. The Carotid Chemoreceptors and Abnormal Breathing Control in Children

Much has been written elsewhere about the possible roles of the carotid chemoreceptors in disease states affecting human infants and children. However, most of this literature consists of inferences from indirect evidence and direct evidence that is sometimes conflicting. Although there is no question that disorders such as bronchopulmonary dysplasia (64,145–147) or prematurity (64,148) are associated with marked abnormalities in ventilatory or arousal responses to hypoxia, it is less clear how much this involves abnormal carotid chemoreceptor function per se versus abnormal CNS processing of chemoreceptor inputs. Alvaro and Rigatto discuss breathing control in premature infants in chapter 10.

Pathological conditions, such as sudden infant death syndrome (SIDS), bronchopulmonary dysplasia and apparent life threatening events (ALTE) may be associated with chronic or recurrent hypoxia. Therefore, it is noteworthy that chronic hypoxia, from birth, markedly blunts carotid chemoreceptor maturation. Using the alternating breathing technique to assess peripheral chemoreflex strength, Hanson et al. reported that kittens born into and reared in F_{IO_2} 0.13 to 0.15 exhibited marked impairment of arterial chemoreflex maturation during the first two weeks of life (149). Similarly, chronic hypoxia from birth in rats has been shown to attenuate the maturation of CO_2-O_2 interaction at the carotid body (138). These results are consistent with reports that glomus cells from rats reared in hypoxia do not depolarize in response to acute hypoxia (109) and do not exhibit $[Ca^{2+}]_i$ responses to acute hypoxic challenge (112). Although the mechanisms remain to be worked out, it is clear that chronic hypoxia may profoundly affect maturation of carotid chemoreceptor sensitivity. Further work is needed to determine the precise role(s) played by carotid chemoreceptor abnormalities in disorders such as SIDS, ALTE, bronchopulmonary dyspepsia, and prematurity.

Chronic or chronic intermittent hypoxia has been implicated in SIDS, although the cause or causes of SIDS remain unknown (150). Involvement of the carotid bodies in the pathogenesis of SIDS is controversial; several investigators have reported specific carotid body abnormalities in SIDS victims (151–153), while others have not found any abnormalities (153,154). Reported abnormalities, such as reduction of dense cytoplasmic granules of the carotid chemoreceptor cells, reduction of glomus cell number and size (152), and 10-fold higher concentrations of dopamine compared with carotid bodies from age-matched control infants (153), may result from chronic hypoxia or from postmortem artifact and do not necessarily implicate the carotid bodies in the pathogenesis. Other studies looking for similar abnormalities in structure and catecholamine levels did not find differences between SIDS victims and controls (154,155). In any case, impairment of carotid chemoreceptor O_2 sensitivity and neural output may not be detectable on postmortem examination. It should also be noted that carotid chemoreceptors need not be abnormal to play a role in SIDS. Normal maturation of carotid body O_2 sensitivity may underlie, in part, developmental vulnerability to stressors such as airway obstruction or asphyxia due to sleeping position or bedding materials covering the infant's face. Carotid chemoreceptor function may start out normal and become blunted by chronic hypoxia (112), which may then further increase vulnerability to hypoxic stress. Finally, chronic intermittent hypoxia may enhance carotid chemoreceptor hypoxia sensitivity (144,156); the higher gain may increase instability of the respiratory control system. Much more work is necessary before conclusions can be reached concerning the role of the carotid chemoreceptors in SIDS.

VII. Summary

The carotid chemoreceptors play a critically important role in numerous aspects of respiratory and cardiovascular control, particularly in defensive responses that are important during sleep. In addition, the effects of carotid chemoreceptor stimulation are complex, with inputs to key brain stem cardiorespiratory cell groups being inhibitory in some cases and stimulatory in others. Complex integrated responses to hypoxia depend on a balance between multiple effects of carotid chemoreceptor stimulation, as well as other effects of hypoxia on cardiorespiratory control centers. Although the carotid chemoreceptors drive vitally important responses such as arousal from sleep in response to hypoxia and the ventilatory response to hypoxia, hypoxia-induced bradycardia, and apnea termination, their chemosensory function is immature at birth and increases with age. As maturation may be impaired by common clinical conditions such as chronic hypoxia or chronic intermittent hypoxia, it is important to understand the numerous key roles played by the carotid chemoreceptors and the changes that occur during postnatal development.

References

1. Nyakas C, Buwalda B, Luiten PG. Hypoxia and brain development. Prog Neurobiol 1996; 49(1):1–51.
2. Hudlicka O, Brown MD. Postnatal growth of the heart and its blood vessels. J Vasc Res 1996; 33(4):266–287.
3. Okubo S, Mortola JP. Control of ventilation in adult rats hypoxic in the neonatal period. Am J Physiol 1990; 259(4 pt 2):R836–R841.
4. Okubo S, Mortola JP. Respiratory mechanics in adult rats hypoxic in the neonatal period. J Appl Physiol 1989; 66(4):1772–1778.
5. Okubo S, Mortola JP. Long-term respiratory effects of neonatal hypoxia in the rat. J Appl Physiol 1988; 64(3):952–958.
6. Marshall JM. Peripheral chemoreceptors and cardiovascular regulation. Physiol Rev 1994; 74(3):543–594.
7. Wasicko MJ, Breitwieser GE, Kim I, et al. Postnatal development of carotid body glomus cell response to hypoxia. Respir Physiol Neurobiol 2006; 154(3):356–371.
8. Kumar P, Hanson MA. Re-setting of the hypoxic sensitivity of aortic chemo-receptors in the newborn lamb. J Dev Physiol 1989; 11(4):199–206.
9. Blanco CE, Dawes GS, Hanson MA, et al. The response to hypoxia of arterial chemoreceptors in fetal sheep and newborn lambs. J Physiol 1984; 351:25–37.
10. Timmers HJ, Wieling W, Karemaker JM, et al. Denervation of carotid baro- and chemoreceptors in humans. J Physiol 2003; 553(pt 1):3–11.
11. Bureau MA, Lamarche J, Foulon P, et al. Postnatal maturation of respiration in intact and carotid body-chemodenervated lambs. J Appl Physiol 1985; 59(3):869–874.
12. Bureau MA, Lamarche J, Foulon P, et al. The ventilatory response to hypoxia in the newborn lamb after carotid body denervation. Respir Physiol 1985; 60(1):109–119.
13. Donnelly DF, Haddad GG. Prolonged apnea and impaired survival in piglets after sinus and aortic nerve section. J Appl Physiol 1990; 68(3):1048–1052.
14. Hofer MA. Lethal respiratory disturbance in neonatal rats after arterial chemo-receptor denervation. Life Sci 1984; 34(5):489–496.
15. Hofer MA. Role of carotid sinus and aortic nerves in respiratory control of infant rats. Am J Physiol 1986; 251(4 pt 2):R811–R817.
16. Kumar P, Bin-Jaliah I. Adequate stimuli of the carotid body: more than an oxygen sensor? Respir Physiol Neurobiol 2007; 157(1):12–21.
17. Nakayama K. Surgical removal of the carotid body for bronchial asthma. Dis Chest 1961; 40:595–604.
18. Dejours P. Chemoreflexes in breathing. Physiol Rev 1962; 42:335–358.
19. Jansen AH, Ioffe S, Russell BJ, et al. Effect of carotid chemoreceptor denervation on breathing in utero and after birth. J Appl Physiol 1981; 51(3):630–633.
20. Herrington RT, Harned HS Jr., Ferreiro JI, et al. The role of the central nervous system in perinatal respiration: studies of chemoregulatory mechanisms in the term lamb. Pediatrics 1971; 47(5):857–864.

21. Cote A, Porras H, Meehan B. Age-dependent vulnerability to carotid chemodenervation in piglets. J Appl Physiol 1996; 80(1):323–331.
22. Hunt CE, Hufford DR, Bourguignon C, et al. Home documented monitoring of cardiorespiratory pattern and oxygen saturation in healthy infants. Pediatr Res 1996; 39(2):216–222.
23. Delacourt C, Canet E, Bureau MA. Predominant role of peripheral chemoreceptors in the termination of apnea in maturing newborn lambs. J Appl Physiol 1996; 80 (3):892–898.
24. Marshall JM. Chemoreceptors and cardiovascular control in acute and chronic systemic hypoxia. Braz J Med Biol Res 1998; 31(7):863–888.
25. Daly MD. Carotid chemoreceptor reflex cardioinhibitory responses: comparison of their modulation by central inspiratory neuronal activity and activity of pulmonary stretch afferents. Adv Exp Med Biol 1993; 337:333–343.
26. Giussani DA, Spencer JA, Moore PJ, et al. Afferent and efferent components of the cardiovascular reflex responses to acute hypoxia in term fetal sheep. J Physiol 1993; 461:431–449.
27. Grogaard J, Kreuger E, Lindstrom D, et al. Effects of carotid body maturation and terbutaline on the laryngeal chemoreflex in newborn lambs. Pediatr Res 1986; 20 (8):724–729.
28. Thach BT. Maturation and transformation of reflexes that protect the laryngeal airway from liquid aspiration from fetal to adult life. Am J Med 2001; 111(suppl 8A):69S–77S.
29. Grogaard J, Lindstrom DP, Stahlman MT, et al. The cardiovascular response to laryngeal water administration in young lambs. J Dev Physiol 1982; 4(6):353–370.
30. Wennergren G, Hertzberg T, Milerad J, et al. Hypoxia reinforces laryngeal reflex bradycardia in infants. Acta Paediatr Scand 1989; 78(1):11–17.
31. Woodson GE, Brauel G. Arterial chemoreceptor influences on the laryngeal chemoreflex. Otolaryngol Head Neck Surg 1992; 107(6 pt 1):775–782.
32. Sladek M, Grogaard JB, Parker RA, et al. Prolonged hypoxemia enhances and acute hypoxemia attenuates laryngeal reflex apnea in young lambs. Pediatr Res 1993; 34(6):813–820.
33. Fleming PJ, Goncalves AL, Levine MR, et al. The development of stability of respiration in human infants: changes in ventilatory responses to spontaneous sighs. J Physiol 1984; 347:1–16.
34. Daristotle L, Berssenbrugge AD, Engwall MJ, et al. The effects of carotid body hypocapnia on ventilation in goats. Respir Physiol 1990; 79(2):123–135.
35. Tehrani FT. A model study of periodic breathing, stability of the neonatal respiratory system, and causes of sudden infant death syndrome. Med Eng Phys 1997; 19(6):547–555.
36. Cleave JP, Levine MR, Fleming PJ. The control of ventilation: a theoretical analysis of the response to transient disturbances. J Theor Biol 1984; 108(2):261–283.
37. Richardson HL, Parslow PM, Walker AM, et al. Maturation of the initial ventilatory response to hypoxia in sleeping infants. J Sleep Res 2007; 16(1):117–127.
38. Fewell JE, Baker SB. Arousal from sleep during rapidly developing hypoxemia in lambs. Pediatr Res 1987; 22(4):471–477.
39. Fewell JE, Konduri GG. Repeated exposure to rapidly developing hypoxemia influences the interaction between oxygen and carbon dioxide in initiating arousal from sleep in lambs. Pediatr Res 1988; 24(1):28–33.

40. Fewell JE, Kondo CS, Dascalu V, et al. Influence of carotid denervation on the arousal and cardiopulmonary response to rapidly developing hypoxemia in lambs. Pediatr Res 1989; 25(5):473–477.
41. Igras D, Fewell JE. Arousal response to upper airway obstruction in young lambs: comparison of nasal and tracheal occlusion. J Dev Physiol 1991; 15(4): 215–220.
42. Fewell JE, Williams BJ, Szabo JS, et al. Influence of repeated upper airway obstruction on the arousal and cardiopulmonary response to upper airway obstruction in lambs. Pediatr Res 1988; 23(2):191–195.
43. Fewell JE, Taylor BJ, Kondo CS, et al. Influence of carotid denervation on the arousal and cardiopulmonary responses to upper airway obstruction in lambs. Pediatr Res 1990; 28(4):374–378.
44. Fewell JE, Kondo CS, Dascalu V, et al. Influence of carotid-denervation on the arousal and cardiopulmonary responses to alveolar hypercapnia in lambs. J Dev Physiol 1989; 12(4):193–199.
45. Lawson EE, Long WA. Central origin of biphasic breathing pattern during hypoxia in newborns. J Appl Physiol 1983; 55(2):483–488.
46. Martin-Body RL. Brain transections demonstrate the central origin of hypoxic ventilatory depression in carotid body-denervated rats. J Physiol 1988; 407:41–52.
47. Frappell P, Saiki C, Mortola JP. Metabolism during normoxia, hypoxia, and recovery in the newborn kitten. Respir Physiol 1991; 86(1):115–124.
48. Mortola JP, Rezzonico R, Lanthier C. Ventilation and oxygen consumption during acute hypoxia in newborn mammals: a comparative analysis. Respir Physiol 1989; 78(1):31–43.
49. Gonzalez C, Almaraz L, Obeso A, et al. Carotid body chemoreceptors: from natural stimuli to sensory discharges. Physiol Rev 1994; 74(4):829–898.
50. Schwieler GH. Respiratory regulation during postnatal development in cats and rabbits and some of its morphological substrate. Acta Physiol Scand Suppl 1968; 304: 1–123.
51. Belenky DA, Standaert TA, Woodrum DE. Maturation of hypoxic ventilatory response of the newborn lamb. J Appl Physiol 1979; 47(5):927–930.
52. Bonora M, Marlot D, Gautier H, et al. Effects of hypoxia on ventilation during postnatal development in conscious kittens. J Appl Physiol 1984; 56(6):1464–1471.
53. Bureau MA, Begin R. Postnatal maturation of the respiratory response to O_2 in awake newborn lambs. J Appl Physiol 1982; 52(2):428–433.
54. Eden GJ, Hanson MA. Maturation of the respiratory response to acute hypoxia in the newborn rat. J Physiol 1987; 392:1–9.
55. Haddad GG, Gandhi MR, Mellins RB. Maturation of ventilatory response to hypoxia in puppies during sleep. J Appl Physiol 1982; 52(2):309–314.
56. Horne RS, Parslow PM, Harding R. Postnatal development of ventilatory and arousal responses to hypoxia in human infants. Respir Physiol Neurobiol 2005; 149 (1–3):257–271.
57. Schramm CM, Grunstein MM. Respiratory influence of peripheral chemoreceptor stimulation in maturing rabbits. J Appl Physiol 1987; 63(4):1671–1680.
58. Long WQ, Giesbrecht GG, Anthonisen NR. Ventilatory response to moderate hypoxia in awake chemodenervated cats. J Appl Physiol 1993; 74(2):805–810.
59. Miller MJ, Tenney SM. Hypoxia-induced tachypnea in carotid-deafferented cats. Respir Physiol 1975; 23(1):31–39.

60. Waites BA, Ackland GL, Noble R, et al. Red nucleus lesions abolish the biphasic respiratory response to isocapnic hypoxia in decerebrate young rabbits. J Physiol 1996; 495(pt 1):217–225.

61. Moore PJ, Ackland GL, Hanson MA. Unilateral cooling in the region of locus coeruleus blocks the fall in respiratory output during hypoxia in anaesthetized neonatal sheep. Exp Physiol 1996; 81(6):983–994.

62. Hertzberg T, Lagercrantz H. Postnatal sensitivity of the peripheral chemoreceptors in newborn infants. Arch Dis Child 1987; 62(12):1238–1241.

63. Hertzberg T, Hellstrom S, Lagercrantz H, et al. Development of the arterial chemoreflex and turnover of carotid body catecholamines in the newborn rat. J Physiol 1990; 425:211–225.

64. Canet E, Kianicka I, Praud JP. Postnatal maturation of peripheral chemoreceptor ventilatory response to O_2 and CO_2 in newborn lambs. J Appl Physiol 1996; 80 (6):1928–1933.

65. Eden GJ, Hanson MA. Effects of chronic hypoxia from birth on the ventilatory response to acute hypoxia in the newborn rat. J Physiol 1987; 392:11–19.

66. Calder NA, Williams BA, Kumar P, et al. The respiratory response of healthy term infants to breath-by-breath alternations in inspired oxygen at two postnatal ages. Pediatr Res 1994; 35(3):321–324.

67. Mulligan E. Carotid chemoreceptor recording in the newborn piglet. In: Eyzaguirre C, Fidone S, Fitzgerald RS, et al, eds. Arterial Chemoreception. New York: Springer-Verlag, 1990:285–289.

68. Carroll JL, Bamford OS, Fitzgerald RS. Postnatal maturation of carotid chemoreceptor responses to O_2 and CO_2 in the cat. J Appl Physiol 1993; 75(6): 2383–2391.

69. Marchal F, Bairam A, Haouzi P, et al. Carotid chemoreceptor response to natural stimuli in the newborn kitten. Respir Physiol 1992; 87(2):183–193.

70. Donnelly DF, Smith EJ, Dutton RE. Neural response of carotid chemoreceptors following dopamine blockade. J Appl Physiol 1981; 50(1):172–177.

71. Biscoe TJ, Purves MJ, Sampson SR. Types of nervous activity which may be recorded from the carotid sinus nerve in the sheep foetus. J Physiol 1969; 202 (1):1–23.

72. Jansen AH, Purves MJ, Tan ED. The role of sympathetic nerves in the activation of the carotid body chemoreceptors at birth in the sheep. J Dev Physiol 1980; 2(5): 305–321.

73. Mulligan E, Lahiri S, Storey BT. Carotid body O_2 chemoreception and mitochondrial oxidative phosphorylation. J Appl Physiol 1981; 51(2):438–446.

74. Mulligan E. Discharge properties of carotid bodies: developmental aspects. In: Haddad GG, Farber JP, eds. Developmental Neurobiology of Breathing. New York: Marcel Dekker, Inc., 1991:321–340.

75. Blanco CE, Hanson MA, Johnson P, et al. Breathing pattern of kittens during hypoxia. J Appl Physiol 1984; 56(1):12–17.

76. Calder NA, Kumar P, Hanson MA. Development of carotid chemoreceptor dynamic and steady-state sensitivity to CO_2 in the newborn lamb. J Physiol 1997; 503(pt 1):187–194.

77. Pepper DR, Landauer RC, Kumar P. Postnatal development of CO_2–O_2 interaction in the rat carotid body in vitro. J Physiol 1995; 485(pt 2):531–541.

78. Bamford OS, Sterni LM, Wasicko MJ, et al. Postnatal maturation of carotid body and type I cell chemoreception in the rat. Am J Physiol 1999; 276(5 pt 1): L875–L884.

79. Kholwadwala D, Donnelly DF. Maturation of carotid chemoreceptor sensitivity to hypoxia: in vitro studies in the newborn rat. J Physiol 1992; 453:461–473.

80. Wolsink JG, Berkenbosch A, DeGoede J, et al. Maturation of the ventilatory response to CO_2 in the newborn piglet. Pediatr Res 1993; 34(4):485–489.

81. McDonald DM, Mitchell RA. The innervation of glomus cells, ganglion cells, and blood vessels in the rat carotid body: a qualitative ultrastructural analysis. J Neurocytol 1975; 4:177–230.

82. Tatsumi K, Pickett CK, Weil JV. Decreased carotid body hypoxic sensitivity in chronic hypoxia: role of dopamine. Respir Physiol 1995; 101(1):47–57.

83. Buttigieg J, Nurse CA. Detection of hypoxia-evoked ATP release from chemoreceptor cells of the rat carotid body. Biochem Biophys Res Commun 2004; 322 (1):82–87.

84. Shirahata M, Balbir A, Otsubo T, et al. Role of acetylcholine in neurotransmission of the carotid body. Respir Physiol Neurobiol 2007; 157(1):93–105.

85. Zapata P. Is ATP a suitable co-transmitter in carotid body arterial chemoreceptors? Respir Physiol Neurobiol 2007; 157(1):106–115.

86. Reyes EP, Fernandez R, Larrain C, et al. Effects of combined cholinergic-purinergic block upon cat carotid body chemoreceptors in vitro. Respir Physiol Neurobiol 2007; 156(1):17–22.

87. Kienecker EW, Knoche H, Bingmann D. Functional properties of regenerating sinus nerve fibres in the rabbit. Neuroscience 1978; 3(10):977–988.

88. Acker H, Lubbers DW, Purves MJ, et al. Measurements of the partial pressure of oxygen in the carotid body of fetal sheep and newborn lambs. J Dev Physiol 1980; 2(5):323–328.

89. Clarke JA, de Burgh DM, Ead HW. Comparison of the size of the vascular compartment of the carotid body of the fetal, neonatal, and adult cat. Acta Anat (Basel) 1990; 138(2):166–174.

90. Moore PJ, Clarke JA, Hanson MA, et al. Quantitative studies of the vasculature of the carotid body in fetal and newborn sheep. J Dev Physiol 1991; 15(4):211–214.

91. Acker H, Degner F, Hilsmann J. Local blood flow velocities in the carotid body of fetal sheep and newborn lambs. J Comp Physiol [B] 1991; 161(1):73–79.

92. Biscoe TJ, Purves MJ. Carotid body chemoreceptor activity in the new-born lamb. J Physiol 1967; 190(3):443–454.

93. Neil E, O'Regan RG. The effects of electrical stimulation of the distal end of the cut sinus and aortic nerves on peripheral arterial chemoreceptor activity in the cat. J Physiol 1971; 215(1):15–32.

94. Band DM, Linton RA. The effect of potassium on carotid body chemoreceptor discharge in the anaesthetized cat. J Physiol 1986; 381:39–47.

95. Donnelly DF, Panisello JM, Boggs D. Effect of sodium perturbations on rat chemoreceptor spike generation: implications for a Poisson model. J Physiol 1998; 511 (pt 1):301–311.

96. Gallego R, Eyzaguirre C, Monti-Bloch L. Thermal and osmotic responses of arterial receptors. J Neurophysiol 1979; 42(3):665–680.

97. Pokorski M, Lahiri S. Effects of naloxone on carotid body chemoreception and ventilation in the cat. J Appl Physiol 1981; 51(6):1533–1538.

98. Joels N, Neil E. The idea of a sensory transmitter. In: Torrance RW, ed. Arterial Chemoreceptors. Blackwell; Oxford, UK: 1968:153–178.

99. Kondo H. An electron microscopic study on the development of synapses in the rat carotid body. Neurosci Lett 1976; 3:197–200.

100. Lopez-Lopez JR, De Luis DA, Gonzalez C. Properties of a transient K+ current in chemoreceptor cells of rabbit carotid body. J Physiol 1993; 460:15–32.

101. Peers C. Hypoxic suppression of K+ currents in type I carotid body cells: selective effect on the Ca2(+)-activated K+ current. Neurosci Lett 1990; 119(2):253–256.

102. Buckler KJ. A novel oxygen-sensitive potassium current in rat carotid body type I cells. J Physiol 1997; 498(pt 3):649–662.

103. Buckler KJ, Vaughan-Jones RD. Effects of hypoxia on membrane potential and intracellular calcium in rat neonatal carotid body type I cells. J Physiol 1994; 476 (3):423–428.

104. Wasicko MJ, Sterni LM, Bamford OS, et al. Resetting and postnatal maturation of oxygen chemosensitivity in rat carotid chemoreceptor cells. J Physiol 1999; 514(pt 2):493–503.

105. Montoro RJ, Urena J, Fernandez-Chacon R, et al. Oxygen sensing by ion channels and chemotransduction in single glomus cells. J Gen Physiol 1996; 107(1):133–143.

106. Rumsey WL, Iturriaga R, Spergel D, et al. Optical measurements of the dependence of chemoreception on oxygen pressure in the cat carotid body. Am J Physiol 1991; 261(4 pt 1):C614–C622.

107. Ganfornina MD, Lopez-Barneo J. Single K+ channels in membrane patches of arterial chemoreceptor cells are modulated by O2 tension. Proc Natl Acad Sci U S A 1991; 88(7):2927–2930.

108. Hatton CJ, Carpenter E, Pepper DR, et al. Developmental changes in isolated rat type I carotid body cell K+ currents and their modulation by hypoxia. J Physiol 1997; 501(pt 1):49–58.

109. Wyatt CN, Wright C, Bee D, et al. O2-sensitive K+ currents in carotid body chemoreceptor cells from normoxic and chronically hypoxic rats and their roles in hypoxic chemotransduction. Proc Natl Acad Sci U S A 1995; 92(1):295–299.

110. Hempleman SC. Increased calcium current in carotid body glomus cells following in vivo acclimatization to chronic hypoxia. J Neurophysiol 1996; 76(3):1880–1886.

111. Peers C, Carpenter E, Hatton CJ, et al. Ca2+ channel currents in type I carotid body cells of normoxic and chronically hypoxic neonatal rats. Brain Res 1996; 739 (1–2):251–257.

112. Sterni LM, Bamford OS, Wasicko MJ, et al. Chronic hypoxia abolished the postnatal increase in carotid body type I cell sensitivity to hypoxia. Am J Physiol 1999; 277(3 pt 1):L645–L652.

113. Pang L, Eyzaguirre C. Different effects of hypoxia on the membrane potential and input resistance of isolated and clustered carotid body glomus cells. Brain Res 1992; 575(1):167–173.

114. Bright GR, Agani FH, Haque U, et al. Heterogeneity in cytosolic calcium responses to hypoxia in carotid body cells. Brain Res 1996; 706(2):297–302.

115. Donnelly DF, Kholwadwala D. Hypoxia decreases intracellular calcium in adult rat carotid body glomus cells. J Neurophysiol 1992; 67(6):1543–1551.

116. Roumy M. Cytosolic calcium in isolated type I cells of the adult rabbit carotid body: effects of hypoxia, cyanide, and changes in intracellular pH. Adv Exp Med Biol 1994; 360:175–177.

117. Sterni LM, Bamford OS, Tomares SM, et al. Developmental changes in intracellular Ca2+ response of carotid chemoreceptor cells to hypoxia. Am J Physiol 1995; 268(5 pt 1):L801–L808.

118. Donnelly DF. Modulation of glomus cell membrane currents of intact rat carotid body. J Physiol 1995; 489(pt 3):677–688.

119. Donnelly DF. Electrochemical detection of catecholamine release from rat carotid body in vitro. J Appl Physiol 1993; 74(5):2330–2337.

120. Donnelly DF, Doyle TP. Developmental changes in hypoxia-induced catecholamine release from rat carotid body, in vitro. J Physiol 1994; 475(2):267–275.

121. Fidone S, Gonzalez C, Yoshizaki K. Effects of low oxygen on the release of dopamine from the rabbit carotid body in vitro. J Physiol 1982 Dec; 333:93–110.

122. Bairam A, Basson H, Marchal F, et al. Effects of hypoxia on carotid body dopamine content and release in developing rabbits. J Appl Physiol 1996; 80(1):20–24.

123. Bairam A, Dauphin C, Rousseau F, et al. Expression of dopamine D2-receptor mRNA isoforms at the peripheral chemoreflex afferent pathway in developing rabbits. Am J Respir Cell Mol Biol 1996; 15(3):374–381.

124. Tomares SM, Bamford OS, Sterni LM, et al. Effects of domperidone on neonatal and adult carotid chemoreceptors in the cat. J Appl Physiol 1994; 77(3): 1274–1280.

125. Hertzberg T, Hellstrom S, Holgert H, et al. Ventilatory response to hyperoxia in newborn rats born in hypoxia: possible relationship to carotid body dopamine. J Physiol 1992 Oct; 456:645–654.

126. Shirahata M, Ishizawa Y, Rudisill M, et al. Presence of nicotinic acetylcholine receptors in cat carotid body afferent system. Brain Res 1998; 814(1–2):213–217.

127. Xu J, Tse FW, Tse A. ATP triggers intracellular Ca2+ release in type II cells of the rat carotid body. J Physiol 2003; 549(pt 3):739–747.

128. Prasad M, Fearon IM, Zhang M, et al. Expression of P2X2 and P2X3 receptor subunits in rat carotid body afferent neurones: role in chemosensory signalling. J Physiol 2001; 537(pt 3):667–677.

129. Bairam A, Joseph V, Lajeunesse Y, et al. Developmental profile of cholinergic and purinergic traits and receptors in peripheral chemoreflex pathway in cats. Neuroscience 2007; 146(4):1841–1853.

130. Zhang M, Zhong H, Vollmer C, et al. Co-release of ATP and ACh mediates hypoxic signalling at rat carotid body chemoreceptors. J Physiol 2000; 525(pt 1): 143–158.

131. Bairam A, Carroll JL. Neurotransmitters in carotid body development. Respir Physiol Neurobiol 2005; 149(1–3):201–15.

132. Bairam A, Joseph V, Lajeunesse Y, et al. Developmental pattern of M(1) and M(2) muscarinic gene expression and receptor levels in cat carotid body, petrosal, and superior cervical ganglion. Neuroscience 2006; 139(2):711–721.

133. Conde SV, Monteiro EC. Hypoxia induces adenosine release from the rat carotid body. J Neurochem 2004; 89(5):148–1156.

134. McQueen DS, Ribeiro JA. Pharmacological characterization of the receptor involved in chemoexcitation induced by adenosine. Br J Pharmacol 1986; 88(3): 615–620.

135. Kobayashi S, Conforti L, Millhorn DE. Gene expression and function of adenosine A(2A) receptor in the rat carotid body. Am J Physiol Lung Cell Mol Physiol 2000; 79(2):L273–L282.

136. Gauda EB, Northington FJ, Linden J, et al. Differential expression of a(2a), A(1)-adenosine and D(2)-dopamine receptor genes in rat peripheral arterial chemoreceptors during postnatal development. Brain Res 2000; 872(1–2):1–10.

137. Carroll JL, Kim I. Postnatal development of carotid body glomus cell O(2) sensitivity. Respir Physiol Neurobiol 2005; 149(1–3):201–215.

138. Landauer RC, Pepper DR, Kumar P. Effect of chronic hypoxaemia from birth upon chemosensitivity in the adult rat carotid body in vitro. J Physiol 1995; 485(pt 2):543–550.

139. Carroll JL. Developmental plasticity in respiratory control. J Appl Physiol 2003; 94(1):75–389.

140. Bavis RW, Russell KE, Simons JC, et al. Hypoxic ventilatory responses in rats after hypercapnic hyperoxia and intermittent hyperoxia. Respir Physiol Neurobiol 2007; 155(3):193–202.

141. Bavis RW. Developmental plasticity of the hypoxic ventilatory response after perinatal hyperoxia and hypoxia. Respir Physiol Neurobiol 2005; 149(1–3):287–299.

142. Bisgard GE, Olson EB, Jr., Bavis RW, et al. Carotid chemoafferent plasticity in adult rats following developmental hyperoxia. Respir Physiol Neurobiol 2005; 145(1):3–11.

143. Peng YJ, Overholt JL, Kline D, et al. Induction of sensory long-term facilitation in the carotid body by intermittent hypoxia: implications for recurrent apneas. Proc Natl Acad Sci U S A 2003; 100(17):10073–10078.

144. Prabhakar NR, Peng YJ, Kumar GK, et al. Altered carotid body function by intermittent hypoxia in neonates and adults: relevance to recurrent apneas. Respir Physiol Neurobiol 2007; 157(1):148–153.

145. Garg M, Kurzner SI, Bautista D, et al. Hypoxic arousal responses in infants with bronchopulmonary dysplasia. Pediatrics 1988; 82(1):59–63.

146. Katz-Salamon M, Jonsson B, Lagercrantz H. Blunted peripheral chemoreceptor response to hyperoxia in a group of infants with bronchopulmonary dysplasia. Pediatr Pulmonol 1995; 20(2):101–106.

147. Katz-Salamon M, Eriksson M, Jonsson B. Development of peripheral chemoreceptor function in infants with chronic lung disease and initially lacking hyperoxic response. Arch Dis Child Fetal Neonatal Ed 1996; 75(1):F4–F9.

148. Katz-Salamon M, Lagercrantz H. Hypoxic ventilatory defense in very preterm infants: attenuation after long term oxygen treatment. Arch Dis Child Fetal Neonatal Ed 1994; 70(2):F90–F95.

149. Hanson MA, Kumar P, Williams BA. The effect of chronic hypoxia upon the development of respiratory chemoreflexes in the newborn kitten. J Physiol 1989; 411:563–574.

150. Gauda EB, Cristofalo E, Nunez J. Peripheral arterial chemoreceptors and sudden infant death syndrome. Respir Physiol Neurobiol 2007; 157(1):162–170.

151. Naeye RL, Fisher R, Ryser M, et al. Carotid body in the sudden infant death syndrome. Science 1976; 191(4227):567–569.

152. Cole S, Lindenberg LB, Galioto FM, et al. Ultrastructural abnormalities of the carotid body in sudden infant death syndrome. Pediatrics 1979; 63(1):13–17.

153. Perrin DG, Cutz E, Becker LE, et al. Sudden infant death syndrome: increased carotid-body dopamine and noradrenaline content. Lancet 1984; 2(8402):535–537.

154. Lack EE, Perez-Atayde AR, Young JB. Carotid bodies in sudden infant death syndrome: a combined light microscopic, ultrastructural, and biochemical study. Pediatr Pathol 1986; 6(2–3):335–350.
155. Perrin DG, Cutz E, Becker LE, et al. Ultrastructure of carotid bodies in sudden infant death syndrome. Pediatrics 1984; 73(5):646–651.
156. Peng YJ, Rennison J, Prabhakar NR. Intermittent hypoxia augments carotid body and ventilatory response to hypoxia in neonatal rat pups. J Appl Physiol 2004; 97 (5):2020–2025.

4

Maturation and Plasticity of Central Components in Cardiovascular and Respiratory Control

DAVID GOZAL
University of Louisville School of Medicine, Louisville, Kentucky, U.S.A.

RONALD M. HARPER
University of California, Los Angeles, Los Angeles, California, U.S.A.

I. Introduction

The ability to rapidly adjust to changes in environmental, state, and/or metabolic conditions while maintaining tightly controlled homeostasis is one of the major adaptive mechanisms underlying survival. In mammalian species, sophisticated systems have evolved to allow for preservation of homeostasis. However, these systems may not be fully integrated or operational during the initial stages of postnatal life, thereby leading to the emergence of vulnerable states under certain circumstances. Examples of such situations include the onset of apnea and/or bradycardia during sleep, which are common problems in the neonate and infant and often result in the need for prolonged hospitalization and home cardiorespiratory monitoring.

It is now quite clear that major differences in respiratory activity exist between wakefulness and sleep. Such differences include a fall in ventilation, a decreased metabolic rate, an increase in alveolar PCO_2, a decrease in responsiveness to ventilatory stimuli, and an increase in airflow resistance (1). Such changes appear to reflect conflicting state-dependent drives (2). However, within sleep states, there is considerable variability in respiratory patterns, such that during non–rapid eye movement (NREM) or slow wave sleep (SWS), respiratory rate decreases and tidal volume may either increase or remain unchanged, while during phasic rapid eye movement (REM) sleep, breathing becomes irregular, rapid, and shallow (3,4). Thus, sleep states exert major effects on moment-to-moment expression of breathing and autonomic control, as well as on evoked responses to specific challenges. The momentary changes are typically far out of proportion to demands dictated by metabolic needs; thus, a portion of the variation associated with state reflects neural processes other than the mechanisms essential for homeostasis and in some instances may compromise vital needs.

A detailed review of each of the central systems underlying homeostatic defense and adaptation during wakefulness and sleep is clearly beyond the scope of this review. Thus, we will focus on three selected and illustrative aspects of maturation in this context: (1) the hypoxic ventilatory response (HVR); (2) central chemosensitivity; and (3) autonomic nervous system tone.

II. Plasticity of Respiratory Control

Until recently, plasticity of respiratory control systems during development was seldom considered as a potential mechanism governing the variance of phenotypic expression within any given species. Thus, development of respiratory control was almost exclusively considered as being strictly governed by genetic influences that laid the framework for a relatively determinate process. However, recent studies have provided a growing body of evidence that has led to a substantial revision of this dogma. It has now become readily apparent that the control of respiration is a dynamic process that is not only dictated by genetic determinates, but is also profoundly influenced through interactions with a multitude of environmental factors. Furthermore, any of these environmental stimuli may elicit entirely disparate respiratory responses depending on the pattern of presentation of the stimulus or the developmental stage at which such environmental stimulus is introduced. For example, a given stimulus may elicit a predictable response when presented to adult mammals, and such response will usually abate on discontinuation of the stimulus or alternatively may persist for only a short period of time after the stimulus is removed. In most if not all cases, the adaptive responses will return to their preexposure characteristics in the mature animal. In contrast, an equivalent perturbation in the developing animal may bring about entirely different adaptive strategies, some of which may persist for extremely prolonged periods of time, namely, the complete lifespan. These alterations in respiratory control that persist as lifelong modifications of the functional properties of the particular respiratory network of interest have led to the concept of ''critical periods'' of susceptibility and have provided unique insights into developmental plasticity. Briefly, the term ''critical period'' as it relates to developmental plasticity refers to a window of time at which structural or functional development of neural networks is uniquely susceptible to environmental influences (5). This period is characterized by accelerated brain growth and synaptogenesis (6,7) as well as developmental regulation of receptors and associated signaling cascades, including neurotransmitters and neuro-modulators (8). Furthermore, this window corresponds to a period of regulated neuronal pruning through tightly controlled apoptotic mechanisms (9). Thus, occurrence of noxious stimuli during this critical period may disrupt the normal maturation of the system and thereby influence its ultimate configuration and function. In contrast, identical exposures that precede or succeed this critical window have minimal effects on normal maturational patterns.

In recent years, various models of developmental plasticity in respiratory control have been identified (5). The majority of these models include environmental stimuli such as sustained hypoxia (SH), hypercapnia, hyperoxia, and intermittent hypoxia (IH) or drugs such as nicotine or cocaine. In addition, models using chemoreceptor denervation and perinatal stress have also been described as exerting profound influences on development. Interestingly, other environmental factors including increased body temperature and sleep deprivation or prenatal factors including maternal smoking, maternal drug use, heavy maternal caffeine consumption, and malnutrition during pregnancy all contribute to postnatal breathing instability (10). Indeed, developmental plasticity occurs in multiple, if not all, neural substrates; however, the focus of our studies will be principally on those underlying control of ventilation with particular emphasis on developmental plasticity induced by IH. Before addressing the effects of chronic intermittent hypoxia (CIH), we will briefly review the acute HVR and the effects of SH on ventilatory development to provide contrasts and similarities in the functional and structural adaptations elicited by the same stimulus, yet presented differently.

A. HVR

The ability to adequately control respiration during a noxious insult is vital at any stage of development; this is especially true for infants in whom maladaptive responses could ultimately lead to mortality [i.e., sudden infant death syndrome (SIDS)]. Thus, an appropriate ventilatory response to an acute hypoxic insult is critical for survival. In mammals, HVR is typically biphasic (Fig. 1), consisting of an initial ventilatory enhancement, also denoted as peak HVR (pHVR), and a subsequent decrease in ventilatory output to levels that are often lower than the early ventilatory increase (11). This later decrease in ventilatory output has been termed hypoxic ventilatory decline (HVD), also "ventilatory roll-off," and is the result of complex interactions between excitatory and inhibitory influences on peripheral chemoreceptors, central respiratory neurons, and metabolic pathways (11).

This early response to hypoxia is initially mediated by activation of peripheral chemoreceptors with the resultant increase in minute ventilation (V_E)

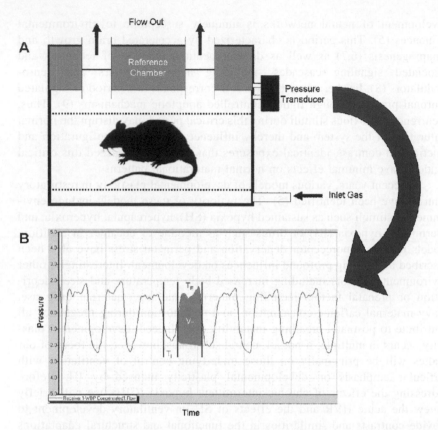

Figure 1A Schematic diagram illustrating WBP in small rodents. Ventilatory measures were conducted in freely behaving rats using conventional flow WBP (Panel A). Changes in recording chamber pressure relative to a reference chamber were amplified and analyzed online using specialized computer software (Panel B). *Abbreviation*: WBP, whole-body plethysmography.

during pHVR. pHVR requires intact central relays within the nucleus tractus solitarii (nTS) and neural transmission of hypoxic afferent input is critically dependent on glutamatergic signaling, particularly the activity of N-methyl-D-aspartate (NMDA) receptors in this critical brain stem region (12–15). The putative mechanism underlying pHVR in the nTS implicates upstream signal transduction involving among other mediators, activation of platelet-activating factor (PAFR) (16–18), which leads to the release of glutamate (Glu) into the synaptic cleft. Upon binding, Glu activates the NMDA receptor and allows the influx of Ca^{2+} into the cell. This process in turn activates many downstream signaling pathways and protein kinases, most notably protein kinase C (PKC) (19–25) and tyrosine kinases (TKs). TK inhibitors modulate the ventilatory response to hypoxia in the conscious rat, and calcium/calmodulin-dependent pathways (CaMKII) are also critically involved in the modulation of peak

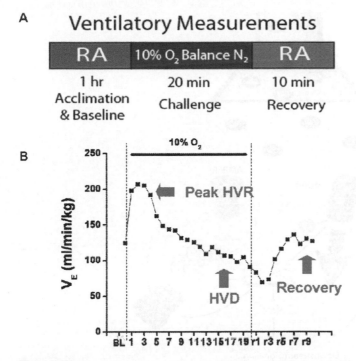

Figure 1B   Acute hypoxic ventilatory challenge. Ventilatory challenges to 10% O_2 were conducted using WBP. Animals were allowed to acclimate to the recording chamber for approximately one hour in room air (30 minutes habituation + 30 minutes baseline), after which a 20-minute acute hypoxia was introduced (Panel A). Analyzed data from one experiment are illustrated in Panel B. *Abbreviation*: WBP, whole-body plethysmography.

hypoxic ventilatory responses (26). CaMKII activity may then act to further modulate the signaling cascade by influencing the translocation of NMDA and α-amino-3-hydroxy-5-methylisoxazole-4-propionic acid (AMPA) receptors to the postsynaptic membrane, the latter of which are tonically involved in the maintenance of ventilation but not necessarily directly involved in acute HVR (27). CaMKII may act through further signal transduction involving neuronal nitric oxide synthase (nNOS) (28–30). Please refer to Figure 2 for a schematic representation of this signaling pathway.

    While glutamatergic mechanisms have been critically implicated in the early component of the minute ventilation ($_E$) enhanced response (12–15), the mechanisms by which HVD occurs remain somewhat unclear. HVD is particularly prominent in developing mammals when compared to mature animals, although clear species-related differences are apparent and relate to the degree of maturity at birth. Depending on the severity of the hypoxic environment and postnatal age of the animal, the early ventilatory enhancement is comparatively reduced. In addition, the sustained ventilatory response in developing mammals may decrease to stable values, which are markedly below those measured in

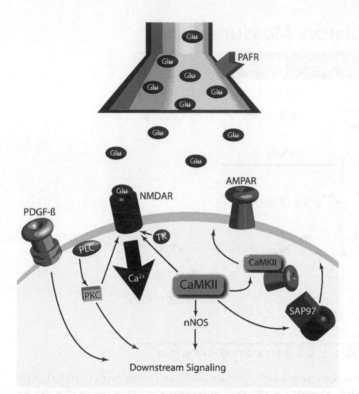

Figure 2 (*See color insert.*) Schematic diagram of a working model for glutamatergic signaling in the nucleus of the solitary tract (nTS) during acute hypoxia. *Abbreviations*: AMPAR, receptor for α-amino-3-hydroxy-5-methylisoxazole-4-propionic acid; CaCMKII, calcium/calmodulin-dependent kinase 2; Glu, glutamate; NMDAR, receptor for *N*-methyl-D-aspartate; nNOS, neuronal nitric oxide synthase; PAFR, platelet activating factor receptor; PKC, protein kinase C; PLC, phospholipase C; PDGF β, receptor for platelet derived growth factor beta; SAP97, one of several PDZ membrane-associated guanylate kinase proteins; TK, tyrosine kinase.

normoxia (31,32). The fall in V_E cannot be accounted for by changes in pulmonary mechanics, altered peripheral chemoreceptor activity, or respiratory muscle fatigue; thus, a central inhibitory process that gradually abates with increasing animal maturation has been postulated (32,33).

Although a comprehensive conceptual framework of the neural signaling during HVD is still lacking, evidence points to an interaction between the withdrawal of excitatory inputs that are expressed during pHVR, and the onset and progressive increase in the expression and function of other mediators, which may participate to impose depressant effects on ventilatory output during HVD. Indeed, studies have shown that decreases in PKC activity temporally coincide with the emergence of HVD (19), while other studies have implicated the involvement of nitric oxide (NO) as a mediator of hypoxic ventilation such that the ability to generate NO correlates with the ability to sustain the ventilatory enhancements recruited during pHVR (28–30). Furthermore, studies have also shown that platelet-derived growth factor-BB (PDGF-BB) will attenuate the acute component of HVR in adult rats and that inhibition of the PDGF-β receptor will attenuate HVD in wild-type mice, while heterozygote PDGF-β receptor mutant mice have reduced magnitudes of HVD (34–37). Other neuromediators of HVD that may operate independently of the above systems have been identified. For example, γ-aminobutyric acid (GABA) signaling within the nTS has been demonstrated to be critically involved in the awake, freely behaving rat (38). Furthermore, the unique role played by adenosine and its cognate receptors in the regulation of HVD and metabolic responses to hypoxia cannot be over-emphasized (39–43). Thus, it would seem that HVD represents the confluence of a complex interplay of both known and possibly yet unknown excitatory and inhibitory signaling pathways whose temporal dynamics and modifications as part of development dictate the characteristics of the individual response.

B. Effects of SH on Respiratory Control

The effect of SH on respiratory control is undoubtedly one of the most exten-sively investigated areas in the field. It has long been established that exposure to environmental hypoxia, such as occurs with exposure to high altitude, leads to time-dependent changes in control of breathing. In adults, exposure to SH enhances the response to subsequent acute hypoxic challenges (37,44–46). The enhanced HVR is brought about by the combination of increased sensitivity of the peripheral chemoreceptors and centrally mediated adaptations within the excitatory networks underlying HVR (37,47,48); however, these effects gradu-ally decrease over time after the humans or animals are removed from the hypoxic environment. In sharp contrast, perinatal sustained hypoxic exposures in every mammalian species thus far studied elicit a progressive decrease in hypoxic ventilatory sensitivity and a relative blunting of HVR (49–51). This reduction in HVR may be accounted in part by reduced O_2 sensitivity of the carotid bodies (52–54). Intriguingly, the blunted sensitivity to hypoxia will consistently persist into adulthood, suggesting that perinatal SH induces devel-opmental plasticity of the HVR despite some evidence that functional recovery of carotid body chemosensitivity may spontaneously occur (50). Consequently, the mechanisms underlying this form of developmental plasticity are currently unknown and still subject to debate. Recent evidence has demonstrated that hypoxic phrenic responses are intact following perinatal hypoxia, supporting the assumption that peripheral chemoreceptor function, as well as related central pathway function are preserved in adult rats following perinatal hypoxia (55). Instead, Bavis et al. (55) proposed that the site of long-term plasticity must reside downstream to the active phrenic motor neurons and therefore be related to neuromuscular transmission, function of respiratory muscles, respiratory mechanics, or feedback control. Furthermore, these investigators also suggest that gender influences are also of importance in perinatal hypoxia-induced respiratory plasticity, with female gender displaying diminished susceptibility for long-term alterations in respiratory output.

In addition to its influence on the abrupt dynamic changes associated with acute hypoxia, i.e. HVR, sustained exposure to environmental hypoxia has also been associated with plasticity in resting normoxic ventilation. In general, SH leads to a progressive time-dependent (days to weeks) increase in resting V_E, which has been termed ventilatory acclimatization to hypoxia (VAH) (56,57), a phenomenon that has been well documented in a variety of mammalian species including humans (58–61). The process of adaptation to hypoxia that results in ventilatory acclimatization appears to involve both ends of the synaptic pathways underlying the ventilatory response, so that development of increased sensitivity of the peripheral chemoreceptors occurs in parallel with enhanced and more efficient integration of afferent inputs and amplification of centrally generated efferent output (46). This process is gradually reduced, and resting V_E reverts to preexposure levels soon after return to normoxia if the exposure occurs after the critical window of development; the duration of this phenomenon is dependent to a certain extent on the preceding duration of the exposure (57). However, in adult mammals, experimental evidence has also revealed that perinatal hypoxia exhibits increases in resting V_E, with some, but not all studies demonstrating that enhanced normoxic ventilation persists into adulthood (>50 days) (55,62,63).

C. Effects of IH on Respiratory Control

Despite the wealth of studies focusing on the contribution of SH to ventilatory plasticity, relatively little is known about the effects of IH on respiratory control. A growing body of evidence suggests that IH is indeed a very different stimulus from SH and may therefore lead to vastly different consequences. It is important to note that IH is a relatively nebulous term that refers to the episodic occurrence of hypoxia and either normoxia or hyperoxia. Obviously, the severity of the hypoxic stimulus, its duration within the cycle, the ramp or square pattern of stimulus presentation, the number of iterations applied, and the overall duration of exposure within the circadian or ultradian period are all important factors that may lead to radically different responses (64). Recently, several studies have been conducted to characterize the effects of varying durations and severity of IH profiles commonly used in experimental protocols (64–70). The consensus reached by these studies is that the presentation and profile of IH exposures are indeed determinants of the physiological responses elicited by IH. Thus, it is important to take into account the type of IH profile used when trying to draw comparisons between different studies. In the following sections, we will consider two discrete categories, namely acute IH (AIH), lasting minutes to hours, and CIH, lasting days to weeks.

D. Effects of AIH on Respiratory Plasticity

In adult anesthetized, vagotomized, paralyzed, mechanically ventilated, isocapnic rats exposed to an AIH stimulus consisting of five minutes of hypoxia ($F_{IO2} = 11\%$) separated by five minutes of hyperoxia ($F_{IO2} = 50\%$) exhibit an

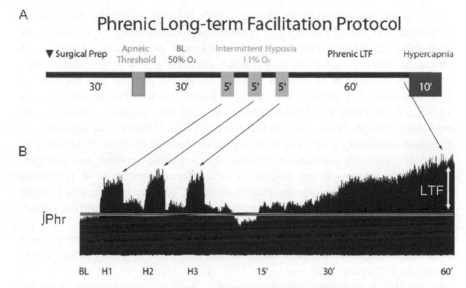

Figure 3 pLTF protocol. Following surgical preparation, phrenic nerve bursting was allowed to stabilize for 30 minutes at which point the apneic threshold was determined. Baseline ETCO$_2$ was set 3 Torr above apenic threshold and strictly maintained throughout the protocol. Three 5-minute bouts of 11% O$_2$ were used as a pLTF induction protocol and nerve bursting was recorded for an additional 60 minutes. Following the 60-minute recording of pLTF, an acute hypercapnic challenge ($\sim$70 Torr ETCO$_2$) was given to determine maximal output (Panel A). Depicted in Panel B is a representative phrenic neurogram demonstrating phrenic output from BL through the end of the 60-minute recording period following the induction protocol. *Abbreviations*: pLTF, phrenic long-term facilitation; ETCO$_2$, end-tidal carbon dioxide; BL, baseline. *Source*: From Ref. 72.

enhancement of phrenic motor output, a phenomenon termed long-term facilitation (LTF) (Fig. 3) (71,72). Furthermore, LTF cannot be elicited by equivalent exposures to noncyclic hypoxia (73). In recent years, Mitchell et al. have reported extensive data implicating involvement of serotoninergic pathways as the critical mediator for this form of neural plasticity (71). According to the proposed model, activation of postsynaptic 5-HT receptors, principally 5-HT$_{2A}$ subtypes, will lead to downstream signaling cascades involving PKC. PKC could then both act directly or indirectly by modulation of other kinases and potentiate the activation of glutamate receptor channels, such as NMDA receptors, thus leading to enhanced phrenic output. More recently, the brain-derived neurotrophic factor (BDNF) has been critically implicated in the initiation and consolidation of LTF and is operational either presynaptically or postsynaptically, through binding to the cognate receptor tyrosine kinase B (TrkB) (74). Other recent studies have pointed to profound genetic as well as gender-related influences in this model (75). However, while our understanding in the adult animal model has considerably advanced, little is known about the effects of IH on phrenic LTF (pLTF) in the early postnatal period, this being largely due to the formidable challenges presented by the surgical preparation. Despite such obstacles, there is some initial evidence suggesting that LTF exhibits age-dependent expression. Indeed, in a study comparing phrenic and hypoglossal LTF in young (3–4 months) and aged (13 months) male Sprague-Dawley rats, significant decreases in LTF emerged in the aged rats, possibly related to age-associated changes in serotonin and its receptors (76). However, the opposite, i.e., increased ventilatory LTF (vLTF) at later ages, appears to occur in female rats, suggesting complex interactions between the respiratory control and estrogen-progesterone systems in the context of AIH-induced phrenic nerve respiratory plasticity (75). Furthermore, the characteristics of phrenic LTF in rats younger than one month and the interactions between development and prepubertal gender-related hormones are currently unknown.

Other models of AIH-induced plasticity have assessed ventilation in freely behaving animals. vLTF represents the enhancement of respiratory output during normoxia following AIH exposures (77). Thus, resting V_E, as measured by whole-body flow-through plethysmography, displays, considerable enhancements of respiratory output following an acute isocapnic IH exposure using a similar stimulation paradigm to that previously used for pLTF. The augmented V_E was primarily accounted for by elevated respiratory frequency without significant contributions from tidal volume (V_T). Interestingly, Olson et al. were unable to demonstrate these ventilatory enhancements after a comparable exposure to continuous hypoxia (77). The excitatory effects of AIH on ventilation have been also confirmed by Ling et al. in rats and have implicated serotoninergic mechanisms (78). Furthermore, altered characteristics of respiratory pattern in the absence of global ventilatory output changes and of chemosensitivity were identified following a small number of brief hypoxic exposures in waking humans (79,80). The presence of LTF was further documented in sleeping men during NREM sleep (81). Subsequent studies have demonstrated that the magnitude of the IH-induced ventilatory increases is amplified by pretreatment with CIH (82). Recent studies have indicated that vLTF is greater in 1-month- versus 2-month-old rats, indicating that younger animals may have an increased capacity for IH-induced ventilatory plasticity (66). Taken together, these studies would suggest that the developmental stage at which the IH paradigm is applied is a major determinant of the overall magnitude and characteristics of the ensuing vLTF.

Studies conducted in the immediate postnatal period, using somewhat different IH paradigms in rabbits (e.g., 10 minutes 10% O_2 followed by 10 minutes 21% O_2, for 5 cycles) (83) or in rats (e.g., 21% O_2 alternating with 5% O_2, 9 cycles over 16 hours, initiated 6 hours after birth) (84,85) demonstrated increased normoxic V_E, i.e., vLTF, mediated primarily through increases in V_T. Under these circumstances, AIH also induced increases in HVR that correlated with increased sensory output from ex vivo carotid bodies harvested from similarly exposed pups (84). Using a different AIH protocol (5 minutes 10% O_2

followed by 10 minutes 21% O_2, for 8 cycles) (65), we were unable to elicit enhancements of the early phase of HVR; however, this AIH protocol revealed attenuations of HVD that correlated with increased expression of nNOS within the caudal brain stem. Thus, pharmacological inhibition of nNOS resulted in normalization of HVD (65).

In summary, incremental evidence suggests that AIH elicits an excitatory form of neuroplasticity that is particularly efficient in the developing animal. However, the respective roles of the various sensory afferent and efferent elements of the functional pathway and the corresponding signaling cascades remain completely elusive, and will undoubtedly be the focus of forthcoming studies.

E. Effects of CIH on Respiratory Plasticity

The technical requirements associated with prolonged IH exposures have somewhat precluded extensive exploration of the effects of CIH. The recent commercial availability of computer-driven servo-controlled environmental systems will undoubtedly allow for quick filling of this knowledge gap.

Indeed, evidence from CIH studies conducted in rats exposed prenatally using 90-second alternations of 10% O_2 and 21% O_2 supports the presence of marked developmental respiratory plasticity (86). Furthermore, it is important to note that when CIH is applied during the prenatal period it leads to lifelong alterations in ventilatory control (87). At the time during which the studies herein were proposed, even fewer studies regarding postnatal CIH and ventilatory plasticity existed in the literature and none directly examined the long-term implications on respiratory plasticity in adult rats. Indeed, Waters et al. found that a CIH profile consisting of 30 minutes a day for 6 days attenuates HVR as demonstrated by diaphragmatic electromyography (EMG) expressed as a function of normoxic baseline activity or as ventilatory output measured using a pneumotachograph in piglets (88–90). Additionally, these investigators reported significant increases in substance-P within the nTS, possibly as a compensatory mechanism for changes in neurokinin-1 (NK1) receptor expression, since the latter appears to be a critical mediator of HVR (91). Unfortunately, little else beyond this is available with regard to early postnatal CIH except for a very recent work from our laboratory showing substantial alterations in both HVR and normoxic ventilation after chronic intermittent hypoxic exposures (92,93), as well as in LTF (94), and also the ability to autoresuscitate from anoxia through gasping mechanisms (95). These alterations display anatomical correlates that merit further investigation in the near future (96).

F. Effect of Sleep on Hypoxic Responses

Developmental changes in ventilatory response patterns to acute hypoxia immediately after birth have been extensively studied. Dynamic changes in the peripheral chemoreceptor sensitivity "set point" to hypoxia during the early postnatal period have been demonstrated in human infants (97,98). Furthermore, it has become evident that the evolution of the hypoxic response over time varies depending on the state of vigilance and the level of maturation at which such challenge is conducted. For example, the preterm infant responds to a mild hypoxic challenge (15% O_2) by sustained ventilatory increments during NREM sleep, progressive ventilatory depression during REM sleep, and the typical biphasic response when awake (99). Similar responses were found in calves, whereby the ventilatory increase associated with application of the hypoxic stimulus lasted longer during quiet sleep compared to active sleep (100). In contrast, studies in mammalian species have found conflicting results with decreased or unchanged hypoxic responses in dogs (101) and even increased responses in rats (102). The mechanisms underlying the resetting of chemoreceptors during postnatal development and the brain regions involved in the transition from transient to sustained increases in ventilation during hypoxia in humans are currently unknown. In addition, sleep states and sleep deprivation, as well as environmental conditions such as ambient PO_2, may independently affect the maturational pattern of one or more of the structures involved in the hypoxic response, and therefore alter the balance between peripheral and central contributions in response to acute hypoxia (103,104).

III. Central Chemosensitivity

Since the early 1960s, areas of the ventrolateral medulla oblongata (VLM) have come to be accepted as the sites of central chemoreception of CO_2 and/or H^+, after Mitchell, Loeschcke et al. reported that localized application of acid or CO_2-saturated solutions to the VLM elicited significant cardioventilatory enhancements (105–107). Since these fundamental studies, several laboratories have expanded on the concept that central chemoreceptors are not restricted to the VLM regions originally described as the sites for central chemoreception and that neurons exhibiting CO_2-chemosensitivity can be found in many other brain regions (108–111). In addition, although the possibility exists that multiple neurotransmitters may be involved in the process of chemosensitivity, the presence of cholinergic muscarinic receptors in those brain stem areas traditionally associated with CO_2 chemosensitivity appears to exert important modulatory roles on the ventilatory response to hypercapnia (112) It remains unclear, however, whether all widely distributed chemosensitive neurons participate in a functionally meaningful fashion on the generation of the ventilatory response to hypercapnia. Furthermore, maturational changes occurring in muscarinic receptor expression and in the functional implications of such chemosensitive sites remain undefined. Indeed, it has been suggested that central CO_2 chemosensory mechanisms may not be fully functional or mature at birth (113); for example, topical application of H^+ to the ventral brain stem is associated with smaller increases in neuronal activity in neonatal cats compared to adult animals (114). However, very few studies have systematically addressed these issues.

It should also be stressed that separation of central and peripheral contributions to the ventilatory response to hypercapnia and/or hypoxia is arduous when testing human subjects. While the ventilatory response to hypercapnia is generally believed to indicate the activity of brain stem chemoreceptors, abrupt elevation of inspired CO_2 concentrations will also elicit a significant contribution of peripheral chemoreceptors (115). Such peripheral contributions to the hypercapnic response are also present in young children, as evidenced from a recent study in preterm infants, which demonstrated larger ventilatory slopes in the response to either endogenous or bolus CO_2 when compared with rebreathing or steady-state methods (116). Independent of such technical considerations, the ventilatory response to hypercapnia in premature infants was lower than that found in term infants, and CO_2 responses increased with postnatal age (117,118). It was further proposed that decreased CO_2 responsivity may underlie determinants of periodic breathing in newborn animals (119) and sleep apnea in preterm infants (120), or even be involved in the pathophysiological mechanisms underlying SIDS (121).

Beyond the infancy period, little is known about the development of central chemoreceptor function. By using rebreathing techniques in awake prepubertal children, Marcus et al. found increased CO_2 ventilatory responses to hypercapnia in the prepubertal children compared with adults, provided that correction of the slopes for body size was performed (122). Similarly, significant developmental differences in CO_2 responses emerged when the CO_2 stimulus was presented in a step or a ramp fashion (123). These findings in older children suggest that some time during the transition from childhood to adulthood, significant changes in the relative contributions of peripheral and central chemoreceptor activity occur. It remains unclear which mechanisms mediate these maturational changes and whether they are operative at the carotid body, neural transmission, or brain stem level.

A. Effect of Sleep on CO_2 Responses

It is now clear that when hypercapnic ventilatory responses are conducted in the adult sleeping subject, CO_2 sensitivity is reduced, especially during REM sleep epochs (124,125). Although studies in infants are not always in close agreement (126,127), it appears that a decrease in central chemosensitivity occurs during REM sleep in the young infants, as it does in adult subjects, when the rebreathing technique is employed (128–130). Thus, the transition from wakefulness to the sleep state will elicit significant reductions in hypercapnic drive, and such changes are further accentuated during REM sleep.

IV. Autonomic Development: Interactions with Breathing and Sleep

Maintenance of homeostasis requires close interaction of autonomic and somatic motor systems, as even gross examination of cardiovascular and respiratory control mechanisms indicates. Transient blood pressure elevation suppresses respiratory activity (preferentially in the upper airway musculature, and thus a particular danger for airway obstruction), slows breath-to-breath timing, and induces arousal (131,132), while lowering blood pressure stimulates ventilation (133). Conversely, respiratory efforts vary cardiac rate, with cardiac acceleration accompanying inspiration and deceleration associated with expiration, resulting from stretch and aortic receptor activity responding to venous return. Both the pressor effects on breathing and respiratory modulation of cardiac rate are accentuated by sleep (132). A large number of motor or vocalization events, central or obstructive apnea during sleep, or increased inspiratory or expiratory loading can initiate large blood pressure changes, which can then reflexively modify subsequent motor events. Hypoxia developing from inadequate ventilation initiates a substantial reorganization of metabolic rate and sympathetic outflow, with consequences to heart rate, blood pressure, and body temperature (134). Acute hypoxia apparently reduces metabolism in the very young, eliciting appropriately diminished ventilation in that classic challenge (135). Thus, any examination of autonomic nervous system development must consider the interactions between brain areas mediating temperature and sympathetic outflow to the cardiovascular system and somatomotor (e.g., respiratory) systems. Overriding all of these interactions are the effects of sleep state, which often result in substantial reorganization of influences of one brain area on another or in near-complete inactivation of systems, e.g., the diminution of hypothalamic influences on temperature-regulating systems and the paralysis of the somatic motor system in REM sleep.

V. Developmental Trends in Cardiovascular and Respiratory Measures

The manner in which infants respond to ventilatory or cardiovascular challenges during sleep bears on a number of critical clinical issues, including SIDS, since SIDS apparently occurs in close temporal relationship with sleep (136). Reactions to provocative challenges are superimposed on levels of background rate and variability, which vary remarkably with age and state. Basal heart rate rises over the first month of life before declining over the next six months (137); overall variability declines during quiet sleep over the first month before rising. The most substantial portion of the variation, i.e., that arising from respiratory sources, follows a similar time course as overall variability (138). The respiratory influences on heart rate variation arise principally from blood pressure and stretch afferent activity exerted by thoracic sources and are mediated primarily by vagal contributions to the heart. Determination of the relative proportion of vagal influences, relative to sympathetic outflow on heart rate variation, has been frequently used to evaluate the development of cardiovascular activity in the infant and has been suggested as a useful index of risk in certain cardiac failure syndromes (139). Infants who later succumb to SIDS, those who are at risk for SIDS, and those afflicted with congenital central hypoventilation syndrome show diminished respiratory-related variation during particular sleep states (138,140). Conversely, infants who later succumb to SIDS also show a diminished incidence of short apnea (141); since such apnea typically arise from blood pressure perturbations resulting from minor movement, the loss of breathing variation might result from a loss of blood pressure influences on cyclic respiratory patterning.

Heart rate responses to head tilt, which induces blood pressure increases and decreases, suggest a substantial effect of age, with younger infants (1–2 days) showing marked increased heart rate compensatory changes to head-up tilt and with older (2–4 months) infants showing either a reduced or no response. Respiratory responses are present at both younger and older ages (Fifer, personal communication). The findings from head-tilt challenge demonstrate a significant role for vestibular and cerebellar input to blood pressure regulation that varies with age. The age dependency of baroreflex responses is an important issue, since at least some SIDS victims succumb to a loss of blood pressure and bradycardia, rather than a respiratory failure (142). Thus, the functional development of neural structures underlying control of blood pressure and slowing of the heart, especially in conditions that could trigger a shock-like reaction, are of interest.

VI. Neural Structures Involved in Autonomic and Respiratory Regulation: Cerebellum and Vestibular Regions

Among the structures mediating the extent of heart rate response to a hypotensive or hypertensive challenge, such as head tilt, are structures within the cerebellum, especially the fastigial nucleus. Bilateral lesions of fastigial nucleus sites abolish the compensatory heart rate responses to blood pressure loss, to the point that the subject may succumb (143). Similarly, the bradycardia accompanying hypertensive challenges is lost with comparable lesions (144). The function of the fastigial nuclei may be that of "dampening" an evoked autonomic response in a fashion comparable to the manner in which the range of certain somatic motor actions is modulated by regions within the cerebellum. Fastigial cerebellar sites, as well as other regions within the cerebellum, also show functional magnetic resonance image (MRI) signal changes to a cold pressor or Valsalva challenge, which elevate blood pressure (145). Although the cerebellum is traditionally associated with aspects of motor rather than autonomic control, its role in cardiovascular action has been known for over 50 years (146), and those functions are now under active investigation (147,148).

Fastigial nuclei also apparently mediate aspects of respiratory control; electrical stimulation induces apnea or tachypnea, depending on frequency of the stimulus (149). Other evidence indicates a role for the cerebellum in respiratory loading (150–152). Both inspiratory and expiratory loading, as well as hypercapnia, activate sites within the cerebellum, as indicated by functional MRI

(153–155). The cerebellar regions activated by loaded breathing may be responsive to both blood pressure and respiratory modulation; contributions of cerebellar influences on breathing and cardiovascular control during development, however, are relatively unexplored.

The potential for cerebellar regions to play a role in limiting the extent of blood pressure responses to a hypotensive challenge is of particular interest when considering the mechanism of failure in the fatal event of SIDS; some infants succumb to bradycardia and hypotension (142). A ventral medullary surface (VMS) site, the arcuate nucleus, has been implicated as being deficient in muscarinic and kainate receptors in a proportion of infants who later succumb to SIDS (101,156). The arcuate nucleus has classically been described to project to the cerebellum, and could well mediate a vestibulo-cerebellar fastigial nucleus-mediated compensatory response to a marked loss of blood pressure. Kinney et al. also report that the arcuate nucleus projects to the caudal midline medullary raphe in humans (157). Excitation of the caudal midline medullary raphe evokes hypotension and bradycardia, although the area contributes little to routine maintenance of blood pressure (158). Thus, reduced muscarinic and kainate receptor binding in the arcuate nucleus may well result in an ineffective ability to compensate to challenges that provoke a profound and sudden loss of blood pressure.

The rapid adjustments in vasomotor activity to body position changes, such as rising from the supine position, or even more-modest body movements indicate that central circulatory compensatory mechanisms other than baroreflexes must be operating. Vestibular systems play an essential role in regulation of blood pressure to head tilt (159), an entirely expected finding, considering the liaisons between vestibular and cerebellar structures. Vestibular nuclei have prominent projections to midline caudal raphe nuclei as well as to the rostral ventrolateral medulla; both regions, in turn, project to the intermediolateral column of the spinal cord, the motor column for sympathetic outflow (for review, see Ref. 160). The conditions under which vestibular nuclei mediate vasomotor tone through the midline caudal raphe, a structure implicated in the sympathoinhibition associated with shock, are not clear. However, the vestibular/caudal raphe relationships are of interest to investigators examining the cardiovascular collapse, which accompanies some cases of SIDS (142). The vestibular system projections to the ventrolateral medulla may also play a critical role in the SIDS event. Any of the potential relationships between structures could be greatly affected by sleep states, a thus-far untested assumption. Sympathetic control, however, is profoundly changed during REM sleep.

VII. Sleep State Effects

Sleep states exert substantial effects on instantaneous cardiac rate variability and vasomotor activity, particularly in REM sleep (161,162). In infants, during quiet sleep, most variation arises from respiratory-related sources, while in REM sleep, variation derives from both respiratory-related sources and marked, longer-term accelerations and decelerations (163). Phasic increases in heart rate and coronary blood flow, accompanied by momentary decreased coronary vasculature resistance, occur during phasic episodes of the REM state in adult animals (164,165), while pauses in heart rate also occur, associated with coronary vasodilation, and these pauses appear to be baroreflex mediated (166). However, bursts of vagally mediated bradycardia, not preceded by tachycardia or blood pressure changes and not accompanied by expected respiratory rate changes, occur in tonic periods of that state (167). The latter finding is significant because the centrally mediated bradycardia points to the existence of state-related mechanisms, which can potentially adversely affect perfusion in the absence of reflex control. The fatal event in some SIDS victims appears to be one circumstance in which bradycardia and hypotension occur, but normal reflexes between heart rate, blood pressure, and breathing apparently are not operative (142).

The vasomotor phenomena that occur during REM sleep present a number of other circumstances that generate concern. In lambs, a substantial increase in systemic vascular resistance occurs during the REM state, preventing a severe loss in blood pressure during that state, and coronary vasculature resistance increases during phasic events, preventing substantial increases in coronary flow (168); the circumstances compromise coronary perfusion at a time when an increasing work load is placed on the heart. Further compromises that could occur in infants, such as hypoxia, might place the individual at risk.

VIII. VMS Activity

The central mechanisms underlying the substantial phasic variation in heart rate, coronary flow, and systemic vascular resistance during the REM state are still unclear, as are the sources for the momentary increases and pauses in breathing. Areas within the rostral VMS, which when cooled induce a loss of blood pressure, show a very large "spontaneous" variation in activity during REM sleep compared with quiet sleep states (169). Intermediate areas of the VMS of the cat show similar phasic changes (170). Correlations between rostral VMS optical activity and momentary arterial pressure suggest that increased activity precedes blood pressure changes and that those correlations preferably occur during REM sleep (171). The findings indicate a more prominent role for regions within the VMS during REM over other states in mediating blood pressure changes, but the nature of that mediation is unknown. In addition to "spontaneous" changes, VMS responses to pressor and ventilatory challenges are also state dependent. The VMS responses to pressor and ventilatory challenges differ markedly in the waking state from anesthetic and sleep states. Elevating blood pressure elicits a widespread, profound decline in VMS activity during both halothane and barbiturate anesthesia, as indicated by optical studies in cats and goats; microelectrode recording from nearby structures in the cat also show marked cell discharge slowing during a similar challenge (172). During waking, however, the response to pressor challenge is only a minor increase in activity (173). Hypoxia increases VMS activity in the anesthetized goat; during waking, the response is dramatically accentuated (174). The response to hypercapnia under anesthesia is a decline in VMS activity; in waking, activity in the rostral VMS increases transiently before declining (175). Cooling a portion of the rostral VMS elicits marked apnea during anesthesia and sleep, but not during waking (176). Changes in state-induced baseline VMS activity may underlie the state-dependent responses to challenges.

A region on the goat VMS ventral to the retrotrapezoid nucleus activates under both anesthesia and waking to a rapid lowering of blood pressure, a challenge that elicits enhanced drive to breathing (133). Cooling this area during anesthesia or sleep elicits apnea (176). Although the rostral VMS areas may not be analogous in both the cat and goat, the response of increased activity to the depressor challenge occurs in both species (173,176,177). Conversely, the decline in VMS activity to blood pressure elevation is associated with a marked loss of respiratory muscle activity and slowing of breathing. Part of the interaction between blood pressure lowering and stimulation of breathing may occur at rostral VMS sites.

Appropriate functioning of the VMS depends on the integrity of vagal and carotid sinus nerve afferents, since carotid nerve transection abolishes VMS responses (a decline in intermediate area activity) to chemoreceptor stimulation by intravenous cyanide (178). Sinus nerve transection also enhances the VMS responses (the response is an activity decline, but the decline is enhanced) to pressor challenge, while vagotomy nearly abolishes the response (179). The findings suggest that carotid sinus chemoreceptor input to the nucleus of the solitary tract (NTS) (which then projects to the VMS) causes the NTS to exert a disfacilitatory or inhibitory influence on intermediate area VMS neurons and that transection releases that influence. Afferent activity from vagal fibers, however, appears to exert an excitatory influence on VMS neurons. Similarly, transient hypoxia challenge (two breaths N_2, to preferentially stimulate peripheral chemoreceptors) increases intermediate area VMS activity, an effect enhanced by sinus nerve section and abolished by vagotomy (179,180). Thus, these data suggest a functionally more excitatory role on the VMS for vagal afferents.

IX. Rostral Brain Influences

Rostral brain structures have the potential to modify respiratory and autonomic patterns in a major fashion and play a particularly large role in mediating sleep-related patterns, alterations induced by affect, or the considerable effects of core temperature manipulation. We define ''rostral structures'' as hypothalamic, limbic, and cortical areas, although a number of other motor regions (e.g., the basal ganglia) and midbrain areas (e.g., the periaqueductal grey) could also be included and almost certainly contribute to both cardiovascular and breathing control during development. The influence of sleep states on descending neural influences on breathing and autonomic control is substantial, with REM sleep normally eliciting near-total suppression of upper airway and thoracic wall respiratory muscle activity as well as sympathetic output; in some syndromes the paralysis of respiratory muscles extends to the diaphragm (181–184). Basal forebrain sites initiate and maintain quiet sleep, whereas pontine mechanisms underlie the major characteristics of REM sleep (185). Although medullary regions maintain respiratory rhythmogenesis and cerebellar/vestibular regions appear to exert dampening effects to minimize variations from homeostasis, descending forebrain influences appear to elicit transient respiratory or cardiovascular changes to particular stimuli or alter background "tone" to provocative challenges.

The descending influences include more than traditional voluntary pathways, since affective "drive" can elicit diaphragmatic movement, bypassing classic pyramidal respiratory control mechanisms, e.g., capsular lesions prevent voluntary diaphragmatic movements that can still be elicited with laughter (186). The latter finding emphasizes the potential for descending affective influences to modify breathing.

The major descending projection systems to structures mediating brain stem respiratory and autonomic control include limbic descending projections from the central amygdala nucleus, the bed nucleus of the stria terminalis and the paraventricular nucleus of the hypothalamus (187–189). The paraventricular hypothalamus projects to the VMS in a wide area just lateral to the pyramids (190) and sends reciprocal projections to the bed nucleus of the stria terminalis and central nucleus of the amygdala. The latter two structures contain respiratory-related neurons (191–193); moreover, the central amygdala nucleus paces breathing by single-pulse stimulation, an effect obliterated by sleep (194), and cooling the central amygdala abolishes conditioned blood pressure responses (195). The paraventricular hypothalamus (as well as the bed nucleus) shows substantial c-fos expression on blood pressure manipulation (196), and the hypothalamus activates to transient respiratory pauses (197) and on stimulation regionally activates the VMS. Since the pathways from rostral sites to midbrain and medullary areas may take a period of time to develop, descending influences may follow a time course of expression; those time courses have yet to be described for most influences.

Functional MRI shows activation of hypothalamic sites, in addition to VMS areas, to loaded breathing (154,155). Since increased airway resistance often accompanies sleep [and is substantial, or near-infinite, in obstructive sleep apnea (OSA)], the responses of these regions to such loading during sleep are of particular interest in determining mechanisms of arousal from obstruction. The hypothalamic activation may result from that structure generating sympathetic influences associated with the blood pressure changes accompanying enhanced airway resistance or with recruitment of cells that project to dorsal pontine areas mediating adrenergic activation.

Descending forebrain systems may be recruited under certain behavioral conditions, such as those associated with stress, vocalization, or affective influences to respiratory control areas. The paraventricular hypothalamus is a major component in pituitary-adrenocortical activation and exhibits cellular activity changes after exposure to stress (198,199). The paraventricular hypothalamus projects to the rostral NTS, to the rat (200) and cat (190) dorsal vagal nucleus, to A1, A2, and A5 noradrenergic brain stem nuclei, and nucleus raphe magnus (201) and sends projections directly to the intermediolateral column of the spinal cord (202); the structure can thus modify both parasympathetic and sympathetic efferent activities.

Respiratory rate and effort are profoundly influenced by core or anterior hypothalamic temperature, an effect that is greatly reduced in REM sleep in both the cat and developing kitten (203,204). Appropriate rapid breathing responses to hypothalamic warming require a period of time to develop in the kitten; very young animals cannot maintain adequate ventilation with such warming and switch intermittently to slower breathing, risking hyperthermic damage (204). Hypothalamic warming effects on breathing are most likely mediated through descending projections to the parabrachial pons, NTS, and periaqueductal grey (190). Thermal influences are important for maintaining breathing early in life, at least for some species; lambs kept apart from maternal warmth show increased apnea (205). REM sleep also abolishes at least some descending rostral influences on autonomic control, including transient hypertension induced by central amygdala nucleus stimulation (191). The near-abolition of descending hypothalamic temperature-related influences on breathing and cardiovascular control by REM sleep poses certain clinical implications; excessively high core temperatures have been found postmortem in SIDS victims (206), and infants with life-threatening events are sometimes found drenched in sweat (207), indicative of intense sympathetic activation. Heat dissipation in the human relies heavily on sympathetic mechanisms by means of sweating and vasodilation; such actions are at least partially mediated through ventral medullary structures (208). Withdrawal of influences from hypothalamic sites during sleep may modulate some of the state-related physiological changes mediated by the VMS.

X. Potential Implications to SIDS

To further illustrate potential integration of some of the mechanisms discussed above to clinical settings, we will briefly discuss a relatively common clinical disorder, namely SIDS, and its potential link to OSA. SIDS is characterized by the sudden death of a seemingly healthy infant that can not be explained following postmortem investigation (209). While the underlying cause of SIDS is still subject to debate, several features are commonly observed in infants who eventually succumb to the disorder. These features include a decreased arousal threshold, an increased sympathovagal balance with concomitant reduction in baroreflex sensitivity, and an increased incidence of OSA (209). The current leading theory regarding the pathogenesis of SIDS directly implicates upper airway resistance along with a spectrum of proposed contributing factors occurring mostly during the late hours of the night during sleep (210). Closer examinations of these associated risk factors reveal that SIDS cases and OSA patients have many common linkages.

The first of these common features is that the overwhelming majority of SIDS deaths are presumed to occur during sleep and OSA is by definition an entirely sleep-dependent disorder (211). Another predisposing factor to SIDS is the presence of viral upper airway infection, such as respiratory syncytial virus (RSV), which itself is known to exacerbate OSA (212–214). Furthermore, craniofacial abnormalities, such as micrognathia, which are contributing factors to OSA, have been documented in many SIDS infants. A family and/or patient history of OSA has also been identified as a risk factor for SIDS in both epidemiological studies (215,216) and prospective polysomnography studies of sleeping infants (209,217). In addition, forensic examinations of SIDS infants have revealed that thymic petechiae consistent with OSA are found in over 70% of SIDS cases (218), and recurrent hypoxic events appear to precede SIDS cases (219). Indeed, further forensic investigation has revealed that brain injury presumably resulting from IH is also common in SIDS infants (220–222). Finally, substantial documented evidence reveals that recovery from OSA is dependent on arousal from sleep, which is known to be impaired by antecedent IH (223–225).

Thus, the strong correlation between OSA and SIDS would suggest that the association between the two is more than coincidental. Furthermore, the possibility arises that if OSA precedes SIDS the pathological sequela of OSA (i.e., IH) may contribute to the pathogenesis of SIDS or perhaps cause the physiological changes in cardio-respiratory control and/or arousability, which ultimately lead to SIDS.

XI. Summary

The multiplicity of central systems whose function is to preserve homeostasis and the elevated number of interdependencies occurring between functionally related structures in the central network usually ensure proper activation of backup defense systems and overall system stability during state transitions. However, perturbations can coincide with normally functioning transitional states and lead to disrupted responses or generation of vulnerable states, e.g., sleep-associated periodic breathing and hypoxemia, bradycardia, or hypotension. Similarly, dynamic changes within individual components in the network and their connectivity to other network elements occur during and even after maturation. The characteristics of such developmental changes are dictated at least in part by environmental, metabolic, state conditions, and overall neuronal activity of each network compartment, thereby creating infinite permutation possibilities in the overall network, i.e., individual and temporal variabilities. Thus, careful consideration of behavioral states and developmental stage must be incorporated in experimental or clinical settings to allow for improved understanding and interpretation of central cardiovascular and respiratory control mechanisms and their responses to particular stimuli.

Acknowledgments

DG is supported by grants from the National Institutes of Health SCOR 2P50-HL-60296 (Project 2), RO1-HL-65270, and RO1-HL-69932, the Children's Foundation Endowment for Sleep Research, and the Commonwealth of Kentucky Challenge for Excellence Trust Fund. RMH is supported by HD-22695.

References

1. Phillipson EA, Bowes G. Control of breathing during sleep. In: Cherniak NS, Widdicombe JG, eds. Handbook of Physiology: Section 3. The Respiratory System, vol 2. Control of Breathing, part 2. Bethesda, Maryland: American Physiological Society, 1986:649–690.

2. Trinder J, Whitworth F, Kay A, et al. Respiratory instability during sleep onset. J Appl Physiol 1992; 73:2462–2469.

3. Douglas NJ, White DP, Pickett CK, et al. Respiration during sleep in normal man. Thorax 1982; 37:840–844.

4. Orem J. The wakefulness stimulus for breathing. In: Saunders NA, Sullivan CE, eds. Sleep and Breathing. 2nd Edition. New York: Marcel Dekker, 1994:113–155.

5. Carroll JL. Developmental plasticity in respiratory control. J Appl Physiol 2003; 94:375–389.

6. Dobbing J, Sands J. Comparative aspects of the brain growth spurt. Early Hum Dev 1979; 3:79–83.

7. Huttenlocher PR. Synapse elimination and plasticity in developing human cerebral cortex. Am J Ment Defic 1984; 88:488–496.

8. Herlenius E, Lagercrantz H. Development of neurotransmitter systems during critical periods. Exp Neurol 2004; 190(suppl 1):S8–S21.

9. Rabinowicz T, de Court , Petetot JM, et al. Human cortex development: estimates of neuronal numbers indicate major loss late during gestation. J Neuropathol Exp Neurol 1996; 55:320–328.

10. Gaultier C, Gallego J. Development of respiratory control: evolving concepts and perspectives. Respir Physiol Neurobiol 2005; 149:3–15.

11. Powell, FL, Milsom, WK, Mitchell GS. Time domains of the hypoxic ventilatory response. Respir Physiol 1998; 112:123–134.

12. Mizusawa A, Ogawa H, Kikuchi Y, et al. In vivo release of glutamate in nucleus tractus solitarii of the rat during hypoxia. J Physiol 1994; 478(pt 1):55–66.

13. Soto-Arape I, Burton MD, Kazemi H. Central amino acid neurotransmitters and the hypoxic ventilatory response. Am J Respir Crit Care Med 1995; 151:1113–1120.

14. Lin J, Suguihara C, Huang J, et al. Effect of N-methyl-D-aspartate-receptor blockade on hypoxic ventilatory response in unanesthetized piglets. J Appl Physiol 1996; 80:1759–1763.

15. Ohtake PJ, Torres JE, Gozal YM, et al. NMDA receptors mediate peripheral chemoreceptor afferent input in the conscious rat. J Appl Physiol 1998; 84:853–861.

16. Simakajornboon N, Graff GR, Torres JE, et al. Modulation of hypoxic ventilatory response by systemic platelet-activating factor receptor antagonist in the rat. Respir Physiol 1998; 114:213–225.

17. Gozal D, Holt GA, Graff GR, et al. Platelet-activating factor modulates cardiorespiratory responses in the conscious rat. Am J Physiol 1998; 275:R604–R611.

18. Reeves SR, Gozal D. Platelet-activating factor receptor and respiratory and metabolic responses to hypoxia and hypercapnia. Respir Physiol Neurobiol 2004; 141:13–20.

19. Gozal D, Gozal E. Hypoxic ventilatory roll-off is associated with decreases in protein kinase C activation within the nucleus tractus solitarius of the rat. Brain Res 1997; 774:246–249.

20. Gozal D, Gozal E, Graff GR. Evidence for a central role of protein kinase C in modulation of the hypoxic ventilatory response in the rat. Adv Exp Med Biol 1998; 450:45–49.

21. Gozal D, Graff GR, Gozal, E, et al. Modulation of the hypoxic ventilatory response by Ca2+-dependent and Ca2+-independent protein kinase C in the dorsocaudal brainstem of conscious rats. Respir Physiol 1998; 112:283–290.

22. Gozal D, Graff GR, Torres JE, et al. Cardiorespiratory responses to systemic administration of a protein kinase C inhibitor in conscious rats. J Appl Physiol 1998; 84:641–648.

23. Gozal E, Roussel AL, Holt GA, et al. Protein kinase C modulation of ventilatory response to hypoxia in nucleus tractus solitarii of conscious rats. J Appl Physiol 1998; 84:1982–1990.

24. Simakajornboon N, Gozal E, Gozal YM, et al. Hypoxia induces activation of an N-methyl-D-aspartate glutamate receptor-protein kinase C pathway in the dorsocaudal brainstem of the conscious rat. Neurosci Lett 2000; 278:17–20.

25. Bandla HP, Simakajornboon N, Graff GR, et al. Protein kinase C modulates ventilatory patterning in the developing rat. Am J Respir Crit Care Med 1999; 159:968–973.

26. Reeves SR, Carter ES, Guo SZ, et al. Calcium/Calmodulin-dependent kinase II mediates critical components of the hypoxic ventilatory response within the nucleus of the solitary tract in adult rats. Am J Physiol Regul Integr Comp Physiol 2005; 289:871–879.

27. Whitney GM, Ohtake PJ, Simakajornboon N, et al. AMPA glutamate receptors and respiratory control in the developing rat: anatomic and pharmacological aspects. Am J Physiol Regul Integr Comp Physiol 2000; 278:R520–R528.

28. Gozal D, Gozal E, Gozal YM, et al. Nitric oxide synthase isoforms and peripheral chemoreceptor stimulation in conscious rats. Neuroreport 1996; 7:1145–1148.

29. Gozal D, Gozal E, Torres JE, et al. Nitric oxide modulates ventilatory responses to hypoxia in the developing rat. Am J Respir Crit Care Med 1997; 155:1755–1762.

30. Torres JE, Kreisman NR, Gozal D. Nitric oxide modulates in vitro intrinsic optical signal and neural activity in the nucleus tractus solitarius of the rat. Neurosci Lett 1997; 232: 175–178.

31. Bureau MA, Zinman R, Foulon P, et al. Diphasic ventilatory response to hypoxia in newborn lambs. J Appl Physiol 1984; 56:84–90.

32. Eden GJ, Hanson MA. Maturation of the respiratory response to acute hypoxia in the newborn rat. J Physiol 1987; 392:1–9.

33. Vizek M, Pickett, CK, Weil JV. Biphasic ventilatory response of adult cats to sustained hypoxia has central origin. J Appl Physiol 1987; 63:1658–1664.

34. Gozal D, Simakajornboon N, Czapla MA, et al. Brainstem activation of platelet-derived growth factor-beta receptor modulates the late phase of the hypoxic ventilatory response. J Neurochem 2000; 74(1):310–319.

35. Vlasic V, Simakajornboon N, Gozal E, et al. PDGF-beta receptor expression in the dorsocaudal brainstem parallels hypoxic ventilatory depression in the developing rat. Pediatr Res 2001; 50(2):236–241.

36. Simakajornboon N, Szerlip NJ, Gozal E, et al. In vivo PDGF beta receptor activation in the dorsocaudal brainstem of the rat prevents hypoxia-induced apoptosis via activation of Akt and BAD. Brain Res 2001; 895(1–2):111–118.

37. Alea OA, Czapla MA, Lasky JA, et al. PDGF-beta receptor expression and ventilatory acclimatization to hypoxia in the rat. Am J Physiol Regul Integr Comp Physiol 2000; 279(5):R1625–R1633.

38. Tabata M, Kurosawa H, Kikuchi Y, et al. Role of GABA within the nucleus tractus solitarii in the hypoxic ventilatory decline of awake rats. Am J Physiol Regul Integr Comp Physiol 2001; 281:R1411–R1419.

39. Richter DW, Schmidt-Garcon P, Pierrefiche O, et al. Neurotransmitters and neuromodulators controlling the hypoxic respiratory response in anaesthetized cats. J Physiol 1999; 514(pt 2):567–578.

40. Kato T, Hayashi F, Tatsumi K, et al. Inhibitory mechanisms in hypoxic respiratory depression studied in an in vitro preparation. Neurosci Res 2000; 38:281–288.

41. Kazemi H, Hoop, B. Glutamic acid and gamma-aminobutyric acid neurotransmitters in central control of breathing. J Appl Physiol 1991; 70:1–7.

42. Gautier H, Murariu C. Neuromodulators and hypoxic hypothermia in the rat. Respir Physiol 1998; 112:315–324.

43. Barros RC, Branco LG. Role of central adenosine in the respiratory and thermoregulatory responses to hypoxia. Neuroreport 2000; 11:193–197.

44. Aaron EA, Powell FL. Effect of chronic hypoxia on hypoxic ventilatory response in awake rats. J Appl Physiol 1993; 74:1635–1640.

45. Dwinell MR, Huey KA, Powell FL. Chronic hypoxia induces changes in the central nervous system processing of arterial chemoreceptor input. Adv Exp Med Biol 2000; 475:477–484.

46. Dwinell MR, Powell FL. Chronic hypoxia enhances the phrenic nerve response to arterial chemoreceptor stimulation in anesthetized rats. J Appl Physiol 1999; 87:817–823.

47. Gamboa A, Leon-Velarde F, Rivera-Ch M, et al. Selected contribution: acute and sustained ventilatory responses to hypoxia in high-altitude natives living at sea level. J Appl Physiol 2003; 94:1255–1262.

48. Leon-Velarde F, Gamboa A, Rivera-Ch M, et al. Selected contribution: peripheral chemoreflex function in high-altitude natives and patients with chronic mountain sickness. J Appl Physiol 2003; 94:1269–1278.

49. Mortola JP, Morgan CA, Virgona V. Respiratory adaptation to chronic hypoxia in newborn rats. J Appl Physiol 1986; 61:1329–1336.

50. Eden GJ, Hanson MA. Effects of chronic hypoxia from birth on the ventilatory response to acute hypoxia in the newborn rat. J Physiol 1987; 392:11–19.

51. Frappell PB, Mortola JP. Hamsters vs. rats: metabolic and ventilatory response to development in chronic hypoxia. J Appl Physiol 1994; 77:2748–2752.

52. Jackson A, Nurse C. Plasticity in cultured carotid body chemoreceptors: environmental modulation of GAP-43 and neurofilament. J Neurobiol 1995; 26:485–496.

53. Sladek M, Parker RA, Grogaard JB, et al. Long-lasting effect of prolonged hypoxemia after birth on the immediate ventilatory response to changes in arterial partial pressure of oxygen in young lambs. Pediatr Res 1993; 34:821–828.

54. Sterni LM, Bamford OS, Wasicko MJ, et al. Chronic hypoxia abolished the postnatal increase in carotid body type I cell sensitivity to hypoxia. Am J Physiol 1999; 277:L645–L652.

55. Bavis RW, Olson EBjr, Vidruk EH, et al. Developmental plasticity of the hypoxic ventilatory response in rats induced by neonatal hypoxia. J Physiol 2004; 557:645–660.

56. Bisgard GE. The role of arterial chemoreceptors in ventilatory acclimatization to hypoxia. Adv Exp Med Biol 1994; 360:109–122.

57. Bisgard GE. Increase in carotid body sensitivity during sustained hypoxia. Biol Signals 1995; 4:292–297.

58. Dempsey JA, Forster HV, doPico GA. Ventilatory acclimatization to moderate hypoxemia in man. The role of spinal fluid (H+). J Clin Invest 1974; 53: 1091–1100.

59. Donoghue S, Fatemian M, Balanos GM, et al. Ventilatory acclimatization in response to very small changes in PO_2 in humans. J Appl Physiol 2005; 98:1587–1591.

60. Eger EI, Kellogg RH, Mines AH, et al. Influence of CO_2 on ventilatory acclimatization to altitude. J Appl Physiol 1968; 24:607–615.

61. Fatemian M, Kim DY, Poulin MJ, et al. Very mild exposure to hypoxia for 8 h can induce ventilatory acclimatization in humans. Pflugers Arch 2001; 441:840–843.

62. Okubo S, Mortola JP. Long-term respiratory effects of neonatal hypoxia in the rat. J Appl Physiol 1988; 64:952–958.

63. Okubo S, Mortola JP. Control of ventilation in adult rats hypoxic in the neonatal period. Am J Physiol 1990; 259:R836–R841.

64. Waters KA, Gozal D. Responses to hypoxia during early development. Respir Physiol Neurobiol 2003; 136:115–129.

65. Gozal D, Gozal E. Episodic hypoxia enhances late hypoxic ventilation in developing rat: putative role of neuronal NO synthase. Am J Physiol 1999; 276: R17–R22.

66. McGuire M, Ling L. Ventilatory long-term facilitation is greater in 1-month-versus 2-month-old awake rats. J Appl Physiol 2004; 98:1195–1201.

67. McGuire M, Zhang Y, White DP, et al. Effect of hypoxic episode number and severity on ventilatory long-term facilitation in awake rats. J Appl Physiol 2002; 93:2155–2161.

68. McGuire, M, Zhang Y, White DP, et al. Chronic intermittent hypoxia enhances ventilatory long-term facilitation in awake rats. J Appl Physiol 2003; 95: 1499–1508.

69. Peng YJ, Prabhakar, NR. Effect of two paradigms of chronic intermittent hypoxia on carotid body sensory activity. J Appl Physiol 2004; 96:1236–1242.

70. Peng YJ, Rennison J, Prabhakar, NR. Intermittent hypoxia augments carotid body and ventilatory response to hypoxia in neonatal rat pups. J Appl Physiol 2004; 97:2020–2025.

71. Fuller DD, Bach KB, Baker TL, et al. Long term facilitation of phrenic motor output. Respir Physiol 2000; 121:135–146.

72. Feldman JL, Mitchell GS, Nattie EE. Breathing: rhythmicity, plasticity, chemosensitivity. Annu Rev Neurosci 2003; 26:239–266.

73. Baker TL, Fuller DD, Zabka AG, et al. Respiratory plasticity: differential actions of continuous and episodic hypoxia and hypercapnia. Respir Physiol 2001; 129: 25–35.
74. Baker-Herman TL, Fuller DD, Bavis RW, et al. BDNF is necessary and sufficient for spinal respiratory plasticity following intermittent hypoxia. Nat Neurosci 2004; 7:48–55.
75. Zabka AG, Behan M, Mitchell GS. Selected contribution: time-dependent hypoxic respiratory responses in female rats are influenced by age and by the estrus cycle. J Appl Physiol 2001; 91:2831–2838.
76. Zabka AG, Behan M, Mitchell GS. Long term facilitation of respiratory motor output decreases with age in male rats. J Physiol 2001; 531:509–514.
77. Olson EB, Jr, Bohne CJ, Dwinell MR, et al. Ventilatory long-term facilitation in unanesthetized rats. J Appl Physiol 2001; 91:709–716.
78. Ling L, Fuller DD, Bach KB, et al. Chronic intermittent hypoxia elicits serotonin-dependent plasticity in the central neural control of breathing. J Neurosci 2001; 21:5381–5388.
79. Morris KF, Gozal D. Persistent respiratory changes following intermittent hypoxic stimulation in cats and human beings. Respir Physiol Neurobiol 2004; 140:1–8.
80. Mateika JH, Mendello C, Obeid D, et al. Peripheral chemoreflex responsiveness is increased at elevated levels of carbon dioxide after episodic hypoxia in awake humans. J Appl Physiol 2004; 96:1197–1205.
81. Babcock M, Shkoukani M, Aboubakr SE, et al. Determinants of long-term facilitation in humans during NREM sleep. J Appl Physiol 2003; 94:53–59.
82. Zabka AG, Mitchell GS, Olson EB, Jr, et al. Selected contribution: chronic intermittent hypoxia enhances respiratory long-term facilitation in geriatric female rats. J Appl Physiol 2003; 95:2614–2623.
83. Trippenbach T. Ventilatory and metabolic effects of repeated hypoxia in conscious newborn rabbits. Am J Physiol 1994; 266(5 pt 2):R1584–R1590.
84. Peng YJ, Prabhakar NR. Reactive oxygen species in the plasticity of respiratory behavior elicited by chronic intermittent hypoxia. J Appl Physiol 2003; 94: 2342–2349.
85. Prabhakar NR, Peng YJ, Kumar GK, et al. Altered carotid body function by intermittent hypoxia in neonates and adults: relevance to recurrent apneas. Respir Physiol Neurobiol. 2007; 157:148–153.
86. Gozal D, Reeves SR, Row BW, et al. Respiratory effects of gestational intermittent hypoxia in the developing rat. Am J Respir Crit Care Med 2003; 167:1540–1547.
87. Gozal D, Reeves SR, Row BW, et al. Respiratory effects of gestational intermittent hypoxia in the developing rat. Am J Respir Crit Care Med 2003; 167:1540–1547.
88. Waters KA, Laferriere A, Paquette J, et al. Curtailed respiration by repeated vs. isolated hypoxia in maturing piglets is unrelated to NTS ME or SP levels. J Appl Physiol 1997; 83:522–529.
89. Waters KA, Tinworth KD. Depression of ventilatory responses after daily, cyclic hypercapnic hypoxia in piglets. J Appl Physiol 2001; 90:1065–1073.
90. Waters KA, Tinworth KD. Habituation of arousal responses after intermittent hypercapnic hypoxia in piglets. Am J Respir Crit Care Med 2005; 171:1305–1311.
91. Wickstrom HR, Berner J, Holgert H, et al. Hypoxic response in newborn rat is attenuated by neurokinin-1 receptor blockade. Respir Physiol Neurobiol 2004; 140:19–31.

92. Reeves SR, Gozal E, Guo SZ, et al. Effect of long-term intermittent and sustained hypoxia on hypoxic ventilatory and metabolic responses in the adult rat. J Appl Physiol 2003; 95:1767–1774.
93. Reeves SR, Gozal D. Respiratory and metabolic responses to early postnatal chronic intermittent hypoxia and sustained hypoxia in the developing rat. Pediatr Res 2006; 60:680–686.
94. Reeves SR, Mitchell GS, Gozal D. Early postnatal chronic intermittent hypoxia modifies hypoxic respiratory responses and long-term phrenic facilitation in adult rats. Am J Physiol Regul Integr Comp Physiol 2006; 290:R1664–R1671.
95. Gozal D, Gozal E, Reeves SR, et al. Gasping and autoresuscitation in the developing rat: effect of antecedent intermittent hypoxia. J Appl Physiol 2002; 92:1141–1144.
96. Reeves SR, Guo SZ, Brittian KR, et al. Anatomical changes in selected cardio-respiratory brainstem nuclei following early post-natal chronic intermittent hypoxia. Neurosci Lett 2006; 402:233–237.
97. Hertzberg T, Lagercrantz H. Postnatal sensitivity of the peripheral chemoreceptors in newborn infants. Arch Dis Child 1987; 62:1238–1241.
98. Walker DW. Peripheral and central chemoreceptors in the fetus and newborn. Ann Rev Physiol 1984; 46:687–703.
99. Rigatto H. Control of ventilation in the newborn. Ann Rev Physiol 1984; 46: 661–674.
100. Jeffrey HE, Read DJC. Reduced lung volume during behavioral active sleep in the newborn. J Appl Physiol 1979; 46:1081–1085.
101. Phillipson EA, Sullivan CE, Read DJC, et al. Ventilatory and waking responses to hypoxia in sleeping dogs. J Appl Physiol 1978; 44:512–520.
102. Pappenheimer J. Sleep and respiration of rats during hypoxia, J Physiol 1977; 266:191–207.
103. Eden GJ, Hanson MA. The effect of chronic hypoxia from birth on the ventilatory response to acute hypoxia in the newborn rat. J Physiol 1987; 392:11–19.
104. Hanson MA, Kumar P, Williams BA. The effect of chronic hypoxia upon the development of respiratory chemoreflexes in the newborn kitten. J Physiol 1989; 411:563–574.
105. Loeschcke HH, Koepchen HP. Versuch fur Lokatisation des Angriffsortes de, Atmungs- und Kreislaufwirkung von Novocain im Liquor cerebrospinalis. Pflugers Arch 1958; 266:623–641.
106. Mitchell RA, Loeschcke HH, Massion WH, et al. Respiratory responses mediated through superficial chemosensitive areas on the medulla. J Appl Physiol 1963; 18:523–533.
107. Schlaefke ME. Central chemosensitivity: a respiratory drive. Rev Physiol Biochem Pharmacol 1981; 90:172–244.
108. Bruce EN, Cherniack NS. Central chemoreceptors. J Appl Physiol 1987; 62: 389–402.
109. Dean JB, Lawing WL, Millhorn DE. CO_2 decreases membrane conductance and depolarizes neurons in the nucleus tractus solitarii. Exp Brain Res 1989; 76: 656–661.
110. Sato M, Severinghaus JW, Basbaum A. Medullary CO_2 chemoreceptor identification by c-fos immunocytochemistry. J Appl Physiol 1992; 73:96–100.
111. Coates EL, Li A, Nattie EE. Widespread sites of brainstem ventilatory chemoreceptors. J Appl Physiol 1993; 75:5–14.

112. Nattie EE, Wood J, Mega A, et al. Rostral ventrolateral medulla muscarinic receptor involvement in central ventilatory chemosensitivity. J Appl Physiol 1989; 66:1462–1470.

113. Moss IR, Scarpelli EM. Generation and regulation of breathing in utero: fetal CO_2 response test. J Appl Physiol 1979; 47:527–531.

114. Whittaker JAC, Trouth CO, Pan Y, et al. Age differences in responsiveness of brainstem chemosensitive neurons to extracellular pH changes. Life Sci 1990; 46:1699–1705.

115. Gabel RA, Kronenborg RS, Severinghaus JW. Vital capacity breaths of 5% or 15% CO_2 in N_2 or O_2 to test carotid chemosensitivity. Respir Physiol 1973; 17:195–208.

116. Rigatto H, Kwiatowski KA, Hasan SU, et al. The ventilatory response to endogenous CO_2 in preterm infants. Am Rev Resp Dis 1991; 143:101–104.

117. Frantz ID III, Alder SM, Thach BT, et al. Maturational effects on respiratory response to carbon dioxide in premature infants. J Appl Physiol 1976; 41:41–45.

118. Rigatto H, Brady JP, de la Torre Verduzco R. Chemoreceptor reflexes in preterm infants. II. The effect of gestational and postnatal age on the ventilatory response to inhaled carbon dioxide. Pediatrics 1975; 55:614–621.

119. Wennergren G, Wennergren M. Respiratory effects elicited in newborn animals via the central chemoreceptors. Acta Physiol Scand 1980; 108:309–311.

120. Gerhardt T, Bancalari E. Ventilatory response to CO_2 in premature infants with apnea. Pediatr Res 1979; 13:534.

121. Kinney HC, Filiano JJ, Sleeper LA, et al. Decreased muscarinic receptor binding in the arcuate nucleus in sudden infant death syndrome. Science 1995; 269:1446–1450.

122. Marcus CL, Glomb WB, Basinski, DJ, et al. Developmental pattern of hypercapnic and hypoxic ventilatory responses from childhood to adulthood. J Appl Physiol 1994; 76:314–320.

123. Gozal D, Arens R, Omlin KJ, et al. Maturational differences in step vs. ramp hypoxic and hypercapnic ventilatory responses. J Appl Physiol 1994; 76:1968–1975.

124. Berthon Jones M, Sullivan CE. Ventilation and arousal responses to hypercapnia in normal sleeping humans. J Appl Physiol 1984; 57:59–67.

125. Douglas NJ, White DP, Weil JV. Hypercapnic ventilatory responses in sleeping adults. Am Rev Resp Dis 1982; 126:758–762.

126. Davi M, Sankaran K, McCallum M, et al. Effect of sleep state on chest distortion and on the ventilatory response to CO_2 in neonates. Pediatr Res 1979; 13:982–986.

127. Haddad GG, Leistner HL, Epstein RA, et al. CO_2-induced changes in ventilation and ventilatory pattern in normal sleeping infants. J Appl Physiol 1980; 48: 684–688.

128. Honma Y, Wilkes D, Bryan MH, et al. Ribcage and abdominal contributions to the ventilatory response to CO_2 in infants. J Appl Physiol 1984; 56:1211–1216.

129. Moriette G, Van Reempts P, Moore M, et al. The effect of rebreathing CO_2 on ventilation and diaphragmatic electromyography in newborn infants. Respir Physiol 1985; 62:387–397.

130. Cohen G, Xu C, Henderson-Smart D. Ventilatory response of the sleeping newborn to CO_2 during normoxic rebreathing. J Appl Physiol 1991; 71:168–174.

131. Marks JD, Harper RM. Differential inhibition of the diaphragm and posterior cricoarytenoid muscles induced by transient hypertension across sleep states in intact cats. Exp Neurol 1987; 95:730–742.

132. Trelease RB, Sieck GC, Marks JD, et al. Respiratory inhibition induced by transient hypertension during sleep. Exp Neurol 1985; 90:173–186.
133. Ohtake PJ, Jennings DB. Ventilation is stimulated by small reductions in arterial pressure in the awake dog. J Appl Physiol 1992; 73:1549–1557.
134. Clark DJ, Fewell JE. Decreased body-core temperature during acute hypoxemia in guinea pigs during postnatal maturation: a regulated thermoregulatory response. Can J Physiol Pharmacol 1996; 74:331–336.
135. Mortola JP, Rezzonico R. Metabolic and ventilatory rates in newborn kittens during acute hypoxia. Respir Physiol 1988; 73:55–67.
136. Beckwith JB. Pathology discussion. In: Bergman AB, Beckwith FB, Ray CG, eds. Sudden Infant Death Syndrome: Proceedings of the Second International Conference on Causes of Sudden Death in Infants. Seattle, Washington: University of Washington Press, 1970:120–122.
137. Harper RM, Leake B, Hodgman JE, et al. Developmental patterns of heart rate and heart rate variability during sleep and waking in normal infants and infants at risk for the sudden infant death syndrome. Sleep 1982; 5:28–38.
138. Kluge KA, Harper RM, Schechtman VL, et al. Spectral analysis assessment of respiratory sinus arrhythmia in normal infants and infants who subsequently died of sudden infant death syndrome. Pediatr Res 1988; 24:677–682.
139. Woo MA, Stevenson WG, Moser DK, et al. Patterns of beat-to-beat heart rate variability in advanced heart failure. Am Heart J 1992; 123:704–710.
140. Woo MS, Woo MA, Gozal D, et al. Heart rate variability in congenital central hypoventilation syndrome. Pediatr Res 1992; 31:291–296.
141. Schechtman VL, Harper RM, Wilson AJ, et al. Sleep apnea in infants who succumb to the sudden infant death syndrome. Pediatrics 1991; 87:841–846.
142. Harper RM, Bandler R. Finding the failure mechanism in the sudden infant death syndrome. Nat Med 1998; 4(2):157–158.
143. Lutherer LO, Lutherer BC, Dormer KJ, et al. Bilateral lesions of the fastigial nucleus prevent the recovery of blood pressure following hypotension induced by hemorrhage or administration of endotoxin. Brain Res 1983; 269:251–257.
144. Chen CH, Williams JL, Lutherer LO. Cerebellar lesions alter autonomic responses to transient isovolaemic changes in arterial pressure in anaesthetized cats. Clin Auton Res 1994; 4:263–272.
145. Harper RM, Bandler R, Alger J, et al. Functional magnetic resonance imaging of hippocampal and cerebellar activation to pressor challenges. Soc Neurosci Abstr 1997; 23:425.
146. Moruzzi G. Paleocerebellar inhibition of vasomotor and respiratory carotid sinus reflexes. J Neurophysiol 1940; 3:20–32.
147. Paton JFR, Spyer KM. Brain stem regions mediating the cardiovascular responses elicited from the posterior cerebellar cortex in the rabbit. J Physiol 1990; 427:533–552.
148. Reis DJ, Golanov EV. Autonomic and vascular regulation. Int Rev Neurobiol 1997; 41:121–149.
149. Williams JL, Everse SJ, Lutherer LO. Stimulating fastigial nucleus alters central mechanisms regulating phrenic activity. Respir Physiol 1989; 76:215–227.
150. Xu F, Frazier DT. Cerebellar role in the load—compensating response of expiratory muscle. J Appl Physiol 1994; 77:1232–1238.

151. Xu F, Owen J, Frazier DT. Cerebellar modulation of ventilatory response to progressive hypercapnia. J Appl Physiol 1994; 77:1073–1080.

152. Huang Q, Zhou D, St. John WM. Cerebellar control of expiratory activities of medullary neurons and spinal nerves. J Appl Physiol 1993; 74:1934–1940.

153. Gozal D, Hathout GM, Kirlew KAT, et al. Localization of putative neural respiratory regions in the human by functional magnetic resonance imaging. J Appl Physiol 1994; 76:2076–2083.

154. Gozal D, Omidvar O, Kirlew KAT, et al. Identification of human brain regions underlying responses to resistive inspiratory loading with functional magnetic resonance imaging. Proc Natl Acad Sci U S A 1995; 92:6607–6611.

155. Gozal D, Omidvar O, Kirlew KAT, et al. Functional magnetic resonance imaging reveals brain regions mediating the response to resistive expiratory loads in humans. J Clin Invest 1996; 97:1–7.

156. Panigrahy A, Filiano JJ, Sleeper LA, et al. Decreased kainate receptor binding in the arcuate nucleus of the sudden infant death syndrome. J Neuropathol Exp Neurol 1997; 56:1253–1261.

157. Zec N, Filiano JJ, Kinney HC. Anatomic relationships of the human arcuate nucleus of the medulla: a DiI labeling study. J Neuropathol Exp Neurol 1997; 56:509–522.

158. Henderson LA, Keay KA, Bandler R. The ventrolateral periaqueductal gray projects to caudal brainstem depressor regions: a functional-anatomical and physiological study. Neuroscience 1998; 82:201–221.

159. Doba A, Reis DJ. Role of the cerebellum and vestibular apparatus in regulation of orthostatic reflexes in the cat. Circ Res 1974; 40:9–18.

160. Yates BJ. Vestibular influences on the autonomic nervous system. In: Highstein SM, Cohen B, Buttner-Ennever JA, eds. New Directions in Vestibular Research, Annals of the New York Academy of Sciences. New York: 1996:458–470.

161. Mancia G, Baccelli G, Adams DB, et al. Vasomotor regulation during sleep in the cat. Am J Physiol 1971; 220:1086–1093.

162. Gassel M, Ghelarducci B, Marchiafava PL, et al. Phasic changes in blood pressure and heart rate during the rapid eye movement episodes of desynchronized sleep in unrestrained cats. Arch Ital Biol 1964; 102:530–544.

163. Harper RM, Schechtman VL. Physiological measurements as predictive tests for SIDS. In: Rognum TO, ed. Sudden Infant Death Syndrome: New Trends in the Nineties. Oslo: Scandinavian University Press 1995:314–319.

164. Kirby DA, Verrier RL. Differential effects of sleep stage on coronary hemodynamic function. Am J Physiol 1989; 256:H1378–H1383.

165. Dickerson LW, Huang AH, Thurnher MM, et al. Relationship between coronary hemodynamic changes and the phasic events of rapid eye movement sleep. Sleep 1993; 16:550–557.

166. Dickerson LW, Huang AH, Nearing BD, et al. Primary coronary vasodilation associated with pauses in heart rhythm during sleep. Am J Physiol 1993; 264: R186–R196.

167. Verrier R, Lau TR, Walloppillai U, et al. Primary vagally mediated decelerations in heart rate during tonic rapid eye movement sleep in cats. Am J Physiol 1998; 274:R1136–R1141.

168. Fewell JE. Influence of sleep on systemic and coronary hemodynamics in lambs. J Develop Physiol 1993; 19:71–76.

169. Rector DM, Gozal D, Forster HV, et al. Imaging of the goat ventral medullary surface activity during sleep-waking states. Am J Physiol Regul Integr Comp Physiol 1994; 267:R1154–R1160.

170. Rector DM, Oguri M, Harper RM. Imaging of ventral medullary surface changes in the freely behaving cat. Soc Neurosci Abstr 1996; 22:852.

171. Harper RM, Rector DM, Poe G, et al. Ventral medullary surface activity changes during momentary blood pressure variation within sleep states. Soc Neurosci Abstr 1995; 21:1015.

172. McAllen RM. Identification and properties of sub-retrofacial bulbospinal neurones: a descending cardiovascular pathway in the cat. J Auton Nerv Syst 1986; 17:151–164.

173. Harper RM, Gozal D, Forster HV, et al. Imaging of ventral medullary surface activity during blood pressure challenges in awake and anesthetized goats. Am J Physiol 1996; 270:R182–R191.

174. Forster HV, Gozal D, Harper RM, et al. Ventral medullary surface activity during hypoxia in awake and anesthetized goats. Respir Physiol 1996; 103:45–56.

175. Gozal D, Ohtake PJ, Rector DM, et al. Rostral ventral medullary surface activity during hypercapnic challenges in awake and anesthetized goats. Neurosci Lett 1995; 192:89–92.

176. Forster HV, Ohtake PJ, Pan LG, et al. Effects on breathing of cooling the ventrolateral medulla (VLM) in anesthetized and awake goats. Proceedings of the International Union of Physiological Science Congress, Glasgow, 1993, 4, 194 (abstr 32).

177. Harper RM, Gozal D, Aljadeff G, et al. Pressor-induced responses of the cat ventral medullary surface. Am J Physiol Regul Integr Comp Physiol 1995; 268: R324–R333.

178. Carroll JL, Gozal D, Rector DM, et al. Peripheral chemoreceptor afferent contributions to the intermediate area of the ventral medullary surface of the cat. Neuroscience 1996; 73:989–998.

179. Gozal D, Aljadeff G, Carroll JL, et al. Afferent contributions to intermediate area of the cat ventral medullary surface during mild hypoxia. Neurosci Lett 1994; 178:73–78.

180. Aljadeff G, Gozal D, Carroll JL, et al. Ventral medullary response to hypoxic and hyperoxic transient ventilatory challenges in the cat. Life Sci 1995; 57:319–324.

181. Severinghaus JW, Mitchell RA. Ondine's curse failure of respiratory automaticity while asleep. Clin Res 1962; 10:122.

182. Harper RM, Sauerland EK. The role of the tongue in sleep apnea. In: Guilleminault G, Dement WC, eds. Sleep Apnea Syndromes. New York: Alan R. Liss, 1978:219–234.

183. Remmers JE, Degroot WJ, Sauerland EK, et al. Pathogenesis of upper airway occlusion during sleep. J Appl Physiol 1978; 44:931–938.

184. Baust W, Weidinger H, Kirchner F. Sympathetic activity during natural sleep and arousal. Arch Ital Biol 1968; 106:379–390.

185. Jouvet M. Recherches sur les structures nerveuses et les mecanismes responsables des differentes phases du sommeil physiologique. Arch Ital Biol 1962; 100:125–206.

186. Munschauser FE, Mader MJ, Ahuja A, et al. Selective paralysis of voluntary but not limbically influenced automatic respiration. Arch Neurol 1991; 48:1190–1192.

187. Holstege G. Anatomical study of the final common pathway for vocalization in the cat. J Comp Neurol 1989; 284:242–252.
188. Holstege G, Meiners L, Tan K. Projections of the bed nucleus of the stria terminalis in the mesencephalon, pons, and medulla oblongata in the cat. Exp Brain Res 1985; 58:379–391.
189. Hopkins DA, Holstege G. Amygdaloid projections to the mesencephalon, pons, and medulla oblongata in the cat. Exp Brain Res 1978; 32:529–547.
190. Holstege G. Some anatomical observations on the projections from the hypothalamus to brainstem and spinal cord: an HRP and autoradiographic tracing study in the cat. J Comp Neurol 1987; 260:98–126.
191. Frysinger RC, Zhang J, Harper RM. Cardiovascular and respiratory relationships with neuronal discharge in the central nucleus of the amygdala during sleep-waking states. Sleep 1988; 11:317–332.
192. Terreberry RR, Oguri M, Harper RM. State-dependent respiratory and cardiac relationships with neuronal discharge in the bed nucleus of the stria terminalis. Sleep 1995; 18:139–144.
193. Zhang JX, Harper RM, Frysinger RC. Respiratory modulation of neuronal discharge in the central nucleus of the amygdala during sleep and waking states. Exp Neurol 1986; 91:193–207.
194. Harper RM, Frysinger RC, Trelease RB, et al. State-dependent alteration of respiratory cycle timing by stimulation of the central nucleus of the amygdala. Brain Res 1984; 306:1–8.
195. Zhang JX, Harper RM, Ni H. Cryogenic blockade of the central nucleus of the amygdala attenuates aversively conditioned blood pressure and respiratory responses. Brain Res 1986; 386:136–145.
196. Li Y-W, Dampney RAL. Expression of Fos-like protein in brain following sustained hypertension and hypotension in conscious rabbits. Neuroscience 1994; 61:613–634.
197. Kristensen MP, Poe GR, Rector DM, et al. Activity changes of the cat paraventricular hypothalamus during phasic respiratory events. Neuroscience 1997; 80:811–819.
198. Coveñas R, de León M, Cintra A, et al. Coexistence of c-Fos and glucocorticoid receptor immunoreactivities in the CRF immunoreactive neurons of the paraventricular hypothalamic nucleus of the rat after acute immobilization stress. Neurosci Lett 1993; 149:149–152.
199. Kristensen MP, Rector DM, Poe GR, et al. Reflectance imaging of the hypothalamic paraventricular region demonstrates biphasic cellular activation patterns in freely behaving cats during noise exposure. First World Congress on Stress, Bethesda, Maryland, 1994:56.
200. Swanson LW, Kuypers HGJM. The paraventricular nucleus of the hypothalamus: cytoarchitectonic subdivisions and organization of projections to the pituitary, dorsal vagal complex, and spinal cord as demonstrated by retrograde fluorescence double labelling methods. J Comp Neurol 1980; 194:555–570.
201. Luiten PGM, ter Horst GJ, Karst H, et al. The course of paraventricular hypothalamic efferents to autonomic structures in medulla and spinal cord. Brain Res 1995; 329:374–378.
202. Saper CB, Loewy AD, Swanson LW, et al. Direct hypothalamo-autonomic connections. Brain Res 1976; 117:305–312.

203. Parmeggiani PL, Azzaroni A, Cevolani D, et al. Responses of anterior hypothalamic-preoptic neurons to direct thermal stimulation during wakefulness and sleep. Brain Res 1983; 269:382–385.
204. Ni H, Schechtman VL, Zhang J, et al. Respiratory responses to preoptic/anterior hypothalamic warming during sleep in kittens. Reprod Fertil Dev 1996; 8:79–86.
205. Johnson P. Airway reflexes and the control of breathing in postnatal life. Ann N Y Acad Sci 1988; 533:262–275.
206. Stanton AN. Overheating and cot death. Lancet 1984; 2:1199–1201.
207. Kahn A, Blum D. Sudden infant death syndrome and phenothiazines. Pediatrics 1983; 71(6):986–988.
208. Lovick TA, Hilton SM. Vasodilator and vasoconstrictor neurones of the ventro-lateral medulla in the cat. Brain Res 1985; 331:353–357.
209. Kahn A, Sawaguchi T, Sawaguchi A, et al. Sudden infant deaths: from epidemiology to physiology. Forensic Sci Int 2002; 130(suppl):S8–S20.
210. Kahn A, Groswasser J, Rebuffat E, et al. Sleep and cardiorespiratory characteristics of infant victims of sudden death: a prospective case-control study. Sleep 1992; 15:287–292.
211. Thach BT. Sleep apnea in infancy and childhood. Med Clin North Am 1985; 69:1289–1315.
212. Thach BT. The role of respiratory control disorders in SIDS. Respir Physiol Neurobiol 2005; 149:343–353.
213. Mitchell EA, Tuohy PG, Brunt JM, et al. Risk factors for sudden infant death syndrome following the prevention campaign in New Zealand: a prospective study. Pediatrics 1997; 100.835–840.
214. Sabogal C, Auais A, Napchan G, et al. Effect of respiratory syncytial virus on apnea in weanling rats. Pediatr Res 2005; 57:819–825.
215. Redline S, Tishler PV, Tosteson TD, et al. The familial aggregation of obstructive sleep apnea. Am J Respir Crit Care Med 1995; 151:682–687.
216. Tishler PV, Redline S, Ferrette V, et al. The association of sudden unexpected infant death with obstructive sleep apnea. Am J Respir Crit Care Med 1996; 153:1857–1863.
217. Kato I, Groswasser J, Franco P, et al. Developmental characteristics of apnea in infants who succumb to sudden infant death syndrome. Am J Respir Crit Care Med 2001; 164:1464–1469.
218. Krous HF, Jordan J. A necropsy study of distribution of petechiae in non-sudden infant death syndrome. Arch Pathol Lab Med 1984; 108:75–76.
219. Jones KL, Krous HF, Nadeau J, et al. Vascular endothelial growth factor in the cerebrospinal fluid of infants who died of sudden infant death syndrome: evidence for antecedent hypoxia. Pediatrics 2003; 111:358–363.
220. Kinney HC, Filiano JJ, Sleeper LA, et al. Decreased muscarinic receptor binding in the arcuate nucleus in sudden infant death syndrome. Science 1995; 269:1446–1450.
221. Sawaguchi T, Franco P, Kato I, et al. From physiology to pathology: arousal deficiency theory in sudden infant death syndrome (SIDS)—with reference to apoptosis and neuronal plasticity. Forensic Sci Int 2002; 130(suppl):S37–S43.
222. Sparks DL, Hunsaker JC, III. Neuropathology of sudden infant death (syndrome): literature review and evidence of a probable apoptotic degenerative cause. Childs Nerv Syst 2002; 18:568–592.

223. Bowes G, Woolf GM, Sullivan CE, et al. Effect of sleep fragmentation on ventilatory and arousal responses of sleeping dogs to respiratory stimuli. Am Rev Respir Dis 1980; 122:899–908.

224. Fewell JE, Williams BJ, Szabo JS, et al. Influence of repeated upper airway obstruction on the arousal and cardiopulmonary response to upper airway obstruction in lambs. Pediatr Res 1988; 23:191–195.

225. Johnston RV, Grant DA, Wilkinson MH, et al. Repetitive hypoxia rapidly depresses cardio-respiratory responses during active sleep but not quiet sleep in the newborn lamb. J Physiol 1999; 519:571–579.

5

Maturation of Breathing During Sleep

CAROL L. ROSEN
Case Western Reserve University School of Medicine, Cleveland, Ohio, U.S.A.

I. Introduction

The objective of this chapter is to describe breathing during sleep in children from infancy to adolescence. Understanding these developmental changes is important for clinicians evaluating common childhood respiratory problems, such as apnea of infancy, apparent life-threatening events (ALTE), obstructive sleep apnea, and other forms of sleep-disordered breathing in children. Knowledge of the range of normative data across the ages is necessary to accurately interpret changes in respiratory parameters during overnight polysomnographic testing. Increasing demand for diagnostic services for children has been stimulated by (1) growth in the number of accredited sleep laboratories, (2) recognition of sleep medicine as an added qualification by the American Board of Medical Specialties, and (3) support of the American Board of Pediatrics for training sleep medicine specialists. New reports of normative data inform the evaluation of sleep-disordered breathing in children and the practice of pediatric sleep medicine since the first edition of this book in 2000 (1).

117

II. Normal Respiration During Sleep: An Overview

During sleep, ventilation decreases compared with wakefulness and varies with sleep state. During non–rapid eye movement (NREM) sleep, the influence of waking/behavioral controls is absent and ventilation is regulated by metabolic factors, primarily carbon dioxide (CO_2). Breathing is regular with a slightly lower respiratory rate and tidal volume, so minute ventilation declines by about 10% (2). This decline, in combination with the supine position and decrease in intercostal muscle tone, results in a decrease in functional residual capacity (FRC) (3). In addition, a sleep-related decrease in upper airway tone and lung volume increases upper airway resistance. During rapid eye movement (REM) sleep, breathing is irregular with variable respiratory rate and tidal volume. Occasional short central respiratory pauses are common during REM sleep in children. Inhibition of tonic activity of the intercostal muscles during REM results in a further decline in FRC (4,5). A relative decrease in upper airway muscle tone when diaphragmatic contractions remain unchanged can predispose to obstructive apnea, especially when the airway is already small or narrow. Finally, hypoxic and hypercapnic ventilatory drives decrease during sleep. During sleep, normal children experience a small increase in the partial pressure of CO_2 and a small decrease in arterial oxyhemoglobin saturation (SpO_2). The magnitude of these changes has not been systematically studied in large pediatric samples of healthy children, but is believed to average 2% for SpO_2 and 4 to 6 mmHg for CO_2. These sleep-related changes in ventilation, upper airway stability, and gas exchange can be exaggerated in children with underlying pulmonary, upper airway, and neuromuscular problems, resulting in increased vulnerability to sleep-disordered breathing. Differences between newborn and adult respiratory systems that make the infant more vulnerable to ventilatory failure are summarized in Table 1. More detailed discussions of developmental changes in various functional components of breathing during sleep, including ventilatory drive, respiratory mechanics, neuromotor activity, and arousability, are presented in Chapters 3 through 6 in this book.

III. Ventilation, Respiratory Patterns, and Apneas

In children, studies of normal respiration during sleep have focused on tabulation of various apnea types and their frequencies, description of respiratory rates and patterns, and summary indices of SpO_2 and CO_2 values. Data on tidal volume and minute ventilation are scarce because they require more invasive measurement strategies that either interfere with sleep or can only be accomplished in sedated subjects. More data are available for preterm and full-term infants in the first months of life than for children and adolescents, but several new reports of normative sleep and breathing data in these age groups have been published (6–8).

Table 1 Difference in the Newborn Compared with the Adult Respiratory System That Increase the Newborn's Vulnerability to Respiratory Failure

Upper airway
  Greater difficulty switching from nasal to oral route of breathing
  Laryngeal reflexes with prominent cardiorespiratory depressant effects
Chest wall properties impairing load compensation
  Increased chest wall compliance
  Circular "barrel-shaped" chest wall with horizontal position of the ribs
  Small diaphragmatic zone of apposition
  Softer, more cartilaginous ribs
  Greater percentage of sleep time in REM when stabilizing intercostal muscles are inhibited
Lower resting FRC
  Low specific lung compliance
  Higher metabolic rate
  Immaturity of respiratory control

Abbreviations: REM, rapid eye movement; FRC, functional residual capacity.

A. Respiratory Frequency

The respiratory rate is high in the neonatal period, then slows down during infancy and early childhood, until it reaches adult values (9,10). This observation is consistent with the well-known inverse relationship between resting respiratory rate and body size across mammalian species. Smaller, younger infants and children have higher respiratory rates per unit body weight than larger, older children. Respiratory rate decreases exponentially with increasing body weight (11). The changes in respiratory frequency with maturation are shown in Table 2. The mean difference between the waking and sleep respiratory rate is greatest in infants and decreases to 1 to 2 breaths per minute in adolescents. In general, the respiratory frequency is higher during REM than during NREM sleep in newborns and infants (12). In children, the respiratory frequency is highest in wakefulness and in stage 1 and lowest during the second half of the night (13). In adolescents, respiratory frequency is highest and most variable during REM sleep and lowest during slow wave sleep (2). These sleep state differences are most prominent in infants, but clinically trivial in children and adolescents.

B. Tidal Volume and Minute Ventilation

Respiration is measured by minute ventilation, defined as the product of respiratory frequency and tidal volume. To increase minute ventilation, a child can either increase the volume of each breath, increase the breathing frequency, or increase both. In the newborn and young child, increasing respiratory rate (rather than tidal

Table 2   Respiratory Rates (Breaths/Min) During Sleep in Children

	Newborn <2 wk	Infant 3–9 mo	Infant 12 mo	Toddler 2 yr	Preschool ~2–6 yr	School age ~7–11 yr	Adolescent ~12–18 yr
Mean		29 (64)					15–16 (2)
Median	40[a] (63)	27–29 (42,63)	24[a] (63)	21 (68)	20 (41)	18 (41)	18 (41)
SD		6 (64)					2 (2,13)
IQR	34–52	22–30 (63)	20–27 (63)		18–21 (41)	17–19 (41)	17–18 (68)
Range				15–31 (68)	14–26 (41)	15–25 (41)	15–22 (68)

References are shown in parentheses.
[a]During quiet sleep.

volume) is the most energy-efficient strategy to cope with higher ventilatory needs (14). This strategy of changing respiratory frequency rather than tidal volume is consistent with data in resting humans showing that both tidal volume and dead space per body weight remain essentially unchanged from birth to adulthood (about 6 mL/kg for tidal volume and 2.2 mL/kg for dead space) (15).

The scant data on tidal volume and minute ventilation during sleep come from the newborn and adolescent age groups (2,12). In general, minute ventilation is slightly higher in REM than in NREM sleep, consistent with the higher respiratory rates in REM. As expected, minute ventilation decreases with age (from 250 mL/kg per minute in newborns to 100 mL/kg per minute in adolescents) and parallels the maturational changes in respiratory frequency and metabolic needs.

C. Apnea Type, Duration, and Frequency

Numerous studies have investigated the frequency and duration of apnea in newborns and infants in the first year of life, with fewer studies in children and adolescents. Variations in sample populations, study methods, measurement conditions, and respiratory event definitions make it difficult to compare data from different studies. Not all studies have characterized sleep states by neurophysiologic criteria (16). Some studies have included children with snoring, but who had low numbers of respiratory events below a certain threshold. In general, central apneas of short duration (less than 10 second) are common in infants and children (17) and occur more often in REM than NREM sleep (18). Mechanisms for the greater respiratory instability in infants during REM compared with NREM sleep include immaturity of central respiratory control and phasic inhibitory-excitatory mechanisms inherent to REM sleep (19).

Apnea in Preterm Infants

Apnea of prematurity has been defined as sudden cessation of breathing that lasts for at least 20 seconds or is accompanied by bradycardia or oxygen desaturation in an infant younger than 37 weeks' gestational age (20). It usually ceases by 37 weeks' postmenstrual age, but may persist for several weeks beyond term, especially in infants born before 28 weeks' gestation (21–23). Extreme episodes lasting ≥30 seconds usually cease at approximately 43 weeks' postmenstrual age (24). A more comprehensive description of breathing during sleep in the premature infant is found in chapter 10. In brief, obstructive and mixed apneas are more frequent in preterm than in full-term infants (25), but there is no consensus regarding the frequency of these events. The difficulty of distinguishing central apneas (no effort, no airflow) from obstructive apneas (effort, no airflow) is technically challenging in these fragile infants (26). Continuous positive airway pressure (CPAP) has been shown to reduce apnea in preterm infants, suggesting that upper airway obstruction is an important contributor to apnea of prematurity (27). Obstructive apnea decreases with increasing postmenstrual age (28). This may be related to the improvement in extrathoracic airway stability with maturation (29). In addition, apneic events may be triggered by chronic hypoxemia or may themselves cause episodic desaturation. In healthy preterm infants, apnea triggered by desaturation decreases over time because of developmental improvements in chest wall stability (30) and in ventilation-perfusion matching (31).

Apnea in Full-Term Infants

In full-term infants, most apneas are central (32). Several studies have shown that obstructive and mixed apneas are rare in healthy infants (32–34). When recorded, obstructive apneas occur mainly during REM sleep (35). The sleeping position (prone or supine) does not alter the incidence, duration, or type of apnea in healthy infants and infants with a history of apnea (36). In this age group, the incidence of both central and obstructive apneas decreases with increasing postmenstrual age (28,32).

Periodic Breathing

Periodic breathing is a common respiratory pattern in preterm infants that is usually not of clinical significance. Older studies suggesting that increased periodic breathing was a marker for increased risk of sudden infant death syndrome (SIDS) have been challenged (37). Periodic breathing is defined as three episodes of apnea lasting longer than 3 seconds, separated by continued respiration of 20 seconds or less. Periodic breathing is more frequent in preterm infants, varies across studies in full-term infants, and decreases during the first two years of life (38,39). Compared with adults, the closeness of eupneic and apneic CO_2 thresholds confers greater vulnerability to the respiratory control system in neonates, because minor oscillations in breathing can bring eupneic CO_2 below threshold, causing apnea (40).

Apnea Beyond the First Year of Life

Central respiratory pauses are part of the normal pattern of breathing during sleep in children and adolescents. The frequency of respiratory pauses (as measured by impedance plethysmography) remains constant from ages 2 to 16 years (41) and is similar to that observed in healthy infants in the first year of life (42). However, the duration of the pauses increases with age. Obstructive apneas of any length are rare in both normal full-term infants and children (6–8,12,16,32,43–45). Obstructive apneas occur mainly in REM and lighter NREM sleep. Normative data for respiratory event indices in studies with at least 40 children beyond the first year of life are summarized in Table 3. Despite the variation in measurement techniques, respiratory event definitions, scoring approach, and sample population, these studies are remarkably similar in their findings: (1) obstructive apneas are extremely rare, and (2) central pauses are occasionally seen, including pauses that last up to 30 seconds.

IV. Gas Exchange

Most of our data about gas exchange during sleep in children comes from noninvasive techniques such as pulse oximetry monitoring of SpO_2, transcutaneous monitoring of partial pressure of oxygen and carbon dioxide (TcO_2 and $TcCO_2$, respectively), and end-tidal CO_2 ($EtCO_2$) monitoring of expired gases. $TcCO_2$ values are helpful as trend data to assess hypoventilation. Available data suggest that gas exchange during sleep improves with advancing postmenstrual age, particularly with respect to transient desaturations in the newborn period. During sleep in normal adults, there is an increase in partial pressure of CO_2 of 3 to 7 mmHg, a decrease in the partial pressure of O_2 of 3 to 9 mmHg, and a decrease in SpO_2 of 2% as compared with wakefulness (46). Similar changes are seen in children. These normal phenomena can be exaggerated in children with lung disease or upper airway obstruction.

A. Oxyhemoglobin Saturation by Pulse Oximetry

Normative data for SpO_2 values from infancy through adolescence are summarized in Table 4. Healthy infants generally have baseline SpO_2 values >95%. The transient, acute decreases correlated with young age, periodic breathing, irregular breathing, and episodic apnea appear to be part of normal breathing and oxygenation behavior in infants (47,48).

Gestational age and sleep state influence the development of stability in arterial oxygenation. Although healthy preterm infants have baseline SpO_2 values in the same range as full-term infants, the variability about the baseline is

Table 3 Pediatric Normative Literature for AI or AHI[a]

Reference	N	Age range (yr)	Obstructive AI	Obstructive AHI	Central AI	Longest central apnea (sec)	Total AHI
8	153	3.2–5.9	0.03 ± 0.10 (0–0.9)	0.08 ± 0.16	0.82 ± 0.73 (0–3.6)		0.90 ± 0.78 (0–3.6)
	388	6.0–8.6	0.05 ± 0.11 (0–0.9)	0.14 ± 0.22	0.45 ± 0.45 (0–3.4)		0.68 ± 0.75 (0–6.6)
57	50	9	0.1 ± 0.2 (0–1.2)	0.1 ± 1.3 (0–1.2)	1.5 ± 1.1 (0–5.1)	30.5	1.6 ± 1.2 (0.1–5.7)
7	66	2.5–9.4	0.01 ± 0.03	0.23 ± 0.31	0.08 ± 0.14		0.37 ± 0.57
6	70	1–15.0	0.1		0.4	20	
17	433	8–11	0.16 ± 1.0	0.75 ± 3.0	0.91 ± 1.6	32	2.7 ± 3.9
69	4	9.7–16.8				30	1.3 ± 1.3 (M) (0.2–6.2) 1.1 ± 0.7 (F) (0–2.8)
16,70	50	1–17.4	0.1 ± 0.5	0.2 ± 0.6 (0–3.4)		26	

[a]Data are presented as mean ± SD and (range), if available.
Abbreviations: AI, apnea indices; AHI, apnea-hypopnea indices.

Table 4 Oxygen Saturation (SpO_2) Values (%) During Sleep in Children

	Infant <1 yr	Preschool ~2–5 yr	School age ~6–12 yr	Adolescent ~13–18 yr
Mean or median SpO_2 value	97–99 (39,48,52,54,64)	99 (7,8,41,54)	96–99 (7,8,41,54–57)	97–99 (2,41,53)
SpO_2 value that is either 2 SD below mean or at the 5th percentile	94–95	95	95	95
Desaturation (≥4%) events/hr (mean ± SD)		0.29 ± 0.35(8)	0.47 ± 0.96(8) 1.2 ± 1.3(56) 0.7 ± 0.9(57)	

References are shown in parentheses.
Abbreviation: SpO_2, oxyhemoglobin saturation.

greater in preterm infants. The frequency of transient desaturation episodes to ≤80% varies considerably with age and between individual patients, with rates being highest in preterm infants, lower in term infants (47–52), and lowest in older children and adolescents. During the regular breathing of quiet or NREM sleep, most infants do not have episodes of desaturation, and when episodes do occur, they are brief. In contrast, during active or REM sleep, the brief apneic pauses are more likely to be associated with desaturation.

In healthy children aged 2 to 16 years, using a desaturation criterion of ≤90% does not show any episodes of desaturation in the majority of children (2,6–8,16,17,53–57). This increased stability in oxygenation may be partially explained by developmental changes in the relationship between lung volume and oxygen consumption. Infants have a highly compliant chest wall, resulting in a FRC that is significantly lower than that of adults when compared on the basis of metabolism (58). Lung volume in infants decreases even further during apneic pauses (59) and during REM sleep (60). Since lung volume at the onset of breath holding is a major determinant of the severity of resulting hypoxemia, the increase in the stability of oxygenation with age is likely due to increased and more stable lung volumes relative to oxygen consumption in the older child.

B. Carbon Dioxide

Both $TcCO_2$ and $EtCO_2$ measurements have been used to noninvasively estimate arterial CO_2 in children. Each method has advantages and disadvantages (61). Basal CO_2 values during sleep are generally between 36 to 42 mmHg in newborns and infants (12). $TcCO_2$ values during sleep change little with postnatal age during the first two years of life (39,62–64). Normal children show an increase in $EtCO_2$ values of 4 to 10 mmHg during sleep (16). Using mass

Table 5 CO_2 Values During Sleep in Children

	Infant <1 yr	Toddler 1–2 yr	Preschool ~3–5 yr	School age ~6–12 yr	Adolescent ~13–18 yr
$TcCO_2$ (mmHg)					
Mean ± SD	40.5 ± 3 (64)				
Median (IQR)	41 (37–44)	42 (40–46)			
	(39, 63)	(39)			
$EtCO_2$ (mmHg)					
Mean ± SD			40.6 ± 4.6	40.7 ± 4.5	40.7 ± 4.5
			(8)	(8)	(8)
Percent total sleep time with $EtCO_2$ > 45 mmHg (%)					
Mean ± SD			20.4 ± 28	1.6 ± 3.8	1.6 ± 3.8
			(8)	(6)	(6)
				6.9 ± 19.1	6.9 ± 19.1
				(16)	(16)
				4.0 ± 15.3	
				(8)	
Percent total sleep time with $EtCO_2$ > 50 mmHg (%)					
Mean ⊥ SD			4.0 ± 15.3	0.29 ±	0.29 ± 0.24
			(8)	0.24 (6)	(6)
				0.5 ± 4.0	0.5 ± 4.0
				(16)	(16)
				2.0 ± 7.1	
				(8)	

References are shown in parentheses.
Abbreviations: CO_2, carbon dioxide; $TcCO_2$, transcutaneous CO_2; $EtCO_2$, end-tidal CO_2.

spectrometer technology in 50 normal children ranging in age from 1 to 17 years showed the mean maximal $EtCO_2$ value during sleep to be 46 ± 4 mmHg (range, 38 to 53) (16). CO_2 values are statistically lower in REM than NREM sleep, but the 1 to 2 mmHg difference is clinically trivial. The limited normative data for CO_2 values measured during polysomnography from infancy to childhood are summarized in Table 5. A recent study (8) describes much higher values during sleep in children than previously reported (6,16).

C. Relationships Between Apnea, Bradycardia, and Desaturation

Bradycardia, apnea, and hypoxemia are closely related in preterm infants. However, the precise mechanisms underlying these relationships, and the level of apnea, bradycardia, and desaturation that constitutes an abnormality, remain controversial. In preterm infants, 83% of bradycardic episodes were associated with apnea and 86% were associated with desaturation (65). Sleep state also influences heart rate changes during apneas in healthy full-term infants studied from one to four months of age in whom a fall in heart rate was more likely to be associated with NREM sleep compared with REM sleep (66). However, a six-month longitudinal cohort study of cardiorespiratory events recorded on home monitors using criteria thought to be clinically useful in the identification of infants at increased risk for SIDS yielded some unexpected findings (24). First, "conventional events" (apnea ≥ 20 second or an age-adjusted bradycardia threshold of a specific duration) were common. Of the 306 healthy term infants, 43% had at least one event that met "conventional criteria," but only 2% had at least one event that met the "extreme" criteria (apnea >30 second or an age-adjusted bradycardia threshold of a specific duration). In general, the degree of desaturation increased with increasing duration of apnea or bradycardia. The frequency of at least one extreme event was similar in term infants in all groups (healthy controls, sibling of SIDS, ALTE), but preterm infants were at increased risk of extreme events until about 43 weeks' postmenstrual age. Of concern, a follow-up study of developmental outcomes in this same cohort in the second year of life showed that ≥ 5 cardiorespiratory events per hour were associated with lower adjusted mean differences in the mental development index of the Bayley Scales of Development in both term and preterm infants (67).

V. Summary

Respiratory adaptation during sleep changes with growth and development as a result of maturation of the mechanics of the respiratory pump and the respiratory control center. In the last five years, new studies have filled many of the gaps in our knowledge of normative respiratory data during sleep beyond the infant age group in nonclinical samples. Although investigators often differed in their measurement approaches, event definitions, and recommended normative thresholds, their findings were remarkably consistent, even across different age groups. The next set of challenges is to better understand the degree to which these abnormal measures are associated with or to predict increased risk for adverse health outcomes, so that treatment can identify the children most likely to benefit from detection, diagnosis, and treatment.

References

1. Rosen CL. Maturation of breathing during sleep: infants through adolescents. In: Loughlin G, Carroll J, Marcus C, eds. Sleep and Breathing in Children. New York: Marcel Dekker, Inc., 2000:181–206.

2. Tabachnik E, Muller NL, Bryan AC, et al. Changes in ventilation and chest wall mechanics during sleep in normal adolescents. J Appl Physiol 1981; 51:557–564.
3. Hudgel DW, Devadatta P. Decrease in functional residual capacity during sleep in normal humans. J Appl Physiol 1984; 57(5):1319–1322.
4. Hudgel DW, Martin RJ, Johnson B, et al. Mechanics of the respiratory system and breathing pattern during sleep in normal humans. J Appl Physiol 1984; 56(1): 133–137.
5. Lopes JM, Tabachnik E, Muller NL, et al. Total airway resistance and respiratory muscle activity during sleep. J Appl Physiol 1983; 54(3):773–777.
6. Uliel S, Tauman R, Greenfeld M, et al. Normal polysomnographic respiratory values in children and adolescents. Chest 2004; 125(3):872–878.
7. Traeger N, Schultz B, Pollock AN, et al. Polysomnographic values in children 2–9 years old: additional data and review of the literature. Pediatr Pulmonol 2005; 40 (1):22–30.
8. Montgomery-Downs HE, O'Brien LM, Gulliver TE, et al. Polysomnographic characteristics in normal preschool and early school-aged children. Pediatrics 2006; 117(3):741–753.
9. Iliff A, Lee V. Pulse rate, respiratory rate and coding temperature of children between two months and eighteen years of age. Child Development 1952; 23: 237–252.
10. Bardella I. Pediatric advanced life support: a review of the AHA recommendations. American Heart Association. Am Fam Physician 1999; 60(6):1743–1750.
11. Gagliardi L, Rusconi F. Respiratory rate and body mass in the first three years of life. The working party on respiratory rate. Arch Dis Child 1997; 76(2):151–154.
12. Gaultier C. Respiratory adaptation during sleep from the neonatal period to adolescence. In: Guilleminault C, ed. Sleep and Its Disorders in Children. New York: Raven Press, 1987:67–98.
13. Carskadon MA, Harvey K, Dement WC, et al. Respiration during sleep in children. West J Med 1978; 128:477–481.
14. Mortola JP. Some functional mechanical implications of the structural design of the respiratory system in newborn mammals. Am Rev Respir Dis 1983; 128(2 pt 2), S69–S72.
15. Polgar G, Weng TR. The functional development of the respiratory system from the period of gestation to adulthood. Am Rev Respir Dis 1979; 120(3):625–695.
16. Marcus CL, Omlin KJ, Basinki DJ, et al. Normal polysomnographic values for children and adolescents. Am Rev Respir Dis 1992; 146(5 pt 1):1235–1239.
17. Tang JP, Rosen CL, Larkin EK, et al. Identification of sleep-disordered breathing in children: variation with event definition. Sleep 2002; 25(1):72–79.
18. Gaultier C. Apnea and sleep state in newborns and infants. Biol Neonate 1994; 65 (3–4):231–234.
19. Haddad GG, Epstein RA, Epstein MAF, et al. Maturation of ventilation and ventilatory pattern in normal sleeping infants. J Appl Physiol 1979; 46:998–1002.
20. Committee on Fetus and Newborn, American Academy of Pediatrics, Apnea, sudden infant death syndrome, and home monitoring. Pediatrics 2003; 111(4 pt 1): 914–917.
21. Henderson-Smart DJ. The effect of gestational age on the incidence and duration of recurrent apnoea in newborn babies. Aust Paediatr J 1981; 17(4):273–276.

22. Eichenwald EC, Aina A, Stark AR. Apnea frequently persists beyond term gestation in infants delivered at 24 to 28 weeks. Pediatrics 1997; 100(3 pt 1):354–359.

23. Darnall RA, Kattwinkel J, Nattie C, et al. Margin of safety for discharge after apnea in preterm infants. Pediatrics 1997; 100(5):795–801.

24. Ramanathan R, Corwin MJ, Hunt CE, et al. Cardiorespiratory events recorded on home monitors: Comparison of healthy infants with those at increased risk for SIDS. JAMA 2001; 285(17):2199–2207.

25. Albani M, Bentele K, Budde C, et al. Infant sleep apnea profile: preterm vs. term infants. Eur J Pediatr 1985; 143(4):261–268.

26. Upton C, Milner A, Stokes G. Upper airway patency during apnoea of prematurity. Arch Dis Child 1992; 67(4 spec no):419–424.

27. Miller M, Carlo W, Martin R. Continuous positive airway pressure selectively reduces obstructive apnea in preterm infants. J Pediatr 1985; 106:91–94.

28. Hoppenbrouwers T, Hodgman JE, Cabal L. Obstructive apnea, associated patterns of movement, heart rate, and oxygenation in infants at low and increased risk for SIDS. Pediatr Pulmonol 1993; 15:1–12.

29. Duara S, Silva Neto G, Claure N, et al. Effect of maturation on the extrathoracic airway stability of infants. J Appl Physiol 1992; 73(6):2368–2372.

30. Heldt GP. Development of stability of the respiratory system in preterm infants. J Appl Physiol 1988; 65(1):441–444.

31. Woodrum D, Oliver T Jr., Hodson W. The effect of prematurity and hyaline membrane disease on oxygen exchange in the lung. Pediatrics 1972; 50(3):380–386.

32. Guilleminault C, Ariagno R, Korobkin R, et al. Mixed and obstructive sleep apnea and near miss for sudden infant death syndrome: 2. Comparison of near miss and normal control infants by age. Pediatrics 1979; 64(6):882–891.

33. Flores-Guevara R, Plouin P, Curzi-Dascalova L, et al. Sleep apneas in normal neonates and infants during the first 3 months of life. Neuropediatrics 1982; 13 (suppl):21–28.

34. Kahn A, Groswasser J, Sottiaux M, et al. Clinical symptoms associated with brief obstructive sleep apnea in normal infants. Sleep 1993; 16(5):409–413.

35. Kahn A, Groswasser J, Rebuffat E, et al. Sleep and cardiorespiratory characteristics of infant victims of sudden death: a prospective case-control study. Sleep 1992; 15 (4):287–292.

36. Kahn A, Groswasser J, Sottiaux M, et al. Prone or supine body position and sleep characteristics in infants. Pediatrics 1993; 91(6):1112–1115.

37. Finer N, Barrington K, Hayes B. Prolonged periodic breathing: significance in sleep studies. Pediatrics 1992; 89(3):450–453.

38. Kelly DH, Riordan L, Smith MJ. Apnea and periodic breathing in healthy full-term infants, 12-18 months of age. Pediatr Pulmonol 1992; 13(3):169–171.

39. Schlüter B, Buschatz D, Trowitzsch E. Polysomnographic reference curves in the first and second year of life. Somnologie 2001; 5:3–16.

40. Khan A, Qurashi M, Kwiatkowski K, et al. Measurement of the CO_2 apneic threshold in newborn infants: possible relevance for periodic breathing and apnea. J Appl Physiol 2005; 98(4):1171–1176.

41. Poets CF, Stebbens VA, Samuels MP, et al. Oxygen saturation and breathing patterns in children. Pediatrics 1993; 92(5):686–690.

42. Poets CF, Stebbens VA, Southall DP. Arterial oxygen saturation and breathing movements during the first year of life. J Dev Physiol 1991; 15(6):341–345.

43. Guilleminault C. Obstructive sleep apnea and its treatment in children: Areas of agreement and controversy. Pediatr Pulmonol 1987; 3:429–436.
44. Kahn A, Blum D, Rebuffat E, et al. Polysomnographic studies of infants who subsequently died of sudden infant death syndrome. Pediatrics 1988; 82(5):721–727.
45. Kahn A, Mozin MJ, Burniat W, et al. Sleep pattern alterations and brief airway obstructions in overweight infants. Sleep 1989; 12(5):430–438.
46. Krieger J. Breathing during sleep in normal subjects. In: Kryger M, Roth T, Dement WC, eds. Principles and Practice of Sleep Medicine. 4th ed. Philadelphia: Elsevier Saunders, 2005:232–244.
47. Stebbens VA, Poets CF, Alexander JR, et al. Oxygen saturation and breathing patterns in infancy. 1: Full term infants in the second month of life. Arch Dis Child 1991; 66(5):569–573.
48. Hunt CE, Corwin MJ, Lister G, et al. Longitudinal assessment of hemoglobin oxygen saturation in healthy infants during the first 6 months of age. Collaborative Home Infant Monitoring Evaluation (CHIME) Study Group. J Pediatr 1999; 135(5): 580–586.
49. Poets CF, Stebbens VA, Alexander JR, et al. Oxygen saturation and breathing patterns in infancy. 2: Preterm infants at discharge from special care. Arch Dis Child 1991; 66(5):574–578.
50. Poets CF, Stebbens VA, Alexander JR, et al. Arterial oxygen saturation in preterm infants at discharge from the hospital and six weeks later. J Pediatr 1992; 120 (3):447–454.
51. Richard D, Poets CF, Neale S, et al. Arterial oxygen saturation in preterm neonates without respiratory failure. J Pediatr 1993; 123(6):963–968.
52. Poets CF, Stebbens VA, Lang JA, et al. Arterial oxygen saturation in healthy term neonates. Eur J Pediatr 1996; 155(3):219–223.
53. Chipps BE, Mak H, Schuberth KC, et al. Nocturnal oxygen saturation in normal and asthmatic children. Pediatrics 1980; 65:1157–1160.
54. Owen G, Canter R. Analysis of pulse oximetry data in normal sleeping children. Clin Otolaryngol Allied Sci 1997; 22(1):13–22.
55. Rosen CL, Larkin EK, Kirchner HL, et al. Prevalence and risk factors for sleep-disordered breathing in 8- to 11-year-old children: association with race and prematurity. J Pediatr 2003; 142(4):383–389.
56. Urschitz MS, Wolff J, Von Einem V, et al. Reference values for nocturnal home pulse oximetry during sleep in primary school children. Chest 2003; 123(1):96–101.
57. Moss D, Urschitz M, Von Bodman A, et al. Reference values for nocturnal home polysomnography in primary schoolchildren. Pediatr Res 2005; 58(5):958–965.
58. Cook C, Cherry R, O'Brien D, et al. Studies on the respiratory physiology of the newborn infant: 1. Observation on normal premature and full-term infants. J Clin Invest 1955; 34(7 pt 1):975–982.
59. Olinsky A, Bryan M, Bryan A. Influence of lung inflation on respiratory control in neonates. J Appl Physiol 1974; 36(4):426–429.
60. Henderson-Smart D, Read D. Reduced lung volume during behavioral active sleep in the newborn. J Appl Physiol 1979; 46(6):1081–1085.
61. Morielli A, Desjardins D, Brouillette RT. Transcutaneous and end-tidal carbon dioxide pressures should be measured during pediatric polysomnography. Am Rev Resp Dis 1993; 148(6 pt 1):1599–1604.

62. Hoppenbrouwers T, Hodgman J, Arakawa K, et al. Transcutaneous oxygen and carbon dioxide during the first half year of life in premature and normal term infants. Pediatr Res 1992; 31(1):73–79.
63. Schäfer T, Schäfer D, Schlafke ME. Breathing, transcutaneous blood gases, and CO_2 response in SIDS siblings and control infants during sleep. J Appl Physiol 1993; 74 (1):88–102.
64. Horemuzova E, Katz-Salamon M, Milerad J. Breathing patterns, oxygen and carbon dioxide levels in sleeping healthy infants during the first nine months after birth. Acta Paediatr 2000; 89(11):1284–1289.
65. Upton C, Milner A, Stokes G. Apnoea, bradycardia, and oxygen saturation in pre-term infants. Arch Dis Child 1991; 66(4 spec no):381–385.
66. Haddad G, Bazzy A, Chang S, et al. Heart rate pattern during respiratory pauses in normal infants during sleep. J Dev Physiol 1984; 6(5):329–337.
67. Hunt CE, Corwin MJ, Baird T, et al. Cardiorespiratory events detected by home memory monitoring and one-year neurodevelopmental outcome. J Pediatr 2004; 145 (4):465–471.
68. Poets CF, Stebbens VA, Alexander JR, et al. Breathing patterns and heart rates at ages 6 weeks and 2 years. Am J Dis Child 1991; 145(12):1393–1396.
69. Acebo C, Millman RP, Rosenberg C, et al. Sleep, breathing, and cephalometrics in older children and young adults. Part I—Normative values. Chest 1996; 109(3): 664–672.
70. Witmans MB, Keens TG, Ward SLD, et al. Obstructive hypopneas in children and adolescents: normal values. Am J Respir Crit Care Med 2003; 168(12):1540.

6

Interaction Between Upper Airway Muscles and Structures During Sleep

SHIROH ISONO
Graduate School of Medicine, Chiba University, Chiba, Japan

I. Introduction

The upper airway is composed of the nose, the pharynx, the larynx, and the extrathoracic trachea. The segment of greatest interest is the pharynx, where partial and/or complete airway obstruction occurs during sleep in patients with the obstructive sleep apnea syndrome (OSAS). Under neural and chemical control, contraction of the pharyngeal muscles surrounding the collapsible conduit of the pharynx modulates its size and stiffness according to the required purpose. The objectives of this chapter are to describe normal pharyngeal airway maintenance achieved by the interaction between the pharyngeal muscles and structures during sleep and to share new information that may relate to the pathophysiology of sleep-disordered breathing.

II. Pharyngeal Maintenance Mechanisms

A. Roles of Pharyngeal Muscles

A simple classification of the pharyngeal muscles greatly aids in understanding the principal role of each muscle for stable respiration. At the level of the pharynx, the surrounding muscles are divided into pharyngeal dilators and constrictors. Major constrictor muscles of the pharynx consist of the superior, middle, and inferior pharyngeal constrictors; however, dilators are numerous. At the level of the oropharyngeal airway (between the tip of the epiglottis and the edge of the soft palate, also known as the retroglossal airway), the genioglossus muscle dilates the airway for respiration, while its fan-like projection of muscle fibers produces complicated movements of the tongue. The genioglossus is the most extensively studied muscle, since reduction of its activity is known to be associated with an increase in upper airway resistance (1). Although contraction of each pharyngeal muscle usually results in unidirectional movement of the structure, the actual movement is determined by the sum of vector forces produced by the group of upper airway muscles participating in the specific function. At the hypopharyngeal airway (between the vocal cords and the tip of the epiglottis), net vector forces of the suprahyoid muscles, which attach superiorly to the hyoid bone (i.e., the geniohyoid and myohyoid), and the infrahyoid muscles, which attach inferiorly to the hyoid bone (i.e., the sternohyoid, thyrohyoid, and omohyoid), determine the position of the hyoid bone and its function in the dilatation of this segment. The position of the hyoid bone and the direction of muscle fibers significantly influence the net vector forces of these muscles. At the level of the velopharyngeal airway (between the edge of the soft palate and the end of the nasal septum), the role of each muscle depends on preference of the breathing route. Contraction of the palatoglossal and palatopharyngeal muscles opens the retropalatal airway, allowing for nasal breathing. These muscles are, therefore, considered to be the dilators during nasal breathing. The tensor veli palatini and the levator veli palatini, which elevate the soft palate, are considered to be the dilators during oral breathing.

Net vector forces of the two antagonistic muscle groups, dilators and constrictors, determine the airway size in the static condition, i.e., during absence of airflow through the airway. Feroah et al. demonstrated that the balance between the stylopharyngeus dilator and the inferior pharyngeal constrictor modulated the isolated pharyngeal airway size in awake goats (2). In addition to regulation of the pharyngeal airway size, recent evidence obtained by electromyographic (EMG) recording of the pharyngeal constrictor suggests another important function of the pharyngeal muscles. Kuna et al. observed that inspiratory phasic activation of the superior pharyngeal constrictor was frequently associated with airway reopening on arousal in patients with OSAS (3). Although their findings appear to disagree with the simple dilator-constrictor model, construction of an extended model of the pharyngeal airway may possibly solve this seeming contradiction. As many dilator muscles exhibit phasic inspiratory activity, especially during mechanical loading (4–7) or chemical stimuli (8,9), inspiration is the most critical phase for airway maintenance since development of negative intraluminal pressure opposes the dilator forces during this period (1,10). Therefore, reciprocal inhibition of the constrictors may be preferable in facilitating dilator muscle function in the simple dilator-constrictor model. However, Kuna's data do not support this idea. One possible interpretation of these data is that contraction of the constrictor muscle results in stiffening of the pharyngeal airway wall, which assists in maintenance of a patent airway reestablished by a burst of the genioglossus upon arousal. Increases in tonic EMG activity, which is often observed in dilator muscles during mechanical loading and chemical stimuli, may also contribute to stiffening of the pharyngeal airway wall. Pharyngeal muscles not only act as dilators or constrictors in controlling the pharyngeal airway size, but also act as stiffeners in regulating compliance of the pharyngeal airway wall.

Recent evidence from electric stimulation of the pharyngeal muscles strongly supports the function of pharyngeal muscles as stiffeners. In anesthetized dogs with an isolated upper airway, Hida et al. measured the static pressure–volume relationship of the upper airway with and without electrical stimulation of the branches of the hypoglossal nerve (11). They demonstrated that compliance of the upper airway, which is the slope of the pressure-volume relationship, was decreased by contraction of the pharyngeal dilators. Fregosi et al. confirmed Hida's observation and further demonstrated that coactivation of tongue protrudors, such as the genioglossus, and retractors, such as the hyoglossus and styloglossus, resulted in stiffening of the upper airway in rats (12,13). In anesthetized patients with sleep-disordered breathing, bilateral electrical stimulation of the tongue musculature, including the protrudor and retractor muscles, decreased the slope of the static pressure-area relationship of the oropharyngeal airway (14). Electrical stimulation at lower airway pressures increased the oropharyngeal cross-sectional area, which indicates that the tongue musculature acts as a dilator when the oropharyngeal airway is small. Contrastingly, electrical stimulation at higher airway pressures resulted in reduction of the oropharyngeal cross-sectional area, indicating that the tongue musculature acts as a "constrictor" when the airway is large. Accordingly, the pharyngeal muscles have two significant functions for respiratory stabilization: one for controlling airway size and the other for regulating airway compliance. The latter function may be particularly important in the child with a small airway.

Although the activation pattern of pharyngeal muscles differs from that of primary inspiratory muscles, evidence of a strong link suggests involvement of the central pattern generator in the regulation of the pharyngeal muscles (15,16). Strohl et al. demonstrated that activation of the alae nasi occurred prior to onset of inspiratory airflow, especially during sleep (90 ms prior to onset of flow during wakefulness vs. 196 ms during sleep) (17). This sequence is considered to act as a stiffener for the collapsible pharynx against the collapsing forces of inspiratory efforts developed by the primary inspiratory muscles. EMG activity of the diaphragm gradually increases during inspiration and peaks in the late inspiratory phase. In contrast, pharyngeal muscle activity peaks in the early inspiratory phase, and higher activity is maintained throughout inspiration.

B. Pharyngeal Muscle Functions for Stable Respiration

The pharyngeal muscle contraction for stable respiration is counteracted by contraction of inspiratory pump muscles (e.g., the diaphragm and external intercostal muscles) that produce negative airway pressure (P_{AW}) and narrow the pharyngeal airway. Considering that the size of the pharyngeal airway is determined by the balance between two antagonistic forces, as proposed by Remmers et al. (1) and Brouillette and Thach (10), and the fact that neural control mechanisms regulate central drives to the pharyngeal and pump muscles, a "neural balance model" is suggested (Fig. 1). In this model, the consciousness level, reflexes, and chemical stimuli interactively modulate the final outputs of the central drives. Moreover, the position of the fulcrum, i.e., the anatomy of the pharynx (structural properties of the pharyngeal airway wall) (18,19), produces variable pharyngeal airway size (anatomical mechanisms). Accordingly, the pharyngeal airway size is determined by interaction between the neural and anatomical mechanisms.

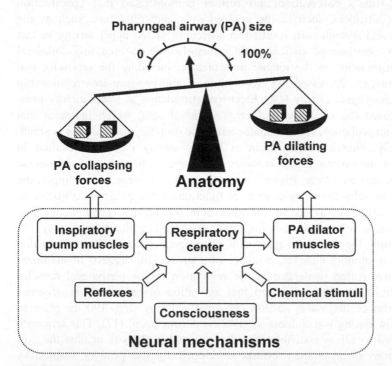

Figure 1 Remmers et al. (1) and Brouillette and Thach's neural balance model (10) for explanation of the interaction between neural and anatomical mechanisms focusing on the neural balance for determining the PA size. *Abbreviation*: PA, pharyngeal airway. *Source*: From Ref. 49.

C. State Dependency of the Neural Mechanisms

Pharyngeal patency during wakefulness is ensured by continual supervision of the higher central nervous system, which regulates and coordinates the action of more than 30 pairs of pharyngeal muscles, in concert with neural and chemical inputs. Serotonergic or noradrenergic neurons are considered to be involved in the wakefulness stimulus to the upper airway motor neuron (20,21). Negative pharyngeal pressure (22), cold air (23), and nasal obstruction (4,24) are known to reflexively augment pharyngeal muscle activity, and these upper airway maintenance reflexes are well maintained during wakefulness. The afferent pathway of the negative pressure reflex is considered to include mechanoreceptors located in the upper airway, and the superior laryngeal nerve, since upper airway anesthesia increases upper airway resistance (25) and sleep-disordered breathing in normal subjects (26). Mezzanotte et al. demonstrated that adult patients with OSAS have significantly greater genioglossal muscle activity compared with normal subjects during wakefulness (27). This does not indicate abnormally augmented neural mechanisms in patients with OSAS. Fogel et al. recently demonstrated no difference in the level of genioglossal activity during wakefulness for a given negative P_{AW} between subjects with and without OSAS, suggesting that the greater genioglossal activity in patients with OSAS is due to structural pharyngeal narrowing (28). In the pediatric population, Gozal and Burnside demonstrated a significant reduction in the pharyngeal cross-sectional area after topical anesthesia of the upper airway (40% reduction in children with OSAS vs. 5% reduction in control children), which most likely depressed the upper airway receptors responsible for the negative pressure reflex (29).

Sleep depresses the higher central nervous system and reduces pharyngeal muscle activity (30,31). The extent of pharyngeal muscle suppression is much greater in rapid eye movement (REM) sleep than in non-REM (NREM) sleep, as with many other skeletal muscles. Indeed, atonia of the upper airway muscle activities is one criterion for staging REM sleep. The negative pressure reflex serves to increase the reduced pharyngeal muscle activity and maintain the pharyngeal airway. The contribution of this reflex may vary depending on the muscles involved, sleep stage, and presence of OSAS. In normal adults, Malhotra et al. demonstrated that the level of peak genioglossal activity was directly associated with the magnitude of negative inspiratory P_{AW} during both wakefulness and NREM sleep, and the slope of the association was greater during wakefulness than NREM sleep (32). This is in accordance with the study reported by Wheatley et al. (33). Shea et al. further reported that negative P_{AW} appeared to regulate the genioglossal activity even within an inspiration, and the responsiveness of the negative pressure reflex was not altered within the physiological range of the chemical stimuli (34,35). Interestingly, the responsiveness was significantly attenuated when negative P_{AW} was produced by an iron lung ventilator during NREM sleep, which eliminated the inspiratory pump muscle activation, suggesting the importance of the influence of the central pattern generator on the reflex (36). While the impairment of the negative pressure reflex is an attractive hypothesis for the pathogenesis of OSAS, no study has succeeded in demonstrating a difference in the EMG responsiveness between subjects with and without OSAS.

Chemical stimuli appear to contribute little to the pharyngeal muscle activity during sleep. Parisi et al. reported that the genioglossal responses to hypoxia and hypercapnia decreased during sleep compared with wakefulness in the goat (awake > NREM > REM) (8,9). The pattern of genioglossus responses to hypoxia was observed to differ significantly from that of the diaphragm, in which the genioglossus was activated only below a Sao_2 threshold, while the diaphragm activity increased monotonously in response to progressive hypoxia. Therefore, the imbalance between the pharyngeal dilating forces and the inspiratory collapsing forces favors pharyngeal narrowing during sleep, as demonstrated by Remmers et al. (1).

The necessity of the pharyngeal muscle contraction for stable breathing during sleep depends on the structural stability of the pharyngeal airway. Henke instituted nasal CPAP in normal young men during NREM sleep to reduce genioglossal activity, then abruptly reduced the mask pressure to atmospheric pressure for a single breath, during which time the suppressed muscle activity was sustained (37). Despite the marked reduction in genioglossal activity, the upper airway resistance did not increase. In complete contrast, as Remmers et al. consistently report, patients with OSAS and anatomical abnormalities of the pharynx require pharyngeal muscle activity in order to maintain a patent airway and thereby stable respiration (38–40).

D. Anatomical Balance of the Upper Airway

Numerous previous reports documented the presence of upper airway structural abnormalities such as a small mandible (41,42), hypertrophied adenoid and tonsils (43), macroglossia (44), and obesity (45,46) in both pediatric and adult patients with OSAS. Isono et al. demonstrated the contribution of abnormal anatomical mechanisms to the increased pharyngeal airway collapsibility (18,19). As illustrated in Figure 2 (47–50), the pharyngeal airway is surrounded by soft tissue such as the tongue and the soft palate, which in turn are enclosed by bony structures such as the maxilla, the mandible, and the vertebra. Accordingly, a simple mechanical model for the pharyngeal airway is that of a collapsible tube surrounded by soft material within a rigid box (48). In this model, the lumen size of the collapsible tube is determined by the mechanical properties of the tube and the transmural pressure (P_{tm}) (47), and the relationship between luminal size and P_{tm} is denoted by the "tube law" of the collapsible tube. P_{tm} is defined as the pressure difference between the pressure inside (P_{lumen}) and outside (P_{tissue}) the tube. For a given P_{lumen}, an increase in P_{tissue} results in reduction of the P_{tm} (i.e., $P_{tm} = P_{lumen} - P_{tissue}$) and consequent lumen narrowing. Structurally, P_{tissue} is determined by the balance between the amount of soft material inside the rigid box and the size of the surrounding rigid box. When the pharyngeal muscles are not contracting, the anatomical balance between the amount of soft tissue inside the bony enclosure and the bony enclosure size determines the pharyngeal airway size (Fig. 3) (49). Obesity, hypertrophied adenoid and tonsils, and macroglossia can increase the amount of soft tissue, producing an increase in P_{tissue} and reduction in airway size. Similarly, midfacial hypoplasia or micrognathia can also increase P_{tissue} and narrow the airway. In a subject with a small mandible, normal growth of the adenoid and tonsils or mild obesity could cause OSAS. In contrast, a subject with normal craniofacial size would not develop OSAS until the adenoid and tonsils hypertrophy abnormally. Pharyngeal muscle contraction can function as a fulcrum of the anatomical balance by changing the tube law of the pharyngeal airway. Accordingly, interaction between the anatomical balance and the neural mechanisms determines the final pharyngeal airway patency. This "anatomical balance model" is an extension of the concept proposed by Shelton et al. who reported that both mandible enclosure size and body weight are important determinants of the apnea hypopnea index (51). It is difficult to measure P_{tissue} in human subjects. In spontaneously breathing pigs, Winter et al. increased P_{tissue} by inflating a balloon inside the mandibular enclosure. They demonstrated a significant increase in upper airway resistance during balloon inflation (52). More recently, Isono et al. measured the pressure between the dorsum of the tongue and soft palate, considered to reflect P_{tissue}, during obstructive apnea induced under general anesthesia (53). The pressure was found to be above atmospheric pressure at end expiration in all patients with OSAS. Kairaitis et al. measured upper airway P_{tissue} in anesthetized rabbits placed in the supine position and reported positive values during spontaneous breathing (54). Limitations of the anatomical balance model do exist, since only two significant anatomical features—the soft tissue surrounding the pharyngeal airway and the bony enclosure size—are included. The validity of the model needs to be assessed in the future and improved, based on an updated knowledge of the pathogenesis of pharyngeal airway maintenance mechanisms.

III. Methodology of Pharyngeal Airway Maintenance Mechanisms

A. Methodological Difficulties and Limitations

Research on pharyngeal airway maintenance mechanisms advances our understanding of the pathogenesis of pharyngeal airway obstruction, which may lead to the establishment of new treatment strategies. As discussed above, pharyngeal airway size is determined by the interaction between anatomical and neural mechanisms, and therefore impairment of either or both mechanism(s) results in pharyngeal airway obstruction (18,55), respectively referred to as the "anatomical hypothesis" and "neural hypothesis" for pharyngeal obstruction. However, due to the complicated interactions between anatomical and neural mechanisms, it is difficult to clearly determine the extent of involvement of each hypothesis in pharyngeal obstruction. Measurement of airway size and evaluation of pharyngeal collapsibility are less valuable when the anatomical mechanisms are not separated from the neural mechanisms. These data are difficult to interpret and may not represent the properties of the pharyngeal airway during sleep when the obstruction is initiated. To date, several experimental techniques have been introduced to suppress or eliminate the neural mechanisms and to allow for the assessment of the purely intrinsic structural properties of the pharyngeal airway ("passive or hypotonic pharynx") (18,38); however, no study has been successful in evaluating the neural mechanisms independently from the anatomical mechanisms.

Inherent methodological limitations for assessment of the neural mechanisms also prevent testing the neural hypothesis. First, electromechanical uncoupling makes the interpretation of changes in EMG activity difficult. For instance, an increase in EMG activity of the genioglossus muscle, a major pharyngeal dilator muscle, does not always imply an increase in the cross-sectional area of the pharyngeal airway. Another limitation in interpreting EMG data is the difficulty in comparison between subjects. For the genioglossus, some researchers have normalized EMG activity using 100% maximum activity obtained by a reproducible procedure, such as swallowing or maximum protrusion of the tongue, although this remains controversial (27). In view of these limitations, several studies have simultaneously measured the EMG activity of several 'representative' muscles during the evaluation of actual mechanical changes of the upper airway, including changes in resistance and airway size, in order to correlate observed changes in EMG activity with mechanical changes (27,56).

B. Assessment of the Passive Pharyngeal Airway

One approach for investigating pharyngeal airway maintenance mechanisms is to assess the purely intrinsic structural properties of the pharyngeal airway (anatomical mechanisms) while eliminating the neural mechanisms. As first reported by Wilson et al., elimination of neural mechanisms was possible through postmortem evaluation (57); however, possible alterations of pharyngeal collapsibility caused by postmortem rigidity strictly limits this study population. For the purpose of assessing the hypotonic pharyngeal airway mechanics during wakefulness, Series et al. proposed a technique to assess dynamic flow profiles in response to negative P_{AW} produced by phrenic nerve stimulation (58). While this method eliminates phasic pharyngeal muscle activity, tonic pharyngeal muscle activation could influence the mechanical properties of the pharyngeal airway.

Application of nasal continuous positive P_{AW} in sleeping patients with OSAS depresses pharyngeal muscle activation, and the suppression persists for at least a breath after an abrupt reduction in nasal P_{AW} (39,59). Depending on the reduced level of P_{AW}, various degrees of inspiratory flow limitation or obstructive apnea are induced in this single breath test.

Several studies have used highly sophisticated techniques allowing for simultaneous measurements of breathing and pharyngeal airway patency, and both the static and dynamic behavior of the passive pharyngeal airway, in humans during sleep (38–40,60). Clinical application of this technique is limited, however, because of its technical difficulty. Schwartz et al. combined the abrupt pressure reduction method and Starling Resistor model to assess the collapsibility of the hypotonic pharyngeal airway (61). Based on the finding that the pharyngeal airway behaves like a Starling resistor model in which cessation of flow and occlusion of the collapsible conduit occur when upstream pressure falls below a critical closing pressure (P_{crit}) (62), Schwartz et al. successfully applied the model to the pharyngeal airway and elegantly accounted for mechanisms of inspiratory flow limitation by the pharynx in sleeping adult humans (62). Marcus et al. extended this application to sleeping children and infants (63,64). The maximum inspiratory flow rate (V_{Imax}) during inspiratory flow limitation is directly related to nasal mask pressure (P_N). According to the linear relationship between V_{Imax} and P_N, P_{crit} is defined as the pressure when $V_{Imax} = 0$. Because of the simplicity and ease of obtaining P_{crit} measurements, this method has become popular as a useful experimental tool for investigating the pathophysiology of pharyngeal obstruction in anesthetized as well as sleeping humans (62–66). The contribution of the neural mechanisms to P_{crit} depends on the pattern of P_N changes during the P_{crit} measurements. Gradual reduction of P_N at 30-second intervals until $V_{Imax} = 0$ or until an arousal occurs allows for recruitment of pharyngeal muscle activation, and therefore P_{crit} possibly reflects the collapsibility of the active pharynx in which the neural mechanisms actively operate (gradual P_{crit}). In contrast, intermittent abrupt reductions of P_N for three to five breaths from a higher P_N to various levels of lower P_N prevents recruitment of the pharyngeal muscle activation during P_{crit} measurements, possibly resulting in a hypotonic pharyngeal airway (intermittent P_{crit}) (61,64). In fact, genioglossal muscle activity is not recruited during intermittent P_{crit} measurements in sleeping adult patients with OSAS (61). However, the applicability of this hypotonic method to subjects without OSAS needs to be validated by demonstrating no recruitment of the upper airway muscle activity in response to abrupt reduction of the P_N, since the neural mechanisms are presumably functioning in these subjects, particularly in sleeping infants and children (5,24,67).

Isono et al. developed a simple method for evaluating solely the anatomical mechanisms, independent of the neural mechanisms (18,19,68). Total muscle paralysis is produced by administration of neuromuscular blockade under general anesthesia to completely eliminate the state-dependent and individual variability of pharyngeal and pump muscle contraction. Under these circumstances, endoscopic evaluation of the static mechanics of the passive pharynx is performed, which is graphically best expressed by plotting the P_{AW} and the pharyngeal cross-sectional area (CSA) relationship. The relationship is

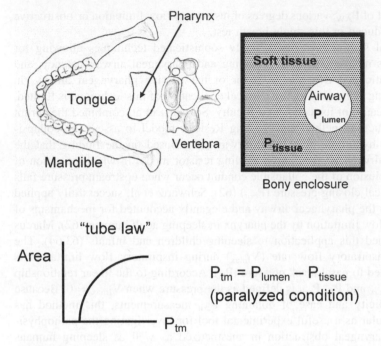

Figure 2 Anatomical arrangements of pharynx, tongue, mandible, and cervical vertebra (*left panel*) and a mechanical model for the structures (*right panel*). In the mechanical model, the luminal size of the collapsible tube is determined by mechanical properties of the tube (tube law) and P_{tm}. P_{tm} is defined as the pressure difference between pressures inside (P_{lumen}) and outside the tube (P_{tissue}). For a given P_{lumen}, an increase in P_{tissue} results in reduction of P_{tm} and therefore narrows the lumen. P_{tissue} is determined by the balance between the amount of soft material inside the rigid box and the size of the surrounding rigid box. *Abbreviations*: P_{tm}, transmural pressure; P_{lumen}, pressure inside the collapsible tube; P_{tissue}, pressure surrounding the collapsible tube. *Source*: From Ref. 50.

fitted by an exponential curve, $CSA = A_{max} - B \exp(-KP_{AW})$, where B and K are constants, and A_{max} denotes maximum CSA. Both the closing pressure of the passive pharynx (P'_{close}) and the K value represent collapsibility of the pharynx. The former determines the position of the exponential curve, and the latter characterizes the shape of the curve. Comparison of these mechanical variables of the passive pharynx between different conditions or populations may clarify conditional or population (age) differences of anatomical mechanisms. For example, Isono et al. demonstrated the contribution of the anatomical hypothesis to the pathogenesis of pediatric and adult OSAS by comparing the variables between controls and patients with OSAS (18,19). The static evaluation of the pharyngeal wall properties, however, does not reveal dynamic processes of pharyngeal obstruction (60). In addition, clinical application is limited because of the need for general anesthesia required for the evaluation.

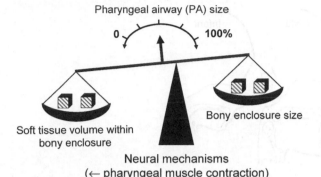

Pharyngeal airway (PA) size

0   100%

Soft tissue volume within
bony enclosure

Bony enclosure size

Neural mechanisms
(← pharyngeal muscle contraction)

Figure 3 Anatomical balance model for explanation of the interaction between neural and anatomical mechanisms focusing on the anatomical balance for determining the PA size. *Abbreviation*: PA, pharyngeal airway. *Source*: From Ref. 49.

IV. Developmental Changes in Pharyngeal Airway Patency

A. Developmental Changes in Anatomical Mechanisms

As illustrated in Figure 4 (49), the craniofacial features of neonates are characterized by a small maxilla and mandible compared with a relatively large cranium. The anatomical balance model, therefore, predicts the presence of upper airway anatomical imbalance and a collapsible pharyngeal airway when the contribution of the neural mechanisms is absent. In fact, Wilson et al. (57) and Reed et al. (69) demonstrated that P'_{close} of the passive pharynx was close to atmospheric pressure in cadaveric neonatal preparations (-0.7 ± 2.0 cmH$_2$O, -0.04 ± 1.5 cmH$_2$O, respectively). Three of nine infants in Wilson's study, and two of five infants in Reed's study had a positive P'_{close}. The results are to be carefully interpreted due to the immaturity of the subjects (mean weight 1420 and 1786 g, respectively) in addition to the cadaveric limitations; however, these studies suggest the necessity of neural mechanisms to maintain patency in the neonatal airway.

The anatomical imbalance in neonates appears to improve during the first year of life in association with the preferential growth of the maxilla and the mandible relative to the cranium. Isono et al. performed pharyngeal endoscopy under general anesthesia with total muscle paralysis in nine normal infants ranging in age from 2 to 12 months, in order to evaluate the anatomical mechanisms during infancy (Fig. 5) (68). They found a direct association between age and A_{max}, reflecting increases in body size. P'_{close} progressively decreases with age during the first year of life (range, 0.7–9.8 cmH$_2$O), decreasing pharyngeal airway collapsibility. Furthermore, a progressive decrease in the K value with maturation indicates a progressive increase in pharyngeal wall

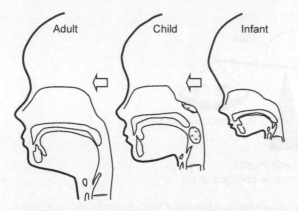

Figure 4 Developmental changes in craniofacial structures from infancy to adulthood are illustrated. Maxillo-mandibular growth, laryngeal descent, and hypertrophy of tonsils and adenoid during development may have significant influences on the PA patency. *Abbreviation*: PA, pharyngeal airway. *Source*: From Ref. 49.

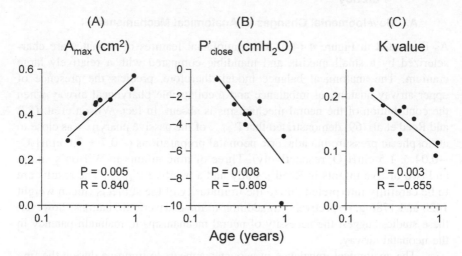

Figure 5 Changes in static mechanics of the passive pharynx within the first year of life. K value represents stiffness of the wall. *Abbreviations*: A_{max}, maximum velopharyngeal area; P_{close}, closing pressure. *Source*: From Ref. 68.

stiffness, which reflects structural changes such as separation of the tip of the epiglottis from the soft palate, downward displacement of the larynx and hyoid bone, and elongation of the pharyngeal airway. These findings indicate that the anatomical properties of the pharynx progressively gain stability in favor of maintaining a patent airway within the first year of life. Using the intermittent

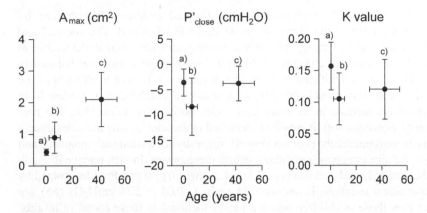

Figure 6 Differences in A_{max}, P'_{close}, and K value among different age groups. **a)** 9 infants (data from Ref. 68), **b)** 13 children (data from Ref. 19), **c)** 17 adults (data from Ref. 18). All data were obtained under general anesthesia with complete paralysis. Closed circles represent mean values and bars indicate SD. *Abbreviations*: A_{max}, maximum velopharyngeal area; P'_{close}, estimated closing pressure. *Source*: From Refs. 68.

P_{crit} technique, Marcus et al. reported that the hypotonic P_{crit} of infants was far below atmospheric pressure (-25 cmH$_2$O) during NREM sleep (64). These observations agree with the polysomnographic observation that obstructive apnea frequency during sleep in infants is highest in weeks 2 to 7 of postnatal age (0.1 events per hour of sleep) and significantly decreases after the seventh week (0 events per hour of sleep) (70).

The pattern of craniofacial growth is determined genetically as well as functionally, and 70% of the growth is completed by 12 years of age (71). During childhood, the preferential growth of the mandible and maxilla continues, increasing the bony enclosure size surrounding the pharynx. In contrast, the concomitant increase in soft tissue volume inside the bony structures, and the hypertrophy of lymphoid tissue such as adenoid and tonsils during childhood, may counteract the beneficial effects of facial growth on pharyngeal airway patency. There is a reduction in the passive P_{close} in children (-7.4 ± 4.9 cmH$_2$O) (19) compared with infants (-3.6 ± 2.7 cmH$_2$O) (Fig. 6) (68), indicating that the anatomical balance favors improvement of pharyngeal patency in most children. Marcus et al. reported that the median value of the hypotonic P_{crit} in sleeping children, determined by the intermittent P_{crit} technique, was -25 cmH$_2$O (64). Notably, the passive P_{close} of children is far below atmospheric pressure and is the lowest among all age groups, which indicates that the pharyngeal airway is open even without neural mechanisms at atmospheric pressure and is anatomically the most stable during childhood. Therefore, obstructive apnea events during sleep are rarely seen in children (less than 1 event per hour of sleep) (72).

The craniofacial development in infants and children, characterized by preferential growth of the mandible, slows down in adulthood. The adenoid and tonsils, which enlarge during childhood, atrophy and are often undetectable in adults. These structural changes are likely to improve the anatomical balance in adults. However, a significant increase in soft tissue is observed in all parts of the body during the transitional period from childhood to adulthood, as is evident from the significant increase in the body mass index during this period (46). The protrusion of submental soft tissue often identified in the adult profile indicates excess soft tissue surrounding the pharynx (Fig. 4), suggestive of anatomical imbalance and pharyngeal airway narrowing without neural mechanisms. In fact, passive P'_{close} in anesthetized and paralyzed adults (-4.4 ± 4.2 cmH$_2$O) (18) and P_{crit} determined by the intermittent technique in anesthetized adults (-0.04 ± 2.74 cmH$_2$O) (65) are higher than those in children and are nearly identical to those found in infants. The differences between children and adults with passive pharyngeal airway collapsibility are in agreement with the fact that the normal values of apnea frequency are much less in children (<1 episode per hour of sleep) than in adults (<5 episodes per hour of sleep) (72,73). However, the differences in anatomical mechanisms alone do not explain why adults have more obstructive apneas than infants, considering that both age groups have a nearly identical mean P'_{close}. The discrepancy between changes in anatomical mechanisms and sleep apnea frequency during development can be explained by the differences in neural mechanisms contributing to pharyngeal airway patency.

B. Developmental Changes in Neural Mechanisms

Pharyngeal EMG studies in sleeping preterm infants demonstrated an immediate and significant augmentation of EMG activity in response to nasal occlusion, indicating that infants have a strong negative pressure reflex (5,24,74). These neural mechanisms in young infants compensate for the relatively high collapsibility of the passive pharyngeal airway described above, resulting in stabilization of pharyngeal airway patency and infrequent obstructive episodes. In fact, Roberts et al. reported that the P'_{close} values obtained during nasal occlusion in sleeping neonates and infants were below atmospheric pressure and were significantly lower than passive P'_{close} values even at the first occluded breath (neonates, -2.8 ± 1.9 cmH$_2$O; infants, -7.7 ± 0.5 cmH$_2$O) (49,75). Active P'_{close} values progressively improved during nasal occlusion, and a direct correlation between genioglossal EMG activity and P'_{close} was observed (Fig. 7) (7).

Jeffries et al. reported that no normal child exhibited phasic inspiratory activity of the genioglossus for more than 50% of sleep time, whereas most children with OSAS showed EMG activity (76). Katz et al. recently measured the genioglossal EMG activity with an intraoral surface electrode in six normal children, and found no reduction in EMG activity during sleep onset (77). One possible interpretation of these data is that normal children do not necessarily operate their neural mechanisms during wakefulness as well as sleep, probably

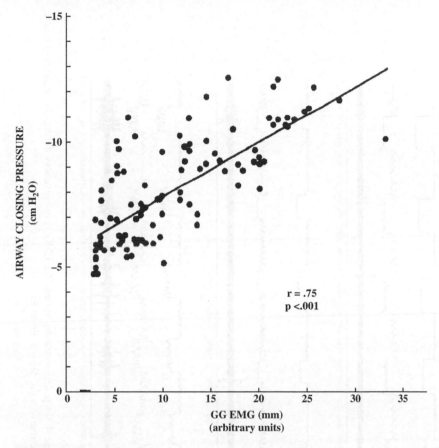

Figure 7   Plot of airway P'_{close} versus amount of GG-EMG activity at time of closure for nasal occlusion during sleep in a neonate with micrognathia. A significant correlation between the variables was evident. *Abbreviations*: P'_{close}, closing pressure; GG-EMG, genioglossal electromyogram. *Source*: From Ref. 7.

due to the stable anatomical structures of the pharyngeal airway. More recently, Katz et al. examined genioglossal EMG responses to negative P_{AW} in 19 normal children during NREM sleep. They found marked variability in individual EMG responsiveness, but it was consistent within subjects (67) (Fig. 8). The overall responsiveness to negative P_{AW} in normal children appears to be intermediate between infants (5,24,74) and adults (4).

Kuna and Smickley measured the genioglossal EMG activity in normal sleeping adults and found that nasal obstruction was associated with only a small increase in the genioglossal EMG activity on the first occluded inspiratory effort

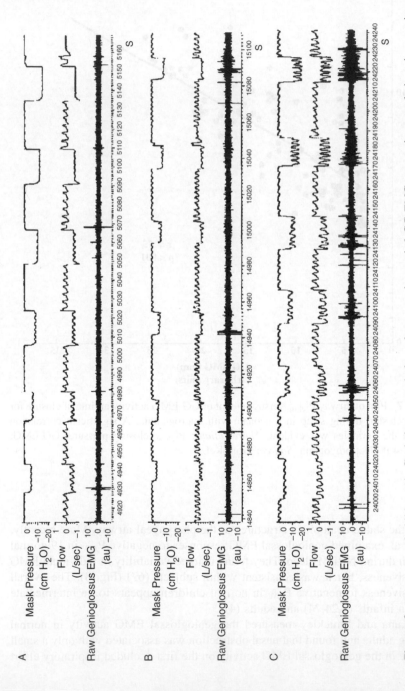

Figure 8 Three normal children (A–C) during stage 4 sleep demonstrating varied GG EMG responsiveness during six negative-pressure challenges. *Abbreviation:* GG EMG, genioglossal electromyogram. *Source:* From Ref. 67.

(4). Increase in the genioglossal EMG activity was proportional to that of the diaphragm activity on the first three occluded efforts. This is in significant contrast to the preferential activation of the upper airway muscles without activation of the diaphragm in infants (24). The negative pressure reflex developed during infancy is believed to diminish later in life, as numerous studies have reported depression of the negative pressure reflex in adults during sleep (32,33). Considering that the pharyngeal airway is equally collapsible in the absence of neural mechanisms in infants and adults (68), adults significantly increase upper airway resistance (78) and develop more obstructive events during sleep than infants, probably due to a different contribution of neural mechanisms to pharyngeal airway maintenance.

V. Mechanical Influences on Pharyngeal Airway Patency

A. Head and Mandible Positions

Within one subject, mandible enclosure size varies with head and mandible positioning changes, resulting in changes in the upper airway anatomical balance (50). The anatomical balance model predicts that neck extension and mandibular advancement increase the mandible enclosure size, favoring maintenance of pharyngeal airway patency, whereas neck flexion and bite opening decrease the mandible enclosure size, narrowing the pharyngeal airway. Thus, pharyngeal airway patency may vary with head and mandible position changes when the neural mechanisms are depressed, particularly during sleep. Although numerous previous studies have reported changes in pharyngeal airway patency in response to head and mandible position changes, studies concerning mechanical influences on anatomical mechanisms for pharyngeal airway maintenance (50,57,69,79) and those examining neural responses to structural changes, particularly during sleep (7,80,81), are few.

Wilson et al. demonstrated a significant influence of head and neck position on the upper airway P_{close} in infants postmortem (57). The P_{close} values in the neutral neck position (-0.7 ± 2.0 cmH$_2$O) increased in a dose-dependent fashion during neck flexion ($+7.4 \pm 4.6$ cmH$_2$O) and decreased during neck extension (-5.2 ± 0.8 cmH$_2$O) (Fig. 9) (57). In anesthetized and paralyzed patients with OSAS, Isono et al. reported a significant increase in the passive P_{close} of approximately 3 cmH$_2$O and reduction of the pharyngeal area during maximal neck flexion, a significant decrease in the passive P_{close} of approximately 4 cmH$_2$O, and an increase in the pharyngeal area during maximal neck extension (50). Notably, stiffening of the pharyngeal airway was also observed during neck extension. Increased upper airway length during neck extension probably increases longitudinal tension of the pharyngeal airway wall, as demonstrated in anesthetized cats with an isolated upper airway (82). Neck flexion appears to have a more profound influence on pharyngeal patency in infants than

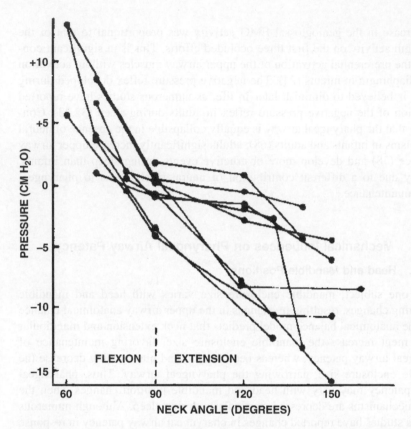

Figure 9 Upper airway P′$_{close}$ plotted against degree of neck flexion or extension (neck angle) for each of nine infants after death. Points for individual infants are connected by straight lines. *Abbreviation*: P′$_{close}$, closing pressure. *Source*: From Ref. 57.

in adults, probably due to the different structural configuration of the upper airway and the different flexibility of the head and neck.

The appropriate use of a pillow produces neck flexion with upper cervical extension. Since the mandible enclosure size is increased by this "sniffing position," the anatomical balance model predicts improvement of pharyngeal airway patency. In fact, Isono et al. demonstrated an increase in the pharyngeal area and a significant decrease in the passive P′$_{close}$ at both the velopharynx and oropharynx of approximately 3 to 4 cmH$_2$O in completely paralyzed and anesthetized adults with OSAS (79). The absence of a significant improvement in disordered breathing frequency with the use of a pillow in patients with severe OSAS may be due to inadequate normalization of pharyngeal collapsibility, concomitant occurrence of bite opening, and/or accidental neck flexion (83).

To maintain airway patency, neural mechanisms need to compensate for pharyngeal anatomical imbalances that result from various mechanical loads. Roberts et al. assessed the response of the genioglossus to experimentally induced neck flexion in sleeping infants with micrognathia (7). They observed that flexion of the neck resulted in upper airway obstruction and that tonic and phasic genioglossal activity progressively increased during the obstruction, with increasing inspiratory drive (Fig. 10). The patent airway and breathing were reestablished immediately after the burst of genioglossal activity. Neural responses should operate better during wakefulness since flexion of the neck during wakefulness does not usually cause flow-limited inspiration or apnea. Bonora et al. suggested reflex mechanisms for regulation of upper airway muscles in response to head position changes (84). They found an instantaneous increase and decrease in genioglossal muscle activity in response to neck flexion and extension in spontaneously breathing awake cats. The responses were diminished but present during breathing through a tracheostomy and were not eliminated by bilateral superior laryngeal nerve section, suggesting little contribution of the reflex from upper airway receptors, and possible involvement of reflexes from vestibular or joint receptors. Variability of both head and mandible positions and the neural responsiveness during sleep may partly account for the variable breathing pattern during sleep within a subject.

Adult patients with OSAS are reported to spend more time with a bite opening greater than 5 mm during sleep ($69 \pm 23\%$) than subjects without OSAS ($11 \pm 12\%$) (85). Isono et al. reported that opening the bite by 1.5 cm increased P'_{close} by 3 cmH_2O in anesthetized and paralyzed patients with OSAS, indicating that bite opening results in upper airway anatomical imbalance (50). EMG activity of both bite opening (lateral pterygoid) and bite closing (masseter) muscles progressively decreased before apneic episodes, and increased at termination of apnea, similar to pharyngeal dilator muscle action (80,81). Interestingly, Hollowell and Suratt noticed inspiratory bite opening both before and after apnea (80). The inspiratory bite opening may be primarily caused by increased negative P_{AW}, which retracts the tongue musculature and rotates the mandible, whereas expiratory bite opening may result from masseter relaxation. Bite opening is also capable of increasing electromechanical uncoupling by changing the vector force direction of the pharyngeal dilator muscles, such as the genioglossus and the geniohyoid. While bite opening induces switching from nasal to oral breathing, bite opening itself is not beneficial for pharyngeal airway maintenance.

Oral appliances, which maintain a forward mandible, are one of the options for treatment of OSAS. A few studies have reported clinical usefulness of the devices in pediatric patients with OSAS (86), although the effectiveness has only been documented in adult patients (87). In anesthetized, paralyzed adult patients with OSAS, Kato et al. reported that mandibular advancement reduced the passive closing pressures at both the velopharynx and the oropharynx in a dose-dependent fashion (88). Interestingly, no improvement in velopharyngeal closing pressure was observed in response to mandibular advancement in anesthetized, obese

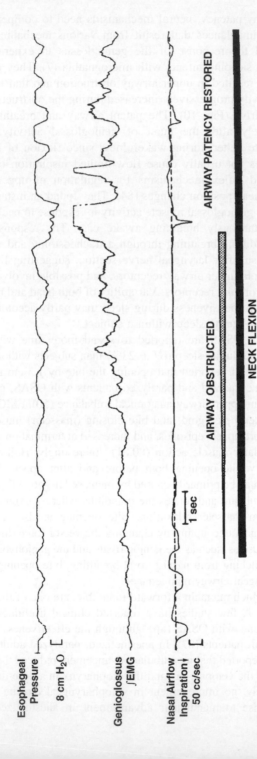

Figure 10 Tracings showing occurrence and resolution of upper airway obstruction associated with experimental neck flexion. During the period of airway obstruction, both inspiratory drive and phasic GG-EMG progressively increased. Despite continued neck flexion, nasal airflow was reestablished in association with increased phasic GG-EMG activity. *Abbreviation:* GG-EMG, genioglossal electromyogram. *Source:* From Ref. 7.

adults, while oropharyngeal P'_{close} was significantly decreased (89). In sleeping adult patients with OSAS, genioglossus muscle activity decreased in response to mandible advancement (Oshima T and Remmers JE, personal communication). Improvement of the anatomical balance by mandibular advancement is likely to diminish the necessity of neural compensatory mechanisms.

B. Body Positions

The gravitational force on the soft tissue around the pharyngeal airway is thought to influence pharyngeal airway maintenance, since the lateral recumbent position and sitting are known to decrease apneic events in patients with OSAS (90,91). Structurally, the large mass of the tongue anteriorly encroaches on the airway within the mandibular enclosure, and only a thin muscular and mucosal layer posteriorly connects the airway with the cervical vertebrae (Fig. 2). Because of this uneven distribution of soft tissue within the bony enclosure, the gravitational impact on the airway may be greatest in the supine position, decreasing in the lateral recumbent and seated positions. In fact, the lateral recumbent position was reported to decrease the P'_{close} of the passive pharynx in patients with OSAS (92). In this context, the prone position is expected to have the smallest gravitational impact on the airway, leading to improvement of pharyngeal airway patency. However, recent observations in anesthetized and paralyzed infants do not support this speculation (93). In agreement with the previous observations by Safar et al. in unconscious adults (94), Ishikawa et al. found that the prone position in fact narrowed the passive pharyngeal airway and increased the P'_{close} of the passive pharynx to above atmospheric pressure, even in normal infants (Fig. 11) (93). Since frequency of apnea in the prone position did not differ from that in the supine position in normal infants, the neural mechanisms should operate to maintain a

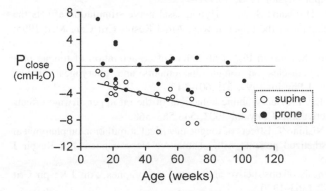

Figure 11 The P_{close} values of the passive pharynx obtained during supine and prone positions are plotted against age for each of 19 infants and small children. The age dependency of P_{close} in the supine position is absent in the prone position. P_{close} was above atmospheric pressure in 10 subjects. *Abbreviation*: P_{close}, closing pressure. *Source*: From Ref. 93.

patent airway even during sleep. However, there have not been any EMG studies to support this speculation. Of note, complete pharyngeal obstruction was confirmed by postmortem CT scan in sudden infant death syndrome victims who were found dead in the prone position (95). Pharyngeal obstruction in the prone position may result from impairment of neural mechanisms, including arousal responses.

References

1. Remmers JE, deGroot WJ, Sauerland EK, et al. Pathogenesis of upper airway occlusion during sleep. J Appl Physiol 1978; 44:931–938.
2. Feroah TR, Forster HV, Pan LG, et al. Reciprocal activation of hypopharyngeal muscles and their effect on upper airway area. J Appl Physiol 2000; 88:611–626.
3. Kuna ST, Smickley JS. Superior pharyngeal constrictor activation in obstructive sleep apnea. Am J Respir Crit Care Med 1997; 156:874–880.
4. Kuna ST, Smickley J. Response of genioglossus muscle activity to nasal airway occlusion in normal sleeping adults. J Appl Physiol 1988; 64:347–353.
5. Cohen G, Henderson-Smart DJ. Upper airway muscle activity during nasal occlusion in newborn babies. J Appl Physiol 1989; 66:1328–1335.
6. Duara S, Rojas M, Claure N. Upper airway stability and respiratory muscle activity during inspiratory loading in full-term neonates. J Appl Physiol 1994; 77:37–42.
7. Roberts JL, Reed WR, Mathew OP, et al. Control of respiratory activity of the genioglossus muscle in micrognathic infants. J Appl Physiol 1986; 61:1523–1533.
8. Parisi RA, Neubauer JA, Frank MM, et al. Correlation between genioglossal and diaphragmatic responses to hypercapnia during sleep. Am Rev Respir Dis 1987; 135:378–382.
9. Parisi RA, Santiago TV, Edelman NH. Genioglossal and diaphragmatic EMG responses to hypoxia during sleep. Am Rev Respir Dis 1988; 138:610–616.
10. Brouillette RT, Thach BT. A neuromuscular mechanism maintaining extrathoracic airway patency. J Appl Physiol 1979; 46:772–779.
11. Hida W, Kurosaswa H, Okabe S, et al. Hypoglossal nerve stimulation affects the pressure-volume behavior of the upper airway. Am J Respir Crit Care Med 1995; 151:455–460.
12. Fuller DD, Williams JS, Janssen PL, et al. Effect of co-activation of tongue protrudor and retractor muscles on tongue movements and pharyngeal airflow mechanics in the rat. J Physiol 1999; 519:601–613.
13. Bailey EF, Fregosi RF. Pressure-volume behaviour of the rat upper airway: effects of tongue muscle activation. J Physiol 2003; 548:563–568.
14. Isono S, Tanaka A, Nishino T. Effects of tongue electrical stimulation on pharyngeal mechanics in anaesthetized patients with obstructive sleep apnoea. Eur Respir J 1999; 14:1258–1265.
15. White DP. Pathogenesis of obstructive and central sleep apnea. Am J Respir Crit Care Med 2005; 172:1363–1370.
16. Horner RL. Impact of brainstem sleep mechanisms on pharyngeal motor control. Respir Physiol 2000; 119:113–121.
17. Strohl KP, Hensley MJ, Hallett M, et al. Activation of upper airway muscles before onset of inspiration in normal humans. J Appl Physiol 1980; 49:638–642.

18. Isono S, Remmers JE, Tanaka A, et al. Anatomy of pharynx in patients with obstructive sleep apnea and in normal subjects. J Appl Physiol 1997; 82:1319–1326.
19. Isono S, Shimada A, Utsugi M, et al. Comparison of static mechanical properties of the passive pharynx between normal children and children with sleep disordered breathing. Am J Respir Crit Care Med 1998; 157:1204–1212.
20. Jelev A, Sood S, Liu H, et al. Microdialysis perfusion of 5-HT into hypoglossal motor nucleus differentially modulates genioglossus activity across natural sleep-wake states in rats. J Physiol 2001; 532:467–481.
21. Fenik VB, Davies RO, Kubin L. REM sleep-like atonia of hypoglossal (XII) motoneurons is caused by loss of noradrenergic and serotonergic inputs. Am J Respir Crit Care Med 2005; 172:1322–1330.
22. Horner RL, Innes JA, Holden HB, et al. Afferent pathway(s) for pharyngeal dilator reflex to negative pressure in man: a study using upper airway anaesthesia. J Physiol 1991; 436:31–44.
23. Basner RC, Ringler J, Berkowitz S, et al. Effect of inspired air temperature on genioglossus activity during nose breathing in awake humans. J Appl Physiol 1990; 69(3):1098–1103.
24. Carlo WA, Miller MJ, Martin RJ. Differential response of respiratory muscles to airway occlusion in infants. J Appl Physiol 1985; 59:847–852.
25. Doherty LS, Nolan P, McNicholas WT. Effects of topical anesthesia on upper airway resistance during wake-sleep transitions. J Appl Physiol 2005; 99:549–555.
26. McNicholas WT, Coffey M, McDonnell T. Upper airway obstruction during sleep in normal subjects after selective topical oropharyngeal anesthesia. Am Rev Respir Dis 1987; 135:1316–1319.
27. Mezzanotte WS, Tanjel DJ, White DP. Waking genioglossal electromyogram in sleep apnea patients versus normal controls: a neuromuscular compensatory mechanism. J Clin Invest 1992; 89:1571–1579.
28. Fogel RB, Malhotra A, Pillar G, et al. Genioglossal activation in patients with obstructive sleep apnea versus control subjects: mechanisms of muscle control. Am J Respir Crit Care Med 2001; 164:2025–2030.
29. Gozal D, Burnside MM. Increased upper airway collapsibility in children with obstructive sleep apnea during wakefulness. Am J Respir Crit Care Med 2004; 169:163–167.
30. Sauerland EK, Harper RM. The human tongue during sleep: electromyographic activity of the genioglossus muscle. Exp Neurol 1976; 51:160–170.
31. Tangel DJ, Mezzanotte WS, White DP. Influence of sleep on tensor palatini EMG and upper airway resistance in normal men. J Appl Physiol 1991; 70:2574–2581.
32. Malhotra A, Pillar G, Fogel RB, et al. Genioglossal but not palatal muscle activity relates closely to pharyngeal pressure. Am J Respir Crit Care Med 2000; 162:1058–1062.
33. Wheatley JR, Tangel DJ, Mezzanotte WS, et al. Influence of sleep on response to negative airway pressure of tensor palatini muscle and retropalatal airway. J Appl Physiol 1993; 75:2117–2124.
34. Shea SA, Akahoshi T, Edwards JK, et al. Influence of chemoreceptor stimuli on genioglossal response to negative pressure in humans. Am J Respir Crit Care Med 2000; 162:559–565.
35. Akahoshi T, White DP, Edwards JK, et al. Phasic mechanoreceptor stimuli can induce phasic activation of upper airway muscles in humans. J Physiol 2001; 531:677–691.

36. Fogel RB, Trinder J, Malhotra A, et al. Within-breath control of genioglossal muscle activation in humans: effect of sleep-wake state. J Physiol 2003; 550:899–910.
37. Henke KG. Upper airway muscle activity and upper airway resistance in young adults during sleep. J Appl Physiol 1998; 84:486–491.
38. Isono S, Morrison DL, Launois SH, et al. Static mechanics of the velopharynx of patients with obstructive sleep apnea. J Appl Physiol 1993; 75:148–154.
39. Launois SH, Feroah TR, Campbell WN, et al. Site of pharyngeal narrowing predicts outcome of surgery for obstructive sleep apnea. Am Rev Respir Dis 1993; 147: 182–189.
40. Morrison DL, Launois SH, Isono S, et al. Pharyngeal narrowing and closing pressure in patients with obstructive sleep apnea. Am Rev Respir Dis 1993; 148: 606–611.
41. Gunn TR, Tonkin SL, Hadden W, et al. Neonatal micrognathia is associated with small upper airways on radiographic measurement. Acta Paediatr 2000; 89:82–87.
42. Jamieson AC, Guilleminault C, Partinen M, et al. Obstructive sleep apneic patients have craniofacial abnormalities. Sleep 1986; 9:469–477.
43. Schechter MS; Section on Pediatric Pulmonology, Subcommittee on Obstructive Sleep Apnea Syndrome. Technical report: diagnosis and management of childhood obstructive sleep apnea syndrome. Pediatrics 2002; 109:e69.
44. Schwab RJ, Pasirstein M, Pierson R, et al. Identification of upper airway anatomic risk factors for obstructive sleep apnea with volumetric magnetic resonance imaging. Am J Respir Crit Care Med 2003; 168:522–530.
45. Kahn A, Mozin MJ, Rebuffat E, et al. Sleep pattern alterations and brief airway obstructions in overweight infants. Sleep 1989; 12:430–438.
46. Redline S, Schluchter MD, Larkin EK, et al. Predictors of longitudinal change in sleep-disordered breathing in a nonclinic population. Sleep 2003; 26:703–709.
47. Isono S. Contribution of obesity and craniofacial abnormalities to pharyngeal collapsibility in patients with obstructive sleep apnea. Sleep Biol Rhythms 2004; 2: 17–21.
48. Watanabe T, Isono S, Tanaka A, et al. Contribution of body habitus and craniofacial characteristics to segmental closing pressures of the passive pharynx in patients with sleep disordered breathing. Am J Crit Care Med 2002; 165:260–265.
49. Isono S. Developmental changes of patency: implications for pediatric anesthesia. Paediatr Anaesth 2006; 16:109–122.
50. Isono S, Tanaka A, Tagaito Y, et al. Influences of head positions and bite opening on collapsibility of the passive pharynx. J Appl Physiol 2004; 97:339–346.
51. Shelton KE, Gay SB, Hollowell DE, et al. Mandible enclosure of upper airway and weight in obstructive sleep apnea. Am Rev Respir Dis 1993; 148:195–200.
52. Winter WC, Gampper T, Gay SB, et al. Enlargement of the lateral pharyngeal fat pad space in pigs increases upper airway resistance. J Appl Physiol 1995; 79: 726–731.
53. Isono S, Tanaka A, Nishino T. Dynamic interaction between the tongue and soft palate during obstructive apnea. J Appl Physiol 2003; 95:2257–2264.
54. Kairaitis K, Parikh R, Stavrinou R, et al. Upper airway extraluminal tissue pressure fluctuations during breathing in rabbits. J Appl Physiol 2003; 95:1560–1566.
55. Kuna S, Remmers JE. Anatomy and physiology of upper airway obstruction. In: Kryger MH, Roth T, Dement WC, eds. Principles and Practice of Sleep Medicine, (3rd edition). Philadelphia: WB Saunders Inc., 2000:840–858.

56. Mortimore IL, Mathur R, Douglas NJ. Effects of posture, route of respiration, and negative pressure on palatal muscle activity in humans. J Appl Physiol 1995; 79:448–454.

57. Wilson SL, Thach BT, Brouillette RT, et al. Upper airway patency in human infant: influence of airway pressure and posture. J Appl Physiol 1980; 48:500–504.

58. Series F, Ethier G. Assessment of upper airway stabilizing forces with the use of phrenic nerve stimulation in conscious humans. J Appl Physiol 2003; 94:2289–2295.

59. Deegan PC, Nolan P, Carey M, et al. Effects of positive airway pressure on upper airway dilator muscle activity and ventilatory timing. J Appl Physiol 1996; 81:470–479.

60. Isono S, Feroah TR, Hajduk EA, et al. Interaction of cross-sectional area, driving pressure and airflow of passive velopharynx. J Appl Physiol 1997; 83:851–859.

61. Schwartz AR, O'Donnell CP, Baron J, et al. The hypotonic upper airway in obstructive sleep apnea: role of structures and neuromuscular activity. Am J Respir Crit Care Med 1998; 157:1051–1077.

62. Schwartz AR, Smith PL, Wise RA, et al. Induction of upper airway occlusion in sleeping individuals with subatmospheric nasal pressure. J Appl Physiol 1988; 64:535–542.

63. Marcus CL, McColley SA, Carroll JL, et al. Upper airway collapsibility in children with obstructive sleep apnea syndrome. J Appl Physiol 1994; 77:918–924.

64. Marcus CL, Fernandes D, Prado LB, et al. Developmental changes in upper airway dynamics. J Appl Physiol 2004; 97:98–108.

65. Eastwood PR, Szollosi I, Platt PR, et al. Comparison of upper airway collapse during general anaesthesia and sleep. Lancet 2002; 359:1207–1209.

66. Rowley JA, Zhou X, Vergine I, et al. Influence of gender on upper airway mechanics: upper airway resistance and Pcrit. J Appl Physiol 2001; 91:2248–2254.

67. Katz ES, Marcus CL, White DP. Influence of airway pressure on genioglossus activity during sleep in normal children. Am J Respir Crit Care Med 2006; 173: 902–909.

68. Isono S, Tanaka A, Ishikawa T, et al. Developmental changes in collapsibility of the passive pharynx during infancy. Am J Respir Crit Care Med 2000; 162:832–836.

69. Reed WR, Roberts JL, Thach BT. Factors influencing regional patency and configuration of the human infant upper airway. J Appl Physiol 1985; 58:635–644.

70. Kato I, Franco P, Groswasser J, et al. Frequency of obstructive and mixed sleep apneas in 1,023 infants. Sleep 2000; 23:487–492.

71. Todd JT, Mark LS, Shaw RE, et al. The perception of human growth. Sci Am 1980; 242:132–134.

72. Marcus CL, Omlin KJ, Basinki DJ, et al. Normal polysomnographic values for children and adolescents. Am Rev Respir Dis 1992; 146:1235–1239.

73. Rosen CL, D'Andrea L, Haddad GG. Adult criteria for obstructive sleep apnea do not identify children with serious obstruction. Am Rev Respir Dis 1992; 146: 1231–1234.

74. Gauda EB, Miller MJ, Carlo WA, et al. Genioglossus response to airway occlusion in apneic versus nonapneic infants. Pediatr Res 1987; 22:683–687.

75. Roberts JL, Reed WR, Mathew OP, et al. Assessment of pharyngeal stability in normal and micrognathic infants. J Appl Physiol 1985; 58:290–299.

76. Jeffries B, Brouillette RT, Hunt CE. Electromyographic study of some accessory muscles of respiration in children with obstructive sleep apnea. Am Rev Respir Dis 1984; 129:696–702.

77. Katz ES, White DP. Genioglossus activity in children with obstructive sleep apnea during wakefulness and sleep onset. Am J Respir Crit Care Med 2003; 168:664–670.

78. Hudgel DW, Martin RJ, Johnson B, et al. Mechanics of the respiratory system and breathing pattern during sleep in normal humans. J Appl Physiol 1984; 56:133–137.

79. Isono S, Tanaka A, Ishikawa T, et al. Sniffing position improves patency in patients with obstructive sleep apnea. Anesthesiology 2005; 103:489–494.

80. Hollowell DE, Suratt PM. Mandible position and activation of submental and masseter muscles during sleep. J Appl Physiol 1991; 71:2267–2273.

81. Yoshida K. A polysomnographic study on masticatory and tongue muscle activity during obstructive and central sleep apnea. J Oral Rehabil 1998; 25:603–609.

82. Thut DC, Schwartz AR, Roach D, et al. Tracheal and neck position influence upper airway airflow dynamics by altering airway length. J Appl Physiol 1993; 75: 2084–2090.

83. Kushida CA, Rao S, Guilleminault C, et al. Cervical positional effects on snoring and apneas. Sleep Res Online 1999; 2:7–10.

84. Bonora M, Bartlett D Jr., Knuth SL. Changes in upper airway muscle activity related to head position in awake cats. Respir Physiol 1985; 60:181–192.

85. Miyamoto K, Ozbek MM, Lowe AA, et al. Mandibular posture during sleep in patients with obstructive sleep apnoea. Arch Oral Biol 1999; 44:657–664.

86. Villa MP, Bernkopf E, Pagani J, et al. Randomized controlled study of an oral jaw-positioning appliance for the treatment of obstructive sleep apnea in children with malocclusion. Am J Respir Crit Care Med 2002; 165:123–127.

87. Schmidt-Nowara W, Lowe A, Wiegand L, et al. Oral appliances for the treatment of snoring and obstructive sleep apnea: a review. Sleep 1995; 18:501–510.

88. Kato J, Isono S, Tanaka A, et al. Dose dependent effects of mandibular advancement on pharyngeal mechanics and nocturnal oxygenation in patients with obstructive sleep apnea. Chest 2000; 117:1065–1072.

89. Isono S, Tanaka A, Tagaito Y, et al. Pharyngeal patency in response to advancement of the mandible in obese anesthetized persons. Anesthesiology 1997; 87:1055–1062.

90. McEvoy RD, Sharp DJ, Thornton AT. The effects of posture on obstructive sleep apnea. Am Rev Respir Dis 1986; 133:662–666.

91. Cartwright RD. Effect of sleep position on sleep apnea severity. Sleep 1984; 7: 110–114.

92. Isono S, Tanaka A, Nishino T. Lateral position decreases collapsibility of the passive pharynx in patients with obstructive sleep apnea. Anesthesiology 2002; 97:780–785.

93. Ishikawa T, Isono S, Aiba J, et al. Prone position increases collapsibility of the passive pharynx in infants and small children. Am J Respir Crit Care Med 2002; 166:760–764.

94. Safar P, Escarraga LA, Chang F. Upper airway obstruction in the unconscious patient. J Appl Physiol 1959; 14:760–764.

95. Rambaud C, Guilleminault C. "Back to sleep" and unexplained death in infants. Sleep 2004; 27:1359–1366.

7

Craniofacial Development and the Airway During Sleep

NALTON F. FERRARO
Children's Hospital, Boston, Massachusetts, U.S.A.

I. Introduction

Patency of the upper airway during sleep is integrally related to craniofacial morphology, but craniofacial structure is only one element that defines airway patency. If a tube is narrow enough, its walls collapsible enough, and the transluminal pressure differential great enough, the tube will fail as a conduit. This happens in the obstructive sleep apnea syndrome (OSAS). This tube, the upper airway, has daunting structural complexity and variability. There are two main intake ports in this tube; internally, it has recesses, multiple valves, movable baffles, and glands that can swell or fill parts of the tube with mucus. The rigidity of the tube can change very quickly secondary to both internal and external control factors; parts of this tube can grow into the lumen (e.g., tonsils). The tube carries multiple fluids, and it works better in certain positions than others. This is the normal human upper airway and functions beautifully most of the time.

To fully understand the upper airway, it will be useful to examine the normal airway, the congenitally abnormal airway (nature's experiments), and therapeutic interventions that attempt to change the airway. In this way, one can gain insight into the impact that structure has on the function of this complex system. Much of what goes on in the upper airway is controlled centrally (1). Neuromuscular control, tone, and central feedback loops are ultimately what determine airway patency, but these crucial factors will not be the focus in this discussion of craniofacial development and anatomy. This structure is, of course, an artifice, because the size and shape of this tortuous tube is under moment-to-moment central nervous system control. This portrait of the craniofacial skeleton is a snapshot, for the sake of clarity, of what is really a moving picture. Marcus and her colleagues have done a great deal to elucidate these neuromuscular mechanisms, particularly during infancy and early childhood. The observation that children snore less frequently than adults and have fewer full obstructive apneas leads to the counterintuitive conclusion that the airway may be less collapsible in children. Studies with subatmospheric pressure loading of the upper airway reveal that the young are more adept at mounting compensatory responses to negative pressure on the airway. Increasing body mass index is an associated factor in this degradation of compensatory responses as one ages (2).

The Johns Hopkins group also analyzed the upper airway pressure-flow relationship in sleep of infants, prepubertal children, and adults. The airway was more collapsible in adults than in infants and children. The infant airway was particularly resistant to collapse and responded to negative pressure loading, whereas the adults' did not (3). These compensatory mechanisms are lessened in OSAS. In general, ventilatory drive may be normal in OSAS despite age; however, upper airway tone and reflexes during sleep are increased in infants and children compared with adults. Tone and reflex vary with age. Arens and Marcus speculate that these mechanisms may be in place to compensate for the relatively narrower airway in infants and children (4).

Using a customized intraoral genioglossus electrode, Katz et al. demonstrated wide variation in neuromuscular compensatory responses. Certain subjects could maintain minute ventilation with negative airway pressure challenges (5). These studies clearly demonstrate how physiological signals can control anatomy.

The airway patency in a retrognathic child, a midface-deficient infant, or even a child with large tonsils is still subject to these central controls, but the structural abnormalities place rather strict limitations on tube patency no matter what the brain tries to do to overcome or compensate. This is a dynamic and everchanging relationship between anatomy and physiology. Sometimes neuromuscular mechanisms can overcome anatomic abnormalities. Sometimes anatomic problems overwhelm any compensatory mechanism that may exist.

Two types of macroglossia illustrate this relationship. In a Boston Children's Hospital series of 14 babies with Beckwith-Wiedemann syndrome and significant macroglossia, only three babies had significant OSAS. Is the lack of OSAS in this group secondary to a large airway (these babies are large), protective neuromuscular tone, or a combination of some other unknown factors? When one studies the picture of the baby with macroglossia (Fig. 1), the lack of OSAS is intriguing and counterintuitive.

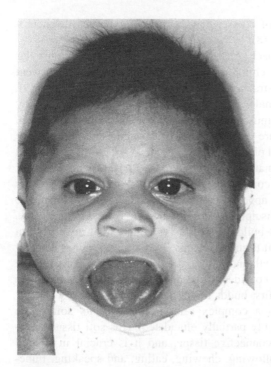

Figure 1 An infant with Beckwith-Wiedemann syndrome. Severe macroglossia and no OSAS.

Sometimes the pathological encroachment by sheer mass in the airway makes it extremely difficult for a child to maintain airway patency despite any compensation. In another Boston Children's Hospital series, lymphatic malformation of the lingual base and floor of mouth required tracheostomy in infancy 58% of the time (6). One cannot be sure that the compensatory mechanisms are intact in these pharyngeal structures that are infiltrated with lymphatic malformation. Surely a "mass" threshold is reached where airway patency is very problematic and no compensatory mechanisms will suffice.

Conversely, when central and neuromuscular controls are malfunctioning, normal structural anatomy cannot alone maintain airway patency. Such a clinical example is a patient with normal craniofacial structure who develops worsening OSA because of a progressive myotonia. The literature is replete with examples of pathological neuromuscular conditions that ultimately cause airway collapse. These examples include conditions such as cerebral palsy (which is generally not progressive) and Duchenne muscular dystrophy (progressive) (7).

A case report about improvement in OSAS after uvulopalatopharyngoplasty and tonsillectomy in a patient with Duchenne muscular dystrophy reveals the interplay between anatomy and neuromuscular tone. Even in a neuromuscular condition, opening the anatomy of the upper airway can shift the equation toward airway patency. This condition, of course, may be temporary, since the neuro-muscular condition is progressive (8).

Another anatomical approach for what is primarily a neuromuscular problem is noted in a study of children with cerebral palsy who underwent mandibular advancement with distraction devices to treat airway obstruction (9). There can be reasonable rationale for treating anatomy when the airway obstruction is primarily of neuromuscular etiology, but great caution is needed. The decision is easier if there are clear-cut anatomical abnormalities that are contributing to the overall clinical picture. If the anatomical structures are normal or near normal, changing the anatomy to compensate for the neuromuscular deficits is a "wager" at best. If continuous positive airway pressure (CPAP) is not possible or if tracheostomy appears even riskier, then trying to open the airway may be reasonable. Interdisciplinary consultation is absolutely necessary.

The two major anatomical building blocks for craniofacial development are the bony elements and the soft tissue elements. Bony growth cannot actually be separated from soft tissue growth and function. For expediency, however, the growth of the bony framework is considered first and the soft tissue elements are added secondarily, much as one first builds the frame for a dwelling.

This bony framework has a complex relationship with its soft tissue envelope, a relationship that is only partially elucidated. This soft tissue enve-lope includes muscle, fat, and connective tissue, and it is crucial in several functions such as breathing, swallowing, chewing, eating, and speaking. Func-tional forces have a profound effect on the craniofacial skeleton. According to the functional matrix theory first proposed by Moss in the 1960s, the develop-ment of the skeletal framework is controlled, at least in part, by the soft tissue envelope and the functional forces to which the skeleton is exposed (10). Such a functional force affecting skeletal growth can be seen in the fetus that has an abnormal lie in utero and on whose developing mandible pressure is exerted, with resultant micrognathia and airway difficulties in infancy. After birth, the deformational forces on the mandible are relieved; the mandible then grows and can "catch up," with resultant improvement in the airway. This process is a rather straightforward demonstration of functional force affecting skeletal growth (11).

Sometimes the situation is less obvious. As noted previously, a baby with Beckwith-Wiedemann syndrome is a large baby with, among other findings, a large tongue. As the child grows, the mandible tends to become large with relative maxillary deficiency, and there may be an anterior open bite. If a significant reduction glossectomy is performed, the open bite closes, but the maxillary/mandibular relationship does not change. This indicates that portions of the facial skeletal changes are "reactive" (the open bite), i.e., secondary to functional forces that are epigenetic. Other skeletal patterns are genetically programmed into the craniofacial skeletal matrix and not the functional matrix (the relative midface hypoplasia and mandibular prognathism). The Treacher Collins syndrome includes a small mandible and a hypoplastic pharynx; these malformations are genetically determined and not controlled to any great extent by manipulation of the functional matrix (12).

A more common example of the functional matrix dilemma is illustrated by the child with "adenoidal facies." This child has a narrow maxilla, anterior open bite, habitually open mouth, and pinched nares. Evaluation reveals significant degree of nasal obstruction from the adenoids and mucosal swelling secondary to allergies or other nasal/nasopharyngeal abnormalities. It is postulated that the nasal obstruction and increased resistance to breathing places forces on the skeleton. This appears to be an obvious example of the functional matrix theory in action. Nasal obstruction shapes the facial skeleton (13). It is legitimate to ask, however, if skeletal development may predispose to nasopharyngeal obstruction. The shape of the facial skeleton results in nasal obstruction. The clinical picture probably develops from multiple contributing factors.

This is probably the safest conclusion because there are studies that support the hypothesis that functional forces such as high nasal resistance from allergies and adenoid hypertrophy change the skeleton (14) and other studies that do not observe this association (15).

Returning to the example of the newborn with micrognathia secondary to external functional forces, "catch up" to some extent can be expected. In the newborn with a syndromic micrognathia that has a genetic basis, "catch up" cannot be expected. Treatment decisions must account for these distinctions. An infant with airway obstruction and a micrognathia that is secondary to deformational forces on the mandible (such as intrauterine pressure on the jaw from positioning) might be expected to anatomically improve. The syndromic infant will not have any major anatomical improvement other than what is provided from surgical or orthodontic treatment. A long-term study in Treacher Collins syndrome illustrates this concept (16).

Elaboration on airway patency related to specific craniofacial anatomic sites follows. The general principles from this introduction that are of paramount importance in understanding the craniofacial skeleton and its relation to OSA include the following:

1. The upper airway is anatomically complex, as is the interplay between craniofacial anatomy and neuromuscular control.
2. The abnormal airways can usually maintain patency because of neural controls, despite markedly deranged facial structure.
3. Conversely, the seemingly adequate anatomical airways can lose patency because of neural control problems.
4. As the upper airway develops from infancy to adulthood, changes include not just a larger framework but also other dynamic and functional changes. Encroachment on the lumen is not static. Tonsils and adenoids can enlarge and shrink, allergies can cause turbinates to swell, airway rigidity changes, and fat depositions fluctuate. The skeleton must be viewed in light of these dynamic changes (13,14,17).

5.   The skeletal framework and the soft tissue envelope have a complex
     interplay. Bone growth itself is affected by soft tissue and functional
     forces, but genetic control of the skeletal matrix is in evidence in many
     syndromes that demonstrate abnormal airways (18,19).

II.   Principles of Craniofacial Growth

The craniofacial structure has a cephalocaudal gradient of growth. The midface
has more postnatal growth potential than the cranium, and the mandible has more
growth potential than the midface. This growth has both vertical and anteroposterior components. In the newborn, the face is dwarfed by and tucked below the
neurocranium. It must grow down and forward (11). In the infant, the tongue is
very close to the soft palate and the depth of the pharynx is small; airway patency
is generally maintained in babies despite this crowded upper airway.

As the maxilla grows, the bony structure elongates and is displaced forward in the anteroposterior plane and downward in the vertical plane. The
mandible follows the same pattern. The net effect is one of a continually
enlarging airway as the soft palate is carried away from the posterior pharyngeal
wall and as the tongue moves forward and inferiorly. The airway should be
continually enlarging. The net result, however, is more complicated. The soft tissues
change as the skeleton grows. The soft palate lengthens and thickens, the tongue
grows, the nasal cavity elongates, but the turbinates enlarge, and so too the
tonsillar and andenoidal tissue hypertrophies (11,13,20,21). The net effect is,
therefore, not as predictable as one might envision.

The bony skeleton itself grows in a complex fashion. There are fields of
bone resorption and bone apposition. Both these processes take place simultaneously, with the downward and forward displacement of the whole skeleton in
space. This bodily displacement is not well understood, but it clearly occurs.

Enlow points out that the nasomaxillary complex relates in a very specific
way to the anterior cranial fossa (11). The anterior margin of the anterior cranial
fossa is the anterior margin of the nasomaxillary complex. The posterior boundaries
of both structures have the same relationship. The configuration of the palate relates
also to the anterior cranial base. The mandibular rami, which are well within the
zygomas in early childhood, grow laterally, so that the adult mandibular rami are
equal to the distance from the lateral edge of one middle cranial fossa to the other.

Development of the brain and the neurocranium controls, to a great degree,
the depth and width of the nasopharyngeal/oropharyngeal airway. The depth of
the pharynx and nasomaxillary complex is a projection of the anterior cranial
fossae. The breadth of the pharynx is a projection of the breadth of the middle
cranial fossae. This nasomaxillary development is inextricably linked to development of the neurocranium, since the midface is attached to the neurocranium.
Enlow notes that there is more variability in mandibular growth than in maxillary
growth, since the mandibular relationship with the neurocranium is not as

intimate as the maxillary relationship. The syndromic midface-deficient growth pattern will highlight this relationship (18,19,22).

Another important concept is basicranial flexure. In other animals, the brain is in line with the spinal column. In humans, the spinal cord comes off the brain at an angle that is somewhat greater than 90°. This allows bipedal activity with the face looking forward; a measurement of this flexure is the anterior cranial base angle. The lines drawn from nasion point to sella to basion (anterosuperior margin of foramen magnum) form this angle. This concept is discussed in detail below. As this angle becomes less obtuse and approaches 90°, it correlates with a shortened anterior cranial base and often lack of pharyngeal depth with airway compromise (19,23–25).

The bony resorptive and appositional fields mentioned above are very active in the growing midface. Bone is resorbed along all the inner nasal walls except for the very top of the nasal vault. The net result is an increase in the nasal airway. At the same time, the nasomaxillary complex displaces anteroinferiorly within the limits of the anterior cranial fossae. This displacement also increases the nasal/nasopharyngeal airway. Transverse maxillary growth occurs under the projectionof the middle cranial fossae, which increases the airway dimensions in width (Fig. 2).

It is of particular interest that the resorptive/deposition fields even involve the bony portion of the intranasal septum, which may respond to some minor buckling of the nasal cartilaginous septum. The bone responds to the cartilaginous functional forces, resulting in a bony deviation in the septum. Increased airway resistance is noted because of the deviated bony and cartilaginous septum and because of deficient support of the nasal tip with an abnormal anterior nasal valve (13,26).

Mandibular growth has generally the same vectors as the nasomaxillary complex. However, there are some important differences. The posterior maxilla can accept bone deposition as it enlarges without any significant structural changes. The mandibular body elongates by encroaching on the territory of the mandibular rami. This is dealt with by an active resorptive field at the anterior ramus and bone deposition at the posterior ramus. The ramus in a manner becomes the mandibular body. This lengthening of the body is important to accommodate the tongue. Vertical mandibular growth is also crucial; this carries the tongue base inferiorly away from the soft palate (27), which in turn creates more airway room. The mandible also widens laterally as a projection of the breadth of the middle cranial fossae, which also improves airway dimension (11).

Recall that the tongue is attached anteriorly to the mandible. A retrognathic mandible is associated with a retropositioned tongue. Within the confines of that mandible, genioglossus and geniohyoid muscle tone control a great deal of the tongue position during sleep (1).

The very small mandible in the infant is often associated with glossoptosis. The tongue not only is retropositioned but is tipped posteriorly. This postero-superiorly displaced tongue prevents the palatal shelves from achieving their

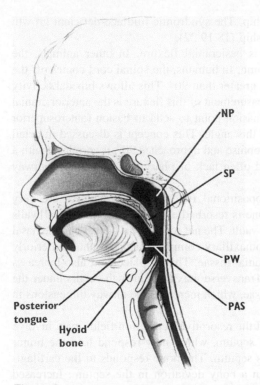

NP

SP

PW

PAS

Posterior
tongue
Hyoid
bone

Figure 2 Sagittal view of normal 10 year old facial skeleton (awake and upright). Note the relationship of the soft palate (SP) to the pharyngeal wall (PW), the depth of the posterior airway space (PAS), the nasopharynx (NP), the relationship of the posterior tongue to the soft palate, and the relationship of the hyoid bone to the mandibular symphysis.

transverse orientation and fusing in utero. As a result, cleft palate is part of the Robin sequence (28,29).

III. Craniofacial Pattern and OSAS

Many groups have characterized the craniofacial features that correlate with OSA in both the pediatric and the adult populations (23,30–33). A straightforward analysis is provided by various measurements on the lateral cephalogram. The lateral cephalogram is a standardized lateral skull radiograph taken with the head in the natural head position (facing straight ahead), and it is used throughout the world to analyze both bony and soft tissue craniofacial relationships. These studies were mainly done with the subject standing and awake, although supine awake lateral cephalogram/OSAS studies have also been performed.

The craniofacial patterns that have correlated with OSAS are provided in the list below and a line tracing of a normal cephalogram is provided as a

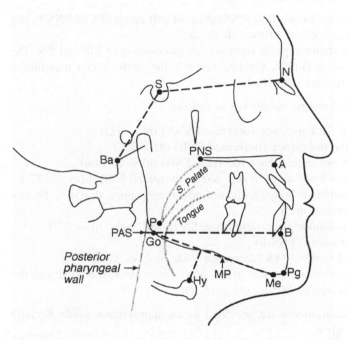

Figure 3 This is a simplified tracing of a lateral cephalogram. The various points have been marked in an obvious fashion for didactic clarity. Various anatomical points may not be as obvious on an actual lateral cephalogram. Straight-line measurements are made from point to point. Angle measurements are constructed by connecting three points. See text for definitions of abbreviations.

reference. The craniofacial patterns noted on the lateral cephalogram that correlate with OSAS include the following (Fig. 3):

1. The sella-nasion-A point (SNA) is an angle that measures maxillary retrusion. The more acute the angle, the more retrusion noted. It is in common usage but there are many exceptions to its predictability.
2. The sella-nasion-B point (SNB) is an angle that measures mandibular retrusion. The statements about SNA apply to SNB also.
3. The nasion-sella-basion (NSBa) is an angle of the anterior cranial base. The less obtuse the angle, the shorter the anterior cranial base. NS (or SN) is a linear measurement of anterior cranial base.
4. The posterior airway space (PAS) is a linear measurement of the radiolucent airway column made along a line from B point through gonial angle (Go).
5. The mandibular plane (MP) to hyoid (Hy) is a linear measurement of the perpendicular from the mandibular plane (roughly the plane of the mandibular inferior border to a tangent at the most superior point of the body of the hyoid).

6. The posterior nasal spine (PNS) to tip of soft palate (P), or PNS-P, is a linear measurement of the soft palate.
7. The mandibular angle is formed from intersection of MP and SN. The steeper the mandible, the less acute is the angle. Steep mandibular angle correlates with OSA.

Some normal cephalometric values are as follows:

*   Maxillary AP deficiency (decreased SNA) (nl = 82°)
*   Mandibular deficiency (decreased SNB) (nl = 79°)
*   Short anterior cranial base (decreased SN) (nl = 71 mm)
*   Less obtuse basicranial flexure angle (decreased NSBa) (nl = 137°)
*   Short mandibular body (decreased pogonion-gonion; Pg-Go < 88 mm men, 79 mm women)
*   Steep mandibular plane (less acute SN to MP angle; nl = 37°)
*   Long soft palate (PNS-P)
*   Decreased sagittal PAS (decreased PAS; nl ≥ 11 mm)
*   Increased distance of the hyoid bone from the mandibular inferior border (decreased MP-H) (nl ≤ 15 mm)

Note: Normal measurements are provided as an approximate guide because variability can be great.

Adenoidal tissue may also be seen on the lateral cephalogram. A recent study reviewed past studies to evaluate and quantify the usefulness of the lateral cephalogram in visualizing adenoidal tissue. The conclusion reached is that the cephalogram view of adenoidal tissue correlates quite well with the adenoidal size. The cephalogram was less suited for estimating the nasopharyngeal airway space (34).

Intranasal structures are not well analyzed on the lateral projection (e.g., turbinates and septal deviations). These structures are best viewed on coronal projections, as are tongue width and soft palatal pharyngeal width. Palatine tonsils, if they are very large, can be viewed as a subtle round density overlying the airway space, but this is not an entirely reliable finding. The correlation between the PAS as measured on the lateral cephalogram and calculated posterior airway volume on computed tomography (CT) is very good (35). One study found good correlation between the size of the functional oropharyngeal airway with mandibular length (Gon-Men), the distance between the third cervical vertebra and the hyoid bone (C3-Hy), and cranial base angle (NSBa). The functional oropharyngeal airway is defined as the minimal sagittal dimension at right angles to the air column (36). One CT study, however, shows variability between predictions from the lateral cephalogram and CT airway volume calculations, when evaluating the nasopharynx (37).

The lateral cephalogram done awake and standing does not necessarily predict the point or points of obstruction during sleep, but this is also true for the awake CT scan. However, analysis of the lateral cephalogram reveals the skeletal patterns and some soft tissue patterns that are known to correlate with OSAS. In our patients with severe facial deformities, the lateral cephalogram provides a quantitative assessment of the deviation of the skeletal complex from the norm and a postsurgical treatment gauge of how normalized the structures have become. An obvious abnormality on a cephalogram, however, should be viewed in the totality of the airway. A very small mandible can certainly coexist with narrowed choanae. The former is obvious on lateral cephalogram; the latter is not.

The two-dimensional and static nature of the lateral cephalogram is a definite limitation. CT scanning and magnetic resonance imaging are techniques that allow volume calculations, three-dimensional imaging of the upper airway, and a more accurate assessment of the soft tissue-skeletal relationships (38,39). The ideal, however, is imaging that can give volumetric data that are not static and can be performed with sleeping subjects. Nasopharyngoendoscopy (asleep and awake) have also been advocated (40–43).

Many groups have systematically evaluated parapharyngeal muscular function in relation to OSAS (1,42). During sleep, the airway narrows across the palate, across the oropharynx posterior to the tongue, and in the hypopharyngeal regions. This narrowing occurs normally but to a greater extent in OSAS subjects. Airway resistance increases. The tensor veli palatini muscle is critical to increased pharyngeal resistance, as its tone decreases during sleep. The tensor veli palatini muscle's decrease in activity during sleep is countered by the increased activity of the genioglossus muscle, which is linked to respiration. At times, the genioglossus muscle can be hypoactive, contributing to the posterior tongue position and airway narrowing. Somnofluoroscopy has been used to view the site of airway narrowing and collapse (20). The collapse can begin at the soft palate and spread caudally. It has been suggested that the soft palate can act as a plug in the oropharynx. With increased resistance and increased transpharyngeal pressures, collapse of the airway propagates downstream.

In awake upright and awake supine subjects, these muscles have relative positions that correlate with skeletal anatomy. The tongue and the genioglussus muscle are retropositioned in the retrognathic subject. The soft palate, which can act more like a plug, and the decreased postural tone of the tensor veli palatini can together produce a more dramatic effect if the nasomaxillary skeletal complex is posteriorly placed and hypoplastic in relation to the posterior pharyngeal wall. The multifactorial nature of OSAS is again underscored (19,24,43,44).

IV. Abnormal Patterns of Craniofacial Growth

Significant maxillary deficiency can predispose to OSAS, as found in the syndromic midface-deficient craniosynostotic disorders (e.g., Apert, Crouzon, and Pfeiffer syndromes). In this group, the soft palate is against the posterior pharyngeal wall, the anterior cranial base is short, and the nasal cavity is small both in the AP plane and vertically. There is an underbite not because of mandibular prognathism but because of marked nasomaxillary deficiency. In fact, the mandible may be smaller than normal; this underscores how deficient the midface can be. In addition, the posterior choanae can be narrow, mucus can occlude the nose, and the palatal shelves can be

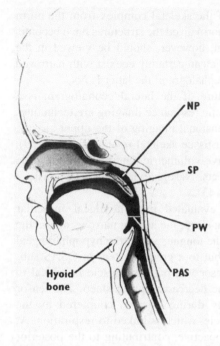

Figure 4 Sagital view of the 10-year old Crouzon or Apert facial skeleton (midface deficiency). Note the closeness of the soft palate to the pharyngeal wall, the lack of depth in the nasopharynx (NP), and the shortness of the anterior cranial base from nasion to sella.

thickened (particularly in Apert syndrome). All of this contributes to a very significant encroachment on the upper airway from a strictly structural standpoint before the neuromuscular issues are even considered (18,19,24,45) (Fig. 4).

Despite all of this, the majority of syndromic midface-deficient patients never require tracheostomy, but there are some critical junctures. For example, the midface-deficient newborn may have some airway difficulty when supine or during feeding but is otherwise well compensated. The work of the pediatric sleep group at Johns Hopkins as described above gives insight into the compensatory mechanisms that keep the severely midface-deficient infant from descending into airway trouble at a lesser frequency than one might expect. This compensated pattern may continue until physiological adenotonsillar hypertrophy occurs and the balance is upset with the development of frank OSAS (often at age 2 or 3 years).

Conversely, an Apert syndrome baby with open cleft palate (30% of Apert infants) may have a compensated airway but then develops OSAS after the palate is repaired. The closed palate encroaches on the small midfacial airway and the function of the tensor veli palatini may be poor. In addition, upper respiratory infections frequently tip these children into an obstructive pattern. Awake, these children may look uncomfortable, breathing with the mouth open and the nasal passages invariably filled with mucus. The resistance in the nasal airway can change from night to night because of the variable factors mentioned above.

In our experience, midface advancements via one stage Le Fort III osteotomy does not predictably result in cure of OSAS in these children (Ferraro, unpublished data, 1997). According to the lateral cephalogram, the nasomaxillary skeletal complex is placed into a "near normal" position. Why is there this unpredictability with this operation? The recurring theme of soft tissue mass, neuromuscular control, tone, and persistent structural abnormalities (e.g., narrow posterior choanae) can foil the obvious skeletal changes made at operation. Distraction osteogenesis, however, offers a remarkable insight into this problem. Distraction osteogenesis of the midface involves the standard osteotomies but the midface is advanced forward over days with distraction devices that are screwed into the bone. The total advancements measured in millimeters are now greater with distraction techniques compared with single-stage advancements. As a result improvement in the airway patency is much more predictable. The threshold to achieve airway patency during sleep with relief of OSAS is now being reached more often. In a 55 patient series, Mathijssen et al. demonstrated excellent improvement in airway function with midface and frontofacial distraction (46).

The child with cleft lip and palate often presents with maxillary hypoplasia; the anterior cranial base is not short as in the syndromic midface-deficient child. The nasal airway, however, may not be normal because of poor anterior nasal valves due to lack of nasal tip support, deviation of the septum, and compromised soft palatal function. If the repaired palate is short in the sagittal plane, however, the airway may actually be benefited, but at significant functional cost of hypernasal speech. The mandible may be normal in size or actually retrognathic (it is rarely hyperplastic) despite the presence of an underbite (26,44,47,48).

A German study reveals that sleep-disordered breathing with a significantly higher respiratory disturbance index and snoring index occurs after closure of the cleft palate. The conclusion is that that primary closure of the palate (a very necessary intervention) causes some airway compromise (49). Fortunately, the child almost always compensates and readjusts to this major change in airway morphology.

Distraction techniques can also treat the maxillary deficiency that is part of the cleft lip/palate clinical picture. A Japanese study correlates this advancement with improvement in upper airway size measured on cephalogram and reduction in nasal resistance measured with rhinomanometry (50).

Mandibular hypoplasia can be syndromic or nonsyndromic, static or progressive. Mild mandibular retrognathia with a class II malocclusion overbite is the commonest abnormal orthodontic pattern seen in the United States. The spectrum's other end includes nonsyndromic infants with Robin sequence and syndromic micrognathia such as Treacher Collins syndrome, Nager syndrome, and Stickler syndrome. Perinatal or childhood trauma, infection, and severe juvenile rheumatoid arthritis can also result in micrognathia with OSA (12,27,28,51–54). A recent study draws a relationship between small mandible and apparent life-threatening events (55).

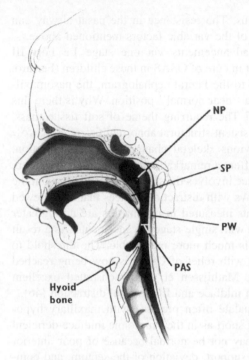

Figure 5 Sagital view of the 10-year old facial skeleton with a micrognathic mandible and normal midface. Note the retropositioned tongue, the small PAS, and the inferior displacement of the hyoid bone with a "clockwise" rotation of the tongue. The tongue then acts as an obstruction from the level of the soft palate to the hypopharynx when muscle tone is decreased during sleep.

Many of these studies confirm the association of the small mandible and OSAS. Reports of correcting OSAS with mandibular reconstruction or advancement are also numerous. The small mandible results in the posterior and superior displacement of the tongue and its base, including the genioglossus muscle. The soft palate, posterior pharyngeal wall, and tongue meet at a very critical point in the airway (Fig. 5). Dental appliances that hold the mandible in a protrusive position are known to treat OSAS in certain subjects. It is clear from many different sources that moving the mandible and tongue away from the posterior pharyngeal wall can improve airway patency during sleep (56,57) (Fig. 6A–C).

A hyoid bone that is at an increased distance from the inferior border of the mandible holds that position because the mandibular rami can be vertically short, the mandibular plane steep, and the tongue posteriorly positioned. Hyoid bone advancement to help open the deep oropharynx/hypopharynx has been proposed. Interestingly, both hyoid advancement toward the mandible and advancement/depression toward the thyroid cartilage are advocated (58,59).

There have been a number of studies documenting the efficacy of mandibular distraction osteogenesis in "opening" the upper airway, treating OSAS,

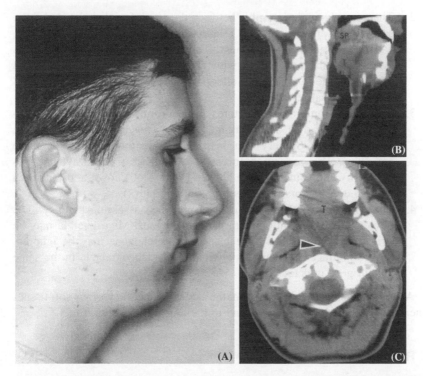

Figure 6 (A) Retrognathic young man with severe OSAS. Note chin position and anterior neck. (B) Same patients spiral CT sagital reconstruction. Tongue (T) and soft palate (SP) from a mass of tissue against the pharyngeal wall. The image is taken supine and awake. (C) CT scan axial view demonstrates a pinpoint airway at the level of the tongue.

and allowing decannulation in children with tracheostomies (60,61). A New York study, however, underscores that advancement to decannulation after mandibular distraction is not an assured result. This reminds one of the multifactorial nature of the airway problem (62).

V. Conclusion

This chapter provides a review of craniofacial development in relation to the airway and airway maintenance during sleep. Certain themes clearly emerge as fundamental.

1. There is a dynamic interplay between anatomy and physiology. It is generally easier to manipulate the anatomy than neuromuscular function. To ignore the neuromuscular reflex and tone components of airway maintenance, however, is perilous.

2. There is a dynamic interplay between the craniofacial skeleton and the associated soft tissue. This relationship changes with growth, age, weight, and intercurrent illness. Three examples: the tongue moves away from the soft palate with skeletal growth; the adenoids and tonsils enlarge in childhood; allergies cause turbinate enlargement and increased nasal resistance.

3. Abnormal craniofacial structures in syndromic children do not normalize on their own. The small mandible in Treacher Collins syndrome remains small. Surgery can help normalize the position of these structures. This repositioning can help improve the airway, but predictability can sometimes be elusive because of known and unknown confounding factors (e.g., neuromuscular control).

4. The whole airway must be considered when assessing patency. The obvious diverts attention from the less obvious. Micrognathia may be strikingly obvious in a patient and narrow choanae may be ignored. Severe midface deficiency is obvious, but tracheomalacia in the same patient goes undetected (63).

Anatomy, neuromuscular function, the skeleton, and the various soft tissues are inextricably linked to each other and to the fourth dimension, time.

References

1. Hudgel DW, Suratt PM. The human airway during sleep. In: Saunders NA, Sullivan CE, eds. Sleep and Breathing. 2nd ed. New York: Marcel Dekker, 1994:191–208.
2. Marcus CL, Lutz J, Hamer A, et al. Developmental changes in response to subatmospheric pressure loading of the upper airway. J Appl Physiol 1999; 87(2):626–633.
3. Marcus CL, Fernandes Do Prado LB, Lutz J, et al. Developmental changes in upper airway dynamics. J Appl Physiol 2004; 97(1):98–108.
4. Arens R, Marcus CL. Pathophysiology of upper airway obstruction: a developmental perspective. Sleep 2004; 27(5):997–1019.
5. Katz ES, Marcus CL, White DP. Influence of airway pressure on genioglossus activity during sleep in normal children. Am J Respir Crit Care Med 2006; 173(8): 902–909.
6. Edwards PD, Rahbar R, Ferraro NF, et al. Lymphatic malformation of the lingual base and oral floor. Plast Reconstr Surg 2005; 115(7):1906–1915.
7. Wilkinson DJ, Balkie G, Berkowitz RG, et al. Awake upper airway obstruction in children with spastic quadriplegic cerebral palsy. J Paediatr Child Health 2006; 42 (1–2):44–48.
8. Sudo A, Fukumizu M, Sugai K, et al. Improvement of obstructive sleep apnea by uvulopalatopharyngoplasty and tonsillectomy in a case of Duchenne muscular dystrophy. No To Hattatsu 2000; 32(4):352–357 (abstr).
9. Preciado DA, Sidman JD, Sampson DE, et al. Mandibular distraction to relieve airway obstruction in children with cerebral palsy. Arch Otolaryngol Head Neck Surg 2004; 130(6):741–745.

10. Moss ML, Salentijn L. The primary role of functional matrices in facial growth. Am J Orthod 1969; 55(6):566–577.
11. Enlow DH. Facial Growth. 3rd ed. Philadelphia: Saunders, 1990.
12. Shprintzen RJ, Croft C, Berkman MD. Pharyngeal hypoplasia in Treacher Collins syndrome. Arch Otolaryngol 1979; 105(3):127–131.
13. Cole P. The Respiratory Role of the Upper Airways. St Louis: Mosby-Year Book, 1993.
14. Weider DJ, Baker GL, Salvatoriello FW. Dental malocclusion and upper airway obstruction: an otolaryngologist's perspective. Int J Otolaryngol 2003; 67(4):323–331.
15. Shanker S, Vig KW, Beck FM, et al. Dentofacial morphology and upper respiratory function in 8-10-year-old children. Clin Orthod Res 1999; 2(1):19–26.
16. Anderson PJ, Netherway DJ, Abbott A, et al. Mandibular lengthening by distraction for airway obstruction in Treacher-Collins syndrome: the long term results. J Craniofac Surg 2004; 15(1):47–50.
17. Ferguson KA, Ono T, Lowe AA, et al. The relationship between obesity and craniofacial structure in obstructive sleep apnea. Chest 1995; 108(2):375–381.
18. Ferraro NF. Dental and oral maxillofacial evaluation and treatment in Apert syndrome. In: Upton J, Zucker RM, eds. Clinics in Plastic Surgery. Apert Syndrome. Philadelphia: Saunders, 1991:291–307.
19. Goldberg JS, Enlow DH, Whitaker LA, et al. Some anatomical characteristics in several craniofacial syndromes. J Oral Surg 1981; 39(7):489–498.
20. Gibson SE, Myer CM III, Strife JL, et al. Sleep fluoroscopy for localization of upper airway obstruction in children. Ann Otol Rhinol Laryngol 1996; 105(9):678–683.
21. Ward SL, Marcus CL. Obstructive sleep apnea in infants and young children. J Clin Neurophysiol 1996; 13(3):198–207.
22. Cistulli PA, Richard GN, Palmisano RG, et al. Influence of maxillary constriction on nasal resistance and sleep apnea severity in patients with Marfan's syndrome. Chest 1996; 110(5):1184–1188.
23. Jamieson A, Guilleminault C, Partinen M, et al. Obstructive sleep apnea patients have craniomandibular abnormalities. Sleep 1986; 9(4):469–477.
24. Peterson-Falzone SJ, Pruzansky S, Parris PJ, et al. Nasopharyngeal dysmorphology in the syndromes of Apert and Crouzon. Cleft Palate J 1981; 18(4):237–250.
25. Steinberg B, Fraser B. The cranial base in obstructive sleep apnea. J Oral Maxillofac Surg 1995; 53(10):1150–1154.
26. Josephson GD, Levine J, Cutting CB. Septoplasty for obstructive sleep apnea in infants after cleft lip repair. Cleft Palate Craniofac J 1996; 33(6):473–476.
27. El-Sheikh MM, Medra AM, Warda MH. Bird face deformity secondary to bilateral temporomandibular joint ankylosis. J Craniomaxillofac Surg 1996; 24(2):96–103.
28. Deegan PC, McGlone B, McNicolas WT. Treatment of Robin sequence with nasal CPAP. J Laryngol Otol 1995; 109(4):328–330.
29. Caouette-Laberge L, Bayet B, Larosque Y. The Pierre Robin sequence: review of 125 cases and evolution of treatment modalities. Plast Reconstr Surg 1993; 93(5): 934–942.
30. Frohberg U, Naples RJ, Jones DL. Cephalometric comparison of characteristics in chronically snoring patients with and without sleep apnea syndrome. Oral Surg Oral Med Oral Pathol 1995; 80(1):28–33.
31. Hochban W, Brandenburg U. Morphology of the viscerocranium in obstructive sleep apnea syndrome—cephalometric evaluation of 400 patients. J Craniomaxillofac Surg 1994; 22(4):205–213.

32. Lowe AA, Santamaria JD, Fleetham JA, et al. Facial morphology and obstructive sleep apnea. Am J Orthod Dentofac Orthop 1986; 90(6):484–491.

33. Miles PG, Vig PS, Weyant RJ, et al. Craniofacial structure and obstructive sleep apnea syndrome—a qualitative analysis and meta-analysis of the literature. Am J Orthod Dentofac Orthop 1996; 109(2):163–172.

34. Major MP, Flores-Mir C, Major PW. Assessment of lateral cephalometric diagnosis of adenoid hypertrophy and posterior upper airway obstruction: a systematic review. Am J Orthod Dentofacial Orthop 2006; 130(6):700–708.

35. Riley RW, Powell NB, Guilleminault C. Obstructive sleep apnea and the hyoid: a revised surgical procedure. Head Neck Surg 1994; 111(6):717–721.

36. Trenouth MJ, Timms DJ. Relationship of the functional oropharynx to craniofacial morphology. Angle Orthod 1999; 69(5):419–423.

37. Aboudara CA, Hatcher D, Nielsen IL, et al. A three-dimensional evaluation of the upper airway in adolescents. Orthod Craniofac Res 2003; 6(suppl 1):173–175.

38. Arens R, McDonough JM, Corbin AM, et al. Linear dimensions of the upper airway structure during development: assessment by magnetic resonance imaging. Am J Respir Crit Care Med 2002; 165(1):117–122.

39. Donnelly LF, Surdulescu V, Chini BA, et al. Upper airway motion depicted at cine MR imaging performed during sleep: comparison between young patients with and those without obstructive sleep apnea. Radiology 2003; 227(1):239–245.

40. Goldberg S, Shatz A, Picard E, et al. Endoscopic findings in children with obstructive sleep apnea: effects of age and hypotonia. Pediatr Pulmonol 2005; 40(3):205–210.

41. Myatt HM, Bechenham J. The use of diagnostic sleep nasoendoscopy in the management of children with complex upper airway obstruction. Clin Otolaryngol Allied Sci 2000; 25(3):200–208.

42. Cistulli PA, Sullivan CE. Pathophysiology of sleep apnea. In: Saunders NA, Sullivan CE, eds. Sleep and Breathing. 2nd ed. New York: Marcel Dekker, 1994:405–448.

43. Miyamoto K, Ozbek MM, Lowe AA, et al. Effect of body position on tongue posture in awake patients with obstructive sleep apnea. Thorax 1997; 52(3):255–259.

44. Chaisrisookumporn N, Stella JP, Epker BN. Cephalometric profile evaluations in patients with cleft lip and palate. Oral Surg Oral Med Oral Pathol 1995; 80(2):137–144.

45. Lauritzen C, Lilja J, Jarlstedt J. Airway obstruction and sleep apnea in children with craniofacial anomalies. Plast Reconstr Surg 1986; 77(1):1–5.

46. Mathijssen I, Arnaud E, Marchac D, et al. Respiratory outcome of mid-face advancement with distraction: a comparison between Le Fort III and frontfacial monobloc. J Craniofac Surg 2006; 17(5):880–882.

47. DeLuke DM, Marchland A, Robles EC, et al. Facial growth and the need for orthognathic surgery after cleft palate repair: literature review and report of 28 cases. J Oral Maxillofac Surg 1997; 55(7):694–697.

48. Orr WC, Levine NS, Buchanan RT. Effect of cleft palate repair and pharyngeal flap surgery on upper airway obstruction during sleep. Plast Reconstr Surg 1987; 80(2):226–232.

49. Rose E, Staats R, Thissen U, et al. Sleep-related obstructive disordered breathing in cleft palate patients after palatoplasty. Plast Reconstr Surg 2002; 110(2):392–396.

50. Mochida M, Ono T, Saito K, et al. Effects of maxillary distraction osteogenesis on the upper airway size and nasal resistance in subjects with cleft lip and palate. Orthod Craniofac Res 2004; 7(4):189–197.

51. Bettega G, Pepin JL, Levy P, et al. Surgical treatment of a patient with obstructive sleep apnea syndrome associated with temporomandibular joint destruction by rheumatoid arthritis. Plast Reconstr Surg 1998; 101(4):1045–1050.
52. James D, Ma L. Mandibular reconstruction in children with obstructive sleep apnea due to micrognathia. Plast Reconstr Surg 1997; 100(5):1131–1138.
53. Perkins JA, Sie KCY, Milczuk H, et al. Airway management in children with craniofacial anomalies. Cleft Palate Craniofac J 1997; 34(2):135–139.
54. Sugahara T, Mori Y, Kawamoto T, et al. Obstructive sleep apnea associated with temporomandibular joint destruction by rheumatoid arthritis: report of case. J Oral Maxillofac Surg 1994; 52(8):876–880.
55. Horn MK, Kinnamon DD, Ferraro NF, et al. Smaller mandibular size in infants with a history of an apparent life-threatening event. J Pediatr 2006; 149(4):499–504.
56. Castro Barbosa R, Aloe F, Travares S, et al. Mandibular-lingual repositioning device-MLRD: preliminary results of 8 patients with obstructive sleep apnea syndrome—OSAS. Sao Paulo Med J 1995; 113(3):888–894.
57. Schmidt-Nowara W, Lowe A, Weigand L, et al. Oral appliances for the treatment of snoring and obstructive sleep apnea: a review. Sleep 1995; 18(6):501–510.
58. Schmitz JP, Bitonti DA, Lemke RR. Hyoid myotomy and suspension for obstructive sleep apnea syndrome. J Oral Maxillofac Surg 1996; 54(11):1339–1345.
59. Riley RW, Powell NB, Guilleminault C. Current surgical concepts for treating obstructive sleep apnea syndrome. J Oral Maxillofac Surg 1987; 45(2):149–157.
60. Lin SY, Halbower AC, Tunkel DE, et al. Relief of upper airway obstruction with mandibular distraction surgery: long term quantitative results in young children. Arch Otolaryngol Head Neck Surg 2006; 132(4):437–441.
61. Steinbacher DM, Kaban LB, Troulis MJ. Mandibular advancement by distraction osteogenesis for tracheostomy-dependent children with severe micrognathia. J Oral Maxillofac Surg 2005; 63(8):1072–1079.
62. Sorin A, McCarthy JG, Bernstein JM. Predicting decannulation outcomes after distraction osteogenesis for syndromic micrognathia. Laryngoscope 2004; 114(10): 1811–821.
63. Mixter RC, David DJ, Perloff WH, et al. Obstructive sleep apnea in Apert and Pfeiffer syndromes: more than a craniofacial abnormality. Plast Reconstr Surg 1990; 86(3):457–463.

8

Breathing and Sleep in Preterm Infants

RUBEN ALVARO and HENRIQUE RIGATTO
University of Manitoba, Winnipeg, Manitoba, Canada

I. Introduction

Breathing and its modulation by sleep have unique characteristics in preterm infants. Our knowledge in this area is recent, having been developed over the past 40 years. There are two reasons for this late emergence: First, preterm infants rarely survived prior to 1950. Only during the second part of the century did survival improve to a point where studies on breathing were feasible. We must not forget that the first rudimentary neonatal intensive care unit was established only as recently as 1964 (1). Second, only after mid-century did the technology become adequate to measure breathing and sleep in these infants. In recent years, we have experienced tremendous advances in the field of respiratory control, and we are now witnessing the initial discovery of several of the genes that control the development and maturation of multiple neurally controlled respiratory functions.

Prematurity profoundly affects breathing, making it highly irregular, with frequent pauses or apneas. We must be aware, however, of major differences in methodology when comparing preterm, term infants, and adults. First, preterm and term infants have always been studied during sleep, since it is not possible to study them during wakefulness. This is relevant because most studies in adult subjects have been performed during wakefulness. Second, babies are almost invariably studied supine whereas adults are more frequently studied seated. Third, babies are usually studied with a nosepiece because they are nose breathers; adults are usually studied using a mouthpiece. These methodological differences have made comparison of breathing in preterm infants with that in adult subjects difficult to interpret. There is currently a major need for studies to be done using similar methodology.

In this chapter, we examine some of the important characteristics of breathing during sleep in preterm infants. Much of the data quoted relate to our own contribution over the last 30 years. An effort has been made to give a comprehensive view of how the knowledge in this area has evolved. Considerations regarding the added effect of sleep on the anatomical and functional limitations of the respiratory system at this age are also presented. Finally, the clinical implications of the effects of sleep on breathing are discussed.

II. History

Prematurity is probably as old as the history of humanity. Newton, for example, is known to have been premature, weighing 1600 g (2). The midwife told his parents that he would not survive; luckily, she was wrong. Accurate assessment of breathing in preterm infants began at the turn of the century. Studies were sporadic for the first half of the 20th century and dealt mostly with simple measurements, such as respiratory frequency and tidal volume (3–7). A more focused investigational effort began in the late forties and early fifties, led by two major groups, the first in Britain with Kenneth Cross (8–12) and Geoffrey Dawes (13) and the second in the United States with Clement Smith and his group at Harvard (14,15). Subsequently, many other centers became interested in neonatal breathing, among them Babies Hospital in New York (Stanley James and colleagues), John Hopkins University (Mary Ellen Avery and colleagues), Vanderbilt University (Mildred Stahlman and colleagues), and Cardiovascular Research Institute in San Francisco (Bill Tooley, John Clements, and colleagues). The initial studies had the objective of characterizing neonatal breathing both in preterm and term infants according to measurements being made in adult subjects. These measurements were primarily related to pulmonary function, such as vital capacity and its components, pulmonary compliance, airway resistance, alveolar ventilation, oxygen consumption, and pulmonary diffusion (14,16–27). At the same time, other investigations related to control of breathing were begun. Responsiveness to different concentrations of oxygen and carbon dioxide were measured, and a more meticulous analysis of breathing pattern emerged (28–32).

The impact of respiratory muscle performance and pulmonary reflexes on breathing was evaluated (10,33–35). At first, all observations were made without regard to sleep state, even though Magnussen in 1944 (36) and Büllow in 1963 (37) had already outlined some of the effects of sleep on breathing. In 1965, Aserinsky (38) first reported the association of periodic breathing and rapid eye movement (REM) sleep in neonates. Today there is a vast literature on the modulatory effect of sleep on breathing in preterm infants (39–44). Two schools in particular, those of Prechtl in Groeningen (41) and Dreyfus-Brisac in Paris (45,46), have made significant contributions to our knowledge of sleep, behavior, and their relationship to breathing. As a result, today most studies on the characteristics of preterm breathing are standardized for sleep state.

III. Classification and Development of Sleep in Preterm Infants

Sleep states and sleep architecture in infants are very different from those of adults and considerable maturation occurs over the first six months of life. In contrast to adult sleep, which is defined solely on physiological criteria, infant sleep states are described in terms of behavioral and physiological characteristics that occur together. Although less differentiated, cyclicity of sleep state has been observed as early as 24 weeks gestation in preterm infants (47,48). Thus, sleep has traditionally been divided into quiet, REM, transitional, and indeterminate states. Quiet sleep is characterized by the absence of REMs coupled with tracé alternans (45–53). REM sleep is defined by the presence of REMs and continuous, irregular, low voltage on the EEG. Transitional sleep represents short epochs lasting 1 to 3 minutes, which are usually observed during the transition from quiet to REM or vice versa. Indeterminate sleep is defined as that state which cannot be described by other definitions. Although breathing activity has been studied in all these states, the majority of physiological studies have been done in quiet and REM sleep. The proportion of quiet sleep increases with age, while the amount of REM decreases with age. The proportion of wakefulness decreases with decreasing gestational age and in very immature infants, it becomes difficult to define wakefulness or arousal (51–53). Normal development of sleeping and waking and sleep organization has a strong biological basis and may correlate well with normal neurological development. Several authors have found that sleep-wake patterns during the preterm period were related to developmental outcomes (54,55)

IV. Sleep States and Arousal from Sleep

Arousal from sleep is considered an important survival response that permits the initiation of both autonomic and behavioral responses that protect from life-threatening events. Spontaneous arousal responses occur periodically and the level of activity is markedly affected by sleep state. Full cortical arousal from sleep is preceded by stereotypical sequence of subcortical events that may serve as protective mechanisms to restore airway patency and/or allow the infants to reposition its head while maintaining sleep efficiency (56–58). The complete sequence of responses usually commenced with an augmented breath, followed by a startle and then cortical arousal (56,57,59). This sequence of events is similar in both sleep states and appears to occur regardless of the type of stimulus or whether the arousal is induced or spontaneous, suggesting that similar brain stem and cortical efferent pathways are involved (56).

It is well known that arousal threshold is altered by sleep state (60,61). Both spontaneous and induced arousals occur more frequently in REM than in quiet sleep, and this has been observed at two to three weeks and two to three months postterm (56). The lower arousal threshold in REM suggests that the excitatory processes that elicit the brain stem and cortical responses may be enhanced during this sleep state (56). Also the development of sleep spindles in quiet sleep at two to three months of age is known to exert inhibitory influences on the reticular formation, inhibiting arousal and maintaining sleep (62).

A. The Effects of Prematurity on Arousal

It has been shown that arousal threshold is also altered by gestational and postnatal age (61). Several authors have found a decrease in arousability with increasing postnatal age in quiet sleep over the first six months of life (63,64). Although Scher et al. reported fewer and shorter arousals and fewer body movements in preterm compared with term infants at similar postconceptional age (65), Horne et al. found that in quiet sleep arousal from sleep was not impaired in preterm infants compared with term infants at the age when sudden infant death syndrome (SIDS) incidence is highest (66). More recently, Tuladhar et al. demonstrated that heart rate responses at arousal were impaired in preterm infants compared with term infants at two to three weeks of corrected age in quiet sleep, suggesting that a reduction or immature autonomic function may contribute to the higher incidence of SIDS in these infants (67).

In preterm infants, the lower arousal threshold in REM sleep is maturationally delayed and does not appear until two to three months postterm. This difference is due to a decrease in the arousal threshold in REM while the threshold in quiet sleep remains unchanged (66). Horne et al. found that while preterm infants with a history of significant apnea had an increase in spontaneous arousals, they were more difficult to arouse to external stimulus than infants without apnea at matched postnatal ages. This suggested that while the neural pathways contributing to spontaneous arousal are intact, or even enhanced in the apneic infants, those mediating arousal in response to trigeminal stimulation appear to be deficient (68).

B. The Effects of Body Position on Sleep and Arousal

We have known for some time that sleep position has a marked influence on sleep architecture and arousal (69–71). A defective arousal response from sleep has been postulated as a likely mechanism to explain why sleeping prone increases the risk of SIDS (64,72,73).

Several studies have found that prone position increases total sleep time and time spent in quiet sleep (64,69,71). In preterm infants, prone position is associated with an increase of 79% of time spent in quiet sleep and an associated decrease of 71% spent in awake (71). Goto el al. have shown also that preterm infants have fewer awakenings lasting longer than 60 seconds in all sleep states when sleeping prone (74).

It is also known that sleeping prone decreases the number and the duration of spontaneous arousal (64) and increases the arousal threshold to air-jet stimulation at two to three weeks and two to three months in term and preterm infants in both sleep states (75). Grosswaser et al. and Myers et al. found that in term and preterm infants, respectively, respiratory arousal following obstructive sleep apneas occurred less frequently in prone position, and that arousal was initiated after a longer time delay from the start of the obstruction (70,71). These impaired arousal responses in prone position seem to disappear by five to six months of age.

V. The Effects of Sleep on the Functional and Mechanical Properties of the Respiratory System in Preterm Infants

The central nervous system is immature in preterm infants and this has a profound influence on breathing. Purpura and Shade (76) have shown that the most significant feature of central nervous system immaturity is the lack of dendritic arborization and axodendritic synaptic connections. It is likely, therefore, that the synaptic excitatory drive exerted on respiratory neurons in both brain stem and spinal cord is much weaker in preterm infants than in either term infants or adult subjects. In addition, axosomatic synaptic connections tend to be inhibitory in nature rather than excitatory, and this induces a powerful suppression of neuronal cell activity (77). In preterm infants, this inhibition is enhanced due to the small size of the synaptic connections and rare arborizations. Because of these neuroanatomical constraints, it is difficult for the preterm infant to sustain a strong respiratory drive over time. REM sleep aggravates the situation, as it induces a strong inhibitory influence on the spinal motor neurons, including the respiratory neurons. This state of affairs makes breathing for preterm infants more difficult, particularly because these infants spend a larger percentage of their time in the REM sleep state. Sleep state also influences the performance of the various components of the chest wall, which in the preterm infant are still unprepared for adequate respiratory activity.

The diaphragm in preterm infants has a relatively small apposition zone; that is, the zone which is in contact with the internal surface of the lower chest wall (78). Because of this, the ability to expand the lower rib cage during inspiration is limited. The compliant chest wall of these infants prevents the expanding influences of the lower rib cage on the upper rib cage unless there is intercostal muscle recruitment. During REM sleep, the intercostal muscles are inactivated, exaggerating the tendency of the upper rib cage to collapse during normal inspiration.

The intercostal muscles are also important for the normal respiratory activity (79). The external intercostal muscles raise the rib cage during inspiration and the internal intercostals lower it during expiration. In the newborn, the ribs are near horizontal, unlike the adult in whom they are angled caudally. This means that the increase in thoracic cross-sectional area induced by lifting the rib cage (the so-called bucket handle mechanism) is less in the preterm infant than in the adult (80). The resulting mechanical disadvantage limits the contribution of rib cage to tidal volume, leading to the common observation that newborns are "abdominal breathers" (81,82). This type of breathing appears to change at about two years of age. As alluded to above, the limited contribution of the external intercostal muscles to tidal volume and chest wall stability is lost during REM sleep (81–84).

The reduced outward recoil of the chest wall (85), which in the preterm infant is close to zero, is by far the most important feature of the immature respiratory apparatus (86). This is mainly due to lack of mineralization of the bones of the chest wall. Gehardt and Bancalari (87) found the chest wall compliance in the preterm infant at 32 weeks of gestation to be 6.4 mL/(cmH$_2$O·kg) as opposed to 4.2 mL/(cmH$_2$O·kg) in the term infant. Because the inward recoil of the lung is just slightly less than that in adult subjects, functional residual capacity (FRC) of small infants is only 10% of vital capacity. This is quite near the closing volume, resulting in significant atelectasis (88,89). On top of all these anatomic limitations, inactivation of intercostal muscles during REM sleep induces a 30% decrease in lung volume (83).

The contractile properties of immature respiratory muscles are also affected in preterm infants. Maxwell et al. (90) measured latent period, time-to-peak isometric tension, one-half relaxation time, and fatigue index (percentage of maximal tension after a series of tetanic stimuli) in diaphragm muscle strips from both preterm and adult baboons. Compared with the adult diaphragm, the latent period, time-to-peak isometric tension, and relaxation time were all longer in the premature muscle. These findings are consistent with the paucity of sarcoplasmic reticulum observed in the fetal diaphragm (90). The relevant clinical correlate of the physiological and histological observations is diaphragmatic fatigue, (decreased tension generated by the muscle when at constant level of neuronal activation), which is not uncommonly observed in neonates, particularly in the preterm infant. Rib cage deformation increases diaphragmatic work, predisposing to fatigue (88). Muller and associates (34) demonstrated a shift in the EMG power spectrum of the diaphragm during breathing with rib cage distortion in infants of 26 to 40 weeks gestational age. The shift was followed by either intercostal muscle recruitment or apnea (91), which suggests that changes in the power spectrum indicated diaphragmatic fatigue. Because chest distortion becomes more intense in REM sleep, fatigue is more likely to occur. Whether this enhances the appearance of apnea became controversial after more recent work. Duara et al. (92) and Mayock et al. (93) suggested that diaphragm fatigue may not be an issue under conditions of increased load in the human and primate infant, and Maxwell et al. in 1983 showed that recovery from fatigue was faster in baboon infants compared with adults. The highly unstable chest wall is also likely to predispose to apnea, although most apneas tend to be central. Knill and Bryan (94) have shown that rib cage deformation induced by airway occlusion or manual compression decreases inspiratory time and tidal volume in newborn infants. In exaggerated form, this reflex (the phrenic inhibitory reflex) may lead to apnea, although this has not been proven experimentally. The reflex is more prominent in REM than in quiet sleep.

The postinspiratory activity of the diaphragm is also affected by sleep state. This activity controls, in part, the duration of the expiratory time (95,96). In neonates, Reis et al. (42) observed that this activity was more pronounced in the lateral than the crural part of the diaphragm, longer in quiet than in REM sleep, and more prolonged in preterm than in term infants (Fig. 1). The length and variability of this activity in preterm infants suggest that these infants use the postinspiratory diaphragmatic activity as an expiratory airflow "braking" mechanism to stiffen the chest wall and/or to increase laryngeal resistance resulting in a dynamically elevated FRC. The role of this mechanism in maintaining lung volume by controlling expiratory time is much more important in preterms than in adults because the former have highly compliant chest wall. This mechanism is enhanced during hypercapnia in premature infants and may be important in maintaining gas exchange in infants with lung disease (97).

Upper airway resistance is also affected by sleep. Harding et al. (98) have shown that the abductor muscles of the larynx (the posterior cricoarytenoid and cricothyroid) contract in phase with the diaphragm irrespective of sleep state. In contrast, the adductors (the thyroarytenoid, lateral cricoarytenoid, and intra-arytenoid) lose their phasic expiratory contraction during REM, resulting in an important increase in upper airway resistance. Studies of the upper airway agree with clinical observations that obstructive apneas occur more frequently in REM than in quiet sleep (89,99). Finally, increased airway resistance, together with the chest wall factors described earlier, contribute to the decreased volumes observed in REM.

The work of breathing is also affected by sleep. REM sleep abolishes intercostal muscle activity and magnifies chest distortion. Luz et al. (100) found that the work of the diaphragm is 40% greater when the respiratory movements are out-of-phase as occurs with distorted breathing in REM.

Pulmonary reflexes are also affected by sleep. Hering and Breuer (101) noted in 1868 that maintained distention of the lungs decreased the frequency of inspiratory effort in anesthetized animals. They showed this effect to be a reflex mediated by afferent vagal fibers (Hering-Breuer reflex or inflation reflex). The receptors for this reflex lie in the smooth muscle and epithelium of airways from trachea to bronchioles. The Hering-Breuer reflex is much more active in the newborn period than in adult life (10,102). Small increases in lung volume cause

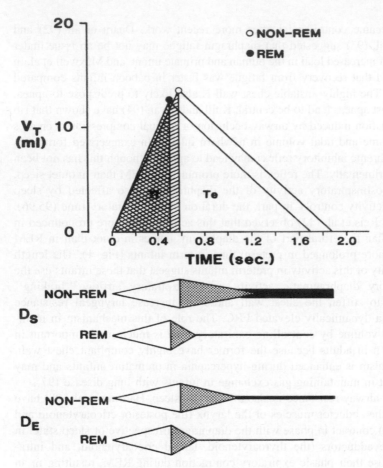

Figure 1 Diagrammatic changes in tidal volume (V_T), "timing" and diaphragmatic EMG in NREM (quiet) and REM (active) sleep. Note that total phasic activity diminishes from NREM to REM sleep. Also, in both sleep states, it is shorter in esophageal (D_E) than in surface EMG (D_S). Expiratory phasic activity as a proportion of total phasic activity decreases significantly from NREM to REM sleep. *Abbreviations*: EMG, electromyogram; V_T, tidal volume. *Source*: From Ref. 42.

apnea. This response is so powerful in the newborn that many researchers have used this inflation to produce apnea and then study the mechanical properties of the respiratory system during the passive expiratory phase after apnea. The action of the stretch receptors is abolished during REM sleep. The irritant receptors use sub-epithelial chemoreceptors located in the trachea, bronchi, and bronchioles. They are designed to detect delicate deformation of the epithelial surface. The irritant receptors are poorly developed in preterm infants, and the reflexes mediated by them are also abolished during REM sleep (33). Therefore, the airway mechanisms responsible for clearing, such as cough, are impaired during REM sleep.

Head described the paradoxical reflex in 1889 (103,104). He observed that in some rabbits, while warming the vagus, inflation of the lung produced a paradoxical effect—a further inspiration rather than inhibition of inspiration. This reflex is one of the earliest examples in physiology of positive feedback. Its function seems to be to provide a deep inspiration and to further allow opening of the alveoli. The paradoxical reflex of Head is commonly observed in the neonate in the form of a sigh (105,106). Many attribute the high prevalence of sighs to the greater need for lung recruitment at this age (44). Sighs are more frequent in REM than in quiet sleep, and also more frequent during periodic than regular breathing (105). Efforts to discover the mechanisms triggering sighs have been fruitless. Asphyxia is important but does not appear to be the only stimulus (105,106).

VI. The Effects of Sleep on the Breathing Pattern

A. Breathing Pattern at Rest

The preterm infant breathes irregularly during sleep. Compared with the term infant and the adult subject, there is a great breath-to-breath variability and long stretches of periodic breathing in which breathing intervals and apneic intervals alternate (107). We have found that the coefficients of variation in minute ventilation decrease with age (36%, 23%, and 10% in preterm, term, and adult subjects, respectively). The greater variation in the preterm infants was related to an increased variability in tidal volume (29% vs. 13%) and respiratory frequency (27% vs. 17%). The major determinant of frequency in preterm infants was expiratory time (71% variability); inspiratory time varied much less (18% variability). Inspiratory flow (V_T/T_i), a measure of central respiratory output, was lower in preterm infants. The "effective" respiratory timing (T_i/T_{tot}) was also lower in preterm infants, inspiratory time occupying only one-third of the duration of the breath in preterm infants versus half the duration of the breath in adult subjects.

Haldane has said that "the surprising fact is not that we breathe regularly but that we do not breathe periodically most of the time"; this observation applies more at this age than at any other (108). This irregularity of breathing is present also during brief episodes of wakefulness, such as those around feeding time, but sleep greatly enhances it.

B. Periodic Breathing and Apnea

Periodic breathing is the alternation between breathing periods and 5- to 10-second apnea. It is commonly seen in preterm infants, occurring in all three states (wakefulness, REM, and quiet sleep) but more commonly in REM sleep (9,109–115). It is frequently stated misconception that in quiet sleep, the infant's breathing is regular. Prechtl (41) and we, however, have clearly shown that periodic breathing is common in quiet sleep (48,113,116). The key difference is that periodic breathing in quiet sleep is regular, that is, the breathing and apneic intervals remain near-constant, whereas periodic breathing is very irregular in REM sleep. The most well-defined periodic breathing in preterm infants is observed in quiet sleep during tracé alternans (Fig. 2). Breathing pattern cannot therefore be used in defining sleep states in preterm infants, in contrast to the conventional criteria applied to sleep definition in adults (117).

Adult subjects normally do not breathe periodically but can be made to do so in quiet sleep with induced hyperventilation (118,119). In infants during sleep, the continuous oscillation in sleep state, from REM to quiet and vice versa, may increase respiratory instability. This observation would agree with our previous findings of maximum incidence of periodic breathing when the rate of change in ventilation was maximal (112). This almost continuous change in resting ventilation during sleep would lead to what Douglas and Haldane (108) called "the hunting of the respiratory center." Sleep can also contribute to periodic breathing and apnea through other mechanisms. For example, chest distortion during REM sleep may trigger a respiratory pause through the intercostal phrenic inhibitory reflex (94). The decrease in FRC during REM sleep decreases the buffering capacity for CO_2 and O_2 and predisposes to instability (83).

Like periodic breathing, apnea is also common in preterm infants, yet we know little about its physiological mechanism. It is probably the most troublesome respiratory problem in preterm infants, now that hyaline membrane disease is largely preventable and treatable.

Apnea means absence of respiratory movements. If apnea persists for 5 to 10 seconds, alternating with normal breathing, the condition is defined as periodic breathing; when apnea is more prolonged, usually greater than 20 seconds, the condition is known simply as apnea (111). Approximately 40–50% of preterm infants breathe periodically during the neonatal period (3,120–123), and the incidence increases significantly with decreasing gestational age. Periodic breathing was thought to be a benign disorder because the respiratory pause is short, but our recent observations suggest that it can be associated with severe desaturation and may predispose to "apparent life-threatening events" (124,125). Apnea, however, has always been considered a serious condition and may lead to brain damage (126).

In early studies, apneas in preterm infants were considered a central event (111,112). Only in subsequent years did it become clear that obstruction of the airway was also frequently present (127–131). Apneas have since been classified into central, obstructive, and mixed. Central apneas are those without associated respiratory efforts; obstructive apneas are those with respiratory efforts, while mixed apneas are those with efforts for part of the apnea. By definition, therefore, airway obstruction occurs only in obstructive and mixed apneas but not in central apneas. Some investigators, however, by directly visualizing the upper airway or measuring the point in the tidal cycle where apnea starts, have suggested that the airway frequently closes during central apnea (127,132). They found that this closure occurs at the beginning of the apnea, raising the possibility that occlusion of the airway per se may be the cause for the apnea. Because respiratory efforts are absent, these apneas are central with "silent obstruction."

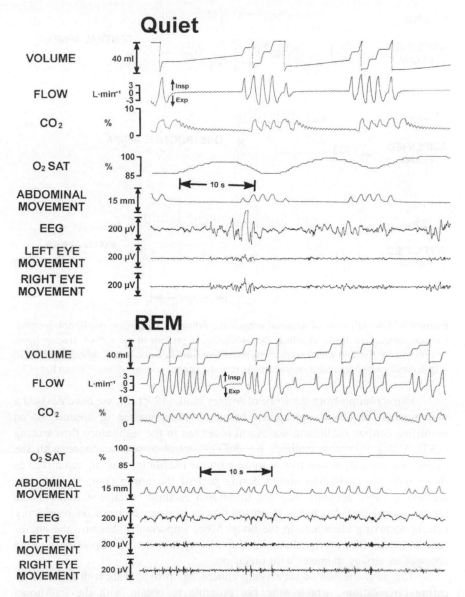

Figure 2 Periodic breathing in one preterm infant during quiet and REM sleep. Note that periodic breathing is more regular, that is, the apneas and breathing intervals are nearly constant, as opposed to the irregular periodicity observed in REM sleep. Also note the presence of sighs in REM sleep.

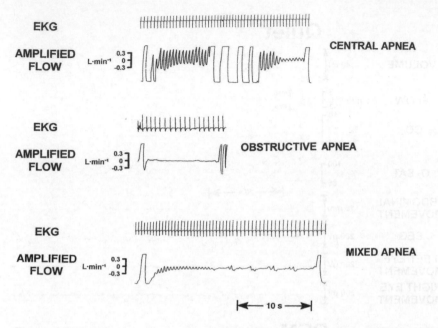

Figure 3 Classification of neonatal apneas according to the cardiac oscillation method. Central apneas are those in which the oscillation is present in the airflow tracing (*top*), obstructive are those in which oscillations are absent (*middle*), and mixed apneas are those in which oscillations are present only during part of the apnea (*bottom*). *Source*: From Ref. 133.

Extrapolating from the work of Milner et al. (127,132), we have devised a new method of classifying apneas based on the presence or absence of an amplified cardiac oscillation waveform observed in the respiratory flow tracing (133). Using this new method, we define central apneas as those with the oscillation present, obstructive as those with the oscillation absent, and mixed as those with the oscillation absent during part of the apnea (Fig. 3). The new method is more accurate than the traditional method because it relies on an airway signal that disappears if obstruction is present, and not on respiratory efforts occurring elsewhere in the body. More importantly, because the amplitude of the oscillation signal is related to airway diameter, it is possible to time changes in airway diameter with precision.

This new method of classifying apneas has provided us with some interesting observations, which were not possible to obtain with the traditional method. First, it allowed us to determine the exact timing of airway closure during apnea. We found that 87% of mixed apneas are associated with an open airway initially, which then closes; in 13% closure of the airway appears first. Second, based on the amplitude of the cardiac oscillation signal, we found that 13% of central apneas are associated with airway narrowing due to instability of the airway (130). This instability appears approximately one second after the onset of apnea. This critical period is similar for apneas of different durations, and the maximal narrowing of the airway lumen always occurs a few seconds after the critical period, usually within nine seconds of the onset of apnea. Such knowledge has important implications in the treatment of apneas since those with an obstructive component may respond better to continuous positive airway pressure (CPAP). Third, we found that in mixed apneas, airway obstruction can occur in the absence of respiratory efforts, suggesting that diaphragmatic contractions are not an essential initial event. In many cases diaphragmatic activity occurred after airway closure (134). Fourth, we found that purely obstructive apneas were almost nonexistent (135). In an analysis of more than 4000 apneas distributed according to duration, we found that apneas became predominantly mixed when they were longer than 10 seconds. Central apneas predominated with durations less than 10 seconds. Purely obstructive apneas were extremely uncommon with apneas of any duration. These findings lend support to the idea that obstruction of the airway may be primarily a central phenomenon resulting in loss of tone of the upper airway musculature.

There has been controversy in the literature on whether periodic breathing and apnea are mechanistically different or whether long apneas are just a step further in the basic respiratory disturbance that induces the short apneas of periodic breathing. In a study carried out in our laboratory we were able to show (1) that a prolonged apnea almost never occurred in the absence of preceding short apneas, and (2) that the risk of a prolonged apnea occurring increased significantly when the preceding period contained an increased number of apneic episodes, increased duration of the longest apneic interval, or increased duration of the apneic time (136). More recently we have shown that the periodic breathing cycles in REM, but not in quiet sleep, were associated with progressive decrease in minute ventilation and oxygenation likely related to the mechanical and chemo-receptor limitations present in this sleep state as mentioned previously (137). We believe that periodic breathing, especially during REM sleep, is a marker for apnea since apneas never occur abruptly in infants breathing regularly, but only in infants whose respiratory pattern is characterized by significant periodicity.

Apneas are more common, longer, and more frequently associated with profound bradycardia during REM sleep than during quiet sleep (39,114,115, 120,138–141). This is true for apneas of all types: central, mixed, and obstructive. Both in infants with and without bronchopulmonary dysplasia (BPD), the prevalence of obstructive apneas was found to be higher in REM than in quiet sleep (99) (Fig. 4). In our analysis of over 4500 cases of apneas, the proportion of central apnea was greater in quiet sleep than in REM or indeterminate sleep (135) (Fig. 5). Although the reason for a higher prevalence of apnea during REM is not entirely clear, the inhibition of spinal motorneurons that occur in this sleep state, acting on a background of poor dendritic arborization and axodendritic synaptic connections, may be very important (76,114). The more inhibitory axosomatic action combined with limited synaptic connections in the preterm infant constitutes an ideal setting for the inhibitory action of REM sleep on the respiratory neurons in otherwise "healthy" preterm infants (114).

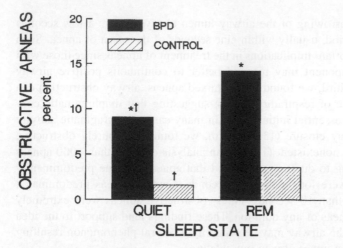

Figure 4 The incidence of obstructive apneas increased in REM sleep in preterm infants with and without BPD (control) ($^{†}p \leq 0.05$ between sleep states). The incidence of obstructive apneas was higher in the BPD group than in the control group in quiet and REM sleep but this was of marginal significance (*$p \leq 0.05$ in relation to control). *Abbreviation*: BPD, bronchopulmonary dysplasia. *Source*: From Ref. 99.

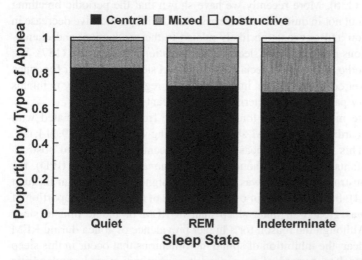

Figure 5 Proportion of central, obstructive, and mixed apneas in the various sleep states. Note that central apneas predominate in quiet sleep and its prevalence decreases toward indeterminate sleep. Concomitantly the prevalence of mixed apneas increased, in a mirror image. Purely obstructive apneas are extremely rare and their prevalence does not change in the various sleep states.

C. Sighs

Sighs are more frequently observed in preterm infants than in adults. On the respiratory tracing they look like a "breath-on-top-of-a-breath." Although there is evidence that sighs play an important role in restoring lung volume, in resetting the mechanical properties of the lung tissue and the airway walls, and in changing the properties of the neurorespiratory control system (142–144), the physiological mechanisms responsible for inducing a sigh and the effects of sighs on the stability of the respiratory system remain unclear.

In preterm infants, a highly compliant chest wall and the presence of apneas contribute to a decrease in lung volume especially during REM sleep (31). In an attempt to maintain or recover lung volume, sighs are then generated. This situation is much more dramatic in the small preterm infant (<1500 g) than in larger infants. In previous studies, we observed an approximate twofold increase in the prevalence of sighs in preterm versus term infants and in REM versus quiet sleep. In the studies we conducted using airway occlusion, in which the presence of a head reflex was detected by deflections on an esophageal pressure catheter, sighs were more frequent on 15% inspired O_2 than on 21% O_2, suggesting that the chemical drive to breathe is also important to induce sighs. The overall findings suggest that, in addition to a decrease in lung volume during REM sleep, the relative hypoxemia of this sleep state plays a role in triggering sighs (105). Several authors have previously observed that in infants, a great percentage of apneas are preceded by sighs (145–148). Studying the morphology of sighs in infants and adult subjects, we have recently found that the sighs in infants are relatively larger than those in adults and that while post-sigh ventilation is usually increased in adults, it is decreased in infants (149). Since the drive to breathe early in life is dependent on increased peripheral chemoreceptor activity, it is conceivable that the sudden increase in arterial Po_2 with sighs, could produce a rapid decline in carotid body afferent discharge leading to hypoventilation and apnea. The other almost instantaneous change that occurs with a sigh includes a decrease in Pco_2. Since the CO_2 apneic threshold is much closer to the baseline CO_2 in neonates compared with adults, the decline in CO_2 below the threshold during a sigh could trigger an apnea or initiate an epoch of periodic breathing in infants with immature respiratory feedback loop (150,151). These findings suggest that although the ability to sigh may be an important mechanism to restore lung volume, sighs have the potential to destabilize breathing and cause hypoventilation and apnea in infants at risk for inadequate control of breathing (149).

VII. The Effects of Sleep on Ventilation

A. Ventilation at Rest

As with adult subjects, minute ventilation is higher during REM than during quiet sleep in preterm infants (42,49,113,152). This higher ventilation in REM sleep is due to a proportionally higher respiratory frequency with no significant change in tidal volume. Alveolar P_{CO_2} also decreases, indicating alveolar hyperventilation in REM sleep. Oxygen consumption is increased during REM. Arterial oxygen tension and O_2 saturation are lower in REM sleep (49,50). Baseline oscillations in arterial blood gases and O_2 saturation are also greater in REM sleep (113,153). These changes are likely consequences of the loss of intercostal muscle tone, upper airway tone, and decreased FRC. As the lung partially collapses in REM sleep, ventilation is maintained via a faster respiratory rate. The decreased lung volume induces greater intrapulmonary shunt, with decreased oxygenation.

B. Response to CO_2

The newborn infant responds to inhaled CO_2 by increasing ventilation. Per unit body weight, the response of neonates is similar to that of adult subjects, about 0.035 L/(kg·min) per Torr increase in alveolar P_{CO_2} (111). The position of the CO_2 response curve in neonates (i.e., minute ventilation vs. inspired CO_2 concentration) is shifted to the left of that of adult subjects by about 4 Torr. This shift has been traditionally explained on the basis of a lower bicarbonate level in neonates (17,111).

Within the newborn population, preterm infants respond less markedly to CO_2 than term infants (25,154,155). It is not clear whether the decreased response to CO_2 in preterm infants is due to less responsive central chemoreceptors, poor performance of the respiratory "pump," or both. To elucidate this problem we compared a group of preterm infants with a group of term infants using the rebreathing technique (50). Minute integrated diaphragmatic activity ($EMG_{di} \times f$), an index of central output, increased less in response to inhaled CO_2 in preterm than in term infants. However, indices of mechanical effectiveness, such as minute ventilation divided by mean inspiratory diaphragmatic activity (V_E)/(EMG_{di}/T_i) were not different in preterm and term infants, suggesting that the respiratory "pump" effectively transduces the central output into negative intrapleural pressure or volume. It seems, therefore, that the decreased response is likely to be centrally mediated.

Using the steady-state method, we were unable to detect a difference in response to CO_2 in REM versus quiet sleep (49). Our observations using the rebreathing technique, however, suggested that during the "phasic" part of REM sleep the respiratory system is less responsive to CO_2 (50) (Fig. 6). This observation is in accordance with studies in dogs in which the response to CO_2 was also less in REM than in quiet sleep (156,157). The explanation for the discrepancy between steady state and rebreathing is that it is difficult to do a steady-state response in REM sleep, since the epochs of "phasic" REM are too short. The response always includes some tonic REM that obscures the differences.

Since the chest wall of preterm infants distorts with great ease, particularly during the phasic periods of REM sleep, it has been suggested that this distortion may contribute to the altered CO_2 response curve. However, we have found that

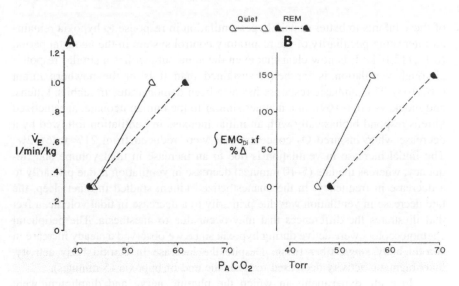

Figure 6 The ventilatory response to CO_2 rebreathing in neonates. Note that preterm infants show a decreased response to CO_2 in phasic REM as compared with quiet sleep. *Source*: From Ref. 50.

if the response to CO_2 in quiet sleep is standardized by fixing the duration of distorted and nondistorted breaths, the response to CO_2 becomes indistinguishable in both states (100). These findings suggest that the decreased CO_2 response in REM as compared to quiet sleep is not due to the possible mechanical disadvantage of chest distortion during REM sleep. It is more likely that the combination of a high and variable respiratory frequency and small tidal volumes in REM sleep are less effective in generating an increase in ventilation during inhaled CO_2.

Considerable interest has been generated by the notion that behavioral activity, such as phonation, can override, within limits, the chemical control of breathing. Phillipson et al. (158) have shown that the response to inhaled CO_2 during speech mimics that seen in active sleep: it is quite scattered and decreased. We have found that the ventilatory response to CO_2 was reduced during suckling. The decreased response was related primarily to changes in "effective" respiratory timing, that is, inspiratory time as a fraction of total respiratory cycle (T_i/T_{tot}), rather than in mean inspiratory flow (V_T/T_i) (159).

In summary, the response of the neonate ventilation to CO_2 is affected by sleep and behavior. These factors may be important in the response to chemical stimuli, especially when the ability to arouse is impaired.

C. Response to Low O_2

In response to low O_2, preterm infants ultimately decrease their ventilation (8,12,112,160). This decrease in ventilation is primarily related to a decrease in frequency with no change or slight increase in tidal volume (112). The inability of these infants to better sustain hyperventilation in response to hypoxia remains an interesting peculiarity of the respiratory control system in the neonatal period (8,12,112,161). It is now clear that even the adult subject has a similar response although ventilation is far better sustained than it is in the newborn infant (162,163). This biphasic response has also been demonstrates in rabbits, kittens, and monkeys (164–169). In a manner similar to the human neonate, anesthetized kittens respond biphasically with an initial increase in ventilation followed by a decrease when inspired O_2 concentrations were reduced from 21% to 6–12%. The initial increase in ventilation is due to an increase in tidal volume and frequency, whereas the late (5–10 minutes) decrease in ventilation is due primarily to a decrease in frequency. In the unanesthetized kitten, studied in quiet sleep, the late decrease in ventilation was due primarily to a decrease in tidal volume, a fact that illustrates the differences that may occur due to anesthesia. The peripheral chemoreceptors were active during hypoxia since we observed a steady increase in carotid body single-fiber firing. Despite the increase in carotid body activity, diaphragmatic activity decreased towards the end of hypoxia (5 minutes).

In acute experiments in which the phrenic nerve and diaphragm were recorded simultaneously, there was an initial increase in activity to a peak level at about one minute, followed by a decrease, usually in frequency, but at times in peak activity as well (141). There was no distinction between the phrenic and diaphragmatic electrical activity. These latter findings, together with those showing an increase in carotid nerve firing, which was maximal at the time respiratory efforts were about to stop, suggest that the late decrease in ventilation during hypoxia is due to inhibition at the central level as originally suggested by Cross (8). This line of thinking is consistent with the inhibition of breathing present in the fetal sheep and released by midcollicular section (170).

Cross et al. (8,12) suggested that a decrease in metabolism could be the basis for the ultimate decrease in ventilation. Many studies have demonstrated a decrease in metabolism during hypoxia, both in animals (171,172) and in humans (12). A decrease in metabolism could induce a corresponding decrease in ventilation mediated through a decrease in CO_2 production (167). This decrease in metabolism is present in various species at various ages (166). It appears to be a uniform defense mechanism that mammals rely on to compensate for the reduced availability of O_2 in the atmosphere. This decrease in metabolism was present in preterm infants in studies performed in our laboratory during quiet sleep, although it did not affect the biphasic shape of the response to hypoxia (169).

The argument for a central inhibitory effect of hypoxia following initial hyperventilation is compelling if one considers the following lines of evidence. First, there is a clear ontogenetic evolution in the response to hypoxia with maturation: hypoxia invariably abolishes breathing in the fetus (173), stimulates and depresses it in the neonate (8,12,112,122), and also stimulates and depresses it in the adult, but less so than in the neonate (163,174). The evolution is therefore one of gradually diminishing the magnitude of depression. Second, although adult subjects clearly show a biphasic response to hypoxia, the ventilatory depression last longer than the duration of hypoxia (163). This has been attributed to the release of inhibitory neurotransmitters, of which adenosine (175), endothelin (176), endorphins (177), and gamma aminobutyric acid (123) are good potential candidates. Third, in the paralyzed piglet model, the central neural output in response to hypoxia was not sustained despite a constant end tidal PCO_2, suggesting that it is not the metabolic rate that determines the late decrease in ventilation (178). The findings of Fung et al. (179) in paralyzed newborn rats also suggest that the ventilatory decrease during hypoxia is mediated via its action on brain stem mechanisms. Fourth, central sites responsible for this depression have been suggested to exist in the upper medulla by Cross et al. (11) or above the midcolliculi by Dawes et al. (170). In the experiments of Dawes et al. (170), hypoxia stimulated breathing in the midcollicular transected fetal sheep, suggesting the possibility of an inhibitory action of hypoxia on a center located rostral to the section level. Finally, Gluckman and coworkers (180,181) have localized a specific area in the rostral lateral pons, in the region of the lateral parabrachial and Kolliker-fuse nuclei that appears to be involved in the central inhibition of breathing during hypoxia in the fetal lamb. After electrolytic lesions of this area, hypoxemia stimulated rather than abolished breathing in the fetus. This appears likely to be site of action for neurotransmitters, which inhibit breathing and are released by hypoxia. Lesions of the red nucleus (182) and cooling of the locus coeruleus (183) also have been shown to block the fall in respiratory output with hypoxia.

Other researchers and we have speculated on the possible release of neuromediators during hypoxia as the primary mechanism for the late decrease in ventilation. Endogenous opiates have been suggested as mediators. In the newborn rabbit, Grunstein et al. (184) were able to prevent the late decrease in ventilation by administration of naloxone, an endogenous opiate antagonist. Hazinski et al. (185) showed an increase in ventilation of anesthetized rabbits in response to naloxone during the first four days of life. Observations in the newborn infant suggest that naloxone inhibits, at least in part, the late decrease in ventilation during hypoxia (177). Observations in the fetus are conflicting, with some studies showing a response and others no response to naloxone (186).

Adenosine has been considered a candidate in the newborn as it decreases ventilation mainly through changes in respiratory frequency. Adenosine has a depressant action on neural activities in many areas of central nervous system (187). Even brief exposure to hypoxia is known to increase brain adenosine concentrations (188). Because of its respiratory depressant activity and increased concentration during hypoxia, adenosine is a potential mediator of late ventilatory depression during hypoxia. Since aminophylline pretreatment only attenuates but does not completely eliminate hypoxic ventilatory depression, adenosine may not be the predominant neurotransmitter responsible for late hypoxic ventilatory depression in adults (174).

Sleep affects the response to low oxygen. The increase in ventilatory response to hypoxia is better sustained during quiet than during REM sleep or

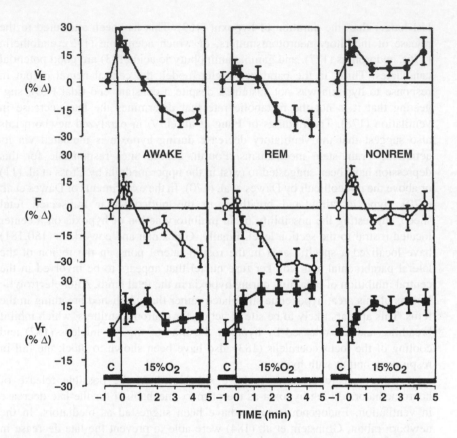

Figure 7 The ventilatory responses to 15% O_2 in preterm infants during wakefulness, REM, and NREM sleep; in NREM sleep or quiet sleep hyperventilation is more sustained. This more sustained ventilation was related primarily to a more sustained respiratory rate in quiet sleep. *Source*: From Ref. 113.

wakefulness (113) (Fig. 7) Jeffery and Read (189) also found a more sustained increase in ventilation during quiet as compared to REM sleep in calves. The results imply that the biphasic response to hypoxia is altered, in part, by behavioral influences on breathing, which are more pronounced during REM sleep and wakefulness.

Because the fetus stops breathing in response to hypoxia (173), and the neonate has a poorly sustained initial hyperventilation with a late decrease in ventilation, we hypothesized that perhaps infants with low birth weight (<1500 g) would only hypoventilate in response to hypoxia (153). This was true in both sleep states although the response was more pronounced in REM sleep. The decrease in ventilation was primarily related to a decrease in frequency, tidal volume remaining practically unchanged.

In summary, the biphasic ventilatory response to mild hypoxia in preterm infants is significantly affected by sleep state, being more sustained in quiet sleep. This effect is likely mediated through the action of a specific neuro-mediators. Since many of these mediators are presently unknown, the discovery of how sleep modulates this response may give us interesting insights into the manner in which the respiratory system is controlled during hypoxia.

VIII. Clinical Conditions Affected by Sleep

There is an important drive to breathe associated with wakefulness. During sleep, this drive ceases. Breathing is then more vulnerable, sustained primarily by brain stem structures and becoming prone to "oscillations." The following is a description of some clinical conditions in the preterm infant that are affected by sleep.

A. Periodic Breathing and Apnea

Although prematurity per se, with its inherent physiological limitations, is crucial to induce respiratory periodicity and apnea, respiratory instability is exaggerated by REM. Medications like theophylline increase central respiratory drive and muscular contractility (190–192). Although usually overlooked, it also affects sleep state, making it lighter, much closer to wakefulness. In general, all medications or maneuvers that tend to wake the infant appear to be effective in reducing apnea, since breathing tends to become more regular with the increased drive produced by arousal.

B. Acute Respiratory Disease and Ventilatory Strategy

The modern use of ventilators, with major efforts toward completely synchronized ventilation, involves great knowledge of the respiratory pattern under baseline conditions. Because this baseline pattern is profoundly affected by sleep, the corresponding effects of sleep must be thoroughly understood. We now know that mechanical ventilation at high and low lung volumes may cause ventilator-induced lung injury (193). Early initiation of CPAP, brief intubation for surfactant administration, "gentle ventilation," and permissive hypercapnia may help to reduce the risk for chronic lung disease. In these tiny infants, for example, the best ventilation is provided with short inspiratory times of the order of 0.25 to 0.35 seconds. Previously these infants were ventilated with inspiratory times equal or greater than 0.5 seconds. Interfering with the normal pattern of ventilation in the nonparalyzed state increases the risk of pneumothorax and intraventricular bleeding (194,195). Furthermore, because of the low FRC in these infants, particularly in REM sleep, it is important to ventilate them with positive end expiratory pressures which are known to recruit lung volume and retain the distal alveolar units open.

C. Chronic Respiratory Disease

With advances in neonatal care and technology, smaller and more immature infants are now surviving. These extremely premature infants who have often received antenatal steroids, postnatal surfactant, and perhaps less mechanical ventilation than 15 years ago, very commonly develop a form of chronic lung disease characterized by decreased alveolarization and diminished lung vascular development (the so-called new BPD) (196). This disorder of lung parenchymal development may lead to important abnormalities in lung function that persist for many years. Infants with this condition have a profile of high carbon dioxide tension and lower arterial Po_2 during the neonatal period. This respiratory insufficiency is greatly aggravated during REM sleep. With the absence of intercostal muscle activity, the lung collapses and baseline arterial gases deteriorate. The residual airway disease, commonly present in infant with bronchopulmonary dysplasia, and the lack of response of the pulmonary irritant reflexes during REM sleep may further compromise clearing of the airway. This is particularly true in situations where there is chronic airway infection, repeated aspirations, or both.

It has been widely cited that infants with chronic lung disease are at high risk for SIDS (197). Studies performed in infants with BPD have shown a "blunted" chemoreflex respiratory response that may predispose them to subsequent respiratory failure (198,199). This impaired chemoreflex response could be the result of chronic hypoxia which modifies the dopaminergic neurotransmission in the peripheral chemoreceptors. As a result, reduced stimulus to breathe and arouse in response to asphyxia during apnea and upper airway obstruction could occur. The blunted chemosensitivity and diminished central respiratory control could play a role in the pathogenesis of life-threatening events or sudden death (199).

D. SIDS

Although the incidence of SIDS has significantly decreased since the introduction of nonprone sleeping campaigns worldwide, it is still the leading cause of death during the postneonatal period (66). The incidence of SIDS has been found to be consistently higher in preterm and low birth weight infants and this increase is inversely related to gestational age (66,200,201).

Because SIDS infants die during sleep, it has been assumed that the vulnerability of sleep is an important factor in their death, although there is no definitive proof that this is so. It is the view of the majority of investigators in this area [at least in those cases in which parental abuse has been ruled out (202)] that dysfunctional development of the respiratory controllers, medical conditions, and environmental factors contribute to SIDS independently or in combination (203). These factors appear to lead to a common final pathway, which is a decreased propensity to arouse from sleep during periods of suffocation, when the face is buried in soft mattresses or pillows. Arousal under these circumstances, allowing the infant to move its head and breathe fresh air, becomes a more important defense mechanism than any possible chemical stimulus to breathe.

Kato et al. found that victims who would succumb to SIDS in the future tended to arouse less by the end of the night with more frequent and longer subcortical activations and fewer cortical arousal than the matched control infants (204). This finding suggested that arousal from sleep could play a crucial role in the occurrence of SIDS. Thach suggested that although arousal failure likely plays a critical role in the events leading to SIDS, it may not be the primary event (205). Since data from infants who died at home suggested that complete airway obstruction occurred immediately before death in most SIDS cases, it is conceivable that repeated episodes of hypoxemia can blunt the arousal responses. This possibility is supported by the study of Waters and Tinworth, who found that the experience of intermittent asphyxia during development led to impair arousal responses in piglets (206).

E. Central Congenital Hypoventilation

In no other neonatal problem is the importance of sleep more dramatic than in the syndrome of central congenital hypoventilation (Ondine's curse) (207). In this syndrome infants are born with the inability to sustain breathing, particularly during sleep. Respiration is overall vulnerable, but usually these infants have some ability to sustain ventilation while awake. This ability is lost during sleep and breathing becomes ineffective. Ventilatory support is frequently necessary until phrenic pacing can be instituted. The success of this treatment is somewhat limited though. In the last few years we have isolated cells from the upper medulla in the fetal rat, located 2 mm rostral to the obex, which have a respiratory phenotype (208). These are pacemaker cells uniquely responsive to CO_2 (Fig. 8). Although work needs to be done to define the respiratory specificity of these cells, we suggest that these cells are responsible for the generation of breathing. Central congenital hypoventilation has recently been highlighted as one of a growing spectrum of disorders of autonomic nervous system dysregulation. Recently, Amiel et al. reported on the identification of Polyalanine expansion mutations in the paired-like homeobox 2b (*PHOX2B*) gene located on chromosome 4p12, as the disease-defining mutation in congenital central hypoventilation syndrome (CCHS), with a small subset of patients having other mutations in *PHOX2B* (209). The size of this mutation is correlated with the severity of the phenotype in CCHS. This discovery has been confirmed by other groups of investigators (210,211).

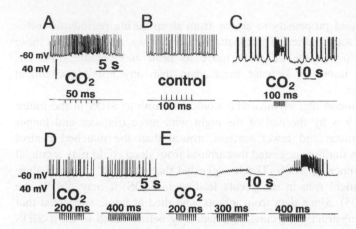

Figure 8 Representative tracing illustrating the changes in electrical activity of a pacemaker-like cell in response to administration of trains of pulses of medium equilibrated with high CO_2 and low pH. (**A**) Single beating cell responded to pulses of CO_2 of 50 and 100 milliseconds with an increase in frequency and a decrease in amplitude. (**B**) Administration of a control solution had no effect on spontaneous electrical activity. (**C**) A bursting neuron also responded to CO_2 pulses of 50 to 100 milliseconds with an increase in spike frequency and a decrease in amplitude; some degree of depolarization was also seen. (**D**) An irregular beating cell did not respond to high pulses of CO_2. (**E**) A silent cell show some depolarization but firing activity was only present with very high CO_2 pulses of 400 milliseconds. *Source*: From Ref. 208.

IX. Conclusions

The history of the influence of sleep on breathing is relatively young (36,37). Only 40 years ago the relationship of REM sleep and periodic breathing was first reported (38). Since then, numerous studies have tried to determine the influence of the various states of sleep on breathing. The fact that the fetus has breathing activity only during REM and not in quiet sleep shows how powerful this influence can be (44).

The effects of sleep on breathing in preterm infants are many. REM sleep increases the incidence of periodic breathing and apnea (40,47,113–115,140), increases minute ventilation (47,113), decreases the ventilatory response to CO_2 (48,156), enhances the late decrease in ventilation with hypoxia (113), increases the rate of sighs (105), increases chest distortion leading to muscle fatigue and increased oxygen consumption (34,47,91,100), inhibits pulmonary reflexes (33,105), and decreases upper airway tone and postinspiratory activity of the diaphragm leading to partial lung collapse during expiration (42,98,100). Sleep is also likely to have a very important role in conditions such as SIDS (212,213) and CCHS (205).

Little is understood presently on exactly how sleep interacts with breathing. Efforts to elucidate this are likely to have priority during this new century. Unraveling this mechanism may hold the key to understanding how breathing is generated and regulated.

References

1. Comroe JH Jr. Premature Science and Immature Lung. Part III. The attack on immature lungs. In: Retrospectroscope: Insights into Medical Discovery. Von Gehr Press, Menlo Park, CA, 1977.
2. Newton Sir Isaac. In: Debus AG, ed. World Who's Who in Science. Chicago: Marquis-Who's Who Inc., 1968:1252.
3. Bouterline-Young HJ, Smith CA. Respiration of full-term and of premature infants. AMA Am J Dis Child 1950; 80:753–766.
4. Deming J, Hanner JP. Respiration in infancy. II. A study of rate, volume and character of respiration in healthy infants during the neonatal period. Am J Dis Child 1936; 51:823–831.
5. Deming J, Washburn AH. Respiration in infancy. Method of studying rates, volume and character of respiration with preliminary report of results. Am J Dis Child 1935; 49:108–124.
6. Murphy DP, Thorpe ES Jr. Breathing measurements on normal newborn infants. J Clin Invest 1931; 10:545–558.
7. Shaw LA, Hopkins FR. The respiration of premature infants. Am J Dis Child 1931; 42:335–341.
8. Cross KW, Oppé TE. The effect of inhalation of high and low concentrations of oxygen on the respiration of the premature infant. J Physiol (Lond) 1952; 117:38–47.
9. Cross KW. Respiratory patterns. In: Wolfe H, ed. Mechanisms of Congenital Malformation. Proceedings of the Second Scientific Conference, Association for the Aid of Crippled Children, New York, 1954:99–105.
10. Cross KW, Klaus M, Tooley WH, Weisser K. The response of the newborn baby to inflation of the lungs. J Physiol (Lond) 1960; 151:551–565.
11. Cross KW, Hooper JMD, Lord JM. Anoxic depression of the medulla on the new-born infant. J Physiol 1954; 125:628–640.
12. Cross KW, Tizard JPM, Tryhall DAH. The gaseous metabolism of the new-born infant breathing 15% oxygen. Acta Pediatr 1958; 47:217–237.
13. Dawes GS. Foetal and Neonatal Physiology. Chicago: Yearbook Medical Publishers, Inc., 1968.
14. Nelson NM, Prod'hom LS, Cherry RB, et al. Pulmonary function in the newborn infant. I. Methods: ventilation and gaseous metabolism. Pediatrics 1962; 30:963–974.
15. Smith CA, Nelson NM. The physiology of the newborn infant. In: Thomas CC, ed., 4th ed. Springfield, Illinois: 1976:1–281:chap 4.
16. Bryan MH. The work of breathing during sleep in newborns. Am Rev Respir Dis 1979; 119(suppl):137–138.
17. Avery ME, Chernick V, Dutton RE, et al. Ventilatory response to inspired carbon dioxide in infants and adults. J Appl Physiol 1963; 18:895–903.
18. Chu JS, Dawson P, Klaus M, et al. Lung compliance and lung volume measured concurrently in normal full term and premature infants. J Pediatr 1964; 34:525–532.
19. Cook CD, Sutherland JM, Segal S, et al. Studies of respiratory physiology in the newborn infant. III. Measurements of the mechanics of respiration. J Clin Invest 1957; 36:440–448.
20. Doershuk CF, Matthews LW. Airway resistance and lung volume in the newborn infant. Pediatr 1969; 3:128–134.
21. Howard PJ, Bauer AR. Irregularities of breathing in the newborn period. Am J Dis Child 1949; 77:592–609.

22. Howard PJ, Bauer AR. Respiration of the newborn infant. Am J Dis Child 1950; 79:611–622.
23. Koch G. Alveolar ventilation, diffusion capacity and A-a PO_2 difference in the newborn infants. Respir Physiol 1968; 4:168–192.
24. Krauss AN, Klain DB, Dahms B, et al. Vital capacity in premature infants. Am Rev Respir Dis 1973; 108:1361–1366.
25. Krauss AN, Klain DB, Waldman S, et al. Ventilatory response to carbon dioxide in newborn infants. Pediatr Res 1975; 9:46–50.
26. Nelson NM. Neonatal pulmonary function. Pediatr Clin North Am 1966; 13:769–799.
27. Wohl ME, Stigol L, Mead J. Resistance of the total respiratory system in healthy infants and infants with bronchitis. Pediatrics 1969; 43:495–509.
28. Graham BD, Reardon HS, Wilson JI, et al. Physiologic and chemical response of premature infants to oxygen-enriched atmosphere. Pediatrics 1950; 6:55–71.
29. Stahlman M. Ventilation control in the newborn: carbon dioxide tension and output. Am J Dis Child 1961; 101:617–627.
30. Stahlman M, Shepard F, Gray J, et al. The effects of hypoxia and hypercapnia on the circulation in newborn lambs. J Pediatr 1964; 65:1091–1092.
31. Thibeault DW, Wong MM, Auld PAM. Thoracic gas volume changes in premature infants. Pediatrics 1967; 40:403–411.
32. Wilson JL, Long SB, Howard PJ. Respiration of premature infants. Response to variation of oxygen and to increased carbon dioxide in inspired air. Am J Dis Child 1942; 63:1080–1085.
33. Fleming PJ, Bryan AC, Bryan MH. Functional immaturity of pulmonary irritant receptors and apnea in newborn preterm infants. Pediatrics 1978; 61:515–518.
34. Müller N, Gulston G, Cade D, et al. Diaphragmatic muscle fatigue of the newborn. J Appl Physiol 1979; 46:688–695.
35. Polgar G, Weng TR. The functional development of the respiratory system. From the period of gestation to adulthood. Am Rev Respir Dis 1979; 120:625–695.
36. Magnussen G. Studies on the respiration during sleep. London: Lewis, 1944.
37. Bülow K. Respiration and wakefulness in man. Acta Physiol Scand 1963; 59(suppl 209):1–110.
38. Aserinsky E. Periodic respiratory pattern occurring in conjunction with eye movement during sleep. Science 1965; 150:763–766.
39. Curzi-Dascalova L, Christove GE. Respiratory pauses in normal prematurely born infants. A comparison with full-term newborns. Biol Neonate 1983; 44:325–332.
40. Guilleminault C, Ariagno R, Korobkin R, et al. Mixed and obstructive sleep apnea and near miss for sudden infant death syndrome: 2. Comparison of near miss and normal control infants by age. Pediatrics 1979; 64:882–891.
41. Prechtl H. The behavioural states of the newborn infant (a review). Brain Res 1974; 76:185–212.
42. Reis FJC, Cates DB, Vandriault LV, et al. I. Diaphragmatic activity and ventilation in preterm infants—the effects of sleep state. Biol Neonate 1994; 65:16–24.
43. Stern E, Parmelee AH, Akiyama Y, et al. Sleep cycle characteristics in infants. Pediatrics 1969; 43:65–70.
44. Rigatto H. Control of breathing during sleep in the fetus and neonate. In: Ferber R, Kryger MH, eds. Principles and Practice of Sleep Medicine in the Child: Philadelphia, W.B. Saunders Company, Pennsylvania 1995:29–43:chap 4.

45. Dreyfus-Brisac C. Ontogenesis of brain bioelectrical activity and sleep organization in neonates and infants. In: Falkner F, Tanner JM, eds. Human Growth. Vol 3. London: Plenum Press, 1979:157.
46. Dreyfus-Brisac C. Ontogenesis of sleep in human prematures after 32 weeks of conceptional age. Dev Psychobiol 1970; 3:91–121.
47. Curzi-Dascalova L, Figueroa JM, Eiselt M, et al. Sleep state organization in premature infants of less than 35 weeks' gestational age. Pediatr Res 1993; 34(5):624–628.
48. Lehtonen L, Johnson MW, Bakdash T, et al. Relation of sleep state to hypoxemic episodes in ventilated extremely-low-birth-weight infants. J Pediatr 2002; 141 (3):363–368.
49. Davi M, Sankaran K, MacCallum M, et al. Effect of sleep state on chest distortion and on the ventilatory response to CO_2 in neonates. Pediatr Res 1979; 13:982–986.
50. Moriette G, Van Reempts P, Moore M, et al. The effect of rebreathing CO_2 on ventilation and diaphragmatic electromyography in newborn infants. Respir Physiol 1985; 62:387–397.
51. Curzi-Dascalova L, Challamel MJ. Neurophysiological basis of sleep development. In: Loughlin GM, Carroll JL, Marcus CL, eds. Sleep and Breathing in Children. A Developmental Approach. New York: Marcel Dekker, 2000:3–37.
52. Hoppenbrouwers T, Hodgman J, Arakawa K, et al. Sleep and waking states in infancy: normative studies. Sleep 1988; 11(4):387–401.
53. Lehtonen L, Martin RJ. Ontogeny of sleep and awake states in relation to breathing in preterm infants. Semin Neonatol 2004; 9(3):229–238.
54. Borghese IF, Minard KL, Thoman EB. Sleep rhythmicity in premature infants: implications for development status. Sleep 1995; 18(7):523–530.
55. Gertner S, Greenbaum CW, Sadeh A, et al. Sleep-wake patterns in preterm infants and 6 month's home environment: implications for early cognitive development. Early Hum Dev 2002; 68(2):93–102.
56. McNamara F, Lijowska AS, Thach BT. Spontaneous arousal activity in infants during NREM and REM sleep. J Physiol 2002; 538(1):263–269.
57. McNamara F, Wulbrand H, Thach BT. Characteristics of the infant arousal response. J Appl Physiol 1998; 85(6):2314–2321.
58. Sforza E, Jouny C, Ibanez V. Cardiac activation during arousal in humans: further evidence for hierarchy in the arousal response. Clin Neurophysiol 2000; 111(9): 1611–1619.
59. Lijowska AS, Reed NW, Chiodini BA, et al. Sequential arousal and airway-defensive behavior of infants in asphyxial sleep environments. J Appl Physiol 1997; 83(1): 219–228.
60. Loy CS, Horne RSC, Cranage SM, et al. Immunisation has no effect on arousal from sleep in the newborn infant. J Paediatr Child Health 1998; 34:349–354.
61. Read PA, Horne RSC, Cranage SM, et al. Dynamic changes in arousal threshold during sleep in the human infant. Pediatr Res 1998; 43(5):697–703.
62. Hoppenbrouwers T. Sleep in infants. In: Guilleminault C, ed. Sleep and Its Disorders in Children. New York: Raven Press, 1997:1–15.
63. Campbell AJ, Bolton DP, Taylor BJ, et al. Responses to an increasing asphyxia in infants: effects of age and sleep state. Respir Physiol 1998: 112(1):51–58.
64. Horne RS, Ferens D, Watts AM, et al. The prone sleeping position impairs arousability in term infants. J Pediatr 2001; 138:811–816.

65. Scher MS, Steppe DA, Dahl RE, et al. Comparison of EEG sleep measures in healthy full-term and preterm infants at matched conceptional ages. Sleep 1992; 15(5):442–448.
66. Horne RS, Sly DJ, Cranage SM, et al. Effects of prematurity on arousal from sleep in the newborn infant. Pediatr Res 2000; 47(4 pt 1):468–74.
67. Tuladhar R, Harding R, Michael Adamson T, et al. Comparison of postnatal development of heart rate responses to trigeminal stimulation in sleeping preterm and term infants. J Sleep Res 2005; 14(1):29–36.
68. Horne RS, Andrew S, Mitchell K, et al. Apnoea of prematurity and arousal from sleep. Early Hum Dev 2001; 61(2):119–133.
69. Kahn A, Groswasser J, Sottiaux M, et al. Prone and supine body position and sleep characteristics in infants. Pediatrics 1993; 91(6):1112–1115.
70. Groswasser J, Simon T, Scaillet S, et al. Reduced arousals following obstructive apnoeas in infants sleeping prone. Pediatr Res 2001; 49:402–406.
71. Myers MM, Fifer WP, Schaeffer L, et al. Effects of sleeping position and time after feeding on the organization of sleep/wake states in prematurely born infants. Sleep 1998; 21(4):343–349.
72. Franco P, Pardou A, Hassid S, et al. Auditory arousal thresholds are higher when infants sleep in the prone position. J Pediatr 1998; 132(2):240–243.
73. Galland BC, Bolton DPG, Taylor BJ, et al. Ventilatory sensitivity to mild asphyxia: prone versus supine sleep position. Arch Dis Child 2000; 83(5):423–428.
74. Goto K, Mirmiran M, Adams MM, et al. More awakenings and heart rate variability during supine sleep in preterm infants. Pediatrics 1999; 103(3):603–609.
75. Horne RS, Franco P, Adamson TM, et al. Effects of body position on sleep and arousal characteristics in infants. Early Hum Dev 2002; 69(1–2):25–33.
76. Purpura DP, Schade IP. Growth and maturation of the brain. In: Progress in the Brain Research. Amsterdam: Elsevier Publishing Co., 1964.
77. Eccles IC. The inhibitory pathways of the central nervous system. Liverpool: Liverpool University Press, 1969:101–104.
78. Hershenson MB. The respiratory muscles and chest wall. In: Becherman RC, Brouillette RT, Hung CE, eds. Respiratory Central Disorders in Infants and Children. Baltimore: Williams and Wilkins, 1992:28.
79. Hagan RAC, Bryan CA, Bryan MH, et al. The effect of sleep state on intercostal muscle activity and rib cage motion. Physiologist 1976; 19:214.
80. Oppenshaw P, Edwards S, Helms P. Changes in rib cage geometry during childhood. Thorax 1984; 39(8):624–627.
81. Hershenson MB, Stark AR, Mead J. Action of the inspiratory muscles of the rib cage during breathing in infants. Am Rev Respir Dis 1989; 139(5):1207–1212.
82. Hershenson MB, Colin AA, Wohl MEG, et al. Changes in the contribution of the rib cage to tidal breathing during infancy. Am Rev Respir Dis 1990; 141(4 pt 1):922–925.
83. Henderson-Smart DJ, Read DJ. Reduced lung volume during behavioral active sleep in the newborn. J Appl Physiol 1979; 46(6):1081–1085.
84. Thach BT, Abroms IF, Frantz ID, et al. Intercostal muscle reflexes and sleep breathing patterns in the human infant. J Appl Physiol 1980; 48(1):139–146.
85. Agostoni E, Mead J. Statics of the respiratory system. In: Fenn WO, Rahn H, eds. Handbook of Physiology, Section 3: Respiration. Washington, DC: American Physiological Society; 1964: 387–409.
86. Agostoni E. Volume-pressure relationships of the thorax and lung in the newborn. J Appl Physiol 1959; 14:909–913.

87. Gerhardt T, Bancalari E. Chest wall compliance in full-term and premature infants. Acta Paediatr Scand 1980; 69(3):359–364.
88. Heldt GP, McIlroy MB. Distortion of the chest wall and work of the diaphragm in preterm infants. J Appl Physiol 1987; 62(1):164–169.
89. Kosch PC, Stark AR. Dynamic maintenance of end-expiratory volume in full-term infants. J Appl Physiol 1984; 57(4):1126–1133.
90. Maxwell IC, McCater RJ, Kuehl TJ, et al. Development of histochemical and functional properties of baboon respiratory muscles. J Appl Physiol 1983; 54(2):551–561.
91. Lopes JM, Muller NL, Bryan MH, et al. Synergistic behavior of inspiratory muscles after diaphragmatic fatigue in the newborn. J Appl Physiol 1981; 51(3):547–551.
92. Duara S, Silva Neto G, Claure N. Role of respiratory muscles in upper airway narrowing induced by inspiratory loading in preterm infants. J Appl Physiol 1994; 77(1):30–36.
93. Mayock DE, Standaert TA, Watchko JF, et al. Ventilatory failure during resistive loaded breathing in the newborn primate. Pediatr Pulmonol 1998; 26(5):312–318.
94. Knill R, Bryan AC. An intercostal-phrenic inhibitory reflex in human newborn infants. J Appl Physiol 1976; 40(3):352–356.
95. Remmers JE, Bartlett JR. Reflex control of expiratory airflow and duration. J Appl Physiol 1977; 42(1):80–87.
96. Remmers JE, DeGroot WJ, Sauerland EK, et al. Pathogenesis of upper airway occlusion during sleep. J Appl Physiol 1978; 44(6):931–938.
97. Eichenwald EC, Ungarelli RA, Stark AR. Hypercapnia increases expiratory braking in preterm infants. J Appl Physiol 1993; 75(6):2665–2670.
98. Harding R, Johnson P, McClelland ME. Respiratory function of the larynx in developing sheep and the influence of sleep state. Respir Physiol 1980; 40(2):165–179.
99. Fajardo C, Alvarez J, Wong A, et al. The incidence of obstructive apneas in preterm infants with and without bronchopulmonary dysplasia. Early Hum Dev 1993; 32(2–3):197–206.
100. Luz J, Winter A, Cates D, et al. Effect of chest breathing and abdomen uncoupling on ventilation and work of breathing in the newborn during sleep. Pediatr Res 1982; 16:296A.
101. Hering E, Breuer J. Dir Selbsteurung der athmung durch den nervus vagus-sitzber akadwiss wien 1868; 57:672–677.
102. Olinsky A, Bryan AH, Bryan AC. Influence of lung inflation on respiratory control in neonates J Appl Physiol 1974; 36(4):426–429.
103. Head H. On the regulation of respiration. II. Theoretical. J Physiol 1889; 10:279–290.
104. Head H. On the regulation of respiration. I. Experimental. J Physiol 1889; 1:1–70.
105. Alvarez JE, Bodani J, Fajardo CA, et al. Sighs and their relationship to apnea in the newborn infant. Biol Neonate 1993; 63(3):139–146.
106. Thach BT, Tauesch HW. Sighing in human newborn infants: role of inflation-augmenting reflex. J Appl Physiol 1976; 41(4):502–507.
107. Al-Hathlol K, Idiong N, Hussain A, et al. A study of breathing pattern and ventilation in newborn infants and adult subjects. Acta Paediatr 2000; 89(12):1420–5.
108. Douglas CG, Haldane JS. The causes of periodic or Cheyne-Stokes breathing. J Physiol 1908–1909; 38(5):401–419.
109. Fenner A, Schalk V, Hoenicke H, et al. Periodic breathing in premature and neonatal babies: incidence, breathing pattern, respiratory gas tensions, response to changes in the composition of ambient air. Pediatr Res 1973; 7(4):174–183.
110. Hornbein TF. The puzzle of periodicity. Pediatrics 1972; 50(2):183–185.

111. Rigatto H, Brady JP. Periodic breathing and apnea in preterm infants. I. Evidence for hypoventilation possibly due to central respiratory depression. Pediatrics 1972; 50(2):202–218.

112. Rigatto H, Brady JP. Periodic breathing and apnea in preterm infants. II. Hypoxia as a primary event. Pediatrics 1972; 50(2):219–228.

113. Rigatto H, Kalapesi Z, Leahy F, et al. Ventilatory response to 100% and 15% O_2 during wakefulness and sleep in preterm infants. Early Hum Dev 1982; 7(1):1–10.

114. Gabriel M, Albani M, Schulte FJ. Apneic spells and sleep state in preterm infants. 1976; 57(1):142–147.

115. Schulte FJ, Busse C, Eichhorn W. Rapid eye movement sleep, motoneurone inhibition, and apneic spells in preterm infants. Pediatr Res 1977; 11(6):709–713.

116. Kalapesi Z, Durand M, Leahy FAN, et al. Effect of periodic or regular respiratory pattern on the ventilatory response to low inhaled CO_2 in preterm infants during sleep. Am Rev Respir Dis 1981; 123(1):8–11.

117. Rechtshaffen A, Kales A. A Manual of Standardized Terminology Techniques and Scoring System for Sleep Stages in Human Subjects. NIH publication No. 204. Washington, DC: US Government Printing Office, 1978.

118. Dempsey JA, Skatrud JB. A sleep-induced apneic threshold and its consequences. Am Rev Respir Dis 1986; 133(6):1163–1170.

119. Younes M. The physiologic basis of central apnea and periodic breathing. Curr Pulmonol 1989; 10:265–365.

120. Glotzbach SF, Ariagno RL. Periodic Breathing. In: Beckerman RC, Brouillette RT, Hunt CE, eds. Respiratory Control Disorders in Infants and Children. Baltimore: Williams and Wilkins, 1992:142–160.

121. Rigatto H. Apnea—Symposium on the Newborn. Pediatr Clin North Am 1982; 29 (5):1105–1116.

122. Rigatto H. Control of breathing in the fetus and newborn. In: Spitzer AR, ed. Intensive Care of the Fetus and Newborn. New York: Mosby Yearbook Publishing Co., 1995:458–469.

123. Young RSK, During JM, Donnelly DF, et al. Effect of anoxia on excitatory amino acids in brain slices of rats and turtles: in vitro microdialysis. Am J Physiol 1993; 264 (4 pt 2):716–719.

124. Hussain A, Idiong N, Lin Y-J, et al. The profile and significance of periodic breathing in preterm infants. Pediatr Res 1997; 41:255A.

125. Lin Y-J, Idiong N, Kwiatkowski K, et al. Periodic breathing in term infants—is it benign? Pediatr Res 1997; 41:161A.

126. Bacola E, Behrle FC, De Schweinitz L, et al. Perinatal environmental factors in late neurogenic sequelae. II. Infants having birth weight from 1500 to 2500 grams. Am J Dis Child 1966; 112(4):359–369.

127. Milner AD, Boon AW, Saunders RA, et al. Upper airway obstruction and apnoea in preterm babies. Arch Dis Child 1980; 55(1):22–25.

128. Thach BT. The role of pharyngeal airway obstruction in prolonging infantile apneic spells. In: Tilden JT, Roeder LM, Steinschneider A, eds. Sudden Infant Death Syndrome. New York: New York Academic Press, 1983:279–292.

129. Dransfield DA, Spitzer AR, Fox WW. Episodic airway obstruction in premature infants. Am J Dis Child 1983; 137(5):441–443.

130. Lemke RP, Idiong N, Al-Saedi S, et al. Evidence of a critical period of airway instability during central apneas in preterm infants. Am J Respir Crit Care Med 1998; 157(2):470–474.

131. Thach BT, Stark AR. Spontaneous neck flexion and airway obstruction during apneic spells in preterm infants. J Pediatr 1979; 94(2):275–281.

132. Ruggins NR, Milner AD. Site of upper airway obstruction in preterm infants with problematical apnoea. Arch Dis Child 1991; 66(7 spec no):787–792.

133. Lemke RP, Al-Saedi S, Alvaro R, et al. Use of a magnified cardiac waveform oscillation to diagnose infant apnea: a theoretical and clinical evaluation. Am Rev Respir Crit Care Med 1996; 154(5):1537–1542.

134. Idiong N, Lemke R, Lin Y-J, et al. Airway closure during mixed apneas in preterm infants: is respiratory effort necessary? J Pediatr 1998; 133(4):509–512.

135. Idiong N, Cates DB, Lemke RP, et al. Profile and significance of the various types of apnea in preterm infants. Pediatr Res 1996; 39:328A.

136. Al-Saedi SA, Lemke RP, Haider AZ, et al. Prolonged apnea in the preterm infant is not a random event. Am J Perinatol 1997; 14:195–200.

137. Ali I, Alallah J, Kwiatkowski K, et al. Morphology of periodic breathing (PB) in quiet (Q) and REM sleep and its role on the control of breathing in preterm infants. Pediatr Res 2006 (abstract E-PAS2006:59:2635.7).

138. Albani M, Bentele KHP, Budde C, et al. Infant sleep apnea profile: preterm vs. term infants. Eur J Pediatr 1985; 143(4):261–268.

139. Flores-Guevara R, Plouin P, Curzi-Dascalova L, et al. Sleep apneas in normal neonates and infants during the first 3 months of life. Neuropediatrics 1982; 13(suppl):21–28.

140. Hoppenbrouwers T, Hodgman JE, Harper RM, et al. Polygraphic studies of normal infants during the first six months of life: III. Incidence of apnea and periodic breathing. Pediatrics 1977; 60(4):418–425.

141. Rigatto H. Control of ventilation in the newborn. Ann Rev Physiol 1984; 46:661–674.

142. Baldwin DN, Suki B, Pillow JJ, et al. Effect of sighs on breathing memory and dynamics in healthy infants. J Appl Physiol 2004; 97(5):1830–1839.

143. Davis GM, Moscato J. Changes in lung mechanics following sighs in premature newborns without lung disease. Pediatr Pulmonol. 1994; 17(1):26–30.

144. Ferris BG Jr., Pollard DS. Effect of deep and quiet breathing on pulmonary compliance in man. J Clin Invest 1960; 39:143–149.

145. Ardila R, Yunis K, Bureau MA. Relationship between infantile sleep apnea and preceding hyperventilation event. Clin Invest 1986; 9:A151.

146. Curzi-Dascalova L, Plassart E. Respiratory and motor events in sleeping infants: their correlation with thoracico-abdominal respiratory relationships. Early Hum Dev. 1978; 2(1):39–50.

147. Hoppenbrouwers T, Hodgman JE, Harper RM, et al. Polygraphic studies of normal infants during the first six months of life. Pediatrics 1977; 60(4):418–425.

148. Weintraub Z, Alvaro R, Mills S, et al. Short apneas and their relationship to body movements and sighs in preterm infants. Biol Neonate 1994; 66(4):188–194.

149. Qurashi MJ, Khalil M, Kwiatkowski K, et al. Morphology of sighs and their role on the control of breathing in preterm infants, term infants and adult subjects. Pediatric Res 2005; (abstr no. 1252).

150. Khan A, Qurashi M, Kwiatkowski K, et al. Measurement of the CO_2 apneic threshold in newborn infants: possible relevance for periodic breathing and apnea. J Appl Physiol. 2005; 98(4):1171–1176.

151. Bradley TD. Crossing the threshold: implications for central sleep apnea. Am J Respir Crit Care Med 2002; 165(9):1203–1204.

152. Krieger J, Turlot J-C, Mangin P, Durtz D. Breathing during sleep in normal young and elderly subjects: hypopneas, apneas, and correlated factors. Sleep 1983; 6(2):108–120.
153. Alvaro R, Alvarez J, Kwiatkowski K, et al. Small preterm infants (<1500 g) have only sustained decrease in ventilation in response to hypoxia. Pediatr Res, 1992; 32 (4):403–406.
154. Frantz ID III, Adler SM, Thach BT, et al. Malnutritional effects on respiratory response to carbon dioxide in premature infants. J Appl Physiol 1976; 41:41–45.
155. Rigatto H, Brady JP, de la Torre Verduzco R. Chemoreceptor reflexes in preterm infants. I. The effect of gestational and postnatal age on the ventilatory response to inhalation of 100% and 15% O_2. Pediatrics 1975; 55(5):604–613.
156. Phillipson EA, Kozar LF, Rebuck AS, et al. Ventilatory and waking responses to CO_2 in sleeping dogs. Am Rev Respir Dis 1977; 115(2):251–259.
157. Sullivan CE, Murphy E, Kozar LF, et al. Ventilatory responses to CO_2 and lung inflation in tonic versus phasic REM sleep. J Appl Physiol 1979; 47(6):1304–1310.
158. Phillipson EA, McLean PA, Sullivan CE, et al. Interaction of metabolic and behavioral respiratory control during hypercapnia and speech. Am Rev Respir Dis 1978; 117(5):903–909.
159. Durand M, Leahy FAN, MacCallum M, et al. Effect of feeding on the chemical control of breathing in the newborn infant. Pediatr Res 1981; 15(12):1509–1512.
160. Brady JP, Ceruti E. Chemoreceptor reflexes in the newborn infant. Effects of varying degrees of hypoxia on heart rate and ventilation in a warm environment. J Physiol 1966; 184(3):631–645.
161. Miller HC, Small NW. Further studies on the effects of hypoxia on the respiration of newborn infants. Pediatrics 1955; 16(1):93–103.
162. Weil JV, Zwillich CW. Assessment of ventilatory response to hypoxia: methods and interpretation. Chest 1976; 70(1 suppl):124–128.
163. Easton PA, Slykerman LJ, Anthonisen NR. Ventilatory response to sustained hypoxia in normal adults. J Appl Physiol 1986; 61(3):906–911.
164. Schwieler GH. Respiratory regulation during postnatal development in cats and rabbits and some of its morphological substrate. Acta Physiol Scand 1968; 304(suppl):1–123.
165. Woodrum DE, Standaert TA, Mayock DE, et al. Hypoxic ventilatory response in the newborn monkey. Pediatr Res 1981; 15(4 pt 1):367–370.
166. Haddad GG, Gandhi MR, Mellins RB. Maturation of ventilatory response to hypoxia in puppies during sleep. J Appl Physiol 1982; 52(2):309–314.
167. Mortola JP, Matsuoka T. Interaction between CO_2 production and ventilation in the hypoxic kitten. J Appl Physiol 1993; 74(2):904–910.
168. Rigatto H, Wiebe C, Rigatto C, et al. Ventilatory response to hypoxia in unanesthetized newborn kittens. J Appl Physiol 1988; 64(6):2544–2551.
169. Rehan V, Haider AZ, Alvaro R, et al. The biphasic response to hypoxia in preterm infants is not solely due to a decrease in metabolism. Pediatr Pulmonol 1996; 22(5): 287–294.
170. Dawes GS, Gardner WN, Johnston BM, et al. Breathing in fetal lambs: the effect of brainstem transection. J Physiol 1983; 335:535–553.
171. Gershan WM, Forster HV, Lowry TF, et al. Effect of metabolic rate on ventilatory roll-off during hypoxia. J Appl Physiol 1994; 76(6):2310–2314.
172. Mortola JP, Rezzonico R, Lanthier C. Ventilation and oxygen consumption during acute hypoxia in newborn mammals: a comparative analysis. Respir Physiol 1989; 78(1):31–48.

173. Boddy K, Dawes GS, Fisher R, et al. Fetal respiratory movements, electrocortical and cardiovascular responses to hypoxaemia and hypercapnia in sheep. J Physiol 1974; 243(3):599–618.

174. Easton PA, Anthonisen NR. Ventilatory response to sustained hypoxia after pretreatment with aminophylline. J Appl Physiol 1988; 64(4):1445–1450.

175. Lopes JM, Davis GM, Mullahoc K, Aranda JV. The role of adenosine on the hypoxic ventilatory response of the newborn piglets. Pediatr Pulmonol 1994; 17(1):50–55.

176. Dreshraj IA, Haxhiu MA, Miller MJ, et al. Endothelin-1 (ET1) acting on central chemosensitive areas causes respiratory depression in piglets. Pediatr Res 1993; 33: A1923.

177. DeBoeck C, Van Reempts P, Rigatto H, et al. Naloxone reduces decrease in ventilation induced by hypoxia in newborn infants. J Appl Physiol 1984; 56(6):1507–1511.

178. Lawson EE, Long WA. Central origin of biphasic breathing pattern during hypoxia in newborns. J Appl Physiol. 1983; 55(2):483–488.

179. Fung ML, Kang W, Darnall RA. Characterization of ventilatory responses to hypoxia in neonatal rats. Respir Physiol 1996; 103(1):57–66.

180. Gluckman PD, Johnston BM. Lesions in the upper lateral pons abolish the hypoxic depression of breathing in unanesthetized fetal lambs in utero. J Physiol 1987; 382:373–383.

181. Johnston BM, Gluckman PD. Peripheral chemoreceptors respond to hypoxia in pontine-lesioned fetal lambs in utero. J Appl Physiol 1993; 75(3):1027–1034.

182. Waites BA, Ackland GL, Noble R, et al. Red nucleus lesions abolish the biphasic respiratory response to isocapnic hypoxia in decerebrate young rabbits. J Physiol 1996; 495(pt 1):217–225.

183. Moore PJ, Ackland GL, Hanson MA. Unilateral cooling in the region of locus coeruleus blocks the fall in respiratory output during hypoxia in anaesthetized neonatal sheep. Exp Physiol 1996; 81(6):983–994.

184. Grunstein MM, Hazinski TA, Schlueter MA. Respiratory control during hypoxia in newborn rabbits: implied action of endorphins. J Appl Physiol 1981; 51(1):122–130.

185. Hazinski TA, Grunstein MM, Schlueter MA, et al. Effect of naloxone on ventilation in newborn rabbits. J Appl Physiol 1981; 50(4):713–717.

186. Moss IR, Scarpelli EM. Generation and regulation of breathing in utero: fetal CO_2 response test. J Appl Physiol 1979; 47(3):527–532.

187. Phillis JW, Wu PH. The role of adenosine and its nucleotides in central synaptic transmission. Prog Neurobiol 1981; 16(3–4):187–239.

188. Winn HR, Rubio R, Berne RM. Brain adenosine concentration during hypoxia in cats. Am J Physiol 1981; 241(2):H235–H242.

189. Jeffery HE, Read DJC. Ventilatory responses of newborn calves to progressive hypoxia in quiet and active sleep. J Appl Physiol 1980; 48(5):892–895.

190. Shannon DC, Gotay F, Stein IM, et al. Prevention of apnea and bradycardia in low birth weight infants. Pediatrics 1975; 55:589–594.

191. Davi M, Rigatto H. Apnea. In: Nelson NM, ed. Current Therapy in Neonatal-Perinatal Medicine. Hamilton, ON: BC Decker, 1985–1986:147–149.

192. Uauy R, Shapiro DL, Smith B, et al. Treatment of severe apnea in prematures with orally administered theophylline. Pediatrics 1975; 55(5):595–598.

193. Dreyfuss D, Saumon G. Ventilator-induced lung injury: lessons from experimental studies. Am J Respir Crit Care Med 1998; 157(1):294–323.

194. Perlman JM, McMenamin JB, Volpe JJ. Fluctuating cerebral blood-flow velocity in respiratory-distress syndrome. Relation to the development of intraventricular hemorrhage. N Engl J Med 1983; 309(4):204–209.

195. Burnard ED, Grattan-Smith P, Picton-Warlow CG, et al. Pulmonary insufficiency in prematurity. Aust Paediatr J 1965; 1:12–38.

196. Coalson JJ. Pathology of new bronchopulmonary dysplasia. Semin Neonatol 2003; 8(1):73–81.

197. American Thoracic Society Documents. Statement on the care of the child with chronic lung disease of infancy and childhood. Am J Respir Crit Care Med 2003; 168 (3):356–396.

198. Katz-Salamon M, Jonsson B, Lagercrantz H. Blunted peripheral chemoreceptor response to hyperoxia in a group of infants with bronchopulmonary dysplasia. Pediatr Pulmonol 1995; 20(2):101–106.

199. Calder NA, Williams BA, Smyth J, et al. Absence of ventilatory responses to alternating breaths of mild hypoxia and air in infants who have had bronchopulmonary dysplasia: implications for the risk of sudden infant death. Pediatr Res 1994; 35(6):677–681.

200. Grether JK, Schulman J. Sudden infant death syndrome and birth weight. J Pediatr 1989; 114(4 pt 1):561–567.

201. Malloy MH, Hoffman HJ. Prematurity, sudden infant death syndrome and age of death. Pediatrics 1995; 96(3 pt 1):464–471.

202. Southall DP, Plunkett MCB, Banks MW, et al. Covert video recordings of life-threatening child abuse: lesions for child protection. Pediatrics 1997; 100(5):735–760.

203. Kahn A, Groswasser J, Franco P, et al. Sudden infant death: stress, arousal and SIDS. Early Hum Dev 2003; 75(suppl):S147–S166.

204. Kato I, Franco P, Groswasser J, et al. Incomplete arousal processes in infants who were victims of sudden death. Am J Respir Crit Care Med 2003; 168(11):1298–1303.

205. Thach BT. The role of respiratory control disorders in SIDS. Respir Physiol Neurobiol 2005; 149(1–3):343–353.

206. Waters KA, Tinworth KD. Habituation of arousal responses after intermittent hypercapnic hypoxia in piglets. Am J Respir Crit Care Med 2005; 171(11): 1305–1311.

207. Mellins RB, Balfour HH, Turino GM, et al. Failure of the automatic control of ventilation (Ondine's curse). Medicine 1970; 49(6):487–504.

208. Rigatto H, Fitzgerald SF, Willis MA, et al. In search of the central respiratory neurons: II. Electrophysiologic studies of medullary fetal cells inherently sensitive to CO_2 and low pH. J Neurosci Res 1992; 33(4):590–597.

209. Amiel J, Laudier B, Attie-Bitach et al. Polyamine expansion and frameshift mutations of the paired-like homeobox gene *PHOX2B* in congenital central hypoventilation syndrome. Nat Genet 2003; 33(4):459–461.

210. Trang H, Dehan M, Beaufils F, et al. The French congenital central hypoventilation syndrome registry: general data, phenotype, and genotype. Chest 2005; 127(1):72–79.

211. Trochet D, O'Brien LM, Gozal D, et al. *PHOX2B* genotype allows for prediction of tumor risk in congenital central hypoventilation syndrome. Am J Hum Genet 2005; 76(3):421–426.

212. Shannon DC, Kelly DH. SIDS and near-miss SIDS. N Engl J Med 1982; 306: 959–1028.

213. Kelly DH, Shannon DC. Periodic breathing in infants with near-miss sudden infant death syndrome. Pediatrics 1979; 63(3):355–360.

9

Apnea During Infancy

JEAN M. SILVESTRI and ALOKA L. PATEL
Rush University Medical Center, Chicago, Illinois, U.S.A.

I. Introduction

Apnea during infancy remains a difficult problem in pediatrics: what is physiologic and what is pathologic? To address this quandary, this chapter will first attempt to describe what is considered the spectrum of normal breathing for a "healthy" term infant from the gold standard of polysomnography as well as multichannel recordings in the hospital and at home. This review will then examine the challenging chief complaint of an apparent life-threatening event (ALTE). ALTE was defined by a National Institutes of Health expert panel in 1986 as "an episode that is frightening to the observer and that is characterized by some combination of apnea (central and occasionally obstructive), color change (usually cyanotic or pallid but occasionally erythematous or plethoric), marked change in muscle tone (usually marked limpness), choking, or gagging" (1). In the subsequent 20 years there has been improved understanding in the epidemiology, diagnosis, and management of this heterogeneous group of patients with diverse underlying pathophysiology. This chapter focuses on examining the cardiorespiratory abnormalities of those infants who have been

211

identified as idiopathic ALTE, specifically those infants in whom no underlying diagnosis was found.

Infants with idiopathic ALTE were previously termed in the literature as "aborted crib death" or "near-miss SIDS," which implied a direct association with sudden infant death syndrome (SIDS), although there is no consensus regarding the relationship between idiopathic ALTE and SIDS. In addition, premature infants represent a proportion of infants who present with ALTE; their specific vulnerabilities are extensively reviewed in other chapters and an attempt will be made to separate these infants from the term infant with idiopathic ALTE. Obstructive sleep apnea syndrome (OSAS) also occurs during infancy and is thoroughly reviewed in other chapters as well. The focus of this chapter is to examine those infants whose ALTE is unexplained; although a proportion of infants with ALTE may have obstructed breathing but may not have been identified as suffering from OSAS.

II. Normative Data in Healthy Term Infants

In reviewing the following studies, one must be aware of the impact of technology and study design on data collection and the ability to make comparisons. Factors include but are not limited to (1) the environment in the laboratory or at home, adjustments for temperature, light, noise, and the ability to make continuous observations; (2) breath detection and the ability to detect obstructed breathing by differing methods, such as use of transthoracic impedance (TTI), respiratory inductance plethysmography (RIP), oral/nasal thermistor, or end-tidal carbon dioxide sensor; (3) scoring algorithms and inter-rater reliability; (4) time of day; (5) duration of recording; and (6) infant sleep position. Normative cardiorespiratory data on healthy term infants were initially obtained from in-hospital nap or overnight polygraphic recordings during sleep and many of the earliest studies were of small sample size. Further data were obtained from two-channel recordings of breathing and heart rate recorded both in hospital and at home initially for only 12 to 24 hours. With the advent of memory monitoring, long-term recording of breathing and heart rate have allowed for longitudinal recording of longer, more representative data and observation of maturation.

Monitors typically used for home recordings do not detect obstruction when TTI is used for breath detection. With TTI, amplitude changes with diaphragm contraction are detected regardless of inspired tidal volume and therefore only central apnea and obstruction can be identified. RIP technology provides a signal that is proportional to tidal volume and can detect obstructed breaths as well as central apneas. This technology, although not typically used at home, was used in the Collaborative Home Infant Monitoring Evaluation (CHIME) monitor for home recording. Polysomnography is considered the standard for apnea detection using multichannel recording (including RIP) with direct observation in a controlled environment. A study comparing apnea identified by the CHIME home monitor using RIP alone versus simultaneously recorded polysomnography in order to identify obstructed breaths within an apnea demonstrated that episodes of apnea and obstruction recorded by RIP were generally confirmed by end-tidal carbon dioxide monitoring or thermistor during polysomnography (2). However, approximately half of the apneas identified on polysomnography were not identified by the RIP monitor alone, highlighting the fact that examining the full range of apnea requires the ability to detect single or multiple obstructed breaths. Technology other than RIP or polysomnography may underestimate the length of an apnea event and not detect obstructed breaths within the apnea event.

A final caveat in reviewing the normative data is that one also has to ask how healthy are the "healthy term controls"? The familial aspect of sleep-disordered breathing (3) and the impact of smoking on respiratory control (4) have been recognized only recently. This history, therefore, has not always been systematically included in the screening of healthy term infants for participation in studies. However, a negative family history of SIDS, ALTE, and apnea has typically been identified.

A. Normative Data from Polysomnography

Overnight longitudinal polysomnographic data recorded from the first week of life and then at 1, 2, 3, 4 and 6 months of age in nine term infants demonstrated that apnea ≥ 6 seconds in duration was common but apnea >20 seconds in duration was uncommon, occurring only in the first week of life (5). Apnea >15 seconds in duration was not observed after 1 month of age. Using a similar design in 22 patients, short apneas of <10 seconds' duration were abundant (6). Apneas >10 seconds duration were more frequent in the first week of life than at subsequent ages. Recording duration substantially affected apnea counts.

In a large cross-sectional study performed from 1988 to 1994, polysomnography was performed on 2073 healthy infants at a postconceptional age of 34 to 91 weeks (median, 55.6 weeks) (7). Central apnea was frequent and generally not associated with bradycardia or oxyhemoglobin desaturation. The 90th percentile for number of central apneas per hour was 5.8 in non–rapid eye movement (NREM) sleep and 12.9 in rapid eye movement (REM) sleep. In addition, three apneas per hour were preceded by a sigh; the frequency of sighs decreased with age. The 90th percentile for duration of central apnea in NREM sleep was 7.5 seconds and 6.2 seconds in REM sleep. No central apnea exceeded 20 seconds and the frequency of central apneas decreased with postconceptional age. Some central apneas were associated with decreases in heart rate and oxyhemoglobin saturation (Spo$_2$), but these decreases were unrelated to apnea duration. Mixed and obstructive apneas were less frequent and of shorter duration. There were 0.05 ± 0.23 obstructive apneas per hour in NREM sleep and 0.46 ± 1.0 obstructive apneas per hour in REM sleep, and even fewer mixed apneas. In another large multicenter study from the same center from 1992 to

1993, polygraphic recordings in 1053 healthy term infants in the first 27 weeks of life demonstrated a small number of mixed and obstructive apneas, decreasing from a mean of 0.2/hr of total sleep time (range, 0–3.9/hr) at 2 to 7 weeks of age to 0 (range, 0–2.8/hr) by 24 to 27 weeks (7). In both populations, short apnea was common and obstructive apnea was rare, especially after the early weeks of life.

From a prospective study of 4100 healthy infants who underwent overnight polysomnography at a median age of nine weeks (range, 5–20), a subset of 100 infants (2.4% of infants) were identified with brief obstructive apnea [median of 1.4 apneas per hour (range, 1.2–1.8)] and were compared with 300 infants without obstructive apnea (8). The median duration of obstructive apneas was 10 seconds (8 infants with apneas >10 seconds), with the longest apnea of 21 seconds. Central apneas were similar in both groups. The only physiologic compromise was a deceleration in heart rate noted with obstructive apneas. Symptoms which differentiated the two groups were a greater frequency of breath holding spells (22% in the apnea group vs. 16% without apnea), fatigue with feeding (28% vs. 16%), profuse sweating during sleep (15% vs. 7%), snoring (26% vs. 23%), and noisy breathing (44% vs. 25%). There were no differences between the groups regarding parental cigarette smoking, but the prenatal versus postnatal exposure was not detailed in the study. These data attempt to correlate clinical symptoms with polysomnographic findings in infants who on entry were thought to be ''normal,'' but were found to have obstructed breathing. The clinical significance of these findings can be only realized by observing the maturation of these infants to determine subsequent development of OSAS.

The same investigators examined another aspect of normal among 550 healthy infants, the majority (72%) of which were studied with overnight polysomnography at a median age of 11 weeks (range, 5–29) and the rest within 1 week of age (4). Comparisons were made between infants based on the maternal smoking history: nonsmokers ($n = 400$); light smokers, whose mothers smoked one to nine cigarettes per day during pregnancy ($n = 37$); and smokers, whose mothers smoked more than 10 cigarettes per day during pregnancy ($n = 72$). The proportion of infants identified with obstructive apneas increased with increased smoke exposure from 41% in nonsmokers to 49% in light smokers, and 65% in smokers. The frequency of obstructive apneas (≥ 3 seconds) also increased from a median of 0 apneas per hour (range, 0–1.8) among nonsmokers to 0.5 (range, 0–1.3) among smokers. In addition, duration of obstructive apneas was longer among smokers at 7 seconds (range, 3–19) versus light smokers and nonsmokers at 4.5 seconds (range, 3–14). The number of central apneas identified was the same across all groups with a median number of 10/hr and median duration of 9 seconds (range, 3–22). Despite the limitations of this study such as recall bias of mothers of under- or over-reporting smoke exposure and quantification of exposure pre- and postnatally, these data again demonstrate that central apnea is common among infants and that a very small amount of obstructive apnea occurs in a normal healthy population, although occurring more frequently in infants with smoke exposure during pregnancy. However, the clinical significance is yet to be determined and will require correlation with other clinical symptoms and longitudinal physiologic recordings.

B. Normative Data from up to 24-Hour Multichannel Recordings in Hospital or at Home

In hospital, overnight recordings of respiratory pattern with TTI and ECG were performed in 46 full-term infants in the newborn period with 65% subsequently studied at home at one and three months of age (9). No infant had central apnea >15 seconds. Using similar methods in a larger study of 250 healthy term infants, in-hospital recordings over the first 3 days of life demonstrated that 27% of infants had apnea for >15 seconds and 5% had long central apneas from 20 to 32 seconds (10). Bradycardia to <80 bpm occurred in 32%, often associated with central apnea >15 seconds and seldom occurred without central apnea.

Breathing patterns of 110 healthy term infants were recorded in hospital and at home at 2 to 6 weeks and 3 and 6 months of age (11). Short apneas of 3.6 to 6 seconds duration were frequent and decreased after 4 weeks of age. Apnea >18 seconds duration was not seen after 7 days of age; however, apnea of 12 to 18 seconds was seen across all age groups and also decreased with age.

In another home study recording with TTI and ECG in 56 healthy infants, overnight recordings were obtained at mean ages of 4 and 14 weeks (for 79% of infants studied at 4 weeks) (12). The longest central apnea was 15 seconds and short apneas were numerous. Using similar technology, another group studied 123 healthy term infants and found only two apneas >12 seconds, lasting 13 seconds and 14 seconds each (13). Short apneas were frequent with 13.8% of infants having apnea of 10 to 12 seconds duration. There was no apparent decrease in the number of apneas >10 seconds duration over the first year of life.

C. Normative Data from Longitudinal Multichannel Recording

With the use of memory monitors with recording capability, normative data could be established over longer observation periods. One study (12) used a TTI/ECG memory monitor in the home that was triggered to record any central apnea of 14 seconds or more, which was measured peak to peak (14). Hemoglobin saturation data was recorded only at the time of an apnea or bradycardia. Over 78,000 hours of monitor use and >10,000 days of data were obtained in 88 healthy term infants at 1 to 19 weeks of age. Of the 1809 central apneas >13 seconds duration, 2.2% were >19 seconds; most occurred in the first three weeks (the longest was 36 seconds in week 1), but two occurred in weeks 16 and 17. The median frequency of apnea of 14 to 19 seconds duration was eight per infant (range, 1–272). Of all apneas, 22% were associated with baseline SpO_2 values <90% and 1% with values <81%. The three longest episodes of apnea were associated with a single-chest wall movement in the middle of the central apnea. If those respiratory efforts were counted as breaths then the apnea duration would be shortened and the longest apnea would be 25 seconds. However, these single respiratory efforts, although recorded with TTI, may be comparable to those observed with recordings using RIP which identified the efforts within a central apnea as obstructed breaths in these healthy infants (2).

Extending these observations using RIP technology with the CHIME monitor, normative longitudinal hemoglobin saturation data was obtained in addition to the breathing and heart rate data during the first three minutes of each hour (thus recording was not triggered by an apnea or bradycardia event) of monitor use in 64 healthy full-term infants who were monitored for ≥ 50 hr/mo for ≥ 3 months (15). The median and 10th percentile for baseline SpO_2 were 97.9% and 95.2%, respectively. An acute decrease in SpO_2 (a decrease of ≥ 10 saturation points from baseline and remaining below 90% for ≥ 5 seconds) was identified at least once in 59% of infants with a median number of decreases of 4 (range, 1–71) and median lowest SpO_2 83% (10th and 90th percentiles, 78% and 87%, respectively). The median time $<90\%$ was 6.3 seconds (10th and 90th percentiles, 6.0 and 9.8 seconds, respectively) and the median time $<80\%$ was 3.5 seconds (10th and 90th percentiles, 1.9 and 6.0 seconds, respectively). A respiratory pause was associated with 95% of the acute decreases: 79% during periodic breathing and 16% during an apnea 5 to 15 seconds in duration. In the remaining 5% of acute decreases, the timing of the recording could not be determined. Overall, this phenomenon decreased with age. Therefore, healthy infants may have episodes of oxyhemoglobin desaturation associated with apneas as a part of normal breathing, frequently in conjunction with periodic breathing.

The CHIME study included longitudinal normative data on 306 healthy term infants as compared with infants at higher risk of SIDS during the first 6 months of life, with a mean of 373 hours per infant (16). Healthy term infants had no family history of ALTE or SIDS; however, 16% of mothers smoked cigarettes during pregnancy in this group. Recording using RIP for breath detection identified obstructed breaths as well as central apnea. Conventional events were defined as: (1) apnea ≥ 20 seconds; (2) if <4 weeks, heart rate <60 bpm for at least 5 seconds, or <80 bpm for at least 15 seconds; (3) if ≥ 4 weeks, heart rate <50 bpm for at least 5 seconds, or <60 bpm for at least 15 seconds. Extreme events were defined as: (1) apnea ≥ 30 seconds, (2) if <4 weeks, heart rate <60 bpm for at least 10 seconds; (3) if ≥ 4 weeks, heart rate <50 bpm for ≥ 10 seconds. Adjusting for variable monitoring durations, for healthy term infants the cumulative incidence was 43% for ≥ 1 conventional events but just 2.3% for ≥ 1 extreme events. There was a high frequency of obstructed breathing with 50% of conventional events with apnea of at least 20 seconds and 70% of extreme events with apnea greater than 30 seconds, including at least three obstructed breaths.

In reviewing the normative data presented above, the variability seen in the <24-hour hospital and home recording studies and longitudinal recordings compared with the polysomnographic studies may in part be related to sample size, scoring criteria, duration of recording, incomplete longitudinal follow-up, heterogeneity of the study populations, as well as the inability to distinguish sleep from quiet wakefulness. Although differences in recording technique and lack of detailed scoring definitions in all studies do not allow for direct comparisons, the normative data in healthy term infants demonstrate that central apnea is common and includes obstructed breaths. The frequency of a sigh preceding apnea has not been systematically studied but is an integral part of this phenomenon. Depending on the methodology used for breath detection and scoring, and duration of observation, apnea durations >20 seconds and occasionally >30 seconds do occur in healthy term infants. Since many of the longer apneas include ≥1 obstructed breaths, the measured duration is longer than in the normative home studies that are unable to detect obstructed breaths. The detailed clinical characteristics of the infants also play a role in defining normative data and contribute to the variability seen.

III. Idiopathic ALTE

In reviewing the ALTE literature, one must remember that ALTE has been ill defined in that it is not a specific diagnosis, but a chief complaint to seek medical attention. In addition, an episode of lifelessness primarily associated with apnea and color change has been reported in 3–5.3% of healthy infants (17,18). Defining ALTE is limited by the fact that the clinical presentation is subjective and typically sourced from a medically naïve observer and therefore difficult to determine accurately. Although there are no reliability data concerning parental reporting of ALTE, one could extrapolate from the data of the reliability of parental reports of apnea occurrence in infants on home monitoring which demonstrate that there may be considerable error in reporting (19).

In a large prospective case series, the most common presenting symptoms for ALTE were apnea, cyanosis, hypotonia, unresponsiveness, labored breathing, and lethargy (20). Once an infant is identified, a diagnostic work up is initiated to determine the underlying etiology. This process to identify the diagnosis and management of the chief complaint has been comprehensively reviewed (21). The possible underlying causes of ALTE are numerous and the most frequent diagnoses are gastrointestinal problems, typically gastroesophageal reflux, and neurologic problems, such as seizures, and respiratory and infectious causes (20,22). From a systematic review of multiple case series of ALTE, a cause could not be identified in up to 83% of cases (23). From the NIH Consensus report the term "apnea of infancy" was defined as an unexplained cessation of breathing for 20 seconds or longer or a shorter respiratory pause associated with bradycardia, cyanosis, pallor and/or marked hypotonia, and generally refers to infants who are older than 37 weeks of gestational age at the onset (1). Further, apnea of infancy should be reserved for those infants for whom no specific cause can be identified. In other words, these are infants whose ALTEs are idiopathic. Confusion in the literature in examining this specific subgroup of infants relates in part to the change in terminology from near-miss SIDS prior to the consensus statement. In addition, those infants who are identified with apnea of infancy or idiopathic ALTE are not always clearly characterized. This chapter focuses on the review of the cardiorespiratory characteristics of idiopathic ALTEs through polysomnography and home recording technology and to discuss potential for recurrence, mechanisms for these findings, and to discuss mortality and morbidity. To help identify the historical perspective of a study, (near-miss) will be used to identify studies that classified infants as near-miss SIDS who would now be classified as "idiopathic ALTE."

A. Polysomnography of Infants with Idiopathic ALTE

Overnight polysomnography of 25 idiopathic ALTE infants (near-miss) was performed at a mean age of 13 ± 5 weeks and a similar distribution of central apnea was found between ALTE infants and controls; however, the duration was longer among ALTE infants as compared with controls [median 11 seconds (range, 3–19) vs. 6.5 seconds (range, 3–10)] (24). All obstructive apneas (scored for >2 seconds) were less than 10 seconds with more obstructive apneas occurring in ALTE infants (6 of 25) as compared with control infants (3 of 15). Drops in transcutaneous oxygen pressure were seen in proportion to the duration of both central and obstructive apneas, but to a significantly greater degree with obstructive apneas.

A subsequent large study from the same center identified 1084 of 2779 referred infants with an idiopathic ALTE and divided the group on the basis of severity of resuscitation: 695 who required gentle stimulation and 389 who required vigorous and intensive resuscitation (25). Only 5% of the 1084 polysomnographic studies gave abnormal results. However, among the subgroup of infants requiring vigorous resuscitation, 61% of infants had obstructive apnea >3 seconds, central apnea >15 seconds, and increased periodic breathing.

The effects of maternal smoking were examined among 270 infants referred for idiopathic ALTE: 85 infants were of mothers who smoked before and after pregnancy compared with 185 infants whose mothers did not smoke at either time (26). Infants of smoking mothers presented and underwent overnight polysomnography at a younger age (10.2 ± 8.5 weeks vs. 13.4 ± 13.9 weeks). Smoking during and after pregnancy was associated with an increased frequency of central apneas. Smoking after pregnancy, rather than during pregnancy, had a positive relationship with frequency of obstructive apneas.

B. Correlation of Polysomnography and Home Monitoring

A number of polysomnographic studies were performed and home monitoring prescribed to identify ALTE infants who may be at risk for subsequent morbidity and sudden death and attempted to correlate polysomnographic abnormalities with home monitoring. Among 29 term infants with idiopathic ALTE (near-miss) who underwent 12 to 24 hours polysomnography between 3 weeks and

6 months of age, no difference was found with regard to the number of central apneas as compared with 30 healthy control infants (27). Mixed and obstructive apneas longer than three seconds were greater among ALTE infants, and the peak incidence was at six weeks of age. Overall apneas greater than 15 seconds were rare. Subsequent events occurred in 27 of 29 ALTEs who were all monitored at home; however, this was before the memory-monitoring era to validate alarms.

Polysomnography performed among 422 infants with idiopathic ALTE was used to determine a subset of infants to be followed with home memory monitoring (28). Normal polysomnography was found in 411 infants and 11 had abnormal studies as defined by obstructive apnea >15 seconds, bradycardia <60 bpm for >3 seconds, and desaturation of oxygen<80% for >5 seconds. Infants with a normal polysomnography who did not require resuscitation ($n = 272$) were not monitored and all survived. Infants with only central apnea >15 seconds on the polysomnogram ($n = 110$) were monitored with non-recording monitors and all of them survived. Infants with severe ALTE needing resuscitation but who had a normal polysomnogram ($n = 27$) were placed on memory monitoring and had no further events. Among 13 infants with an abnormal polysomnogram who had memory monitoring, four had no events and seven had subsequent events with bradycardia <50 bpm, but the associated respiratory pattern with the events was not described despite use of memory monitoring. However, by using polysomnography a small subset of patients may be identified as at higher risk of subsequent documented events.

C. Home Monitoring of Infants with Idiopathic ALTE

A number of studies were performed using home monitoring for idiopathic ALTE, prior to the consistent use of memory monitoring. Among five studies that evaluated infants with a near-miss event or an idiopathic ALTE who subsequently had home monitoring, 26–68% of infants had subsequent events (29–33). As noted before, the reliability of parental interpretation of alarms as significant events is questionable (19), and given that up to 92% of alarms may be false or movement-loose lead events (34), it is unclear from these studies how many of the recurrent events were documented events versus false alarms. Without memory monitoring, efforts were made to distinguish infants requiring mild stimulation versus intense stimulation and resuscitation. In a study of 200 infants with idiopathic ALTE monitored at home without memory monitoring (25), although 88% of infants had alarms and required stimulation, only 10% had serious events, which is less than that observed in prior studies (29–33). However, without memory monitoring, clinical correlation is tenuous.

These observations are important in that home memory monitoring has been useful in identifying an underlying pathology in infants with recurrent ALTEs when the initial evaluation was unremarkable and was determined as idiopathic ALTE (35,36). In two case series of infants with recurrent severe

ALTEs, monitoring not only for ECG and breathing movement but also additional channels to monitor oxygenation allowed for the further diagnosis of seizures, suffocation, and fabrication (Munchausen syndrome by proxy). This demonstrates how memory monitoring can better elucidate underlying mechanisms and help to clarify the natural history and frequency of recurrence of ALTE in infants.

In a monitor program using memory monitors, events during the initial hospital investigation for ALTE predicted subsequent events recorded at home (37). Significant events were defined as a central apnea >20 seconds, a central apnea <20 seconds associated with age-corrected bradycardia >5 seconds, or age-corrected bradycardia >5 seconds without central apnea. Subsequent significant events occurred in 24 (33%) of the 73 ALTE infants of which 88% were idiopathic ALTE. Significant events were recorded in 48% of ALTE infants within the first month of monitoring. Of note, compliance was exceptional with 80% using the monitor at least 12 hr/day for infants <6 months, allowing for longer observation periods to capture events. Of the total recorded events among the ALTE group, 35% were apneas >20 seconds in 15 infants, and 65% were age-related bradycardia ≥5 seconds in 13 infants (the majority associated with irregular breathing). Among 22 ALTE infants there were 144 clinical events at the time of monitor alarms, of which 8 infants had 88 significant events validated (61% correlation). Among 16 infants with ALTE who had 134 significant events, 60% of those significant events had no report of clinical symptoms. This study helps to further describe the natural history of ALTE and identifies infants who may have further events which are typically within a month of the initial event. This study again stresses the difficulty in correlating recorded significant events and clinical events as observed by the caregivers.

Data from the CHIME study, as described earlier, included longitudinal data on 1079 infants that included not only healthy term infants but also siblings of infants who died of SIDS, symptomatic (having clinically apparent apnea or bradycardia episodes) and asymptomatic preterm infants with birth weight <1750 g, and idiopathic ALTEs (16). Idiopathic ALTE infants were divided into term ($n = 107$) and preterm ($n = 45$). The frequency of cigarette use in pregnancy was highest in the term ALTE infants (43.4%), as compared with the preterm ALTE infants (34.9%) and healthy term infants (16.3%). The majority of events recorded that exceeded conventional and extreme thresholds were apnea without bradycardia. Among infants in whom hemoglobin saturation data were available, the degree of hypoxemia increased with increasing duration of apnea and bradycardia. Conventional events were associated with median decreases in SpO_2 of 20–30% or more. Of all extreme events, only 25% were associated with a decrease in SpO_2 of <10%, with the remaining associated with a greater than 10% desaturation. Adjusting for variable monitoring durations, among ALTE infants who were term, the cumulative incidence was 34.4% for ≥1 conventional events and 13.1% for ≥1 extreme events, as compared to 43.2% and 2.3%, respectively, for healthy term infants. Among the ALTE infants who were preterm the cumulative incidence was 58.5% for ≥1 conventional events and 19.2% for ≥1 extreme events. Although all infants being monitored for an idiopathic ALTE had an increased risk for repeated extreme episodes, the difference was statistically significant only for the preterm ALTE infants. Among the 116 term and preterm infants who had at least one extreme event, 51.7% had a second event, 57.3% had a third event, and 80% had a fourth event (*n* = 28). Most subsequent events occurred within six weeks of the prior event. This large longitudinal study further adds to the natural history of infants with cardiorespiratory events, and challenges the concept of what has been determined as "pathologic" in the past as actually being relatively common. The settings for extreme events were set at a level where all investigators felt there would be physiologic compromise; however, the definitive answer to determine the extent of abnormality to cause injury is undetermined.

D. Physiologic Studies in Idiopathic ALTE

Interest in performing physiologic studies among different populations of infants with ALTE was initially conceived to provide some insight into the underlying pathophysiology of SIDS. Without a consensus regarding the association of SIDS with ALTE, further studies were performed to provide a better understanding of the mechanisms that initiate and terminate the frightening event that is typically apnea. Physiologic studies have been hampered by sample size and the ability to have a well-defined group of infants with idiopathic ALTE in comparison with normal infants matched not only for age, gestation, sex, cigarette smoke exposure but also with a negative family history of SIDS, ALTE, obstructive apnea, or other respiratory control disorder. Altered ventilatory and arousal responses to hypercarbia have been reported for severe ALTE compared to control infants (38–41). Both increased and normal ventilatory responses to hypercarbia have been demonstrated. In some cases, although exhibiting a response, ALTE infants exhibited a significantly decreased response strength and response time compared to controls (41). In addition, hypercarbic ventilatory response studies were unable to identify the subgroup of 23 of 65 infants with idiopathic ALTE who would have subsequent events (39). Altered ventilatory and arousal responses to hypoxia have also been reported among some idiopathic ALTE infants with increased episodes of periodic breathing (38,42). Response to hyperoxia has also been examined (41). Although demonstrating a comparable decrease in ventilation, ALTE infants took longer to respond compared to control infants.

Heart rate response to different physiologic challenges has been examined to identify differences among ALTE infants, and to identify infants at risk of subsequent events. Whether using the perturbation of head-upright tilt test or response to hypercarbia, infants with idiopathic ALTE have demonstrated altered or attenuated heart rate responses even when there was no difference in ventilatory response to hypercarbia between severe ALTE infants and control infants (43,44). These studies support that among some ALTE infants, disordered autonomic control may play a key role in their clinical presentation and risk for subsequent events.

E. Morbidity and Mortality of Idiopathic ALTE

As noted in the cited studies, the risk of recurrent events is variable depending on whether one is determining recurrence based on parent reports, alarms, or documented events and their correlation with clinical events. Clinical characteristics at the time of the presentation such as skin color, tone, behavioral state, or degree of resuscitation were not significant factors influencing the recurrence risk of a subsequent documented prolonged event (45). No study has adequately evaluated the risk of recurrence in a well-defined group of infants. However, events identified in hospital at the time of evaluation are associated with subsequent events (37), and if events recur they typically do so within four to six weeks of the initial event (16,37).

Neurodevelopmental sequelae are the concern of a significant ALTE. The question has been at what level does the duration, frequency, or severity of the apnea, bradycardia, or hypoxia have to be to cause neurologic damage. Early studies of the follow-up of 41 (near-miss) infants demonstrated a high percentage of abnormalities of tone, which improved with age; however, only 60% of children from 10 months to 2 years were normal compared with 94% of control infants (46). A smaller but longer 10 year follow-up study of 26 infants with idiopathic ALTE who were followed with home monitoring demonstrated only minor behavioral problems at a mean age of 2.7 years and had no differences in behavior or IQ at a mean age of 7 years (range, 6–10) (47).

Data from the CHIME study have begun to answer the question as to the degree of severity that is needed to alter neurodevelopmental outcome. Term infants who had adequate compliance with monitoring and returned for the Bayley Scales of Infant Development assessment at one year of age demonstrated a lower adjusted means for mental development with an increasing number of recorded events (48). Among the 138 term infants evaluated, 38% had no conventional events and 90% had no extreme events. Within the term group, 107 had idiopathic ALTE. A dose effect is suggested in that term infants having 0, 1 to 4, and 5+ conventional events were associated with unadjusted mean mental developmental index (MDI) values of 103.6 ± 10.6, 104.2 ± 10.7, and 97.7 ± 10.9, respectively. The adjusted mean difference in MDI for term infants having 5+ conventional events compared with no events was 5.6 points lower in term infants. A similar trend was seen for the Psychomotor Developmental Index, but it did not achieve statistical significance. Although ALTE infants were a subgroup of this population, these data imply that more frequent events which include both central and obstructive events, some associated with hypoxia, may cause sequelae in the developing infant. One may question whether these findings are the direct result of the events or combinations of the events or some underlying cause in the infant. Longitudinal studies are necessary to determine if the impact of these events is short lived or will herald other problems in the spectrum of sleep-disordered breathing later in life.

The overall risk of mortality among ALTE infants is also difficult to determine because of the heterogeneous group of infants reported. Among the series cited in this chapter, mortality for idiopathic ALTE is 0–13% (29–33). However, an even higher mortality of 30% is cited among a subset of idiopathic ALTE infants with severe recurrent events requiring vigorous stimulation and resuscitation (32). Some of these deaths were sudden and unexpected and occurred prior to the performance of a consistent death scene investigation. SIDS and ALTE have been associated in that infants who have had an ALTE may have up to three to five times higher risk of SIDS by some reports (49). Although no definitive rates are known, the incidence of a prior ALTE has been reported in 5–9% of SIDS infants; however, the majority of SIDS infants do not have a preceding event. Another factor which argues against a relationship is that the majority of ALTE infants are younger (8 weeks) than the age of peak incidence for SIDS infants (18 weeks) (22). Smoking was the only risk factor that was found to overlap for infants with SIDS and ALTE in a prospective population based study (22). Risk reduction strategies have been effective in reducing the incidence of SIDS; however, the rate of ALTE has remained unchanged in a similar time period (22,50).

IV. Summary

Term normal infants have occasional central and obstructive apneas, some associated with oxyhemoglobin desaturation, rarely with bradycardia. This improves with time postnatally over the first year of life. Prenatal and postnatal smoke exposure increases the frequency of these apnea events. In clinical practice it is often difficult to define what degree of apnea is normal with certainty or to define absence of pathology with confidence. Home memory monitors have become a diagnostic tool to assist the clinician in assessment of an infant with questionable apnea symptoms or a significant ALTE and in identifying a patient who may require further evaluation. A longer recording period (days to weeks) will allow for better identification of cardiorespiratory abnormalities or reassurance of normalcy. Infants with idiopathic ALTE have been poorly characterized and studies are subject to recall bias, parental unreliability, and lack of memory monitors in early studies. Events are frequently associated with oxyhemoglobin desaturation.

Memory monitoring provides the clinician with data to review. However, how does the clinician decide what to do with these data; what is considered normal for an infant? Should monitoring continue? Is further evaluation or intervention required? From the normative data reviewed in this chapter, it is difficult to determine an absolute threshold of frequency and severity of apneas that are considered normal and monitor data must be interpreted in the context of the clinical situation. Currently many apnea monitors are set with an apnea alarm threshold of 20 to 25 seconds and alarms may be extended when there are no physiologic sequelae of oxyhemoglobin desaturation or bradycardia (which would trigger further evaluation) and after reassurance that no underlying pathology has been identified. However, a degree of uncertainty has been raised regarding these criteria. Data from the CHIME study suggests an additive effect of multiple apneas on neurodevelopmental outcome. However, it remains unclear what the alternative therapy would be and whether that therapy reducing the number of apnea episodes would have a beneficial or harmful result. Clearly more research is needed to better understand this difficult clinical problem.

Among patients with an ALTE, potential mechanisms include decreased ventilatory response to hypercarbia, altered ventilatory and arousal responses to hypoxia, and possibly disordered autonomic control. Infants being monitored for an idiopathic ALTE had an increased risk for repeated extreme episodes, usually within 6 weeks. CHIME study data imply that more frequent cardiorespiratory events may be associated with neurodevelopmental sequelae in the developing infant. Mortality for idiopathic ALTE is 0–13%, but may be higher for idiopathic ALTE infants with severe recurrent events requiring resuscitation. SIDS and ALTE have an unclear association. The time course of the two differ and risk reduction strategies that have been effective in reducing SIDS have not altered the rate of ALTE. Most SIDS deaths are not preceded by an ALTE. Although ALTE infants may have an increased risk of death, there is no evidence that the mechanism is the same as in SIDS. Further study is needed to better characterize infants with idiopathic ALTE compared with a well-defined normative population of healthy infants. This will assist in identifying underlying mechanisms and natural history, potentially identifying a genetic component to the etiology of ALTE, as well as identifying infants who are at risk for neurodevelopmental morbidity, with the intention of possible intervention and prevention.

References

1. National Institutes of Health Consensus Development Conference on Infantile Apnea and Home Monitoring, Sept 29 to Oct 1, 1986. Pediatrics 1987; 79:292–299.
2. Weese-Mayer DE, Corwin MJ, Peucker MR, et al. and The CHIME Study Group. Comparison of apnea identified by respiratory inductance plethysmography with that detected by end tidal CO_2 or thermistor. Am J Crit Care Med 2000; 162:471–480.
3. Tishler PV, Redline S, Ferrette V, et al. The association of sudden unexpected infant death with obstructive sleep apnea. Am J Respir Crit Care Med 1996; 153: 1857–1863.
4. Kahn A, Groswasser J, Sottiaux M, et al. Prenatal exposure to cigarettes in infants with obstructive sleep apnea. Pediatrics 1994; 93:778–783.
5. Hoppenbrouwers T, Hodgman JE, Harper R, et al. Polygraphic studies of normal infants during the first six months of life. III: Incidence of apnea and periodic breathing. Pediatrics 1977; 60:418–425.

6. Hoppenbrouwers T, Hodgman JE, Arakawa K, et al. Respiration during the first six months of life in normal infants III: computer identification of breathing pauses. Pediatr Res 1980; 14:1230–1233.
7. Kahn A, Franco P, Kato I, et al. Breathing during sleep in infancy. In: Loughlin GM, Carroll JL, Marcus CL, eds; Lenfant C, exec. ed. Sleep and Breathing in Children: Lung Biology in Health and Disease. New York: Marcel Dekker, Inc., 2000:405–423.
8. Kahn A, Groswasser J, Sottiaux M, et al. Clinical symptoms associated with brief obstructive apnea in normal infants. Sleep 1993; 16:409–413.
9. Stein IM, White A, Kennedy JL Jr., et al. Apnea recordings of healthy infants at 40, 44, and 52 weeks postconception. Pediatrics 1979; 63:724–730.
10. Stein IM, Fallon M, Merisalo RL, et al. The frequency of apnea and bradycardia in a population of healthy, normal infants. Neuropediatrics 1983; 14:73–75.
11. Richards JM, Alexander JR, Shinebourne EA, et al. Sequential 22-hour profiles of breathing patterns and heart rate in 110 full-term infants during their first 6 months of life. Pediatrics 1984; 74:763–777.
12. Hunt CE, Brouillette RT, Hanson D, et al. Home pneumograms in normal infants. J Pediatr 1985; 106:551–555.
13. Kelly DH, Stellwagen LM, Kaitz E, et al. Apnea and periodic breathing in normal full-term infants during the first twelve months. Pediatr Pulmonol 1985; 1:215–219.
14. Hunt CE, Hufford DR, Bourgignon C, et al. Home documented monitoring of cardiorespiratory pattern and oxygen saturation in healthy infants. Pediatr Res 1996; 39:216–222.
15. Hunt CE, Corwin MJ, Lister G, et al., and The CHIME Study Group. Longitudinal assessment of hemoglobin oxygen saturation in healthy infants during the first six months of age. J Pediatr 1999; 134:580–586.
16. Ramanathan R, Corwin MJ, Hunt CE, et al., and The Collaborative Home Infant Monitoring Evaluation (CHIME) Study Group Cardiorespiratory events recorded in the home: comparison of healthy infant with those at increased risk for SIDS. JAMA 2001; 285:2199–2207.
17. Mitchell EA, Thompson JMD. Parental reported apnoea, admissions to hospital, and sudden infant death syndrome. Acta Paediatr 2001; 90:417–422.
18. Fleming P, Blair P, Platt MW, et al. The case control study: results and discussion. In: Fleming P, Bacon C, Blair P, et al., eds. Sudden Unexpected Deaths in Infancy: The CESDI SUDI Studies 1993–1996. London: The Stationary Office, 2000:13–96.
19. Steinschneider A, Santos V. Parental reports of apnea and bradycardia: temporal characteristics and accuracy. Pediatrics 1991; 88:1100–1105.
20. Altman RL, Brand DA, Forman S, et al. Abusive head injury as a cause of apparent life-threatening events in infancy. Arch Pediatr Adolesc Med 2003; 157:1011–1015.
21. DeWolfe CC. Apparent life-threatening event: a review. Pediatr Clin North Am 2005; 52:1127–1146.
22. Kiechl-Kolendorfer U, Hof D, Peglow UP, et al. Epidemiology of apparent life threatening events. Arch Dis Child 2004; 90:297–300.
23. McGovern MC, Smith MBH. Causes of apparent life threatening events in infants: a systematic review. Arch Dis Child 2004; 89:1043–1048.
24. Kahn A, Blum D, Waterschoot P, et al. Effects of obstructive sleep apneas on transcutaneous oxygen pressure in control infants, siblings of sudden infant death

syndrome victims, and near miss infants: comparison with effects of central sleep apneas. Pediatrics 1982; 70:852–857.

25. Kahn A, Rebuffat E, Sottiaux M, Blum D. Problems in the management of infants with an apparent life-threatening event. Ann N Y Acad Sci 1988; 533:78–88.

26. Toubas PL, Duke JC, McCaffree MA, et al. Effects of maternal smoking and caffeine on infantile apnea: a retrospective study. Pediatrics 1986; 78:159–163.

27. Guilleminault C, Ariagno R, Korobkin R, et al. Mixed and obstructive sleep apnea and near miss sudden infant death syndrome: 2. comparison of near miss and normal control infants. Pediatrics 1979; 64:882–891.

28. Daniels H, Naulaers G, Deroost F, et al. Polysomnography and home documented monitoring of cardiorespiratory pattern. Arch Dis Child 1999; 81:434–436.

29. Ariagno RL, Guilleminault C, Korobkin R, et al. 'Near-miss' for sudden infant death syndrome infants: a clinical problem. Pediatrics 1983; 71:726–730.

30. Duffty P, Bryan MH. Home apnea monitoring in 'near-miss' sudden infant death syndrome and in siblings of SIDS victims. Pediatrics 1982; 70:69–74.

31. Dunne K, Matthews T. Near-miss sudden infant death syndrome: clinical findings and management. Pediatrics 1987; 79:889–893.

32. Oren J, Kelly D, Shannon DC. Identification of a high-risk group for sudden infant death syndrome among infants who were resuscitated for sleep apnea. Pediatrics 1986; 77:495–499.

33. Sivan Y, Kornecki A, Baharav A, et al. Home monitoring for infants at high risk for sudden infant death syndrome. Isr J Med Sci 1997; 33:45–49.

34. Weese-Mayer DE, Brouillette RT, Morrow AS, et al. Assessing validity of infant monitor alarms with event recording. J Pediatr 1989; 115:702–708.

35. Samuels MP, Poets CF, Noyes JP, et al. Diagnosis and management after life threatening events in infants and young children who received cardiopulmonary resuscitation. BMJ 1993; 306:489–492.

36. Poets CF, Samuels MP, Noyes JP, et al. Home event recordings of oxygenation, breathing movements, and heart rate and rhythm in infants with recurrent life-threatening events. J Pediatr 1993; 123:693–701.

37. Côté A, Hum C, Brouillette RT, et al. Frequency and timing of recurrent events in infants using home cardiorespiratory monitors. J Pediatr 1998; 312:783–789.

38. van der Hal AL, Rodriguez AM, Sargent CW, et al. Hypoxic and hypercapnic arousal responses and prediction of subsequent apnea in apnea of infancy. Pediatrics 1985; 75:848–854.

39. Coleman JM, Mammel MC, Reardon C. Hypercarbic ventilatory response in infants at risk for SIDS. Pediatric Pulmonology 1987; 3:226–230.

40. Katz-Salamon M, Milerad J. The divergent ventilatory and heart rate response to moderate hypercapnia in infants with apnoea of infancy. Arch Dis Child 1998; 79:231–236.

41. Katz-Salamon M. Delayed chemoreceptor responses in infants with apnoea. Arch Dis Child 2004; 89:261–266.

42. Milerad J, Hertzberg T, Wennergren C, et al. Respiratory and arousal responses to hypoxia in apnoeic infants reinvestigated. Eur J Pediatr 1989; 148:565–570.

43. Edner A, Katz-Salamon M, Lagercrantz H, et al. Heart rate response profiles during head upright tilt test in infants with apparent life threatening events. Arch Dis Child 1997; 76:27–30.

44. Harrington C, Kirjavainen T, Teng A, et al. Altered autonomic and reduced arousability in apparent life-threatening event infants with obstructive sleep apnea. Am J Respir Crit Care Med 2002; 165:1048–1054.
45. Steinschneider A, Richmond C, Ramaswamy V, et al. Clinical characteristics of an apparent life-threatening event and the subsequent occurrence of prolonged apnea and prolonged bradycardia. Clin Pediatr 1998; 37:223–230.
46. Korobkin R, Guilleminault C. Neurologic abnormalities in near miss for sudden infant death syndrome infants. Pediatrics 1979; 64:369–374.
47. Kahn A, Sottiaux M, Appelboom-Fondu J, et al. Long-term development of children monitored as infants for an apparent life-threatening event during sleep: a 10-year follow-up study. Pediatrics 1989; 83:668–673.
48. Hunt CE, Corwin MJ, Baird T, et al., and The CHIME Study Group. Cardiorespiratory events detected by home memory monitoring and one-year neurodevelopmental outcome. J Pediatr 2004; 145:465–471.
49. Hunt CE, Hauck FR. Sudden infant death syndrome. CMAJ 2006; 174(13): 1861–1869.
50. Gershon WM, Besch NS, Franciosi RA, et al. A comparison of apparent life-threatening events before and after the back to sleep campaign. Wisconsin Med J 2002; 101:39–45.

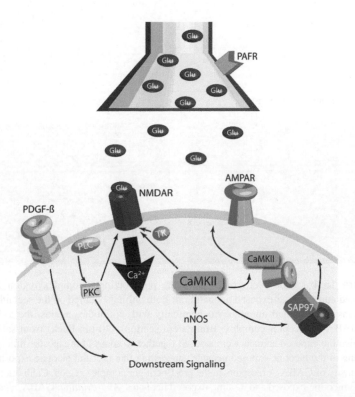

Figure 4.2 Schematic diagram of a working model for glutamatergic signaling in the nucleus of the solitary tract (nTS) during acute hypoxia. *Abbreviations*: AMPAR, receptor for α-amino-3-hydroxy-5-methylisoxazole-4-propionic acid; CaCMKII, calcium/calmodulin-dependent kinase 2; Glu, glutamate; NMDAR, receptor for *N*-methyl-D-aspartate; nNOS, neuronal nitric oxide synthase; PAFR, platelet activating factor receptor; PKC, protein kinase C; PLC, phospholipase C; PDGF β, receptor for platelet derived growth factor beta; SAP97, one of several PDZ membrane-associated guanylate kinase proteins; TK, tyrosine kinase.

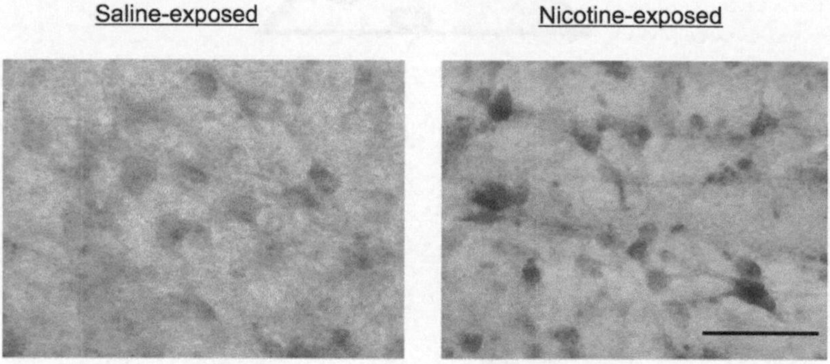

Saline-exposed   Nicotine-exposed

Figure 15.4 Photomicrographs from the pre-Botzinger complex region in a saline-exposed and nicotine-exposed neonatal rat; both animals studied on the second day of life. Sections were stained immunocytochemically with antibodies against the α-3 subunit of the GABA-A receptor complex. Brain stem sections (40-μm thick) from saline-exposed and nicotine-exposed animals were assayed together to control for exposure time. Note darker staining in the nicotine-exposed neonate, suggesting that prenatal nicotine exposure increases the density of GABA-A receptors in the pre-Botzinger complex region. Calibration bar 50 μm. $N = 3$ nicotine-exposed and 3 saline-exposed neonates. *Abbreviation*: GABA, γ-aminobutyric acid. *Source*: From Luo, McMullen, and Fregosi, unpublished observations.

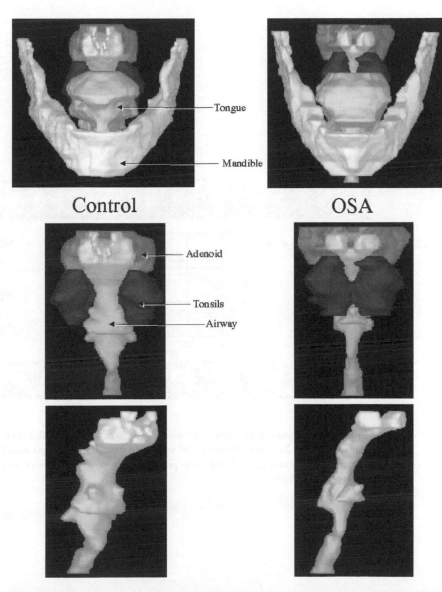

Figure 19.2 Three-dimensional reconstruction of airway (light blue), adenoid (orange) and tonsils (red), tongue (pink), and mandible (white) in a normal child and a child with obstructive sleep apnea syndrome. Note differences in airway size and shape. *Source*: From Ref. 63.

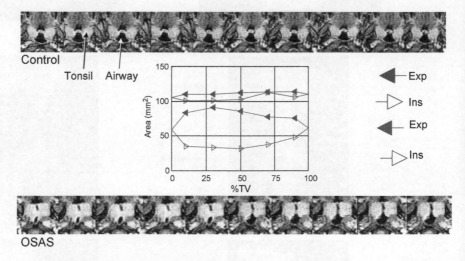

Figure 19.3 Dynamic changes in cross-sectional area at midtonsillar level during tidal breathing (TV) at 20% increments of tidal volume (5 increments in inspiration [Ins] and 5 in expiration [Exp]) in a control child (*top panels*) and a child with obstructive sleep apnea syndrome (*bottom panels*).

10

Apparent Life-Threatening Events: Pathogenesis and Management

MARTIN P. SAMUELS
Keele University and University Hospital of North Staffordshire, Staffordshire, U.K.

I. Introduction

An apparent life-threatening event (ALTE) is the term used to describe a clinical presentation that involves a sudden, unexpected change in an infant's behavior that is frightening to parents or caregivers but does not lead to death or persistent collapse. Thus, an ALTE is an episode with a beginning and an end, the latter having come about either spontaneously or as a result of vigorous stimulation or cardiopulmonary resuscitation. The infant is usually described by the observer of the event as having had a disturbance of at least two of the following: breathing, color, consciousness, movement, or muscle tone. ALTE therefore describes symptoms and is not a diagnosis of specific condition.

Although such episodes may occur in children older than 12 months, the majority of patients are less than 1 year and predominantly under 6 months of age (1). This age distribution and the fear engendered in the observer provide support to the possibility that such episodes, if undetected, may lead to the sudden and unexpected death of the infant (crib or cot death).

Such episodes will be accompanied by the parent or caregiver being sufficiently concerned to take action at the time the infant was found. They will

229

have thought the infant was at risk or in the process of dying or actually dead and their actions will usually reflect this. The emergency services will have been contacted and urgent admission to hospital arranged. The decision of parents or caregivers to resuscitate an infant is dependent on their perception of the situation, as well as their knowledge and skills in performing resuscitative measures. Institution of resuscitation usually reflects a more severe event than the one in which no resuscitation is given. However, it is possible that parents react very differently to events of similar severity.

II. Relationship to Sudden Infant Death

The commonest category of death in infancy is that which is sudden and unexplained, despite a thorough autopsy, examination of the scene of death, and review of the case history (sudden infant death syndrome, SIDS). The mechanisms that cause sudden and unexpected death in an infant are probably similar in part to some of the mechanisms which cause ALTE. This observation is supported by the fact that whereas most studies report survival in infants who have had an ALTE, a small proportion of infants who suffer recurrent ALTE progress to sudden and unexpected death (2). It has also been identified that a small proportion of infants who die of SIDS have a history of a previous ALTE or apnea: 7% in the National Institute of Child Health and Development Cooperative Epidemiological Study of SIDS in the United States (3) and 8.8% in an Australian series (4).

For these reasons, infants who suffer ALTE have been considered an "at risk" group (for sudden death), and their study has been of particular interest with regard to the mechanisms for sudden infant death. This approach helps our understanding of the pathophysiology of events in living infants that may result in sudden death, and compliments the approaches from pathological and epidemiological studies.

III. Definition

The National Institutes of Health Consensus Development Conference on Infantile Apnea (1987) defined an ALTE as an episode that is frightening to the observer and is characterized by a combination of apnea, skin color change, marked change in muscle tone, choking, and gagging (3). Such episodes were previously known as "near-miss SIDS." However, the majority of infants who suffer an ALTE survive and are not at high risk of sudden death—this term has therefore been abandoned. The definition includes identification of the caregivers' reaction to the event; thus, infants whose caregivers underreact may not come to the attention of health professionals or be characterized as having suffered an ALTE, even though they may have had some combination of these symptoms. Conversely, benign physiological events in babies may sometimes have excessive intervention by parents, particularly those who are anxious, attention seeking, or suffer abnormal illness behavior. Such infants may thereby receive unnecessary hospital admission and investigations. Clinicians need to be aware of the spectrum of parental reactions as these often determine management pathways, and it is important that the clinicians maintain an objective view to avoid inappropriate investigations and treatment.

In addition to above situations, there are others in which it can be difficult to decide whether an infant is classified as having suffered an ALTE. For example, some infants with ALTE may only recover in part and thus continue to remain unwell when in hospital. In such infants, initial investigations and management will be guided by the ongoing symptoms and signs. In such cases, the finding of an abnormality (e.g., a positive blood culture, a nasopharyngeal aspirate positive for respiratory syncytial virus, or an underlying metabolic disorder) will be followed by the diagnosis in the infant being reclassified from ALTE to a more specific illness or condition, e.g., septicemia, bronchiolitis, or inborn error of metabolism. Nevertheless, the parents may have as their greatest concern the presenting event. Such families may continue to require support along similar lines as if the infant had suffered an unexplained ALTE.

In some situations an infant collapses unexpectedly at home and remains severely ill, sometimes without adequate explanation. In some cases recalcitrant shock and death follow, but their presentation may be akin to an ALTE. Conversely, the infant may spontaneously and fully recover with the parents demonstrating less concern and reporting the event only at some later time to health professionals. The fear an event causes in parents or caregivers is assessed by their verbal reports and their actions. Therefore, whether such infants constitute ALTE is debatable. Finally, infants who have recurrent ALTE may be classified as suffering from apnea of infancy. This reclassification merely renames a clinical problem, does not define its cause, and confuses the definition, as not all ALTE necessarily involve cessation of breathing.

IV. The Evidence Base

Most studies relating to ALTE, near-miss SIDS, or near death episodes are at a low level of evidence (grade 2 and lower)—they involve a retrospective review of a series of cases and the results of usually selective investigations. Another group of studies examines the physiology of infants who have suffered ALTEs, often performed on the basis that they are a group at high risk for SIDS. Such studies aim to determine susceptible mechanisms in infants, which may provide answers to the mechanisms for sudden unexplained infant death. However, studies are difficult to compare because the populations of infants may differ widely among the studies. This is because (1) there is no single accepted definition by which infants were included in studies (see above) and (2) clinical practices and diagnostic labeling differ even within a single health facility. Presentation and initial management of infants who present with ALTEs vary between regions and countries, partly as a result of different health care systems.

Most published case series of ALTE infants come from clinicians within specialist or teaching centers who have a special interest in the assessment of ALTE infants—such data may not represent the pathophysiology or appropriate management pathways for infants presenting with ALTE in other populations, particularly those that are community based. Case series may also be biased depending on whether the publications are from units who have a particular subspecialist interest, e.g., gastroenterology or neurology. In addition to these biases in the published literature, there is a lack of adequate descriptive studies in populations, such as the incidence of ALTE and its outcome. There is a wide variation between units, regions and countries in the assessment, investigation, and management of such infants.

V. Epidemiology

Wennergren et al., in a prospective epidemiological multicenter study over 24 months, found an incidence for attacks of lifelessness of 0.46/1000 live births in Sweden (1). This was half the rate for SIDS (0.94/1000 live births). Studies have also shown that infants who suffer from ALTE are most likely to present in the day time (rather than during the night) (1,5). If such episodes do occur at night, those infants who are unable to arouse or compensate may die and be classified as SIDS. In the Swedish study, the age distribution for ALTE was similar to that of SIDS cases, with a peak around six to eight weeks of age. Such episodes may occur in the neonatal period (6–8).

Myerberg et al. have estimated that 6/1000 full-term infants and 86/1000 preterm infants may suffer from ALTE (total 11/1000 live births) (9). In South Australia, with 20,000 births per year, ALTE resulted in hospital admission in 13.7/1000 live births (10); in North Staffordshire, England (population, 480,000), with 6500 live births per year, a prospective study, in 1995, identified 30 infants presenting to hospital who had suffered ALTE in a year (4.6/1000) (unpublished observations); and in Sheffield, England, in 1997, there were 76 ALTEs out of 6022 births in one year (rate, 12.6/1000) (Primhak R, personal communication). Thus, incidence rates for ALTE vary roughly from 0.5 to 14 per 1000 live births, a more than 20-fold difference. This variability is likely to be related to different case definition and ascertainment.

VI. Causes

Infants who present with ALTE are a varied group, ranging from parents who are overly concerned about a benign or physiological event to those where the infant is truly in a life-threatening situation (11). Published case reviews have identified a large number of different causes for the clinical presentation of ALTE (Table 1). A systematic review of diagnosed causes of ALTE has described 728 different diagnoses (12). The relative prevalence of each condition depends on

Table 1 Causes of ALTE

Respiratory
    Infection—e.g., respiratory syncytial virus, pertussis, pneumonia
    Upper airway obstruction—e.g., retrognathia (120,157,165–167)
    Lower airway obstruction or closure—e.g., tracheobronchomalacia
    Intrapulmonary shunting, e.g., cyanotic breath holding (17,54,88)
Neurological
    Epileptic—seizure induced (26,96–98)
    Intracranial hemorrhage—vitamin K deficiency, child abuse
    Central hypoventilation—congenital, drugs, neurological disease
    Neuromuscular disease
Infective
    Septicemia, urinary tract infection, gastroenteritis
    Meningoencephalitis
Autonomic
    Vasovagal
    Gastroesophageal reflux
    Skin pallor changes
Child Abuse (18,104–118)
    Illness fabrication
    Attempted suffocation
    Poisoning
Cardiac
    Tachyarrhythmias—Wolfe-Parkinson White (133–134) and Long QT syndromes
    Congenital heart disease
Inborn areas of metabolism (129–132)
Miscellaneous
    Carbon monoxide poisoning (168)
    Cat smothering (169)
    Abnormal infant holding practices (170)
    Hemorrhagic shock encephalopathy syndrome (171)
Unknown

the method of ascertainment, which varies from consecutive admissions to an accident and emergency (A&E) department (13,14) to infants referred for evaluation at a tertiary sleep center. The range of investigations performed for ALTE is wide: 0 to 26, mean 15.5 in one study (15), with a low yield contributing to diagnosis (5.9% of 3776 investigations or 33.5% of positive tests).

Clinical management of such infants does not require, therefore, an exhaustive list of investigations, but needs a careful and focused clinical assessment of each case commencing with history, examination, and usually a period of inpatient observation. It is important to appreciate that the finding of an abnormal investigation does not automatically imply it to be the cause of the infant's event. Abnormalities on investigation may be the result of the ALTE (particularly if it was severe) or simply represent homeostatic instability, autonomic dysfunction, or an unrelated finding. Studies that have investigated large numbers of ALTE infants have shown that there is a failure to find a cause in   40–50% of cases (16,17). However, there is probably a wide variation in practice as some infants who present with ALTE and in whom an investigation is found to be abnormal, e.g., pernasal swab positive for pertussis, may be diagnosed as pertussis, rather than "ALTE-caused pertussis." Such issues confound the case ascertainment from one study to another.

VII.   History and Examination

Health professionals should listen carefully to the parents' observations as well as their reactions or feelings to it. In this way, the professional may become more aware of the real and perceived risks of the episode. A clear description of the event should be noted including who was present, what each person observed, and what their actions were. The timing of the event should be noted, including whether the infant was awake or asleep and what activity he or she was performing. It can help to determine how it was discovered that the event was occurring in the infant. Sometimes parents or caregivers discover such cases by chance.

A record of the infant's position should be made, whether there was movement and how the infant was holding itself. The color of the infant should be noted—this may include red, blue, purple, pale, gray, or white. It may be possible to observe whether color change has occurred on the face as a whole (central cyanosis), just around the eyes and mouth, or in the limbs. The presence of vomit or blood from the nose and mouth should be recorded. This may be a marker for trauma and an event that is intentionally induced [odds ratio, 41 (18)]. The presence or absence of breathing movements should be asked but it may be difficult for observers to reliably report this finding. Even nurse observations of the presence or absence of breathing in infants receiving hospital neonatal care may correlate poorly with recorded breathing patterns (19–21). In these studies, nurses failed to detect naturally occurring episodes in preterm infants on conventional bedside breathing movements and ECG monitors: 46–67% of episodes documented on multichannel recordings went undetected. The actions of the observers should be noted and also the response of the infant to these. The time scale for these actions and the recovery of the infant should be noted and whether any similar event had happened in the past.

A general pediatric history of the mother's pregnancy and delivery, the infant's birth, and neonatal progress should be obtained. A history of feeding, weight gain, development, and recent minor symptoms should be noted. A detailed family medical history and social history should also be obtained. The latter should include who else is at home, other medical problems within the family, and any contact with psychiatric or social services.

Infants who are historically at particular risk of subsequent events or sudden death may be identified: these include those who were born prematurely, who may be suffering subclinical hypoxemia (22), and those who had bleeding from the mouth and nose, which may indicate trauma or child abuse (18).

A full clinical examination with the infant completely undressed should be performed. The height, weight, and head circumference should be recorded and plotted on a growth chart. Particular attention should be paid to examination of the upper airway, respiratory, and cardiovascular systems. Neurodevelopmental assessment is important because a number of neurological conditions may present with apnea. To detect trauma, fundoscopy should be performed. All infants should undergo initial spot measurement of arterial oxygen saturation (Spo$_2$) and in infants who were preterm or may have a respiratory prodrome, a longer period of monitoring of Spo$_2$ should be undertaken.

VIII. Initial Management and Investigations

Parents of an infant who has suffered an ALTE may be extremely anxious and concerned that their infant is dying. For this reason alone, it is probably appropriate to admit all infants who have suffered a first ALTE. This allows time for a full assessment, a period of observation, and discussion with the family.

A recurrence rate for severe ALTE has been reported to be as high as 68% (23), and for all ALTEs, episodes are more likely to recur in the few days after the first event (1). These provide further support for initial hospital admission. Some ALTEs may be recurrent within a short period of time (hours to a few days). These subsequent events may be observed and a diagnosis made by clinical observation, e.g., infantile spasms. In addition, clinical physiological monitoring or recording allows documentation of any further events and the findings from this may indicate a diagnosis (4,17,24). Both respiratory illnesses, such as respiratory syncytial virus (RSV) and pertussis (25), and epileptic seizures (26) may cluster in this way.

Some infants may initially be seen some days after the episode either in the pediatric office, admissions room, or outpatient clinic. In such cases, admission may not be required if it is agreed the infant has had no further events and is clinically well.

No study has identified any single investigation as having a high positive predictive value for detecting an abnormality that will alter the outcome (15). There is, thus, much controversy on which initial investigations should be undertaken in an infant presenting with a first ALTE. In most cases, it is reasonable to check serum sodium, potassium, calcium, renal and liver function, full blood picture, blood and urine cultures, throat or pharyngeal swabs, and chest X ray (Table 2).

If the infant is examined very soon after the event, an arterial blood gas may help provide documentation of the severity of the episode (18). Other markers of metabolic disturbance such as blood glucose, lactate, and ammonia could also be taken at this time. Continued observation, particularly for the development of respiratory infection, fever, or other signs of sepsis should be undertaken with a low threshold for treating sepsis in infants younger than four weeks of age. Nose swabs and pharyngeal aspirates should be collected for viral

Table 2 Investigations in Infants Presenting with ALTE

First-line investigations
  Hemoglobin
  White cell count
  Blood culture
  Urine culture
  Nasopharyngeal aspirate for viral immunofluorescence and culture
  Pernasal swab for pertussis
  Chest X ray
  Biochemical screen
Second-line investigations (severe/recurrent events)
  Multichannel physiological recordings/event recording[a]
  Blood sugar[b]
  Arterial blood gas[b]
  Lactate[a]
  Ammonia[b]
  Serum and urine metabolic studies (e.g., for amino/organic acids)
  Urinary toxicology screen
  EEG
  Cranial imaging (CT, MRI)
  ECG
  Esophageal pH monitoring
  ENT examination of the airway under anesthetic
  Echocardiogram
  Skeletal survey
  Covert video surveillance

---

[a]Of particular value for documenting pathophysiology during subsequent event.
[b]If close to event/still unwell.

immunofluorescence and culture and pertussis culture. Urine should be collected for microscopy, bacterial culture, and antibiotic sensitivities, and specimens saved for urinary and blood metabolic screens (27). Urine and blood should be collected and held for toxicology screens. Parents or caregivers may not always give complete information about medicines given to the infants, some of which may be inadvertent and some deliberate.

A majority of infants suffer a single event only and survive. Adverse outcomes are more likely with infants who have had recurrent events or where there is a family history of SIDS. In the absence of these, investigations should be kept to a minimum in an otherwise well infant. However, if the infant remains unwell, develops new symptoms, has recurrent episodes, or there is a family history of SIDS, further investigations should be undertaken. The most common diagnoses from some recent studies are shown in Table 3. The role of multi-channel physiological recording or esophageal pH recording as a routine in ALTEs is more complex and discussed in the next sections.

Table 3 Diagnostic Categories for ALTE and Proportions Found
for Each Category

Diagnostic categories (range of %)	Proportions (Ref.)
Breathing problems (5–25%)	13/64 (59)
	60/857 (128)
	17/340 (4)
	40/157 (17)
Epilepsy (7–25%)	4/59 (59)
	78/857 (128)
	25/340 (4)
	7/46 (161)
	10/157 (17)
	6/65 (14)
Gastroesophageal reflux (24–62%)	72/117 (61)
	263/857 (128)
	211/340 (4)
	12/50 (59)
	9/17 (63)
Induced or fabricated illness (2–16%)	5/340 (4)
	25/157 (17)
	3/128 (116)
Metabolic (2–8%)	5/65 (27)
	14/857 (128)
Vasovagal (11%)	95/857 (128)
Unknown (23.51%)	281/857 (128)
	80/157 (17)
	15/65 (14)

IX. Physiology

Physiological studies in infants who have suffered ALTE have not shown any particular test with a high positive predictive value for an adverse outcome. Studies have identified subgroups of infants who suffer from abnormal hypoxemia or esophageal acidity, and in these recurrent events have reduced or stopped after intervention such as oxygen therapy (17) or treatment for reflux (28). Most physiological studies have looked at groups of infants suffering from ALTE and identified group differences from healthy controls. However, there is usually a large overlap between normal and ALTE infants that makes the usefulness of physiological testing limited in identifying an individual's susceptibility to further events. Such studies, therefore have little role in clinical management. That is, they do not help predict recurrence or risk for sudden death in individual patients.

Respiratory studies have identified the presence of increased apneic pauses (29–31), obstructive apnea (32), periodic breathing (33–34), higher heart and respiratory rates (35), and abnormalities in waking and ventilatory responses to carbon dioxide (36–38). These abnormalities have not always been borne out by other studies (39,40). Decreased specific airway conductance (41,42) and abnormalities in diaphragm strength (43) have also been identified in ALTE infants. Whether these are cause, effect, or associated phenomena in relation to the ALTE are unknown.

Studies suggest that there may be an abnormality in autonomic function in infants who have had ALTE, as identified by increased sweating at night (44), heart rate variability abnormalities (45), changes in sleep state (46) and blood pressure responses (47). Neurological studies, such as brain stem auditory evoked responses (48,49), have not shown differences from controls.

X. Multichannel Recordings

Case series show an enormous variation in the proportion of infants who demonstrate abnormalities on pneumograms, sleep studies, or multichannel physiological recordings. Such studies have different methodologies and definitions of abnormality. They have not been found to be predictive of recurrence of events (35,50). Event recordings in infants during further events and in those who subsequently die of SIDS do not indicate apneic pauses (central apnea) as being a primary abnormality (51,52). Bradycardia has been identified in event recordings during death or near death episodes (51), but this too may be secondary, e.g., to hypoxemia (52). Event recordings that focus on alarms based on apnea or bradycardia criteria have identified most events as being artifactual (53). However, when recordings are made of clinical events, hypoxemia has been identified as one of the main abnormalities (52).

This hypoxemia was due to varied causes, including respiratory events due to intrapulmonary shunting (54), epileptic seizure induced events (26), and intentional attempted suffocation (18). The "shunt" events were manifested as hypoxemic episodes in association with chronic lung disease of prematurity, respiratory infections, or cyanotic breath holding, and when recurrent, treatment with additional inspired oxygen helped reduce or stop events (17). The particular susceptibility of preterm infants to subclinical chronic lung disease and clinically undetected hypoxemia may put these infants at increased risk of hypoxemic episodes, ALTE, and sudden death. Additional oxygen therapy appeared to be therapeutic in reducing cyanotic-apnea episodes in this group of infants (22).

Although recognition and treatment of hypoxemia in ex-preterm infants may be important in reducing subsequent events (55), standard recordings looking for apneic events (cessation of breathing or airflow) have been shown not to be predictive of future events (35,56). There is also no gain from routine multichannel recordings in subsequent siblings of ALTE infants (57).

XI. Medical Causes

A. Gastroesophageal Reflux

Gastroesophageal reflux is commonly considered to be a cause of ALTE. Initial reports of the finding of reflux suggested it had a major role in producing life-threatening events, and its treatment is mandatory when identified (28,58–59).

Reflux is more common during active sleep (60) and has been considered to act via reflex effects on central respiratory control (61,62) or in some cases induce epileptic seizures (63). However, as outlined below, it is likely that reflux is more commonly incidentally found than is a cause of events.

In two cohorts of ALTE infants referred to sleep units, the prevalence of reflux was 62% of 340 infants (diagnosed by barium swallow or milk scan) (4) and 20% of 3799 infants (diagnostic methods not stated) (64). A systematic search for reflux in 130 infants with ALTE presenting to an emergency room found 26% to have reflux (14). However, the detection of reflux is highly dependent on the methodology used (65,66), and studies based on contrast studies or scintigraphy cannot be relied upon (67). Increasing the combination of techniques used for detecting reflux, e.g., with esophageal pH monitoring for 24 hours, barium swallow, and radionuclide milk scans, will result in an increasing prevalence of gastroesophageal reflux found in infants who have suffered ALTE (59). However, the true prevalence of reflux in ALTE may be less important than the susceptibility of some infants to react adversely to it.

Controlled studies suggest that the association between ALTE and gastroesophageal reflux is weak. Acid reflux to the proximal esophagus did not increase in 18 ALTE infants compared with 120 controls (68), or in 50 infants with ALTE compared with another 50 without ALTE (69).

Furthermore, there is poor evidence of temporal association between reflux episodes and pathophysiological events (70–74). In 21 infants with ALTE with polygraphically demonstrated apneas and episodes of acid reflux, apnea and reflux were seldom temporally associated; where they were associated, the apnea generally preceded the reflux episode (74). A study of 26 infants with ALTE found reflux in 19, but no temporal association between reflux and cardiorespiratory events on polygraphic monitoring. In addition, in three out of five infants who underwent fundoplication, the apneas persisted (71). Another study of 17 infants with ALTE found five who had reflux episodes associated with apnea; however, in two of these infants both the reflux and the apnea were preceded by a seizure, which was felt to be the primary etiology (63).

Two studies have demonstrated temporal associations. In one study of 15 infants with a history of awake apnea, 13 had more than one episode of reflux preceding airway obstruction during polygraphic monitoring (75). In a second study of 16 ALTE infants, reflux was followed by a fall in Spo_2 despite normal recordings of breathing movements and ECG (76).

Hypoxemia and apnea may occur in association with feeds but without evidence of gastroesophageal reflux (77). This may have arisen because of the effects of sucking and swallowing on breathing, through reduced diaphragmatic activity, or autonomic effects. It may also be possible that gastroesophageal reflux is one consequence of active expiratory muscle activity in infants prone to respiratory events, rather than the cause of them. Infants may produce active expiratory activity to overcome decreased airway conductance (41,42) and thus increase intra-abdominal pressure. However, this has not been formally examined.

Recently, a study of intraluminal impedance monitoring for reflux in 22 infants has found that only 22% of reflux demonstrated by this technique would be detected by pH monitoring, and that 30% of apneas documented by polygraphy were associated temporally with reflux on impedance monitoring (78). However, this patient group contained less than 12 patients with ALTE or apnea history. Using esophageal intraluminal impedance rather than esophageal pH, a study in preterm infants found that while cardiorespiratory events and reflux were common, there was little evidence for a temporal association (79).

Although gastroesophageal reflux features strongly in lists of causes of ALTE, it is debated whether all ALTE should have investigation to detect reflux, given the difficulty in knowing whether, even when found, it is the cause of the disease. Some suggest that only infants with ALTE and a history of vomiting, poor weight gain, feed refusal, etc should be investigated for reflux (80). Future work will hopefully examine more closely why some infants respond adversely to reflux with abnormal hypoxemic or apneic episodes. It may be that we will be able to use an investigation like the modified Bernstein's test to determine which infants respond to physical and chemical stimuli within the esophagus or upper airway (81).

Thus, a causative association between gastroesophageal reflux and ALTE is yet to be firmly established. Furthermore, there are no randomized controlled trials of the effect of treatment of gastroesophageal reflux on ALTE. There is undoubtedly a need for improvement in the methodology of reflux detection, as well as a better understanding of the susceptibility in individual infants to the effects of reflux. In patients presenting with recurrent apnea or ALTE, it would be prudent to document, where possible, evidence of the temporal association of the events with gastroesophageal reflux before undertaking surgical treatment for the reflux.

B. Breath Holding

Breath-holding attacks are commonly reported by parents (82) and onset may be in infancy (83). They may present to a health professional as an ALTE. There are no agreed diagnostic criteria for these events. The outcome of breath-holding spells is generally thought to be benign (84–87), but some researchers have questioned this, reporting deaths occurring as a result of repeated breath holding (88–92).

Iron therapy has been found to reduce breath-holding attacks in a randomized controlled trial in 67 children with a high prevalence of iron deficiency and of consanguinity; the response to treatment was greater in those with iron deficiency (93). A randomized controlled trial of the putative nootropic drug, piracetam, showed a reduction in the frequency of breath-holding attacks, and a reported 92% of patients with complete resolution after two months treatment, compared with 30% in the placebo group (94). Thus, if an ALTE is considered to be due to a breath-holding event, treatment with iron should be considered, particularly if there is evidence of iron deficiency. Further trials of the safety and efficacy of piracetam should be undertaken before this drug can be recommended in such episodes.

C. Epilepsy

Apnea or ALTE may be a presentation of partial epilepsy (26,95–98). In ALTEs presenting to emergency departments, epilepsy has been found in 7–25% of cases (13,14).

Infants and children may present with no obvious signs apart from episodes of apnea, cyanosis, and change in heart rate. In addition, electroencephalography (EEG) between seizures may be normal (26,96,97,99,100). Hypoxemic episodes from nonepileptic ALTEs can also result in secondary and prolonged epileptic seizures (101,102). Continuous recordings are needed to document an event and should include simultaneous measurements of ECG, respiratory effort and airflow, oxygenation, EEG, and video to determine whether seizure activity precedes or follows the clinical symptoms (26,103).

D. Child Abuse

Apnea, cyanotic episodes, and ALTE have been reported as presenting symptoms of child abuse, through mechanisms, such as intentional suffocation, intentional head injury, and fabricated events (18,104–118). Child abuse has been found to be a cause of 3/128 (2.3%) of ALTE cases (116). In a case-control study comparing 33 ALTEs due to child abuse (confirmed by covert video surveillance) with 40 control children who required cardiopulmonary resuscitation for ALTE, risk factors for child abuse included petechiae, bleeding from the mouth or nose, and one or more siblings with ALTE or sudden unexplained death (18). Physiological recordings taken during episodes may suggest imposed upper airway obstruction (18,110), but a definitive diagnosis is best achieved by the use of covert video surveillance (18,110–112,117,118); failure to do so may lead to either inability to protect the child or inappropriate allegations of abuse. Hence, it is extremely important that a multiagency approach to assessment and investigation is taken when this possibility is considered.

E. Intrinsic Upper Airway Obstruction

A polysomnogram-based study of 29 ALTE and 30 control infants found a significant increase in obstructive apneas in the ALTE group (32). In contrast, a study of 107 term ALTEs using documenting cardiorespiratory monitors and oximetry did not observe a significant difference in apneic events in the subsequent 16 weeks compared to 306 healthy term infants (119).

A subgroup of patients with ALTEs found to have obstructive sleep apnea (OSA) on polysomnography had relatives with a higher risk of sleep-related breathing disorders and smaller upper airways than those of ALTE children with normal polysomnograms (120).

Nasal continuous positive airway pressure (CPAP) has been used successfully to treat infants with recurrent ALTE who were found to have upper airway obstruction (121) and has also been shown to normalize autonomic function in these infants (122). In the absence of randomized controlled trials and given the favorable prognosis of most ALTEs, this intervention should be reserved for infants with proven OSA and severe and recurrent symptoms.

F. Central Hypoventilation Syndrome

Congenital central hypoventilation syndrome (CCHS) involves an infant's inability to provide effective spontaneous alveolar ventilation, particularly during sleep (123–125). In cases where CCHS is present with cyanotic-apneic episodes, or changes in color, muscle tone, and conscious level, the infant usually remains unwell. Although case reports of CCHS do describe some cases initially presenting with an episode of apnea or ALTE, the condition is rare and does not present itself in case series of ALTE.

If undiagnosed, CCHS will lead to death (126–127). Diagnosis involves assessment of the infant's response to carbon dioxide in different sleep stages (123) and investigation for the paired-like homeobox 2b (PHOX2B) mutation (125). Cases of ALTE should undergo assessment to ensure that they are not hypoventilating and as this condition is rare, confirmation of the diagnosis and initiation of treatment requires specialist facilities.

G. Inborn Errors of Metabolism

Inborn errors of metabolism may present as ALTE, having been found in 2–8% of case series (27,128,129). In addition, these errors may also cause sudden death (130–132). Consideration should be given to this diagnosis, particularly where there is a family history of sudden death, muscle, or metabolic disorder. Diagnosis can be made by appropriate biochemical tests and effective treatment can be given to reduce the risk of further collapses for some diagnoses.

H. Cardiac Dysrhythmias

A case series of six patients with cardiac dysrhythmias presenting as ALTE has been reported (133); although in a series of patient with ALTE, identified dysrhythmias account for less than 1% of cases (14,64). Arrhythmias may also be a presenting feature of metabolic disease (129). A study of 24-hour ECG recording in 100 infants with ALTE found 62% with one or more dysrhythmias and 30 with a QTc interval above the 97th percentile (134). No control group was studied; the only two patients treated had sinus node dysfunction and no subsequent adverse events were seen in this cohort.

An ECG of 305 infants referred for ALTE did not find dysrhythmia or ECG abnormalities (135). Thus, it seems that cardiac dysrhythmias are a rare cause of ALTE and the benefit of routinely measuring the QTc interval in infants with ALTE has not been established. Nevertheless, it is a simple investigation to perform and may just reveal rare cases of other cardiac involvement as part of metabolic disease (136), muscle disorder (137), or myocarditis (138) presenting as ALTE.

XII. Psychological Assessment

Families who have had infants with ALTE see their infants more negatively than those with healthy infants, and mothers report feeling less attachment (139). Whether these are directly the result of the apnea or characterize the families whose infants present with ALTE is unknown. It is possible that some families present with infants with ALTE because they are more stressed or have different personality characteristics prior to the event. In view of the fact that parental anxiety, depression, and lack of parenting skills are detrimental to the emotional development of infants, psychosocial assessment is warranted and support provided where possible.

Mothers who present infants with recurrent ALTE that are either fabricated or induced have adverse psychosocial backgrounds, mostly demonstrating personality disorders (18). Diagnosis may be aided by close examination of maternal and family responses to the infant, antecedent psychosocial history, and whether abnormal illness behavior exists within the family. Covert video surveillance may be needed to detect ALTE due to child abuse (18).

XIII. Discharge Planning and Home Monitoring

The plans for follow-up of infants and their families need to be individualized and depend on the underlying diagnosis, severity of the event, and views of parents, doctors and community staff. Infants with a single mild episode or definite diagnosis, e.g., bronchiolitis, require minimal follow-up. This may in turn be reassuring to the families. Those with recurrent episodes require further investigation and follow up. There is an increased risk of death in infants with subsequent events (140), so greater surveillance and more extensive investigation may be required to reach a diagnosis. This may include the long-term use of hospital or home-based multichannel recordings (17). Because of increased risks of death, special care needs to be taken in planning the discharge of infants who have had ALTE that received cardiopulmonary resuscitation (140), in infants who were born very premature (141,142), and in those where possible child protection concerns exist (107).

The results of some studies suggest home monitoring may prevent deaths in certain high-risk groups (2,23,143,144). However, there has been no randomized controlled trial performed to show monitors reduce mortality, and they should not be provided on this basis (145).

Practices for offering home monitoring vary widely from those who consider that home monitoring has no role to play to those in whom it is offered to all families. Cardiorespiratory monitoring using impedance pneumography and ECG has not been clinically validated to detect potentially severe apneic-hypoxemic episodes or ALTE, and thus their use has been criticized (146). This is in contrast to monitors detecting abnormal oxygenation, which pick up 90–100% of serious hypoxemic-apneic episodes (52,147). Cardiorespiratory monitors have a high rate of false alarms (53) and may not detect events, deaths having occurred on such monitors (148,149). In the United Kingdom, apnea monitors that work by detection of body movements alone are used. These monitors have a poor ability to detect potentially life-threatening, hypoxemic events (147), and deaths have occurred on these monitors too (150). There is also a theoretical risk in older infants of strangulation from such monitors (151). It does not seem appropriate to monitor for events due to upper or lower airway obstruction by use of monitors that detect respiratory pauses—more appropriate monitors would involve detection of hypoxemia, using pulse oximetry or transcutaneous pO_2 (147).

An advance in monitor technology in recent years has been the ability to record monitor use and the physiological signals prior to an alarm. Cardiorespiratory monitors have shown bradycardia rather than cessation of breathing movements to precede death or near-death episodes (152). Although oxygenation was not recorded in these studies, another study recording near-death episodes has shown hypoxemia as the initial changing parameter (52).

Our own practice has been to offer home oxygen monitoring to infants with recurrent events, in whom cardiopulmonary resuscitation has been required, or where there is increased anxiety, e.g., because of prematurity or a previous infant death due to SIDS (147). Such monitoring should ideally have the ability to record compliance and store prolonged periods of data, to include at least 15 to 20 minutes of data around any clinically significant events (52). The signals ideally would include: oxygenation, breathing movements, pulse waveform, ECG, and time when triggered by parents, whether or not an alarm has occurred. Such equipment would allow the diagnostic process to continue at home, but unfortunately current devices do not meet these criteria.

Documented monitoring shows parents use monitoring devices with variable compliance (153,154). Furthermore, they may increase or lower parental anxiety (155,156). Ongoing support is likely to be needed for many parents, particularly those who undergo home physiological monitoring. At the time of hospital discharge, parents require a clear account of what has happened, the observations, investigations and results while in hospital, and the level of medical understanding for the infant's event. This may or may not include a diagnostic label, but health professionals should be cautious in applying diagnostic labels without good objective evidence. This caution will avoid the escalation of treatments for a recurrent condition that appears unresponsive to treatment. For example, infants with recurrent ALTE should avoid fundoplication (even if they have reflux), unless esophageal monitoring has objectively documented reflux as the trigger for events. Similarly, such infants should avoid a label of epilepsy and escalating anticonvulsant therapy, unless objectively documented primary epileptic discharges have been captured on EEG during events (26).

If infants are discharged home without ongoing physiological monitoring, they should spend some time in hospital without monitors attached. Usually a period of observation of at least 24 hours while the infant is well will be required before discharge. This should be undertaken when the family feels confident and health professionals are happy with the infant's condition.

XIV. Specific Management for Recurrent ALTE

Specific treatments may be administered to those infants in whom a diagnosis of a specific condition has been found to account for the recurrent events; single events are less reliably categorized as being due to an associated medical problem and early institution of treatments should be avoided.

Infants with recurrent events and findings of a small upper airway due to, e.g., retrognathia or Pierre Robin sequence may benefit from CPAP (157). Hypoxemic-apneic episodes in infections such as RSV and pertussis may also benefit from lung distending measures including CPAP or continuous negative extrathoracic pressure (158). In preterm infants with baseline hypoxemia, additional inspired oxygen may be an effective therapy for recurrent cyanotic-apneic episodes (22) and may be of value in other episodes involving sudden intrapulmonary shunting (17). Oxygen therapy not only increases the baseline arterial Spo_2 from which any respiratory event occurs, thus prolonging the time taken for the development of hypoxemia, but may also be therapeutic by improving airway conductance and pulmonary vasodilation (54).

For recurrent events that begin in the presence of a caregiver, consideration should be given to the possibility of imposed upper airway obstruction or attempted suffocation (18,107). This is one manifestation of illness induction; other abnormal illness behavior may feature in the parent or caregiver or other children. Because this involves serious, life-threatening child abuse, measures must be taken to investigate it through usual child protection procedures, liaising early with statutory agencies, such as the police and social services. Early communication with parents who perform this abuse may place an infant at risk of further abuse due to failure to obtain evidence to protect the child. Covert video surveillance may be needed to confirm the diagnosis and must be undertaken in consultation with other agencies that are responsible for child protection, such as the police and social services (18,112).

Apneic pauses and periodic breathing are reduced in term infants by the use of theophylline (31). However, treatment of these pneumographic findings probably has little clinical relevance—their presence does not predict sudden death (159,160). Furthermore, methylxanthine medication increases the tendency toward gastroesophageal reflux and lowers the seizure threshold. Such medications reduce alarms from monitors, which detect apneic pauses, but these are of dubious pathological importance. Diagnosis and treatment of epilepsy will be important in infants and will require further neurological assessment to determine the underlying cause (161).

Pacemakers have been inserted into infants with profound bradycardia or sinus pauses in events (51), but such findings should be confirmed as primary cardiac electrophysiological abnormalities (133) and not secondary to hypoxemia from epileptic seizures (26), sleep related upper airway obstruction (120,121), or attempted suffocation (110).

XV. Outcome

In three cohort studies of ALTEs presenting to emergency departments (13,14,162), there were 2/359 subsequent deaths—a subsequent mortality of 0.6%. Three further studies report complete cohorts of infants with ALTE referred to sleep units (4,64,163): 2/1503 (0.13%) infants subsequently died. A systematic review selecting studies with adequate causal investigations found 5 deaths in 643 infants followed for 6 to 18 months (0.8%) (12). These deaths occurred in infants with severe gastroesophageal reflux (2 infants) and rare congenital metabolic disorders (3 infants). These data suggest that the risk of subsequent death after ALTE is less than 1%. Despite a number of case reports of individual fatalities after ALTE, these data suggest that the outlook is generally reassuring, although serious underlying conditions must be taken into account. Infants who need repeated vigorous resuscitation appear to be at higher risk of subsequent death (17,140). Follow-up into preadolescence has found no significant differences in behavior or IQ between ALTE infants and matched controls (164).

Thus, while reassurance that there is a low risk for subsequent sudden death can be given to parents of infants suffering a single, mild ALTE, infants with recurrent events require specialist assessment and follow-up, particularly with regard to detection of causes that are either rarer (epileptic seizure induced apnea) or more difficult to diagnose (attempted suffocation using covert video surveillance).

References

1. Wennergren G, Milerad J, Lagercrantz H, et al. The epidemiology of sudden infant death syndrome and attacks of lifelessness in Sweden. Acta Paediatr Scand 1987; 76:898–906.
2. Kelly DH, Shannon DC, O'Connell K. Care of infants with near-miss sudden infant death syndrome. Pediatrics 1978; 61:511–514.
3. Infantile Apnea and Home Monitoring. Report of a consensus development conference 1987. U.S. Department of Health and Human Services. Public Health Service, National Institutes of Health Publication No. 87-2905, 1987.
4. Rahilly PM. The pneumographic and medical investigation of infants suffering apparent life threatening episodes. J Paediatr Child Health 1991; 27:349–353.

5. Khan A, Blum D, Hennart P, et al. A critical comparison of the history of sudden death infants and infants hospitalised for near-miss for SIDS. Eur J Pediatr 1984; 143:102–107.

6. Grylack LJ, Williams AD. Apparent life-threatening events in presumed healthy neonates during the first three days of life. Pediatrics 1996; 97:349–351.

7. Burchfield DJ, Rawlings J. Sudden deaths and apparent life-threatening events in hospitalised neonates presumed to be healthy. Am J Dis Child 1991; 145:1319–1322.

8. Rodriguez-Alarcón J, Melchor JC, Linares A, et al. Early neonatal sudden death or near death syndrome. An epidemiological study of 29 cases. Acta Paediatr 1994; 83:704–708.

9. Myerberg DZ, Carpenter RG, Myerberg CF, et al. Reducing post-neonatal mortality in West Virginia: state wide intervention program targeting risk identified at and after birth. Am J Public Health 1995; 85:631–637.

10. Ponsonby AL, Dwyer T, Couper D. Factors related to infant apnoea and cyanosis: a population-based study. J Paediatr Child Health 1997; 33:317–323.

11. DeWolfe CC. Apparent life-threatening event: a review. Pediatr Clin N Am 2005; 52:1127–1146.

12. McGovern MC, Smith MBH. Causes of apparent life threatening events in infants: a systematic review. Arch Dis Child 2004; 89:1043–1048.

13. Gray C, Davies F, Molyneux E. Apparent life-threatening events presenting to a pediatric emergency department. Pediatr Emerg Care 1999; 15:195–199.

14. Davies F, Gupta R. Apparent life threatening events in infants presenting to an emergency department. Emerg Med J 2002; 19:11–16.

15. Brand DA, Altman RL, Purtill K, et al. Yield of diagnostic testing in infants who have had an apparent life-threatening event. Pediatrics 2005; 115:885–893.

16. Kahn A, Groswasser J, Sottiaux M, et al. Clinical problems in relation to apparent life-threatening events in infants. Acta Paediatr Suppl 1993; 82(suppl 389):107–110.

17. Samuels MP, Poets CF, Noyes JP, et al. Diagnosis and management after life threatening events in infants and young children who received cardiopulmonary resuscitation. BMJ 1993; 306:489–492.

18. Southall DP, Plunkett MCB, Banks MW, et al. Covert video recordings of life threatening child abuse: lessons for child protection. Pediatrics 1997; 100:735–760.

19. Peabody JL, Volpe JJ. Episodes of apnea and bradycardia in the preterm infant: impact on cerebral circulation. Pediatrics 1985; 76:333–338.

20. Southall DP, Levitt GA, Richards JM, et al. Undetailed episodes of porlonged apnea and bradycardia in preterm infants. Pediatrics 1983, 72:541–551.

21. Muttitt SC, Finer NN, Tierney AJ, et al. Neonatal apnea: diagnosis by nurse versus computer. Pediatrics 1988; 82:713–720.

22. Samuels MP, Poets CF, Southall DP. Abnormal hypoxemia after life threatening events in infants born before term. J Pediatr 1994; 125:441–446.

23. Ariagno RL, Guilleminault C, Korobkin R, et al. "Near miss" for sudden infant death syndrome infants: a clinical problem. Pediatrics 1983; 71:721–730.

24. Guilleminault C, Ariagno RL. Why should we study the infant 'near miss for Sudden Infant Death'? Early Hum Dev 1978; 2(3):207–218.

25. Anas N, Boettrich C, Hall CB, et al. The association of apnea and respiratory syncytial virus infection in infants. J Pediatr 1982; 101:65–68.

26. Hewertson H, Poets CF, Samuels MP, et al. Epileptic seizure induced hypoxemia in infants with apparent life threatening events. Pediatrics 1994; 94:148–156.

27. Arens R, Gozal D, Williams JC, et al. Recurrent apparent life-threatening events during infancy: a manifestation of inborn errors of metabolism. J Pediatr 1993; 123:415–418.

28. Herbst JJ, Book LS, Bray PF. Gastroesophageal reflux in the "near miss" sudden infant death syndrome. J Pediatr 1978; 92:73–75.

29. Guilleminault C, Peraita R, Souquet M, et al. Apneas during sleep in infants; possible relationships with sudden infant death syndrome. Science 1975; 190:677–679.

30. Haidmayer R, Kurz R, Kenner T, et al. Physiological and clinical aspects of respiration control in infants with relation to the sudden infant death syndrome. Klin Wochenschr 1982; 60:9–18.

31. Hunt CE, Brouillette RT, Hanson D. Theophylline improves pneumogram abnormalities in infants at risk of sudden infant death syndrome. J Pediatr 1983; 103:969–974.

32. Guilleminault C, Ariagno R, Korobkin R, et al. Mixed and obstructive sleep apnea and near miss for sudden infant death syndrome: 2. Comparison of near miss and normal control infants by age. Pediatrics 1979; 64:882–891.

33. Kelly DH, Shannon DC. Periodic breathing in infants with near miss sudden infant death syndrome. Pediatrics 1979; 63:355.

34. Brady JP, Ariagno RL, Watts JC, et al. Apnea, hypoxemia and aborted sudden infant death syndrome. Pediatrics 1978; 62:686–691.

35. Oren J, Kelly DH, Shannon DC. Pneumogram recordings in infants resuscitated for apnea of infancy. Pediatrics 1989; 83:364–368.

36. Anwar M, Marotta F, Fort MD, et al. The ventilatory response to carbon dioxide in high risk infants. Early Hum Dev 1993; 35:183–192.

37. Haddad GG, Leistner HL, Lai TL, et al. Ventilation and ventilatory pattern during sleep in aborted sudden infant death syndrome. Pediatr Res 1981; 15:879–883.

38. McCulloch K, Brouillette RT, Guzzetta AJ, et al. Arousal responses in near-miss sudden infant death syndrome and in normal infants. J Pediatr 1982; 101:911–917.

39. Ariagno R, Nagel L, Guilleminault C. Waking and ventilatory responses during sleep in infants near-miss for sudden infant death syndrome. Sleep 1980; 3:351–359.

40. Parks YA, Paton JY, Beardsmore CS, et al. Respiratory control in infants at increased risk for sudden infant death syndrome. Arch Dis Child 1989; 64:791–797.

41. Kao LC, Keens TG. Decreased specific airway conductance in infant apnea. Pediatrics 1985; 76:232–235.

42. Hartmann H, Seidenberg J, Noyes JP, et al. Small airway patency in infants with apparent life threatening events. Eur J Pediatr 1998; 157:71–74.

43. Scott CB, Nickerson BG, Sargent CW, et al. Developmental patterns of maximal transdiaphragmatic pressure in infants during crying. Pediatr Res 1983; 17:707–709.

44. Kahn A, Van de Merckt C, Dramaix M, et al. Transepidermal water loss during sleep in infants at risk for sudden death. Pediatrics 1987; 80:245–250.

45. Leistner HL, Haddad GG, Epstein RA, et al. Heart rate and heart rate variability during sleep in aborted sudden infant death syndrome. J Pediatr 1980; 97:51.

46. Haddad GG, Walsh EM, Leistner HL, et al. Abnormal maturation of sleep states in infants with aborted sudden infant death syndrome. Pediatr Res 1981; 15:1055–1057.

47. Fox GP, Matthews TG. Autonomic dysfunction at different ambient temperatures in infants at risk of sudden infant death syndrome. Lancet 1989; 2:1065–7.

48. Gupta PR, Guilleminault C, Dorfmann LJ. Brainstem auditory evoked potentials in near-miss sudden infant death syndrome. J Pediatr 1981; 98:791–794.
49. Lüders H, Orlowski JP, Dinner DS, et al. Far-field auditory evoked potentials in near-miss sudden infant death syndrome. Arch Neurol 1984; 41:615–617.
50. Hodgman JE, Hoppenbrouwers T, Geidel S, et al. Respiratory behavior in near-miss sudden infant death syndrome. Pediatrics 1982; 69:785–792.
51. Kelly DH, Pathak A, Meny R. Sudden severe bradycardia in infancy. Pediatr Pulmonol 1991; 10:199–204.
52. Poets CF, Samuels MP, Noyes JP, et al. Home event recordings of oxygenation, breathing movements, and heart rate and rhythm in infants with recurrent life-threatening events. J Pediatr 1993; 123:693–701.
53. Weese-Mayer DE, Morrow AS, Conway LP, et al. Assessing clinical significance of apnoea exceeding fifteen seconds with event recording. J Pediatr 1990; 117:568–574.
54. Poets CF, Samuels MP, Southall DP. Potential role of intrapulmonary shunting in the genesis of hypoxemic episodes in infants and young children. Pediatrics 1992; 90:385–391.
55. Gray PH, Rogers Y. Are infants with bronchopulmonary dysplasia at risk for sudden infant death syndrome? Pediatrics 1994; 93(5):774–777.
56. Barrington KJ, Finer N, Li D. Predischarge respiratory recordings in very low birth weight newborn infants. J Pediatr 1996; 129:934–940.
57. Duke JC, Sekar KC, Toubas PL, et al. Apnea in subsequent asymptomatic siblings of infants who had an apparent life-threatening event. J Perinatol 1992; 12:124–128.
58. Leape LL, Holder TM, Franklin JD, et al. Respiratory arrest in infants secondary to gastresophageal reflux. Pediatrics 1977; 60:924–928.
59. Jeffery HE, Rahilly P, Read DJC. Multiple causes of asphyxia in infants at high risk for sudden infant death. Arch Dis Child 1983; 58:92–100.
60. Jeffery HE, Reid I, Rahilly P, et al. Gastro-esophageal reflux in "near-miss" sudden infant death infants in active but not quiet sleep. Sleep 1980; 3:393–399.
61. de Bethmann O, Couchard M, de Ajuriaguerra M, et al. Role of gastro-esophageal reflux and vagal overactivity in apparent life-threatening events: 160 cases. Acta Paediatr Suppl 1993; 82(suppl 389):102–104.
62. Beyaert C, Marchal F, Dousset B, et al. Gastroesophageal reflux and acute life-threatening episodes: role of a central respiratory depression. Biol Neonate 1995; 68:87–90.
63. Tirosh E, Jaffe M. Apnea of infancy, seizures, and gastroesophageal reflux: an important but infrequent association. J Child Neurol 1996; 11:98–100.
64. Kahn A, Rebuffat E, Franco P, et al. Apparent life threatening events and apnea of infancy. In: Beckerman R, Brouillette R, Hunt C, eds. Respiratory Control Disorders in Infants and Children. Baltimore: Williams & Wilkins, 1992:178–189.
65. Graff MA, Kashlan F, Carter M, et al. Nap studies underestimate the incidence of gastroesophageal reflux. Pediatr Pulmonol 1994; 18:258–260.
66. MacFadyen UM, Hendry GMA, Simpson H. Gastro-esophageal reflux in near-miss sudden infant death syndrome or suspected recurrent aspiration. Arch Dis Child 1983; 58:87–91.
67. Rudolph CD, Mazur LJ, Liptak GS, et al. GER Guideline Committee of the North American Society for Pediatric Gastroenterology and Nutrition. Pediatric GE reflux clinical practice guidelines. J Pediatr Gastroenterol Nutr 2000; 32:S1–S31.

68. Arana A, Bagucka B, Hauser B, et al. PH monitoring in the distal and proximal esophagus in symptomatic infants. J Pediatr Gastroenterol Nutr 2001; 32:259–264.

69. Kahn A, Rebuffat E, Sottiaux M, et al. Lack of temporal relation between acid reflux in the proximal esophagus and cardiorespiratory events in sleeping infants. Eur J Pediatr 1992; 151:208–212.

70. Ariagno RL, Guilleminault C, Baldwin R, et al. Movement and gastresophageal reflux in awake term infants with 'near miss' SIDS, unrelated to apnea. J Pediatr 1982; 100:894–897.

71. Rosen CL, Frost JD, Harrison GM. Infant apnea: polygraphic studies and follow up monitoring. Pediatrics 1983; 71:731–736.

72. Paton JY, Nanayakkara CS, Simpson H. Observations on gastro-esophageal reflux, central apnoea and heart rate in infants. Eur J Pediatr 1990; 149:608–612.

73. Newell SJ, Booth IW, Morgan MEI, et al. Gastro-esophageal reflux in preterm infants. Arch Dis Child 1989; 64:780–786.

74. Arad-Cohen N, Cohen A, Tirosh E. The relationship between gastroesophageal reflux and apnea in infants [see comments]. J Pediatr 2000; 137:321–326.

75. Spitzer AR, Boyle JT, Tuchman DN, et al. Awake apnea associated with gastro-esophageal reflux: a specific clinical syndrome. J Pediatr 1984; 104:200–205.

76. See CC, Newman LJ, Berezin S, et al. Gastroesophageal reflux-induced hypoxemia in infants with apparent life-threatening event(s). AJDC 1989; 143:951–954.

77. Guilleminault C, Coons S. Apnea and bradycardia during feeding in infants weighing >2000 gm. J Pediatr 1984; 104:932–935.

78. Wenzl TG, Schenke S, Peschgens T, et al. Association of apnea and nonacid gastroesophageal reflux in infants: investigations with the intraluminal impedance technique. Pediatr Pulmonol 2001; 31:144–149.

79. Peter CS, Sprodowski N, Bohnhorst B, et al. Gastroesophageal reflux and apnea of prematurity: no temporal relationship. Pediatrics 2002; 109:8–11.

80. Puntis JW, Booth IW. ALTE and gastro-oesophageal reflux [see comment]. Arch Dis Child 2005; 90:653; author reply 653.

81. Friesen CA, Streed CJ, Carney LA, et al. Esophagitis and modified Bernstein tests in infants with apparent life-threatening events. Pediatrics 1994; 94:541–544.

82. Bridge E, Livingstone S, Tietze C. Breath-holding spells. Their relationship to syncope, convulsions and other phenomena. J Pediatr 1943; 23:539–561.

83. Bhatia MS, Singhal PK, Dhar NK, et al. Breath holding spells: an analysis of 50 cases. Indian Pediatr 1990; 27:1073–1079.

84. Abe K, Oda N, Amatomi M. Natural history and predictive significance of head-banging, head-rolling and breath-holding spells. Dev Med Child Neurol 1984; 26:644–648.

85. Lombroso CT, Lerman P. Breathholding spells (cyanotic and pallid infantile syncope). Pediatrics 1967; 39:563–581.

86. Laxdal T, Gomez MR, Reiher J. Cyanotic and pallid syncopal attacks in children (breath-holding spells). Dev Med Child Neurol 1969; 11:755–763.

87. Stephenson JB. Blue breath holding is benign [see comment]. Arch Dis Child 1991; 66:255–257.

88. Southall DP, Samuels MP, Talbert DG. Recurrent cyanotic episodes with severe arterial hypoxemia and intrapulmonary shunting: a mechanism for sudden death. Arch Dis Child 1990; 65:953–961.

89. Paulson G. Breath-holding spells: a fatal case. Dev Med Child Neurol 1963; 5: 246–251.
90. Southall D, Stebbens V, Shinebourne E. Sudden and unexpected death between 1 and 5 years. Arch Dis Child 1987; 62:700–705.
91. Samuels MP, Talbert DG, Southall DP. Cyanotic 'breath holding' and sudden death. Arch Dis Child 1991; 66:257–258.
92. Taiwo B, Hamilton AH. Cardiac arrest: a rare complication of pallid syncope? Postgrad Med J 1993; 69:738–739.
93. Daoud AS, Batieha A, al-Sheyyab M, et al. Effectiveness of iron therapy on breath-holding spells. J Pediatr 1997; 130:547–550.
94. Donma MM. Clinical efficacy of piracetam in treatment of breath-holding spells. Pediatr Neurol 1998; 18:41–45.
95. Donati F, Schaffler L, Vassella F. Prolonged epileptic apneas in a newborn: a case report with ictal EEG recording. Neuropediatrics 1995; 26:223–225.
96. Nunes ML, Appel CC, da Costa JC. Apparent life-threatening episodes as the first manifestation of epilepsy. Clin Pediatr 2003; 42:19–22.
97. Ramelli GP, Donati F, Bianchetti M, et al. Apneic attacks as an isolated manifestation of epileptic seizures in infants. Eur J Paediatr Neurol 1998; 2:187–191.
98. Singh B, Al Shahwan SA, Al Deeb SM. Partial seizures presenting as life-threatening apnea. Epilepsia 1993; 34:901–903.
99. Watanabe K, Hara K, Hakamada S, et al. Seizures with apnea in children. Pediatrics 1982; 70:87–90.
100. van Rijckevorsel K, Saussu F, de Barsy T. Bradycardia, an epileptic ictal manifestation. Seizure 1995; 4:237–239.
101. Emery ES. Status epilepticus secondary to breath-holding and pallid syncopal spells [see comment]. Neurology 1990; 40:859.
102. Aubourg P, Dulac O, Plouin P, et al. Infantile status epilepticus as a complication of 'near-miss' sudden infant death. Dev Med Child Neurol 1985; 27:40–48.
103. Carmant L, Kramer U, Holmes GL, et al. Differential diagnosis of staring spells in children: a video-EEG study. Pediatr Neurol 1996; 14:199–202.
104. Alexander R, Smith W, Stevenson R. Serial Munchausen syndrome by proxy. Pediatrics 1990; 86:581–585.
105. Berger D. Child abuse simulating "near-miss" sudden infant death syndrome. J Pediatr 1979; 95:554–556.
106. Kravitz RM, Wilmott RW. Munchausen syndrome by proxy presenting as factitious apnea. Clin Pediatr 1990; 29:587–592.
107. Meadows R. Suffocation, recurrent apnoea and sudden infant death. J Pediatr 1990; 117:351–357.
108. Morris B. Child abuse manifested as factitious apnea. South Med J 1985; 78: 1013–1014.
109. Minford AM. Child abuse presenting as apparent "near-miss" sudden infant death syndrome. BMJ (Clin Res Ed) 1981; 282:521.
110. Samuels MP, McClaughlin W, Jacobson RR, et al. Fourteen cases of imposed upper airway obstruction. Arch Dis Child 1992; 67:162–170.
111. Rosen CL, Frost JD Jr., Bricker T, et al. Two siblings with recurrent cardiorespiratory arrest: Munchausen syndrome by proxy or child abuse? Pediatrics 1983; 71:715–720.

112. Hall DE, Eubanks L, Meyyazhagan LS, et al. Evaluation of covert video surveillance in the diagnosis of munchausen syndrome by proxy: lessons from 41 cases. Pediatrics 2000; 105:1305–1312.

113. Truman TL, Ayoub CC. Considering suffocatory abuse and Munchausen by proxy in the evaluation of children experiencing apparent life-threatening events and sudden infant death syndrome. Child Maltreat 2002; 7:138–148.

114. Rosen C, Frost J, Glaze D. Child abuse and recurrent infant apnea. J Pediatr 1986; 109:1065–1067.

115. Altman RL, Brand DA, Forman S, et al. Abusive head injury as a cause of apparent life-threatening events in infancy. Arch Pediatr Adolesc Med 2003; 157:1011–1015.

116. Pitetti RD, Maffei F, Chang K, et al. Prevalence of retinal hemorrhages and child abuse in children who present with an apparent life-threatening event. Pediatrics 2002; 110:557–562.

117. Byard RW, Burnell RH. Covert video surveillance in Munchausen syndrome by proxy. Ethical compromise or essential technique? Med J Aust 1994; 160:352–356.

118. Epstein MA, Markowitz RL, Gallo DM, et al. Munchausen syndrome by proxy: considerations in diagnosis and confirmation by video surveillance. Pediatrics 1987; 80:220–224.

119. Ramanathan R, Corwin MJ, Hunt CE, et al., The Collaborative Home Infant Monitoring Evaluation Study Group. Cardiorespiratory events recorded on home monitors: comparison of healthy infants with those at increased risk for SIDS. JAMA 2001; 285:2199–2207.

120. Guilleminault C, Heldt G, Powell N, et al. Small upper airway in near-miss sudden infant death syndrome infants and their families. Lancet 1986; 1:402–407.

121. McNamara F, Sullivan CE. Obstructive sleep apnea in infants and its management with nasal continuous positive airway pressure. Chest 1999; 116:10–16.

122. Harrington C, Kirjavainen T, Teng A, et al. nCPAP improves abnormal autonomic function in at-risk-for-SIDS infants with OSA. J Appl Physiol 2003; 95:1591–1597.

123. Gozal D. Congenital central hypoventilation syndrome: an update. Pediatr Pulmonol 1998; 26:273–282.

124. Weese-Mayer DE, Silvestri JM, Menzies LJ, et al. Congenital central hypoventilation syndrome: diagnosis, management, and long-term outcome in thirty-two children. J Pediatr 1992; 120(3):381–387.

125. Weese-Mayer DE, Berry-Kravis EM. Genetics of congenital central hypoventilation syndrome: lessons from a seemingly orphan disease. Am J Respir Crit Care Med 2004; 170:16–21.

126. Oren J, Kelly DH, Shannon DC. Long-term follow-up of children with congenital central hypoventilation syndrome. Pediatrics 1987; 80:375–380.

127. Deonna T, Arczynska W, Torrado A. Congenital failure of automatic ventilation (Ondine's curse). A case report. J Pediatr 1974; 84:710–714.

128. Kahn A, Montauk L, Blum D. Diagnostic categories in infants referred for an acute event suggesting near-miss SIDS. Eur J Pediatr 1987; 146:458–460.

129. Bonnet D, Martin D, Pascale De L, et al. Arrhythmias and conduction defects as presenting symptoms of fatty acid oxidation disorders in children. Circulation 1999; 100:2248–2253.

130. Bonham JR, Downing M. Metabolic deficiencies and SIDS. J Clin Pathol 1992; 45:33–38.

131. Chalmers RA, Stanley CA, English N, et al. Mitochondrial carnitine-acylcarnitine translocase deficiency presenting as sudden neonatal death. J Pediatr 1997; 131: 181–182.

132. Treacy EP, Lambert DM, Barnes R, et al. Short-chain hydroxyacyl-coenzyme A dehydrogenase deficiency presenting as unexpected infant death: a family study. J Pediatr 2000; 137:257–259.

133. Keeton BR, Southall E, Rutter N, et al. Cardiac conduction disorders in six infants with "near-miss" sudden infant deaths. BMJ 1977; 2:600–601.

134. Woolf PK, Gewitz MH, Preminger T, et al. Infants with apparent life threatening events. Cardiac rhythm and conduction. Clin Pediatr 1989; 28:517–520.

135. Southall DP, Janczynski RE, Alexander JR, et al. Cardiorespiratory patterns in infants presenting with apparent life-threatening episodes. Biol Neonate 1990; 57:77–87.

136. Mathur A, Sims HF, Gopalakrishnan D, et al. Molecular heterogeneity in very-long-chain acyl-CoA dehydrogenase deficiency causing pediatric cardiomyopathy and sudden death. Circulation 1999; 99:1337–1343.

137. Fried K, Beer S, Vure E, et al. Autosomal recessive sudden unexpected death in children probably caused by a cardiomyopathy associated with myopathy. J Med Genet 1979; 16:341–346.

138. Khan MA, Das B, Lohe H, et al. Neonatal myocarditis presenting as an apparent life threatening event. Clin Pediatr (Phila) 2003; 42:649–652.

139. Jenkins RL. Indices for maternal/family anxiety and disruption related to infant apnea and home monitoring. Health Care Women Int 1996; 17:535–548.

140. Oren J, Kelly D, Shannon DC. Identification of a high-risk group for sudden infant death syndrome among infants who were resuscitated for sleep apnea. Pediatrics 1986; 77:495–499.

141. Grether JK, Schulman J. Sudden infant death syndrome and birth weight. J Pediatr 1989; 114:561–567.

142. Wariyar V, Richmond S, Hey E. Pregnancy outcome at 24-31 weeks gestation: neonatal survivors. Arch Dis Child 1989; 64:678–686.

143. Kahn A, Blum D. Home monitoring of infants considered at risk for the sudden infant death syndrome. Eur J Pediatr 1982; 139:94–100.

144. Duffty P, Bryan MH. Home apnea monitoring in 'near-miss' sudden infant death syndrome (SIDS) and in siblings of SIDS victims. Pediatrics 1982; 70:69–74.

145. American Academy of Pediatrics. Apnea, sudden infant death syndrome and home monitoring. Pediatrics 2003; 111:914–917.

146. Hodgman JE, Hoppenbrowers T. Home monitoring for sudden infant death syndrome. The case against. Ann N Y Acad Sci 1988; 533:164–175.

147. Poets CF, Samuels MP, Noyes JP, et al. Home monitoring of transcutaneous oxygen tension in the early detection of hypoxemia in infants and young children. Arch Dis Child 1991; 66:676–682.

148. Davidson Ward SL, Keens TG, Chan LS, et al. Sudden infant death syndrome in infants evaluated by apnea programs in California. Pediatrics 1986; 77:451–455.

149. Meny RG, Blackmon L, Fleischman D, et al. Sudden infant death and home monitors. Am J Dis Child 1988; 142:1037–1040.

150. Samuels MP, Stebbens VA, Poets CF, et al. Deaths on infant 'apnoea' monitors. Mat Child Health 1993; 18:262–266.

151. Emery JL, Taylor EM, Carpenter RG, et al. Apnoea monitors and accidental strangulation. BMJ 1992; 304:117.

152. Meny RG, Carroll JL, Carbone MT, et al. Cardiorespiratory recordings from infants dying suddenly and unexpectedly at home. Pediatrics 1994; 93:44–49.

153. Silvestri JM, Hufford DR, Durham J, et al. Assessment of compliance with home cardiorespiratory monitoring in infants at risk of sudden infant death syndrome. J Paediatr 1995; 127:384–388.

154. Gibson E, Spinner S, Cullen JA, et al. Documented home apnea monitoring: effect on compliance, duration of monitoring, and validation of alarm reporting. Clin Pediatr 1996; 35(10):505–513.

155. Ahmann E. Family impact of home apnoea monitoring: an overview of research and its clinical implications. Pediatr Nurs 1992; 18:611–616.

156. Noyes J, Stebbens V, Sobhan G, et al. Home monitoring of infants at increased risk of sudden death. J Clin Nurs 1996; 5:297–306.

157. Guilleminault C, Pelayo R, Clerk A, et al. Home nasal continuous positive airway pressure in infants with sleep-disordered breathing. J Pediatr 1995; 127:905–912.

158. Al-balkhi A, Klonin H, Marinaki K, et al. Review of treatment of bronchiolitis related apnoea in two centres. Arch Dis Child 2005; 90:288–291.

159. Southall DP, Richards JM, Stebbens VA, et al. Cardiorespiratory patterns in 16 full term infants who suffered SIDS. Pediatrics 1986; 78:787–796.

160. Southall DP, Richards JM, Rhoden KJ, et al. Prolonged apnea and cardiac arrhythmias in infants discharged from neonatal intensive care units: failure to predict an increased risk for sudden infant death syndrome. Pediatrics 1982; 70:844–851.

161. Tirosh E, Jaffe M. Apparent life-threatening event: a neurologic perspective. J Child Neurol 1995; 10:216–218.

162. Veereman-Wauters G, Bochner A, Van Caillie-Bertrand M. Gastroesophageal reflux in infants with a history of near-miss sudden infant death. J Pediatr Gastroenterol Nutr 1991; 12:319–323.

163. Ariagno RL, Guilleminault C, Korobkin R, et al. 'Near-miss' for sudden infant death syndrome infants: a clinical problem. Pediatrics 1983; 71:726–730.

164. Kahn A, Sottiaux M, Appelboom-Fondu J, et al. Long-term development of children monitored as infants for an apparent life-threatening event during sleep: a 10-year follow-up study. Pediatrics 1989; 83:668–673.

165. Cozzi DA, Bonanni M, Cozzi F, Villa MP, et al. Recurrent apparent life-threatening event relieved by glossopexy. J Pediatr Surg 1996; 31:1715–1718.

166. Engelberts AC. The role of obstructive apnea in sudden infant death syndrome and apparent life threatening event. Int J Pediatr Otorhinolaryngol 1995; 32(suppl): S59–S62.

167. McMurray JS, Holinger LD. Otolaryngic manifestations in children presenting with apparent life-threatening events. Otolaryngol Head Neck Surg 1997; 116:575–579.

168. Kahn A, Haesaerts D, Blum D. Carbon monoxide and near-miss cot death. Lancet 1985; 1:168–169.

169. Kearney MS, Dahl LB, Stalsberg H. Can a cat smother and kill a baby? BMJ 1982; 285:777.

170. Byard RW, Burnell RH. Apparent life threatening events and infant holding practices. Arch Dis Child 1995; 73:502–504.

171. Levin M, Hjelm M, Kay JDS, et al. Haemorrhagic shock and encephalopathy: a new syndrome with a high mortality in young children. Lancet 1983; 2:64–67.

11

Pathophysiology of Sudden Infant Death Syndrome

BRADLEY T. THACH
Washington University, St. Louis, Missouri, U.S.A.

I. Pathophysiology of Sudden Infant Death Syndrome

There are many hypotheses for the cause of death in sudden infant death syndrome (SIDS). For many of these hypotheses, little or nothing is known about the relevant pathophysiological mechanisms. The use of the term sudden unexplained death in infants (SUDI) is becoming more common as it now seems evident that a number of infants formerly diagnosed as SIDS victims should now be diagnosed with "accidental suffocation," homicide, cardiac arrhythmias, inborn errors of metabolism, or other disorders with differing pathophysiological mechanisms (Table 1). For example, even when death scene findings strongly support a diagnosis of accidental suffocation as the cause of death, it is believed by many that such infants may have brain stem defects that predispose them to suffocation. In such cases it is argued that these deaths are not completely explained by evidence from the death scene and postmortem examination, and so the use of the term SIDS still is appropriate. The following overview is divided into sections where at least some evidence of the pathophysiology has been documented as well as several more prominent theories for causal mechanism where evidence is still lacking.

Table 1 Estimated Frequency of Causes of Sudden Unexpected Deaths in Infancy

		References
Accidental suffocation in crib	20–30%	50
Death during bed sharing	>50%	57
Cardiac arrhythmia (prolonged QT)	4–5%	47
Metabolic errors	3–5%	61
Homicide	6–10%	70

II. Failure to Autoresuscitate from Severe Hypoxia

Several recent studies have analyzed home monitored recordings of cardiac and respiratory activity just prior to deaths in infants diagnosed as SIDS victims, as well as other deaths due to natural causes (1–3). Of the 18 or so SIDS deaths analyzed so far, there have been only two cases in which central apnea occurred before the onset of hypoxic apnea and hypoxic gasping. In these recordings bradycardia occurs abruptly just prior to onset of apnea. This suggests that the preceding hypoxemia was severe and already present during the 15-second period captured on tape just prior to the bradycardia. It is relevant that compared with infants dying of other causes, the SIDS infants showed decreased ability to transiently increase their heart rate or recover eupneic breathing as a result of hypoxic gasping (2). Why autoresuscitation might fail is conjectural. It has been shown that aspiration occurs premortem in at least 15% of SIDS cases, and this could account for the airway obstruction and failure to recover (4).

These studies suggest that central or mixed apnea is not the most frequent immediate precursor to death in the small collection of SIDS home-monitored recordings analyzed so far and more importantly that the "failure to autoresuscitate" hypotheses for SIDS is backed by substantial evidence.

III. Abnormal Chemoreceptor Function Hypothesis

Congenital hypoventilation syndrome (CHS) is a suggested model for SIDS. In infants with CHS, death can rapidly occur during sleep. Carbon dioxide (CO_2) sensitivity in these infants is virtually absent during non–rapid eye movement (NREM) sleep. However, almost all patients are diagnosed within hours or days following birth due to onset of severe hypoventilation. Since SIDS deaths have a peak incidence occurring at two to four months of life in seemingly healthy infants, it is difficult to envision how CHS, per se, could have a significant role in SIDS.

Other SIDS theories concern carotid body function. There is a significant increase in sensitivity of the peripheral chemoreceptors during the first few weeks of life. It has also been shown that carotid body denervation in animal models is followed by hypoventilation and sudden death later on (5–7). However, denervated animals for the most part are markedly symptomatic prior to death. As in the case of CHS, SIDS infants are, by definition, healthy prior to death, and therefore the role of substantial carotid body dysfunction in SIDS remains conjectural. It cannot be ruled out, however, that a partial decrease in sensitivity to hypercapnia or hypoxemia might have a causal role in SIDS.

IV. Obstructive Sleep Apnea and Apnea of Prematurity as a Cause of SIDS and the Potential Role of Viral Infection

Several types of apnea should be considered. The first of these is apnea of prematurity (A of P), which can be subdivided into two primary forms. The second is obstructive sleep apnea (OSA). As there is much circumstantial evidence suggesting a role of sleep apnea in SIDS, infantile apnea will be considered in detail.

A of P can be subdivided into spells that occur in wakefulness and those occurring during sleep (8). The mechanism involved in awake apnea is attributed to the acute hypoventilation associated with breath holding that occurs with or without crying (9,10). Such spells can result in sudden severe hypoxia with secondary hypoxic apnea. Significantly, the mechanism of recovery from these spells is autoresuscitation by gasping (10,11). Precipitating causes are usually pain or emotional stress. Indeed, the hypoventilation associated with ordinary crying has many similarities to clinical breath holding, which is often preceded by crying. With crying or breath holding, intermittent right to left intracardiac shunting of venous blood is partially responsible for the hypoxemia in addition to hypoventilation (12). Arousal from sleep often involves a brief period of breath holding or apnea, and therefore, when an infant is already in a hypoxic environment, arousal may cause a sudden, severe increase in hypoxemia (13). In preterm infants breath holding during arousal is a common cause of oxygen desaturation (9,15). Therefore, although SIDS is believed to occur when infants are presumed to be sleeping, the potential role of brief arousal followed by the sequence of breath holding, desaturation, and failed autoresuscitation cannot be fully excluded as having a causal role in some SIDS deaths.

Other forms of apnea in preterm infants occur primarily during sleep. This potentially includes OSA and reflex apnea caused by laryngeal chemoreflexes (LCR). Airway obstruction in A of P has been attributed to LCR (15,16). Unlike OSA, A of P is predominantly a mixed apnea, consisting of respiratory pauses associated with sporadic obstructed breaths, which is unlike that seen in OSA. A of P is usually associated with swallowing during the spell, a characteristic of LCR apnea but not known to be present in OSA (15).

From the onset of its discovery, the dominant theme in LCR research has been elucidating conditions leading to the prolonged apnea that is associated with stimulation of laryngeal water receptors in neonatal animals. LCR-induced apnea was viewed by Downing and colleagues as a potential explanation for SIDS, a dominant theme that has persisted until the present time (17). Many studies have suggested circumstances in which LCR apnea may be fatal. This contrasts with Johnson and colleagues' original suggestion that the primary function of LCR reflexes is prevention of aspiration (18,19). Under normal circumstances, these reflexes serve as an airway protective function. Clearly, swallowing removes fluids from the pharyngeal airway, adjacent to the larynx, while vocal cord constriction combined with apnea can prevent aspiration.

In studies of sleeping preterm infants, water or physiological saline infused into the pharynx elicited repeated swallowing, apnea, and airway closure, resulting in obstructed inspiratory efforts (15,16). However, with maturation of the nervous system, the apnea becomes less frequent and less prolonged (20). It is relevant that several studies in preterm infants have found that apnea with bradycardia associated with swallowing and intermittent airway obstruction occurs spontaneously during sleep in the absence of any detectable stimulus (15,21,22). Identical episodes can occur with regurgitation of gastric contents into the pharynx in these infants (23). These observations suggest that endogenous stimuli from accumulated pharyngeal secretions or regurgitated gastric fluid can elicit LCR responses in preterm infants and are a significant cause of A of P (20). Other more recent studies have shown that A of P with the hallmark characteristic being mixed apnea can persist after 40 weeks postconceptional age and well into the first two months of life (24).

All in all, A of P as a cause of the initial events leading to hypoxemia in SIDS remains a viable hypothesis. A few of the SIDS death recordings examined so far indicate that central apnea precedes death before the onset of bradycardia, hypoxic apnea, and gasping (1). Therefore, A of P could be the initial event that causes severe hypoxia in some SIDS deaths. The apnea hypothesis is also strengthened by the observation that episodes of A of P continue to occur in preterm infants long after discharge from the hospital (25). Preterm infants are at particularly at increased risk for SIDS. Additionally, in both animal models and in human infants, respiratory syncytial virus (RSV) is associated with increased severity or prolongation of LCR-induced apnea, which in infants often requires mechanical ventilation to prevent death (26). Preterm infants are much more likely to present with apnea secondary to RSV infection than term infants. It should be noted that anemia can greatly prolong the duration of LCR apnea (27). Hence it is relevant to note that a nadir in hematocrit occurs in infants at two to four months of life. Altogether this suggests that the risk of prolonged apnea from LCR reflexes might peak at three to four months when anemia of prematurity peaks as well as an increase in risk for RSV infection. In support of the argument for viral infection as a precursor for at least some SIDS cases, it has been recently shown that there is an increase in interleukins in the cerebrospinal fluid of many victims in contrast with infants dying of other causes (28). In other studies, RSV infection has been associated with increased activity of LCR reflexes associated with an increase in interleukins in the laryngeal mucosa (29). Evidence suggests that these cytokines can be transported to the brain stem from the inflamed upper airway tissues by a hematogenous route or retrograde axonal transport. This evidence comes from animal models and also studies in SIDS infants (30–32). It remains to be seen how increased brain stem interleukins might be a cause of sudden death. Yet, all in all these observations link the theory that subtile infections can cause SIDS to the A of P theory for cause of death in SIDS (33).

As regards SIDS, it must be acknowledged that, in the past, A of P has generally been discounted as causal in SIDS, since a history of such apnea does not increase risk for SIDS (34). However, upper airway viral infection is a primary risk factor for SIDS and also for reoccurrence of apnea in preterm infants (34). Seasonal outbreaks of such infections lasting no more than a few weeks or months are well documented. This is especially true for RSV infection in winter months when SIDS reaches a peak incidence. Furthermore, RSV infection is a common cause of reoccurrence of apnea in preterm infants.

V. OSA, A Cause of SIDS

Upper airway obstruction has long been a leading theory for cause of SIDS. Evidence for this comes from multiple studies. First, the vast majority of SIDS infants are presumed to die during sleep and OSA is entirely a sleep dependent disorder (35). Second, the severity of OSA is increased by increased nasal resistance such as occurs with viral upper airway infection, which is itself a risk factor for SIDS (34,35). Additionally, certain craniofacial morphological features are strongly associated with increased risk for OSA. Significantly, such abnormalities are reportedly increased in SIDS infants (36,37). Furthermore, sudden death from OSA is well documented in infants with these abnormalities, for example, micrognathia (8). Also, a large epidemiological study found that a family history of OSA is a risk factor for SIDS (38). Another important observation is that a prospective polygraphic study of sleeping infants found that brief episodes of obstructive apnea were more common in infants who ultimately died of SIDS compared with survivors (39). In yet another study, the distribution of thymic petechiae in SIDS victims suggests that airway obstruction is a precipitating event in 70% of SIDS cases (40). Moreover, new physiological evidence links OSA with the prone sleep position (41). In this study, compliance of the pharyngeal airway was significantly increased when anesthetized infants were placed prone. That is, the intrinsic compliance of the pharyngeal airway without added muscle support is increased in the prone position. Increased pharyngeal compliance is closely associated with OSA (35). This finding forms a potential link between the increased risk both for OSA and for SIDS in prone-sleeping infants. Finally, recovery from an episode of OSA is entirely dependent on arousal from sleep, and several laboratories have shown that repeated hypoxic episodes such as occur in OSA impair the ability to arouse from sleep (42–45). This can lead to a long lasting arousal deficit due to unique characteristics of the developing nervous system (46).

We conclude that there is strong, albeit indirect, evidence indicating that OSA either predisposes an infant to SIDS or actually acts as the final critical stressor causing death.

VI. Cardiac Hypothesis for SIDS

It has long been proposed that the sudden death of an infant must be caused by either sudden spontaneous respiratory or cardiac failure. For either mechanism there would be no specific postmortem findings. One major theory is that there are inherent cardiac conduction defects in SIDS infants. Specifically, a prolonged QT interval would render the heart susceptible to ventricular fibrillation. Schwartz and colleagues suggested this theory over 20 years ago (47). When ventricular bradycardia or fibrillation occurs as a result of this conduction abnormality, most patients spontaneously recover. However, sudden death is well documented and can occur in the absence of any proceeding cardiac symptoms (48). A number of genetic mutations have been documented in sodium ion or potassium channels in the myocardial cell membrane (49). These are the defects that cause prolongation of the QT interval. Seven gene mutations have been identified. These are found in two-thirds of the families with prolonged QT syndrome. Of relevance to SIDS, certain of these genotypes are associated with death primarily during sleep. The triggering event may be emotional excitement when awake or a loud noise that results in waking from sleep. These events are associated with a rapid change in sympathetic activity that predisposes the heart to arrhythmias. Also relevant to SIDS is the QT interval, which is longest in the first week, shortens with maturation, and then peaks again at two to three months of age. This developmental period coincides with the age of peak risk for SIDS. There is strong evidence supporting prolonged QT interval's causal role in SIDS. First, a prolonged QT interval in the first week of life is strongly associated with SIDS (47). Infants have been reported who died suddenly and unexpectedly and who had a prolonged QT interval prior to death. Additionally, 4.3% of a large case series of SIDS had pathological QT mutations (48). Also, one infant has been reported with ventricular fibrillation and cardiac arrest who was successfully cardioverted and certainly would have died had not intervention been immediate (50). This infant was found to have a very prolonged QT interval. Considering all of these findings, there is very strong evidence that in a minority of SIDS infants, at least, sudden death is caused by genetic mutations resulting in prolongation of the QT interval.

Although the QT syndrome may benefit from therapy with β blockers, it remains highly controversial as to which infants with prolonged QT syndrome should be treated and also as to whether or not all infants should be screened for genetic defects.

VII. Accidental Suffocation and Thermal Stress Theories

Both accidental suffocation and an allied diagnosis, "wedging" or "positional asphyxia" have been widely used by medical examiners for many years. Prior to the emergence of Public Health Safe Sleep Campaigns, these diagnoses were less used than they are today. As the pathophysiology of the various types of infant suffocation has been elucidated, the use of the diagnosis SIDS is used less frequently when the death scene investigation indicates airway compromise at the time of death. It has been estimated that 30% or more of sudden unexplained deaths in infants can be attributed to accidental suffocation when a careful death scene investigation has been performed (51).

There have been many studies of air exchange when an infant's airway is covered by bedding. These include theoretical, mechanical, animal, and living infant models (13,52–54). These studies indicate that expired air is trapped to a greater or lesser extent when the infant's airway is covered by porous bedding (13,52–54). In this situation, the expired air is rebreathed. Over time, the oxygen content of rebreathed air decreases and CO_2 content increases. The thickness of the bedding determines the size of the pool of gas that is oxygen depleted. Therefore, if the bedding beneath the face is thin, then an increase in tidal volume may be sufficient to prevent asphyxia from progressing to dangerous levels (54). Rebreathing can occur if the infant's head is covered by a blanket or quilt, or if the infant is lying prone, facedown, with the face covered by a mattress or other bedding. There are several factors determining the extent of rebreathing (53). These include the degree of softness of bedding beneath the infant's face, which determines the depth of the pocket around the face. The deeper the pocket, the greater the seal around the face and the less likely that there will be side air channels formed allowing access to fresh air. There are many infants who normally sleep facedown. When they do, small channels can be demonstrated in the folds of the bedding that provide access to air and thereby reduce rebreathing (54). Another critical factor determining death or survival when an infant's face is covered is the infant's own airway protective responses (55). These responses are learned through experience (56). Infants who normally sleep prone frequently experience rebreathing in the facedown position during a single night (57). The great majority of infants who normally sleep prone learn to lift and turn their heads to the side. This requires arousal from sleep, due to an increase in blood CO_2 and to a lesser extent reduction in oxygen saturation (55). Infants who have never slept prone often fail to turn their heads to the side to avoid rebreathing when they are in a facedown position. Increasing asphyxia occurs, and although they may lift their heads, this lasts only seconds and asphyxia occurs again as soon as their heads drop down (56).

Once in a rebreathing environment, the rate of progression of severity is highly variable. Slight changes in head position may create new channels through creases in the bedding material, thereby allowing some access to fresh air, which decreases the severity of asphyxia (54). Although in the absence of a change in head position, the progression of asphyxia is usually slow and takes place over several minutes dangerous asphyxia has been noted to happen in seconds if the infant briefly arouses (13). This is because arousal is usually accompanied by a sharp decrease in respiratory frequency. When this is marked, infants may rapidly desaturate to 85% or below. Presumably, they would continue to progressively desaturate if there is no intervention by a caregiver. Once oxygen saturation reaches 20–40%, hypoxic coma occurs and arousal is no longer possible. Even though autoresuscitation by gasping would then occur, this would be ineffective when the infant is already in a hypoxic environment.

Sudden death from the infant's head being wedged between two surfaces is well documented. This form of suffocation occurs when an infant gains the ability to move into an environment with a potential for wedging. These infants usually have not yet developed the motor skills allowing escape. Death can result from rebreathing, chest or nasal compression, or a combination of these. Many of these deaths are diagnosed as SIDS, particularly when a detailed death scene investigation has not been performed.

Compromise of an infant's airway by a sleeping parent during bed sharing has also been well documented. As bed sharing has become more popular, these deaths are increasing. As many as 50% of sudden unexpected infant deaths now occur when infants are sharing a bed, sofa, or sofa chair with others (51,58). The presumed mechanism of death during bed sharing is accidental suffocation resulting from close contact with a cosleeper or suffocation by soft bedding. However, the actual cause of death in this situation is usually very difficult to prove.

With extreme elevations in body temperature there is a risk for fatal heat stroke. The concept that heat stress, in and of itself, can result in SIDS is based on data from countries where it is common to cover infants with quilts and dress them in many outer layers of clothing during winter (34,59,60). Since the face is a major source of heat elimination it has been suggested that infants who are facedown die from heat stress. Proponents of this theory believe that heat stress death may not necessarily be associated with an actual elevation in body temperature.

Several observations weigh against heat stress as a major cause of SIDS. Dangerous asphyxia can occur very soon after an infant turns facedown in bedding. When this happens, it would seem that asphyxia might precipitate death before the heat stress associated with being facedown could take effect. This of course does not rule out that the combination of heat stress and rebreathing may be more lethal than either alone. Additionally, in the United States, SIDS rates do not increase during summer heat waves when there are marked increases in heat related deaths in the general population due to heat stroke (61). This suggests that heat stress is not a major cause of SIDS in the United States. Finally, perhaps the greatest problem with accepting the heat stress theory is that other than extremely elevated body temperature leading to heat stroke, there has been no lethal pathophysiological mechanism identified that could cause sudden death.

VIII. Metabolic Deficiencies Presenting as SIDS

Sudden infant deaths attributed to metabolic disorders technically are not SIDS. Nevertheless, infant deaths resulting from inborn errors of metabolism often have negative histories for illness. When autopsy findings in such cases do not reveal a cause of death, they are diagnosed as SIDS. To date, a number of defects known to cause sudden death have been described. Listed as the most to least common, they include medium-chain and very long chain acyl-CoA dehydrogenize deficiency, glutaric acidemia type 1 and type 2, carnitine palmitoyl transferase type II/translocation deficiencies, severe carnitine deficiency, isovaleric acidemia, 12-methylbutyric-CoA dehydrogenase deficiencies, long-chain hydroxy acyl-CoA dehyrogenase and trifunctional protein deficiencies (62). The great majority of infants with these disorders first present with acute metabolic academia and/or hypoglycemia with a rapid onset and are admitted to the hospital. Once there, they respond well to medical therapy. A period of lack of food intake is often a precipitating factor, since these infants are unable to adequately utilize fat. Fatalities are believed to be the result of cardiac arrhythmias resulting from the effects of elevated carnitine on cardiac pacemaker cells. Most medical examiners are now screening for metabolic defects in samples of bile or blood taken at the postmortem examination. It has been estimated in the past that 3–6% of sudden infant deaths are the result of such metabolic disorders (62). However, since accurate postmortem screening is becoming more routine, the number of deaths diagnosed as SIDS is becoming less frequent.

IX. Brain Stem Pathology and SIDS

The past decade has seen much research on brain stem defects in SIDS infants. Kinney and associates pioneered this work, and their major findings have now been confirmed by others (63,64). Both subtle anatomical changes and receptor deficiencies have been described in brain stem nuclei. It has been shown that certain nuclei have decreased serotonergic receptor sites. These nuclei are believed to be critical for CO_2 sensitivity and arousal mechanisms as well as for cardiorespiratory control. In other research, inherited defects in serotonin transporter genes have been documented in SIDS infants (65,66).

Considering these findings, it appears that most SIDS infants have multiple abnormalities in the brain stem involving serotonin (67). It has been proposed that brain stem receptor abnormalities make infants vulnerable to sudden death. A very recent finding is that the number of neurons that are deficient in serotonin receptors are actually increased in SIDS infants (67). This raises the possibility that the total number of serotonin receptors may not be reduced in the brain stem in which case the increased neurons may represent a compensation for the reduced receptors on individual neurons. As such, it is possible that these infants actually may not have abnormal brain stem function. All in all, it is clear that the brain serotonergic system is altered in many SIDS infants. It is unclear if these alterations are congenital or acquired postnatally. The significance of a possible genetic predisposition to SIDS as suggested by altered serotonin transporter genes is also unclear.

Regarding the physiological functions that might be impaired by these brain stem abnormalities, the focus to date has been on deficiency in arousal and on related CO_2 sensory mechanisms. The theory that decreased CO_2 sensitivity might be causal in SIDS is strengthened by reports of arcuate nucleus hypoplasia in a few SIDS infants (68). The arcuate nucleus is believed to be a major site for CO_2 sensitivity related to respiratory function. However, studies in animal models with agents that block the specific serotonin receptor sites have produced only modest decreases in CO_2 sensitivity (21%) (69). Moreover, the reduced CO_2 response is present in males only (70). Therefore, as far as blunting of the CO_2 response is concerned, it is unclear how a reduction in serotonergic receptor sites could significantly increase the risk for SIDS (71).

In summary, it seems clear that serotonergic systems in the brain stem are abnormal in many SIDS victims. It has been proposed that arousal from sleep, alterations in sleep state cycles, cardiovascular control, or CO_2 responsiveness might result from this abnormality (72). However, at the present time, it remains to be seen how such abnormalities could make infants substantially more vulnerable to SIDS.

References

1. Poets CF, Meny RG, Chobanian MR, et al. Gasping and other cardiorespiratory patterns during sudden infant deaths. Pediatr Res 1999; 45:350–354.
2. Sridhar R, Thach BT, Kelly D, et al. Characterization of successful and failed autoresuscitation in sudden infant death syndrome (SIDS) and other infants dying sudden and unexpectedly. Pediatr Pulmonol 2003; 36:113–122.
3. Meny RG, Carroll JL, Carbone MT, et al. Cardiorespiratory recordings from infants dying suddenly and unexpectedly at home. Pediatrics 1994; 93:44–49.
4. Krous HF, Masoumi H, Haas EA, et al. Gastric aspiration in cases of sudden infant death syndrome for which cardiopulmonary resuscitation was not attempted. J Pediatr 2007; 150:241–246.
5. Bureau MA, Lamarche J, Foulon P, et al. Postnatal maturation of respiration in intact and caroid body-chemodenervated lambs. J Appl Physiol 1995; 59:869–874.
6. Donnelly D, Haddad G. Respiratory changes induced by prolonged laryngeal stimulation in awake piglets. J Appl Physiol 1986; 61(3):1018–1024.

7. Cote A, Porras H, Meehan B. Age-dependent vulnerability to carotid chemo-denervation in piglets. J Appl Physiol 1996; 80:323–331.

8. Thach BT. Sleep apnea in infancy and childhood. In: Thawley ST, ed. Symposium on Sleep Apnea Disorders. Med Clin North AM, 1985; 69(6):1289–315.

9. Abu-Osba YK, Brouillette R, Wilson S. Breathing pattern and transcutaneous oxygen tension during motor activity in preterm infants. Am Rev Resp Dis 1982; 125(4):382–387.

10. Peiper A. Gasping respiration, Breath-holding, Whooping cough attack. In: Consultants Bureau Inc., ed., New York, Cerebral Function in Infancy and Childhood. 1963:327–339, 371–382.

11. Gauk SW, Kidd L, Prichard JS. Mechanisms of seizures associated with breath-holding spells. N Engl J Med 1963; 268:1436–1441.

12. Lind J. Changes in the circulation and lungs at birth. Acta Paediatr Scand 1960; 49:39–52.

13. Patel AL, Paluszynska D, Harris KA. Sudden respiratory decompensation in sleeping infants while rebreathing. Pediatrics 2003; 111(4):e328.

14. Walsh SZ, Meyer WW, Lind J. The Human Fetal and Neonatal Circulation: Function and Structure. Springfield: Charles C Thomas 1974;89–104.

15. Speidel BD. Adverse effects of routine procedures on preterm infants. Lancet 1978; 1(8069):864–866.

16. Pickens DL, Schefft G, Thach BT. Prolonged apnea associated with upper airway protective reflexes in apnea of prematurity. Am Rev Respir Dis 1988; 137:113–118.

17. Davies A, Koenig J, Thach B. Upper airway chemoreflex responses to saline and water in preterm infants. J Appl Physiol 1988; 64:1412–1420.

18. Downing SE, Lee JC. Laryngeal chemosensitivity: A possible mechanism for sudden infant death. Pediatrics 1975; 55:640–649.

19. Johnson P, Salisbury D, Storey A. Apnea induced by stimulation of sensory receptors in the larynx. In: Bosma JF, Showacre J, eds. Symposium on Development of Upper Respiratory Anatomy and Function. Implications for Sudden Infant Death Syndrome. Washington, DC: US Government Printing Office, 1975: 160–183.

20. Harding R, Johnson P, McCelland M. Liquid-sensitive laryngeal receptors in the developing sheep, cat and monkey. J Physiol 1978; 277:409–422.

21. Pickens D, Schefft G, Thach BT. Pharyngeal fluid clearance and aspiration preventive mechanisms in sleeping infants. J Appl Physiol 1989; 66(3):1164–1171.

22. Menon AP, Schefft GL, Thach BT. Frequency and significance of swallowing during prolonged apnea in infants. Am Rev Respir Dis 1984; 130:969–973.

23. Miller MJ, DiFiore JM. A comparison of swallowing during apnea and periodic breathing in premature infants. Pediatr Res 1995; 37:796–799.

24. Menon AP, Scheff GL, Thach BT. Apnea associated with regurgitation in infants. J Pediatr 1985; 106:625–629.

25. Hunt C, Corwin M, Baird T, et al., and Collaborative Home Infant Monitoring Evaluation (CHIME) Study Group. Cardiorespiratory events detected by home memory monitoring and one-year neurodevelopmental outcome. J Pediatr 2004; 145:465–471.

26. Pickens DL, Schefft GL, Thach BT. Characterization of prolonged apneic episodes associated with respiratory syncytial viral infection in infants. Pediatr Pulmonol 1989; 6:195–201.

27. Fagenholz S, Lee J, Downing E. Association of anemia with reduced central respiratory drive in the piglet. Yale J Biol Med 1979; 52:263–270.

28. Vege A, Rognum TO, Aasen AO, Saugstad OD. Are elevated cerebrospinal fluid levels of IL-6 in sudden infant death, infectious deaths, and deaths due to heart/lung in infants and children due to hypoxia? Acta Paediatr. 1998; 84:193–196.

29. Lindgren C, Jing L, Graham B, et al. Respiratory syncytial virus infection reinforces reflex apnea in young lambs. Pediatr Res 1992; 31:381–385.

30. Banks WA, Ortiz L, Plotkin SR, et al. Human interleukin-1a, murine IL-1a and murine IL-1 are transported from blood to brain in the mouse by a shared satiable mechanism. J Pharmacol Exp Ther 1991; 259(3):988–996.

31. Maehlen J, Olsson T, Zachau A, et al. Local enhancement of major histocompatibility complex (MHC) class I and II expression and cell infiltration in experimental allergic encephalomyelitis around axotomized motor neurons. J Neuroimmunol 1989; 23(2):125–132.

32. Kadhim H, Kahn A, Sebire G. Distinct cytokine profile in SIDS brain: a common denominator in a multifactorial syndrome? Neurology 2003; 61:1256–1259.

33. Moscovis SM, Gordon AE, Al Madani OM, et al. Interleukin-10 and sudden infant death syndrome. FEMS Immunol Med Microbiol 2004; 42(1):130–138.

34. Mitchell EA, Scragg R, Stewart AW, et al. Results from the first year of the New Zealand Cot Death Study. N Z Med J 1991; 104:71–76.

35. White D. Pathophysiology of obstructive sleep apnea. Thorax 1995; 50:797–804.

36. Guilleminault C, Partinen M, Hollman K. Familial aggregates in obstructive sleep apnea syndrome. Chest 1996; 107:1545–1551.

37. Siebert JR, Haas JE. Enlargement of the tongue in sudden infant death syndrome. Pediatr Pathol 1991; 11:813–826.

38. Tishler P, Redline S, Ferrette V, et al. The association of sudden unexpected infant death with obstructed sleep apnea. Am J Respir Crit Care Med 1996; 153:1857–1863.

39. Kahn A, Groswasser J, Rebuffat E, et al. Sleep and cardiorespiratory characteristics of infant victims of sudden death: a prospective case-control study. Sleep 1992; 15 (4):287–292.

40. Krous H, Jordan J. A necropsy study of distribution of petechiae in non-sudden infant death syndrome. Arch Pathol Lab Med 1984; 108:75–76.

41. Ishikawa T, Isono S, Aiba J, et al. Prone position increases collapsibility of the passive pharynx in infants and small children. Am J Respir Crit Care Med 2002; 166:760–764.

42. Waters K, Tinworth K. Habituation of arousal responses after intermittent hypercapnic hypoxia in piglets. Am J Respir Crit Care Med 2005; 171:1305–1311.

43. Fewell JE, Williams BJ, Szabo JS. Influence of repeated upper airway obstruction on the arousal and cardiopulmonary response to upper airway obstruction in lambs. Pediatr Res 1988; 23:191–195.

44. Johnston RV, Frant DA, Wilkerson MH, et al. Repetitive hypoxia rapidly depresses arousal from active sleep in newborn lambs. J Physiol 1998; 510:651–659.

45. Bowes G, Woolf GM, Sullivan CE, et al. Effects of sleep fragmentation on ventilatory and arousal responses of sleeping dogs to respiratory stimuli. Am Rev Respir Dis 1980; 122:899–908.

46. Carroll JL. Developmental plasticity in respiratory control. J Appl Physiol 2003; 94:375–389.

47. Schwartz PJ, Stramba-Badiale M, Segantini A, et al. Prolongation of the QT interval and the sudden infant death syndrome, N Engl J Med 1998; 338:1709–1714.
48. Towbin JA, Ackerman MJ. Cardiac sodium channel gene mutations and sudden infant death syndrome. Circulation 2001; 104(10):1092–1095.
49. Wang DW, Desai RR, Crotti L, et al. Cardiac sodium channel dysfunction in sudden infant death syndrome. Circulation. 2007; 115:368–376.
50. Schwartz PJ, Priori JP, Napolitano C, et al. A molecular link between the sudden infant death syndrome and the long-QT syndrome. N Engl J Med 2000; 343: 262–267.
51. Unger B, Kemp JS, Wilkins D, et al. Racial disparity and modifiable risk factors among infants dying suddenly and unexpectedly. Pediatrics 2003; 111:127–131.
52. Chiodini B, Thach BT. Impaired ventilation in infants sleeping face down: potential significance for sudden infant death syndrome. J Pediatr 1993; 123:686–692.
53. Kemp JS, Thach BT. Quantifying the potential of infant bedding to limit CO_2 dispersal and factors affecting rebreathing in bedding. J Appl Physiol 1995; 78:740–745.
54. Patel A, Harris K, Thach BT. Inspired CO_2 and O_2 in sleeping infants rebreathing from bedding: relevance for sudden infant death syndrome. J Appl Physiol 2001; 91:2537–2545.
55. Lijowska A, Reed NW, Mertins-Chiodini BA. Sequential arousal and airway defensive behavior of infants in asphyxial sleep environments. J Appl Physiol 1997; 83:219–228.
56. Paluszynska D, Harris K, Thach BT. Influence sleep position experience on ability of prone sleeping infants to escape from asphyxiating microenvironments by changing head position. Pediatrics 2004; 114:1634–1639.
57. Waters KA, Gonzalez AJC, Morielli A, et al. Face straight down and face-near-straight down position in healthy, prone-sleeping infants. J Pediatr 1998; 128: 616–625.
58. Blair PS, Sidebotham P, Berry PJ, et al. Major epidemiological changes in sudden infant death syndrome: a 20-year population-based study in the UK. Lancet 2006; 367(9507):314–319.
59. Mitchell EA, Tuohy PG, Brunt JM, et al. Risk factors for sudden infant death syndrome following the prevention campaign in New Zealand: a prospective study. Pediatrics 1997; 100:835–840.
60. Fleming PJ, Blair PS, Bacon C, et al. Environment of infants during sleep risk of the sudden infant death syndrome: results from 1993-5 case-control study for confidential inquiry into stillbirths and deaths in infancy. BMJ 1996; 313:191–195.
61. Scheers-Masters J, Schootman M, Thach BT. Heat stress and sudden infant death syndrome incidence a U.S. population based epidemiological study. Pediatrics 2003; 113:E586–E592.
62. Rinaldo P. Metabolic causes of sudden and unexpected death in early life. Available at: http://www.Savebabies.org/NBS/sids-medical report6-98.php.
63. Kinney HC, Filiano JJ, White WF. Medullary serotonergic network deficiency in the sudden infant death syndrome: review of a 15 year study of a single dataset. J Neuropathol Exp Neurol 2001; 60:228–247.
64. Ozawa Y, Okade N. Alteration of serotonergic receptors in the brainstem of human patients with respiratory disorders. Neuropediatrics 2002; 33:142–149.

65. Narita N, Narita M, Takashima S, et al. Serotonin transporter gene variation is a risk factor for sudden infant death syndrome in the Japanese population. Pediatrics 2001; 107:690–692.
66. Maher BS, Marazita ML, Rand C, et al. 3' UTR polymorphism of the serotonin transporter gene and sudden infant death syndrome. Haplotype analysis. Am J Med Genet A 2006; 140:1453–1457.
67. Paterson DS, Trachtenberg FL, Thompson EG, et al. Multiple serotonergic brainstem abnormalities in sudden infant death syndrome. JAMA 2006; 296:2124–2132.
68. Filiano JJ, Kinney HC. Arcuate nucleus hypoplasia in the sudden infant death syndrome. J Neuropathol Exp Neurol 1992; 51(4):394–403.
69. Curran AK, Darnall RA, Filiano JJ, et al. Muscimol dialysis in the rostral ventral medulla reduced the CO_2 response in awake and sleeping piglets. J Appl Physiol 2001; 90:971–980.
70. Pematti EM, Berniker AV, Kereshi B, et al. Ventilatory response to hypercapnia and hypoxia after extensive lesion of medullary serotonergic neurons in newborn conscious piglets. J Appl Physiol 2006; 101:1177–1188.
71. Emery J. Families in which two or more cost deaths have occurred. The Lancet 1986; 327:313–315.
72. Darnall RA, Harris MB, Gill WH. Inhibition of serotonergic neurons in the nucleus paragigantocellularis lateralis fragments sleep and decreases rapid eye movement in the piglet: implications for sudden infant death syndrome. J Neurosci 2005; 25 (36):8322–8332.

12

Sudden Infant Deaths: Risk Factors, Contributory Factors, and Causal Factors

PETER FLEMING and PETER S. BLAIR
University of Bristol, Bristol, U.K.

I. Introduction

Sudden unexpected infant deaths have been recognized since antiquity, but it was not until post-neonatal mortality rates substantially fell in the Western world during the early part of the 20th century that greater attention was paid to the phenomenon of unexpected and unexplained deaths in apparently healthy infants. "Sudden Infant Death Syndrome" or SIDS was proposed in 1969 as a descriptive term for those infant deaths that were unexpected and remained unexplained after thorough investigation. In 1994 a more precise definition of SIDS was proposed (1): "The sudden death of an infant, which is unexplained after review of the clinical history, examination of the circumstances of death, and postmortem examination."

II. Investigation and Classification of Unexpected Infant Deaths

The process of investigation after any unexpected infant death should seek to collect as much information as possible about factors that may have contributed to the death, in order to help understand (and in future possibly prevent) such deaths. It is essential, however, that the investigation be conducted with both thoroughness and sensitivity, bearing in mind that while the great majority of such deaths are natural tragedies, it is equally important to identify those instances in which neglect or abuse may have caused or contributed to the death (2,3).

The precise nature of the investigation and composition of the investigating team will vary according to the requirements of the relevant state or national legislation. In England, regulations introduced under recent legislation have defined these requirements, which will be mandatory from 2008 (3,4). These regulations were based on the conclusions of a national review body, chaired by a senior barrister, and including pediatricians, pathologists, police, coroners, social services, and representatives of the government, the judiciary, and parents' organizations (3). An overview of the requirements of these regulations is given below as an example of the need for thorough and integrated investigations.

A. The English Protocol for Investigation of Unexpected Infant Deaths

The protocol involves emergency first responders, clinical staff, police, pathologists, coroners, social services, and other agencies working together and sharing information to minimize duplication and maximize available information to help identify contributory or causal factors. The initial investigation must include a careful and detailed medical, social, and environmental history, with a thorough review of the circumstances of death, including visiting and carefully examining the scene of death. This home visit with the parents or carers should ideally be conducted jointly by a pediatrician and a child protection police officer whose combined expertise in infant physiology and development and in forensic examination maximizes the potential to recognize both natural and unnatural contributory factors. The pathologist (who must have appropriate pediatric training) should conduct a thorough postmortem examination to an evidence-based protocol (3,5), and should be provided with as full an account as possible of the history, clinical examination of the infant, and scene examination before commencing the procedure. At all stages of the investigation, there must be continual sharing of information by all agencies involved, and—except in those rare instances in which criminal prosecution might be compromised by so doing—the parents must be kept fully informed. Meeting the needs of parents for care and support must be central to the process. Finally, when all investigations are completed, usually two to four months after the death, a multi-agency case review meeting should be convened—usually in the primary care setting. The aim of this meeting is to ensure that all professionals share information; review and, if possible, come to conclusions about the cause of or contributory factors to the death; decide on who is to inform the parents of the results of the investigations (usually the pediatrician plus a member of the primary health care team); and produce a report for the coroner to inform and facilitate the Inquest.

Classification	0	I A	I B	II A	II B	III
Contributory or potentially "causal" Factors	*Information not collected*	*Information collected but no factors identified*	*Factor present but not likely to have contributed to ill health or to death.*	*Factor present, and may have contributed to ill health, or possibly to death*	*Factor present and certainly contributed to ill health, and probably contributed to the death*	*Factor present, and provides a complete and sufficient cause of death*
History: (1)						
Death-scene examination (2)						
Pathology (3)						
Other (specify)						
Other Evidence of Neglect or abuse?						
Overall classification (4)						

(1): To include a detailed history of events leading up to the death, together with medical, social and family history, plus explicit review of any evidence suggesting past neglect or abuse of this child or other children in the family.
(2): Results of detailed review of the scene of death by the paediatrician and police Child Protection officer in the light of the history given by parents or carers.
(3): Pathological investigations to a standardised protocol, including gross pathology, histology, microbiology, toxicology, radiology, clinical chemistry, and any relevant metabolic investigations, including frozen section of liver stained for fat.
(4): This will generally equal the highest individual classification listed above.

Figure 1 The grid is completed at the multidisciplinary case discussion meeting (usually held 8–12 weeks after the death). An entry must be made on the line of each heading line, and a score (0–III) accorded to each line as agreed by all professionals present. The overall score is generally equal to the highest score within the grid. A score of III equates to a complete and sufficient cause of death. Scores of I to IIB meet the definition of SIDS. *Abbreviation*: SIDS, sudden infant death syndrome. *Source*: From Refs. 2 and 3.

Thus, the "cause" of death as finally certified through the coroners' system reflects the full breadth of professional expertise in understanding both natural and possible unnatural contributory or causal factors (2,3).

The careful review of potential contributory factors allows unexpected infant deaths to be separated into those for which no significant contributory factors were identified, those for which one or more factors were found that may have contributed to the death but do not in themselves give a complete explanation (and thus by definition would still be classified as SIDS), and those for which a complete and sufficient explanation was found. Several classifications of unexpected infant deaths using such approaches have been published and allow studies to distinguish between varying degrees of contribution ranging from environmental, infectious, and physiological causes to genetically determined factors in different infants (6), although a standardized international classification system would be more desirable (7).

Figure 1 shows the Avon Clinicopathological classification, which is based on this approach, and has been widely adopted in the United Kingdom (2,3,5,8).

Most epidemiological background factors associated with unexpected but explained infant deaths (i.e., those deaths classified as III in Fig. 1 such as unrecognized overwhelming infection) are very similar in character to those factors found among SIDS victims (i.e., those deaths classified as I to IIB in Fig. 1) (9). Indeed, there is some evidence that improved investigation has led to an increase in the proportion of reported deaths that are explained, in particular deaths due to metabolic disorders (2,3,5,8). Thus, it is important that similar investigation should be applied to all such deaths, and any study of unexpected infant deaths should include all sudden unexpected deaths in infancy (SUDI), and not be restricted to only those classified as SIDS—either by arbitrary assignment at the beginning of the investigative process or at the end of a full investigation (2,3).

Although there has been some reluctance by professionals to fully engage in such a process, on the grounds that it is demanding of both time and energy, and may not be sustainable, recent studies have shown that with minimal additional resources such an approach can be implemented and sustained over many years (8). Certainly, the savings—both financial and emotional—from avoidance of inappropriate criminal charges, together with the recognition of genuine child protection issues, warrant the adoption of a robust and thorough but sensitive investigation in all cases of unexpected infant deaths.

III. The Epidemiology of Unexpected Infant Deaths: Modifiable and Nonmodifiable Risk Factors

In 1904, Willcox (10) and in 1892 Templeman (11) noted the excess of unexpected infant deaths in the poorest families and agreed that the majority of such deaths were due to accidental overlaying while bed sharing, recommending that parents be encouraged to use cribs for their babies to sleep in. One hundred years later, the American Academy of Pediatrics (AAP) made a similar recommendation, though the evidence for this has been the subject of wide debate (12–15).

A. The Diagnosis of SIDS and Subsequent Decline in the SIDS Rate

The diagnosis of SIDS is unique, in that it is not a cause of death but rather a diagnosis of exclusion, arrived at only after thorough investigation as outlined above. Only when recognized causes of infant death have been excluded can the death be labeled SIDS, and there are valid concerns that such labeling could create a "diagnostic dustbin" (16) or, at the very least, attribute too much homogeneity to what might be disparate causes of death (17).

In 1953, a committee formed to investigate sudden death in infancy in the United Kingdom (18) suggested that around 1400 such deaths occurred annually. In the late 1980s, epidemiological evidence from several different countries (19–24) suggested that SIDS could be related to infants sleeping in the prone position. In 1991, the "Back to Sleep" campaign was initiated in the United

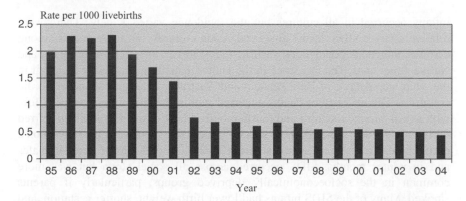

Figure 2 SIDS rate in England and Wales, 1985–2004. *Abbreviation*: SIDS, sudden infant death syndrome. *Source*: Office for National Statistics and the Foundation for the Study of Infant Deaths.

Kingdom to encourage parents to avoid placing their infants on their front and the SIDS rate fell from a peak of 2.3 deaths in 1988 to 0.7 per 1000 live births in 1994 (Fig. 2). Similar dramatic reductions have since been observed in many other countries following such an intervention campaign. The possibility that other modifiable risk factors might be amenable to further interventions in this mysterious group of conditions has led to multiple epidemiological studies of the residual deaths. Further identification of other unsafe infant care practices, particularly within the sleep environment, have led to additional amendments and revision of the initial campaign message and probably helped to reduce the rate further over the last 10 years to 0.4 per 1000 live births. This equates to the prevention of over 10,000 infant deaths in England and Wales since the campaign was first launched, and more than 100,000 worldwide.

The fall in the number of deaths has been accompanied by several major changes in the epidemiological characteristics of SIDS (8), most notably an increased proportion of the deaths occurring in deprived families and while bed sharing. Some pathologists are reluctant to use the label "SIDS" when parents have consumed alcohol or illegal drugs or when the circumstances of death raise the unproven possibility of overlying, preferring to use the term "unascertained" (25). Such labeling causes confusion among parents, makes it difficult to accurately monitor SIDS rates, and does not adequately flag up the concerns of the pathologists. This inappropriate diagnostic shift emphasizes the importance of a detailed multiprofessional review using an accepted classification system in establishing the final allocated "cause" of unexpected infant deaths.

B. Epidemiological Characteristics Prior to the Fall in SIDS

Many studies were conducted prior to 1991 and there was broad agreement on some of the epidemiological findings. The unexpected, unexplained deaths of infants occurred in all cultures but the incidence varied widely. There were relatively fewer SIDS deaths in several Asian cultures, but more deaths among certain indigenous populations such as the Maoris, Australian Aborigines, and Native Americans. The incidence in the United Kingdom was lower than that in the white populations of New Zealand and Australia, but higher than the Nordic countries. The majority of deaths occurred within the first nine months of life, with a peak around the third and fourth month. Many of the deaths also occurred during night sleep, although there was no discernable increase in prevalence on a particular day of the week across studies (26–29). More deaths occurred in males and in winter months. SIDS occurred across all social strata but was more common in the socioeconomically deprived groups, particularly if parents smoked. Many of the SIDS infants had lower birth weight, shorter gestation, and more perinatal problems. There was a strong correlation with young maternal age and higher parity, and the risk increased with multiple births, single motherhood, or a poor obstetric history.

The assumption that these factors were specific to SIDS led to its description as an "epidemiological entity" (30), but many were also closely associated with other infant deaths. A direct comparison of background demographic factors revealed that only the age distribution and high prevalence of tobacco exposure distinguished SIDS infants from infants who died suddenly from identifiable causes (9). Deaths from congenital malformations decrease steadily from an early age, whereas deaths from respiratory or infectious diseases remain relatively constant over the first year of life (31). In general, the highest prevalence of infant deaths is in the first weeks after birth when infants are most vulnerable (32,33). However, few SIDS deaths occur in the first month, with a large peak at three to four months and a steady decline thereafter. The prevalence of smoking during pregnancy is higher among SIDS mothers than control mothers matched for socioeconomic status for all social groups.

It is perhaps in the infant sleeping environment that the epidemiological study of SIDS has had the most success. Prone sleeping was actively encouraged in some Western countries in the 1960s and 1970s (34) to improve infant posture and skeletal growth (35), to prevent flattening of the skull (35,36), and to avoid the perceived risk of aspiration in the supine position (37,38). This was also a time when neonatal intensive care units were expanding and apparent benefits of using the prone position were found among preterm infants, including a discernable increase in quiet sleep (39), better gastric emptying (40), better oxygenation (40,41), and more effective ribcage and abdominal coupling with decreased work of breathing (42). What was best for the relatively small number of preterm infants was not necessarily beneficial for the rest of the infant population. Historical references to infant sleeping position in art and early medical texts suggest that very few, if any, infants were placed prone to sleep before the 20th century (43). Population-based studies identified the prone sleeping position and thermal stress as major factors associated with SIDS. SIDS infants were commonly more warmly wrapped and placed in warmer rooms than surviving control infants (24,44–46). Gilbert found that the combination of viral infection and heavy wrapping was associated with a high relative risk (44), while a study from Tasmania, (45) found that the risk from prone position was potentiated by overnight heating, swaddling, recent infection, and mattress type. Williams confirmed these findings in a study from New Zealand and found a small additive effect if the mother smoked (47).

C. "Back to Sleep" Campaigns

Although positioning and wrapping were not sufficient to fully explain the sudden deaths, they could be linked to some causal chain of events. Intervention campaigns to advise parents against these practices were instigated in many countries from 1990 onward. In all countries in which risk reduction campaigns were conducted, a fall in infant prone sleeping was followed by a fall in SIDS rate. Some campaigns publicized the potential risk of heavy wrapping; studies of control infants in Avon before and after the Back to Sleep campaign (44,48) showed that the thermal resistance (tog value) of bedding and clothing with which normal infants were usually covered fell by almost half after the Back to Sleep campaign. The winter peaks of SIDS deaths have almost disappeared in the United Kingdom, while SIDS is now largely confined to families living in relative or absolute socioeconomic deprivation.

D. Epidemiological Characteristics Since the Fall in Numbers of SIDS

Distal Factors

A longitudinal study conducted in Avon from 1984 to 2003 (8) shows that among SIDS families the proportion from the most disadvantaged socioeconomic groups has risen from 47% to 75%. This change in the socioeconomic distribution of SIDS families has been accompanied by increased proportions of single mothers, younger mothers, mothers who smoke, and lower birth weight infants. The prevalence of maternal smoking during pregnancy among SIDS mothers (80–90%) is twice the level expected among control mothers with similarly deprived socioeconomic backgrounds (49), lending support to the hypothesis that infant exposure to tobacco smoke is some part of a causal mechanism. There is a clear increase in the risk of SIDS, with increasing levels of exposure to tobacco smoke, both in utero and after birth (50–52), and a recent review by Mitchell and Milerad suggests that this risk has grown despite advice against smoking in almost all risk reduction campaigns (53). In recent studies over one-third of SIDS victims were preterm, compared with a U.K. population prevalence of 5% for preterm delivery. For such infants, the effects of other risk factors in combination with the increased risk from prematurity leads to very high risk [e.g., for preterm infants put down on the side, odds ratio = 9.13 (95%, CI 4.93–16.90), and for those put down prone, odds ratio = 62.8 (95%, CI 12.06–327)] (54).

The previously recognized increase in the risk of SIDS with increasing birth order may be changing. The longitudinal study from Avon suggests that SIDS is now most common among firstborn infants (8). These distal factors may have limited use in terms of immediate prevention, but studying the changes in patterns may have implications in terms of potential causal pathways.

Several studies have now shown no evidence that immunization is associated with an increased risk of SIDS, and some evidence that the risk may be reduced (55).

Proximal Factors

New evidence on risks within the infant sleeping environment has changed some of the advice now given to parents.

The Risk of Positioning Infants on the Side to Sleep

Before the Back to Sleep campaign, few studies had looked at the use of the side sleeping position and the findings were inconclusive (46,56–58); the side position with the lower arm extended to avoid infants rolling on their front was suggested as a safe alternative to supine sleeping. More recent studies (48,59–63) suggest that the side position carries a similar degree of attributable risk to being placed prone, mainly because the position is unstable, and some infants who roll from side to prone have difficulty extricating themselves from this position. Certain infants with abnormalities of the upper airway (e.g., Pierre Robin syndrome) may experience airway obstruction if placed supine, and some may benefit from side or occasionally prone positioning for sleep, but many can be safely placed supine. While gastroesophageal reflux is slightly reduced in the prone position compared with the supine, the increased risk of SIDS means that this position should not be used to treat reflux unless this is causing severe symptoms (e.g., growth failure or recurrent aspiration) that have not responded to alternative treatments. Apart from these rare conditions, in most countries the only recommended sleeping position for infants is supine. In some countries, use of the side position may have increased despite knowledge of its potential risks (64,65), with many parents and health care professionals citing either outdated SIDS guidelines or fear of aspiration, cyanosis, or apnea when the infant is placed supine (66–69). These concerns are not supported by either findings from the pathology or epidemiology. A review of 196 infant deaths in South Australia found evidence of aspiration of gastric contents into the airways and alveoli of three infants but all were found face down in the prone position (70). Similar findings linking aspiration with the prone rather than the supine position have been found in the United Kingdom (71), while a large cohort study of over 8000 surviving U.K. infants showed no association between the prevalence of vomiting and infant sleeping position (72). A recent study from New Zealand (73) has linked the increase in sleeping supine with nonsynostotic plagiocephaly, recommending that parents should vary the infant head position when putting them down to sleep and to give their infants five minutes of supervised "tummy time" each day. This may also help reduce the risk of "unaccustomed prone" position, when infants roll into or fall asleep in this position for the first time. In studies in Australia, the United States, and the United Kingdom, supine sleeping was not linked to apnea or cyanosis and no demonstrable increase in symptoms or illness among supine sleeping infants was found (72,74,75).

The Risk of Soft Sleeping Surfaces

Soft mattresses and other malleable surfaces have been associated with an increased risk of SIDS (5,76,77) and there is some evidence that this risk is even higher in combination with established risk factors such as the prone sleeping position (78,79) and infant thermal stress (80). Pillows, cushions, and bean bags have been used not just as a sleep surface but also as a prop to maintain the body position of a sleeping infant or to provide easier access to bottle feeding. This practice presents the additional risk, even to supine sleeping infants, of such objects potentially covering the external airways (81). This includes the adult size V-shaped pillows used to accommodate breast-feeding (82). The current advice is to sleep infants on a firm mattress and away from soft objects.

The Risk of Bedding Covering the Infant

It is not uncommon for SIDS infants to be discovered dead with bedclothes covering the head and face, indeed "accidental mechanical suffocation" was a term used to describe these deaths prior to the SIDS classification (83). However studies in the late 1940s rejected the idea that a child could be suffocated by "ordinary bedclothes" largely based on the lack of postmortem findings to support asphyxia as a cause of death (83–87). Uncontrolled observations from early studies (88–91) suggest that around a fifth of SIDS infants were found with bedding covering the face or head and were thus ignored or interpreted to be part of the agonal struggle just prior to death. Subsequent findings of reduced arousability during the sleep of SIDS infants (92), observations of undisturbed bedding (93), and the lack of such a struggle during recordings of several SIDS infants who died while on a monitor (93) do not support the idea that head covering is just a consequence of the terminal event. While postmortem examination cannot distinguish between the possible mechanisms of airway obstruction, rebreathing, or thermal stress, over 20% of SIDS victims are found with bedding over the head (8,61,63,79,87,94–98), 10 times more than the incidence among age-matched controls and highly significant even after adjusting for other risk factors. Studies have linked head covering to loose bedding (8), infant movement down under the covers (8,99), and the use of duvets (8,99,100) or quilts (101). In 1997, a *Feet to Foot* campaign, subsequently endorsed by the AAP (12,102), was launched in England and Wales by the Foundation for the Study of Infant Death to encourage parents to tuck the bedding in firmly, avoid using duvets or pillows, and place the feet of the infant at the foot of the cot.

The Risk Associated with Unobserved Sleep

Despite a complete absence of supporting evidence, many childcare "experts" in the 1950s to the 1990s recommended that infants should sleep in a room separately from parents (103,104). Throughout history most human infants slept in a consistently rich sensory environment with close and continual contact between mothers and babies and the solitary sleep experience of Western societies was a recent development (105). Reports from New Zealand and the United Kingdom showed that the risk of SIDS was lower if infants shared a bedroom with parents (106–108), and further analysis of the U.K. data suggests that parental supervision for daytime sleep is equally important (109). Parental presence during infant sleep does not guarantee that the infant would be constantly observed nor, indeed, that parental intervention would prevent death from occurring. However, having the sleeping infant nearby during the day may alert parents to circumstances such as young infants rolling from the side to the prone position, or bedclothes covering the infant's head or face.

The Risk Associated with Bed Sharing

Unexpected infant deaths can occur in any sleep environment. Recent case-control studies show that up to half of the deaths occur while infants share a sleep surface ("co-sleep") with an adult (63,79,110,111), a marked rise from studies in the 1980s. This proportional rise in co-sleeping SIDS deaths has led some authorities, including the AAP (12) to recommend against bed sharing. However, longitudinal data from Avon over the last 20 years shows that this apparent rise in prevalence is more due to the effectiveness of intervention campaigns in reducing SIDS deaths in the solitary sleeping environment (80% fall) than to an increase in deaths when bed sharing (8). The proportion of bed-sharing deaths has risen from an average of 16% of all SIDS deaths prior to the Back to Sleep campaign to 34% after, yet the number of SIDS deaths in the parental bed in Avon has almost halved over the same period. Bed-sharing SIDS deaths have fallen but not at the same rate as those occurring in the cot. More worrying is the rise in both prevalence and number of SIDS infants with a parent on a sofa, which carries a markedly increased risk (48,63,108). At least some of these deaths occurred when mothers inadvertently fell asleep while feeding on a sofa during the night.

Bed sharing is perceived to be and is treated as a risk factor in the field of SIDS epidemiology and dealt in this rudimentary way there is ample evidence to advise against such a practice. On closer inspection, however, there are several things to be considered. Adjusting for potential confounders specifically associated with the adult co-sleeping environment, such as recent alcohol consumption, sleep deprivation, overcrowded conditions, and adult-sized duvets renders bed sharing nonsignificant as a risk factor, suggesting that it is not bed sharing itself but the particular circumstances in which bed sharing occurs that puts an infant at risk (108). An intriguing aspect of this debate is that in certain Asian cultures where particular forms of mother–infant co-sleeping (sleeping on futons) is common such as in Japan (112) and Hong Kong (113), the cot death rates are very low; corresponding to findings in the Bangladeshi (114) and Asian (115) communities in the United Kingdom and to the Pacific Island communities in New Zealand (116). Another aspect is that of generalization: the majority of bed-sharing SIDS mothers smoke while the majority of bed-sharing mothers in the population do not. The magnitude of any increase in risk for nonsmoking breast-feeding mothers who are bed sharing on a firm flat surface and who have not taken alcohol or other drugs is unclear, but certainly small (63,107,117–119). There is also the wider debate beyond the field of SIDS in terms of the potential advantages associated with bed sharing. Before the last century and in most non-Westernized cultures today, the normative practice is for the mother to share a sleep surface with the infant (120). Postulated physiological benefits of close contact between infants and caregivers include improved cardiorespiratory stability and oxygenation, fewer crying episodes, better thermoregulation, an increased prevalence and duration of breast-feeding, and enhanced milk production (121,122).

It is becoming clear from recent studies that bed sharing both for infants and mothers results in complex interactions, which are completely different from isolated sleeping and which need to be understood in detail before applying simplistic labels such as "safe" or "unsafe" (123–125). The unusual level of criticism and hostility (13,14) generated by the recent Policy Statement by the AAP against bed sharing (12) is a testament to the current polarized debate. Current advice in the United Kingdom does not advise against bed sharing, but describes particular circumstances when bed sharing should be avoided. Co-sleeping with an infant on a sofa should always be avoided.

The Apparent Protective Effect of Infant Pacifier Use

The current debate on bed sharing holds many parallels with the debate on dummy use (pacifiers). Several studies have examined the prevalence of infant dummy use and shown a reduced risk for SIDS (63,79,111,126–130), one recent study from California (131) going so far as to suggest that the risk of SIDS would be reduced by 90% if all infants used a dummy. Some countries such as Holland and the United States actively encourage such a practice, although, like the advice on bed sharing, this has again been met with criticism (13,132) mainly concerning the potential adverse effects regarding breast-feeding. The evidence of a significant association is not in dispute, but whether this association is causal in itself is still being debated (132). The mechanism by which a pacifier might reduce the risk of SIDS, or by its absence increase the risk, is unknown, but several mechanisms have been postulated. These include avoidance of the prone sleeping position (133), protection of the orophayngeal airway (134,135), reduction of gastroesophageal reflux through non-nutrient sucking (125), or lowering the arousal threshold (136). These mechanisms, however, assume the presence of a pacifier in the infant's mouth, but the observational evidence suggests that pacifiers generally fall out within

30 minutes of the infant falling asleep (136,137), while many of the night time deaths are thought to occur much later during sleep (108,138). Alternatively, dummy use may be a marker for some protective factors that have eluded measurement. The physiology not only of infant dummy use, but also nonuse among routine users and infant thumb sucking, which leads to identical physiological effects but is inhibited by pacifier use (139) deserves further investigation.

Before recommending the use of pacifiers, the potential disadvantages must be considered. There appears to be a clear relationship between frequent or continuous pacifier use and a reduction in breast-feeding (140–143) and a significantly higher risk of otitis media (144,145) and oral yeast infection (146). Other potential disadvantages include accidents (airway obstruction) (147), strangulation by cords tied to the dummy (148), eye injuries (149), and dental malocclusion (150).

IV. Infant Physiology and the Pathophysiology of Unexpected Death

While the final sequence of events leading to death is not known for the great majority of unexpected infant deaths, and there is no reason to presume that there is a single mechanism involved, a number of studies have been published of unexpected infant deaths that have occurred while the infant was undergoing physiological recordings (151). These recordings have shown a range of physiological events leading up to the final collapse and death, but in some infants there was an initial period in which there was normal respiratory activity but a relative tachycardia. In several infants, the final event was one of profound bradycardia, with respiratory activity continuing until a late stage. In many of these recordings, despite the carers having been alerted to the bradycardia by audible alarms, and having attempted resuscitation, this was not successful. This sequence of events is more suggestive of a cardiovascular rather than a respiratory event as the primary trigger for the final collapse. One possible physiological explanation for such a pattern might be a catastrophic fall in blood pressure as a consequence of sudden peripheral vasodilatation—e.g., in response to toxins or as a consequence of heat stress (152).

Several population-based case-control studies have shown that infants who died unexpectedly were more heavily wrapped, and more likely to be sleeping in warm rooms than age and community-matched controls (5,24,119). The increased risk of SIDS from heavy wrapping was greatest for the older infants (more than three months of age), and was especially high for those infants with evidence of an acute viral upper respiratory tract infection (44). In a study of the metabolic response to acute viral upper respiratory tract infection, we observed that younger infants (less than 3 months of age) commonly showed a fall in metabolic rate with infection, while those over three months usually showed an increase, commonly accompanied by fever (153). The metabolic rate of infants during sleep rises over the first few months after birth, such that by three months of age, healthy infants excrete up to 50% more heat per unit surface area than in the first week after birth (154). Thus, infants over three months of age might be more at risk from heavy wrapping that compromised their ability to lose heat, particularly at the time of an acute minor viral infection. In recent studies we have shown that there is little if any further rise in metabolic rate per unit surface area between three and six months of age (155).

In a population-based observational study of infant thermal care at home, we showed that most mothers accurately achieved conditions of predicted thermal neutrality for their infants at home, but the young mothers, those who smoked and those who did not breast-feed, were more likely to wrap their infants more heavily (156). In a prospective longitudinal laboratory study of mothers and infants sharing a room or sharing a bed for overnight sleep we showed that, despite a much warmer microenvironment, infants thermoregulated more effectively, with a slightly greater diurnal fall in rectal temperature when bed sharing with their mother than when sleeping in a cot adjacent to the mother's bed (125). The development of the diurnal fall in core temperature occurs at ages between approximately three and four months, occurring earlier in girls and breast-fed infants than in boys or bottle-fed infants (157).

In a study of infants in Mongolia, comparing the use of traditional swaddling with the use of infant sleeping bags, in a population in which bed sharing and very heavy wrapping is virtually universal, we showed that infants of families living in "Ger" (traditional circular tents) maintained normal thermoregulation despite extremes of indoor environmental temperature, sometimes ranging from $-3°C$ to $+25°C$ within a single 24-hour period (158). Infants living in modern apartment blocks (in which indoor temperatures were comparable to those we have observed in the United Kingdom) were wrapped similarly to those in the much colder traditional dwellings, and showed some evidence of heat stress, with elevated core temperature, particularly during the daytime. These infants showed smaller diurnal falls in core temperature than infants sleeping in traditional dwellings, suggesting that their warmer environment may have led to delay in the development of the normal diurnal fall in core temperature at night (159).

Associations have been described between the risk of SIDS and polymorphisms of genes involved in the development of the autonomic nervous system (160), various cardiac channelopathies (161), and the serotonergic system in the brain stem (162) (see chap. 13). This latter group is of particular interest in the light of recent histological evidence of abnormalities of serotonergic neurons in the brain stem of SIDS victims, though it remains unclear whether these represent primary developmental abnormalities or consequences of earlier (possibly in utero) events (163).

Blackwell and Morris have each shown the potential importance of toxigenic Staphylococci as contributory agents to circulatory collapse and sudden death in infancy (164,165). Toxin production in such Staphylococci increases with increasing environmental temperature and is minimal below 37°C (164). SIDS victims have increased nasopharyngeal colonization with staphylococci compared with healthy age and community-matched controls (152). In the prone position, or with head covering (particularly in the presence of potential rebreathing), nasopharyngeal temperature is likely to rise above the normal value of 32°C, with resultant increase in toxin production by any toxigenic staphylococci present on the mucosal surface (166). Transmucosal absorption of toxin might thus lead to circulatory collapse and death without the need for invasive infection to occur.

Elevated levels of interleukin 6 in the cerebrospinal fluid of SIDS victims compared to age-matched controls dying of known causes raised the possibility of a vigorous pro-inflammatory response being part of the pathophysiology of SIDS (167).

Drucker has recently shown that common polymorphisms leading to high levels of pro-inflammatory cytokines (e.g., interleukin 6, VEGF) or low levels of anti-inflammatory cytokines (e.g., interleukin 10) are associated with increased risk for unexpected deaths in infants (168). A high pro-inflammatory response to infection, with vigorous sympathetic activity including peripheral vasoconstriction and pyrexia might indirectly lead to further toxin production in the nasopharynx.

The relationship between the pro-inflammatory cytokine IL1-β and the risk of SIDS is complex, and Moscovis (168) has shown potentially important ethnic differences in the patterns of gene polymorphisms. In both Aboriginal Australian and Bangladeshi infants a particular polymorphism (TT) is found, that is uncommon in infants of European origin. This polymorphism is associated with a marked increase in IL1-β production, and increased pro-inflammatory responses on exposure to tobacco smoke. This may partially explain the major difference between aboriginal Australian infants with high maternal smoking rates and high SIDS rate, and Bangladeshi infants who are genetically similar with regard to IL1-β, but have very low rates of maternal smoking and very low SIDS rates.

The potential interaction between genetic and environmental factors is further exemplified by the anti-inflammatory cytokine IL10, production of which is markedly decreased by exposure to tobacco smoke (168).

V. The "Triple Risk" Hypotheses and Prospects for Prevention of SUDI

As noted above, there is considerable evidence that SIDS could be a consequence of a wide range of infant-environment interactions.

The triple risk hypothesis, which envisages SIDS occurring as a result of a final insult (one which is not usually fatal on its own) that affects a baby with an intrinsic vulnerability (arising from genetic or early developmental factors), at a potentially vulnerable stage of physiological development (e.g., immunological, respiratory, cardiovascular, thermal), has been proposed in various forms by a number of authors over the past 15 years (169).

The recent developments in our knowledge of environmental, immunological, genetic, and physiological factors in infants, and recognition of the changes in all these systems that occur during the first few months after birth, as outlined above, strongly support a triple risk model of causation for most unexpected infant deaths, including some for which a partial or even a complete "explanation" can be identified on thorough investigation.

This approach to understanding the pathophysiological processes that may contribute to unexpected infant deaths holds great promise for targeted interventions to further reduce the number of such deaths.

VI. Current Recommendations

The scientific rigor with which data is gathered is not easily applied to the dissemination of the results, and formulating advice can be a subjective exercise of weighing up the available evidence and constrained by attempts to simplify the message. The debate on the safety, advantages, and disadvantages of infant care practices must be informed not just by epidemiological evidence from one narrow field but from many disciplines from different fields if it is to become more than the exchange of mere opinion. The advantages of getting the advice right are evident in the dramatic fall in SIDS deaths after advice against the prone sleeping position, but it should be remembered that adoption of the prone position was initially largely a consequence of medical advice.

References

1. Rognum TO, Willinger M. The story of the "Stavanger definition" In: Rognum TO, ed. Sudden Infant Death Syndrome: New Trends in the Nineties. Oslo: Scandinavian University Press, 1995:21–25.
2. Fleming PJ, Blair PS, Sidebotham P, et al. Investigating sudden unexpected deaths in infancy and childhood and caring for bereaved families: an integrated multi-agency approach. BMJ 2004; 328:331–334.
3. Kennedy H, Epstein J, Fleming PJ, et al. Sudden unexpected death in infancy. A multi-agency protocol for care and investigation. The report of a working group convened by the Royal College of Pathologists and the Royal College of Paediatrics and Child Health. RCPath & RCPCH, London, 2004. Available at: www.rcpch.ac.uk.
4. Working Together to Safeguard Children. A Guide to Inter-Agency Working to Safeguard and Promote the Welfare of Children. 2006. Department for Education and Skills, UK. Available at: http://www.everychildmatters.gov.uk/search/IG00060/.
5. Fleming PJ, Blair PS, Bacon C, et al. Sudden unexpected death in infancy. The CESDI SUDI Studies 1993–1996. London: The Stationery Office, 2000.
6. Krous HF, Beckwith B, Byard R, et al. Sudden infant death and unclassified sudden infant deaths: a definitional and diagnostic approach. Pediatrics 2004; 114:234–238.

7. Bajanowski T, Vege A, Byard R, et al. Sudden infant death (SIDS)—standardised investigations and classification: recommendations. Forensic Sci Int 2007; 165: 129–143.

8. Blair PS, Sidebotham P, Berry PJ, et al. Major changes in the epidemiology of sudden infant death syndrome: a 20-year population based study of all unexpected deaths in infancy. Lancet 2006; 367:314–319.

9. Leach CEA, Blair PS, Fleming PJ, et al. Sudden unexpected deaths in infancy: similarities and differences in the epidemiology of SIDS and explained deaths. Pediatrics 1999; 104:e43. Available at: http://www.pediatrics.org/cgi/content/full/4/e43.

10. Willcox WH. Infantile mortality from "overlaying". BMJ 1904; September 24:1–7.

11. Templeman C. Two hundred and fifty eight cases of suffocation of infants. Edinb Med J 1892; 38:322–329.

12. American Academy of Pediatrics Policy Statement. The changing concept of sudden infant death syndrome: diagnostic coding shifts, controversies regarding the sleeping environment, and new variables to consider in reducing risk. Pediatrics 2005; 116:1245–1255.

13. Gessner BD, Porter TJ. Bed sharing with unimpaired parents is not an important risk factor for sudden infant death syndrome. Pediatrics 2006; 117:990–991.

14. Kattwinkel J, Hauck F, Moon RY, et al. In reply. Pediatrics 2006; 117:994–996.

15. Krous HF. The international standardised autopsy protocol for sudden unexpected infant death. In: Rognum TO, ed. Sudden Infant Death Syndrome: New Trends in the Nineties. Oslo: Scandinavian University Press, 1995:81–85.

16. Emery JL. Is sudden infant death syndrome a diagnosis? Or is it just a diagnostic dustbin? BMJ 1989; 299:1240.

17. Huber J. Sudden infant death syndrome: the new clothes of the emperor. Eur J Pediatr 1993; 152:93–94.

18. Limerick SR. Sudden infant death in historical perspective. J Clin Pathol 1992; 45 (11 suppl):3–6.

19. Beal S, Blundell H. Sudden infant death syndrome related to position in the cot. Med J Aust 1978; 2:217–218.

20. Saturnus KS. Plötzlicher Kindstod—eine Folge der Bauchlage? In: Festschrift Professor Leithoff, ed. Kriminalstatistik. Verlag: Heidelberg, 1985:67–81.

21. Davies DP. Cot death in Hong Kong: a rare problem? Lancet 1985; 2:1346–1349.

22. de Jonge GA, Engleberts AC, Koomen-Liefting AJ, et al. Cot death and prone sleeping position in the Netherlands. BMJ 1989; 298:722.

23. Mitchell EA, Scragg R, Stewart AW, et al. Results from the first year of the New Zealand cot death study. N Z Med J 1991; 104:71–76.

24. Fleming PJ, Gilbert R, Azaz Y, et al. Interaction between bedding and sleeping position in the sudden infant death syndrome: a population based case-control study. BMJ 1990; 301:85–89.

25. Limerick SR, Bacon CJ. Terminology used by pathologists in reporting on sudden infant deaths. J Clin Pathol 2004; 57(3):309–311.

26. Froggatt P, Lynas MA, MacKenzie G. Epidemiology of sudden unexpected death in infants ('cot death') in Northern Ireland. Br J Prev Soc Med 1971; 25:119–134.

27. Fedrick J. Sudden unexpected death in infants in the Oxford Record Linkage area. An analysis with respect to time and space. Br J Prev Soc Med 1973; 27:217–224.

28. Rintahaka PJ, Hirvonen J. The epidemiology of sudden infant death syndrome in Finland in 1969–80. Forensic Sci Int 1986; 30:219–233.

29. McGlashan ND. Sudden deaths in Tasmania, 1980–1986: a seven year prospective study. Soc Sci Med 1989; 29:1015–1026.
30. Daltveit AK, Øyen N, Skjærven R, et al. The epidemic of SIDS in Norway 1967–93: changing effects of risk factors. Arch Dis Child 1997; 77:23–27.
31. Bouvier-Colle MH, Inizan J, Michel E. Postneonatal mortality, sudden infant death syndrome: factors preventing the decline of infant mortality in France from 1979 to 1985. Paediatr Perinat Epidemiol 1989; 3:256–267.
32. Kraus JF, Greenland S, Bulteys M. Risk factors for sudden infant death syndrome in the US collaborative perinatal project. Int J Epidemiol 1989; 18:113–119.
33. Wagner M, Samson-Dollfus D, Menard J. Sudden unexpected infant death in a French county. Arch Dis Child 1984; 59:1082–1087.
34. Beal SM. Sleeping position and SIDS: past, present and future. In: Rognum TO, ed. SIDS: New Trends in the Nineties. Oslo: Scandinavian University Press, 1995: 147–151.
35. Editorial. Prone or Supine? BMJ 1961; 1304.
36. Greene D. Asymmetry of the head and face in infants and in children. Am J Dis Child 1930; 41:1317–1326.
37. Abramson H. Accidental mechanical suffocation in infants. J Pediatr 1944; 25: 404–413.
38. Masterson J, Zucker C, Schulze K. Prone and supine positioning effects on energy expenditure and behaviour of low birthweight neonates. Pediatrics 1987; 89: 689–692.
39. Martin RJ, Herrell N, Rubin D, et al. Effect of supine and prone positions on arterial tension in the preterm infant. Pediatrics 1979; 63:528–531.
40. Yu V. Effect of body positioning on gastric emptying in the neonate. Arch Dis Child 1975; 50:500–504.
41. Schwartz FCM, Fenner A, Wolfsdrop J. The influence of body position on pulmonary function in low birth babies. S Afr Med J 1975; 49:79–81.
42. Fleming PJ, Muller N, Bryan MH, et al. The effects of abdominal loading on ribcage distortion in premature infants. Pediatrics 1979; 64:425–428.
43. Hiley C. Babies' sleeping position. BMJ 1992; 305:115.
44. Gilbert R, Rudd P, Berry PJ, et al. Combined effect of infection and heavy wrapping on the risk of sudden unexpected infant death. Arch Dis Child 1992; 67:171–177.
45. Ponsonby A-L, Dwyer T, Gibbons LE, et al. Thermal environment and sudden infant death syndrome: case-control study. BMJ 1992; 304:277–282.
46. Klonnoff-Cohen HS, Edelstein SL. A case-control study of routine and death scene sleep position and sudden infant death syndrome in Southern California. JAMA 1995; 273:790–794.
47. Williams S, Taylor B, Mitchell E. Sudden infant death syndrome: insulation from bedding and clothing and its effect modifiers. Int J Epidemiol 1996; 25:366–375.
48. Fleming PJ, Blair PS, Bacon C, et al. Environment of infants during sleep and risk of the sudden infant death syndrome: results from 1993–5 case-control study for confidential inquiry into stillbirths and deaths in infancy. BMJ 1996; 313:191–195.
49. Fleming PJ, Blair PS, Ward Platt M, et al. Sudden infant death syndrome and social deprivation: assessing epidemiological factors after post-matching for deprivation. Paediatr Perinat Epidemiol 2003; 17:272–280.
50. Mitchell EA, Ford RPK, Stewart AW, et al. Smoking and the sudden infant death syndrome. Paediatrics 1993; 91:893–896.

51. Klonoff-Cohen HS, Edelstein SL, Lefkowitz ES, et al. The effect of passive smoking and tobacco exposure through breast milk on sudden infant death syndrome. JAMA 1995; 273:795–798.

52. Blair PS, Fleming PJ, Bensley D, et al. Smoking and the sudden infant death syndrome: results from 1993–5 case-control study for confidential inquiry into stillbirths and deaths in infancy. BMJ July 1996; 313:195–198.

53. Mitchell EA, Milerad J. Smoking and the sudden infant death syndrome. Rev Environ Health 2006; 21(2):81–103.

54. Blair PS, Ward Platt MP, Smith IJ, et al. Sudden infant death syndrome and sleeping position in pre-term and low birthweight infants: an opportunity for targeted intervention. Arch Dis Child 2006; 91(2):101–106.

55. Fleming PJ, Blair PS, Ward Platt M, et al. The accelerated immunisation programme in the UK and sudden unexpected death in infancy. BMJ 2001; 322:822–825.

56. Kahn A, Blum D, Hennart P. A critical comparison of the history of sudden-death infants and infants hospitalised for near-miss for SIDS. Eur J Pediatr 1984; 143:103–107.

57. Tonkin SL. Infant mortality. Epidemiology of cot deaths in Auckland. N Z Med J 1986; 99:324–326.

58. Mitchell EA, Taylor BJ, Ford RPK, et al. Four modifiable and other major risk factors for cot death: the New Zealand study. J Paediatr Child Health 1992; 28 (suppl):S3–S8.

59. Skadberg BT, Morild I, Markestad T. Abandoning prone sleeping: effect on the risk of sudden infant death syndrome. J Pediatr 1998; 132(2):340–343.

60. Scragg RK, Mitchell EA. Side sleeping position and bed sharing in the sudden infant death syndrome (review). Ann Med 1998; 30(4):345–349.

61. L'Hoir MP, Engleberts AC, van Well GT, et al. Risk and preventive factors for cot death in the Netherlands, a low-incidence country. Eur J Pediatr 1998; 157 (8):681–688.

62. Li DK, Petitti DB, Willinger M, et al. Infant sleeping position and the risk of sudden infant death syndrome in California, 1997–2000. Am J Epidemiol 2003; 157(5):446–455.

63. Carpenter PR, Irgens PL, Blair PS, et al. Sudden unexplained infant death in 20 regions in Europe: case control study. Lancet 2004; 363(9404):185–191.

64. Cullen A, Kiberd B, McDonnell M, et al. Sudden infant death syndrome—are parents getting the message? Ir J Med Sci 2000; 169(1):40–43.

65. Kiechl-Kohlendorfer U, Peglow UP, Kiechl S, et al. Epidemiology of sudden infant death syndrome (SIDS) in the Tyrol before and after an intervention campaign. Wein Klin Wochenschr 2001; 113(1–2):27–32.

66. Rose M, Murphy M, Macfarlane JA, et al. 'Back to sleep': the position in Oxfordshire and Northampton. Paediatr Perinat Epidemiol 1998; 12(2):217–227.

67. Nelson EAS, Serra A, Cowan S, et al. Maternity advice survey: sleeping position in Eastern Europe. Arch Dis Child 2000; 83:304–306.

68. Hein HA, Pettit SF. Back to sleep: good advice for parents but not for hospitals? Pediatrics 2001; 107(3):537–539.

69. Pastore GM, Guala A, Zaffaroni M. Back to sleep: risk factors for SIDS as targets for public health campaigns. J Pediatr 2003; 142(4):453–454.

70. Byard RW, Beal SM. Gastric aspiration and sleeping position in infancy and early childhood. J Paediatr Child Health 2000; 36(4):403–405.

71. Fleming PJ, Stewart A. What is the ideal sleeping position for infants? Dev Med Child Neurol 1992; 34:916–919.

72. Hunt L, Fleming P, Golding J, et al. Does the supine sleeping position have any adverse effects on the child?:I. Health in the first six months. Pediatrics 1997; 100 (1):e11.

73. Hutchison BL, Thompson JM, Mitchell EA. Determinants of nonsynostotic pla-giocephaly: a case-control study. Pediatrics 2003; 112(4):e316.

74. Ponsonby AL, Dwyer T, Couper D. Sleeping position, infant apnoea, and cyanosis: a population-based study. Pediatrics 1997; 99(1):e3.

75. Hunt CE, Lesko SM, Vezina RM, et al. Infant sleep position and associated health outcomes. Arch Pediatr Adolesc Med 2003; 157:469–474.

76. Mitchell EA, Scragg J, Clements M. Soft cot mattresses and the sudden infant death syndrome. N Z Med J 1996; 109:206–207.

77. Geib LT, Nunes NL. The incidence of sudden death syndrome in a cohort of infants. J Pediatr (Rio J) 2006; 82(1):21–26.

78. Flick L, White DK, Vemulapolli C, et al. Sleep position and the use of soft bedding during bed sharing among African American infants at increased risk for sudden infant death syndrome. J Pediatr 2001; 138(3):338–343.

79. Hauck FR, Herman SM, Donovan M, et al. Sleep environment and the risk of sudden infant death syndrome in an urban population: the Chicago Infant Mortality Study. Pediatrics 2003; 111(5 pt 2):1207–1214.

80. Sawczenko A, Fleming PJ. Thermal stress, sleeping position, and the sudden infant death syndrome. Sleep 1996; 19(10 suppl):S267–S270.

81. Scheers NJ, Dayton CM, Kemp JS. Sudden infant death with external airways covered: case-comparison study of 206 deaths in the United States. Arch Pediatr Adolesc Med 1998; 152(6):540–547.

82. Byard RW, Beal SM. V-shaped pillows and unsafe infant sleeping. J Paediatr Child Health 1997; 33(2):171–173.

83. Abramson H. Accidental mechanical suffocation in infants. J Pediatr 1944; 25: 404–413.

84. Wooley PV. Mechanical suffocation during infancy. J Pediatr 1945; 26:572–575.

85. Davison WH. Accidental infant suffocation. BMJ 1945; 25:251–252.

86. Werne J, Garrow I. Sudden deaths of infants allegedly due to mechanical suffo-cation. Am J Public Health 1947; 37:675.

87. Bowden K. Sudden death or alleged accidental suffocation in babies. Med J Aust 1950; 1:65–72.

88. Nelson EAS, Taylor BJ, Weatherall IL. Sleeping position and infant bedding may predispose to hyperthermia and the sudden infant death syndrome. Lancet 1989; 1(8631):199–201.

89. Nelson EAS, Taylor BJ, Mackay SC. Child care practices and the sudden infant death syndrome. Aust Paediatr J 1989; 25(4):202–204.

90. Bass M, Kravath RE, Glass L. Death scene investigation in sudden infant death. N Engl J Med 1986; 315:100–105.

91. Wilson CA, Taylor BJ, Laing RM, et al. Clothing and bedding and its relevance to sudden infant death syndrome: further results from the New Zealand Cot Death Study. J Paediatr Child Health 1994; 30(6):506–512.

92. Beal SM. Sudden infant death syndrome in South Australia 1968–97. Part 1: Changes over time. J Paediatr Child Health 2000; 36:540–547.

93. Poets CF. Apparent life-threatening events and sudden infant death on a monitor. Paediatr Respir Rev. 2004; 5(suppl A):S383–S386.

94. Horne RS, Oarslow PM, Ferens D, et al. Arousal responses and risk factors for sudden infant death syndrome. Sleep Med 2002; 3(suppl 2):S61–S65.

95. Dix J. Homicide and the baby-sitter. Am J Forensic Med Pathol 1998; 19(4):321–323.

96. Thach BT. Sudden infant death syndrome: old causes rediscovered? N Engl J Med 1986; 315(2):126–128.

97. Schellscheidt J, Ott A, Jorch G. Epidemiological features of sudden infant death after a German intervention campaign in 1992. Eur J Pediatr 1997; 156(8):655–660.

98. Nelson T, To K-F, Wong Y-Y, et al. Hong Kong case-control study of sudden unexpected infant death. N Z Med J 2005; 118(1227):U1788.

99. L'Hoir MP, Engelberts AC, van Well GT, et al. Case-control study of current validity of previously described risk factors for SIDS in The Netherlands. Arch Dis Child 1998; 79(5):386–393.

100. Markestad T, Skadberg B, Hordvik E, et al. Sleeping position and sudden infant death syndrome (SIDS): effect of an intervention programme to avoid prone sleeping. Acta Paediatr 1995; 84:375–378.

101. Ponsonby A-L, Dwyer T, Couper D, et al. Association between use of a quilt and sudden infant death syndrome: case-control study. BMJ 1998; 316(7126):195–196.

102. Foundation for the Study of Infant deaths. BabyZone leaflet. Available at: http://www.sids.org.uk/fsis/fsid.

103. Spock B, Rothenberg MB. Baby and Child Care. New York: Pocket Books, 1985: 219.

104. Leach P. Baby and Child. London: Michael Joseph, 1980:93–94.

105. McKenna J. An anthropological perspective on the sudden infant death syndrome (SIDS): the role of parental breathing cues and speech breathing adaptations. Med Anthropol 1986; 10:9–91.

106. Scragg RKR, Mitchell EA, Stewart AW, et al. Infant room-sharing and prone sleep position in sudden infant death syndrome. Lancet 1996; 347:7–12.

107. Tappin D, Ecob R, Brooke H. Bedsharing, roomsharing, and sudden infant death syndrome in Scotland: a case-control study. J Pediatr 2005; 147(1):32–37.

108. Blair PS, Fleming PJ, Smith IJ, et al., and the CESDI SUDI research group. Babies sleeping with parents: case-control study of factors influencing the risk of sudden infant death syndrome. BMJ 1999; 319:1457–1462.

109. Blair PS, Ward Platt M, Smith IJ, et al. Sudden infant death syndrome and the time of death: factors associated with night-time and day-time deaths. Int J Epidemiol 2006; 35(6):1563–1569.

110. Tappin D, Brooke H, Ecob R, et al. Used infant mattresses and sudden infant death syndrome in Scotland: case-control study. BMJ 2002; 325(7371):1007.

111. McGarvey C, McDonnell M, Chong A, et al. Factors relating to the infant's last sleep environment in sudden infant death syndrome in the Republic of Ireland. Arch Dis Child 2003; 88(12):1058–1064.

112. Takeda KA. A possible mechanism of sudden infant death syndrome (SIDS). J Kyoto Prefecture Univ Med 1987; 96:965–968.

113. Davies DP. Cot death in Hong Kong. A rare problem? Lancet 1985; 2:1346–1347.

114. Gantley M, Davies DP, Murcott A. Sudden infant death syndrome. Links with infant care practices. BMJ 1993; 16:263–282.

115. Farooqi S, Lip GYH, Beevers DG. Bed-sharing and smoking in sudden infant death syndrome. BMJ 1994; 308:204–205.

116. Tuohy PG, Counsell AM, Geddis DC. Sociodemographic factors associated with sleeping position and location. Arch Dis Child 1993; 69:664–666.
117. Wailoo M, Ball H, Fleming PJ, et al. Infants bedsharing with mothers: helpful, harmful or don't know? Arch Dis Child 2004; 89:1082–1083.
118. Fleming PJ, Blair PS, McKenna JJ. New knowledge, new insights and new recommendations: scientific controversy and media hype in unexpected infant deaths. Arch Dis Child 2007; 92:61–64.
119. McGarvey C, McDonnell M, O'Regan M, et al. An eight year study of risk factors for SIDS: bedsharing vs non bedsharing. Arch Dis Child 2006; 91:318–323.
120. Mosko S, McKenna J, Dickel M, et al. Parent-infant co-sleeping: the appropriate context for the study of infant sleep and implications for sudden infant death syndrome (SIDS) research. J Behav Med 1993; 16:589–610.
121. Anderson GC. Current knowledge about skin-to-skin (Kangaroo) care for preterm infants. J Perinatol 1991; 11:216–226.
122. Ludington-Hoe SM, Hadeed AJ, Anderson GC. Physiological responses to skin-to-skin contact in hospitalised premature infants. J Perinatol 1991; 11:19–24.
123. McKenna JJ. Sudden Infant Death Syndrome in Cross-Cultural Perspective. Is Infant-Parent Cosleeping Protective? Ann Rev Anthropol 1996; 25:201–216.
124. Ball HL, Hooker E, Kelly PJ. Where will the babies sleep? Attitudes and practices of new and experienced parents regarding co-sleeping with their new-born infant. Am Anthropol 1999; 101:143–151.
125. Fleming PJ, Young J, Blair PS. The importance of mother-baby interactions in determining night time thermal conditions for sleeping infants: observations from the home and the sleep laboratory. Pediatr Child Health 2006; 11(suppl):7A–11A.
126. Mitchell EA, Taylor BJ, Ford RPK, et al. Dummies and the sudden infant death syndrome. Arch Dis Child 1993; 68:501–504.
127. Fleming PJ, Blair PS, Pollard K, et al. Pacifier use and sudden infant death syndrome: results from the CESDI/SUDI case control study. Arch Dis Child 1999; 81:112–116.
128. L'Hoir MP, Engelberts AC, van Well GT, et al. Dummy use, thumb sucking, mouth breathing and cot death. Eur J Pediatr 1999; 158:896–901.
129. Brooke H, Tappin DM, Beckett C, et al. Dummy use on the day/night of death: case-control study of sudden infants death syndrome (SIDS) in Scotland, 1996–99, sixth SIDS International Conference, Auckland, New Zealand, February 2000 (abstr).
130. Vennemann MMT, Findeisen M, Butterfaß-Bahloul T, et al. Modifiable risk factors for SIDS in Germany: results of GeSID. Acta Paediatr 2005; 94(6):655–660.
131. Li DK, Willinger M, Petitti DB, et al. Use of a dummy (pacifier) during sleep & risk of SIDS: population based case-control study. BMJ 2006; 332(7532):18–22.
132. Blair PS, Fleming PJ. Dummies and SIDS: causality has not been established. BMJ 2006; 332(7534):178.
133. Righard L. Sudden infant death syndrome and pacifiers: a proposed connection could be a bias. Birth 1998; 25:128–129.
134. Cozzi F, Albani R, Cardi E. A common pathophysiology for sudden cot death and sleep apnoea. "The vacuum-glossoptosis syndrome". Med Hypotheses 1979; 5:329–338.
135. Cozzi F, Morini F, Tozzi C, et al. Effect of pacifier use on oral breathing in healthy newborn infants. Pediatr Pulmonol 2002; 33:368–373.

136. Franco P, Scaillet S, Wermenbol V, et al. The influence of a pacifier on infants' arousals from sleep. J Pediatr 2000; 136:775–779.

137. Weiss PP, Kerbl R. The relative short duration that a child retains a pacifier in the mouth during sleep: implications for sudden infant death syndrome. Eur J Pediatr 2001; 160:60–70.

138. Golding J, Limerick S, Macfarlane A. Sudden infant death syndrome. Patterns, Puzzles and Problems. Open Books, 1985:33–35.

139. Pollard K, Fleming PJ, Young J, et al. Night time non-nutritive sucking in infants aged 1 to 5 months: relationship with infant state, breast feeding, and bed- versus room-sharing. Early Hum Dev 1999; 56:185–204.

140. Barros FC, Victora CG, Semer TC, et al. Use of pacifiers is associated with decreased breast-feeding duration. Pediatrics 1995; 95:497–499.

141. Righard L, Alade MO. Breastfeeding and the use of pacifiers. Birth 1997; 24:116–120.

142. Howard CR, Howard FM, Lanphear B, et al. The effects of early pacifier use on breastfeeding duration. Pediatrics 1999; 103:E33.

143. Vogel AM, Hutchison BL, Mitchell EA. The impact of pacifier use on breast-feeding: a prospective cohort study. J Paediatr Child Health 2001; 37:58–63.

144. Warren JJ, Levy SM, Kirchner HL, et al. Pacifier use and the occurrence of otitis media in the first year of life. Pediatr Dent 2001; 23:103–107.

145. Uhari M, Mantysaari K, Niemela M. A meta-analytic review of the risk factors for acute otitis media. Clin Infect Dis 1996; 22:1079–1083.

146. Mattos-Graner RO, de Moraes AB, Rontani RM, et al. Relation of oral yeast infection in Brazilian infants and use of a pacifier. J Dent Child 2001; 68:33–36.

147. Simkiss DE, Sheppard I, Pal BR. Airway obstruction by a child's pacifier—could flange design be safer? Eur J Pediatr 1998; 157:252–254.

148. Feldman KW, Simms RJ. Strangulation in childhood: epidemiology and clinical course. Pediatrics 1980; 65:1079–1085.

149. Stubbs AJ, Aburn NS. Penetrating eye injury from a rigid infant pacifier. Aus N Z J Ophthalmol 1996; 24:71–73.

150. Adair SM, Milano M, Lorenzo I, et al. Effects of current and former pacifier use on the dentition of 24- to 59-month-old children. Pediatr Dent 1995; 17:437–444.

151. Meny R, Carroll J, Carbone MT, et al. Cardiorespiratory recordings from infants dying suddenly and unexpectedly at home. Pediatrics 1994; 93:44–49.

152. Morris JA. The common bacterial toxins hypothesis of sudden infant death syndrome. FEMS Immunol Med Microbiol 1999; 25:11–17.

153. Fleming PJ, Howell T, Clements M, et al. Thermal balance and metabolic rate during upper respiratory tract infection in infants. Arch Dis Child 1994; 70:187–191.

154. Azaz Y, Fleming PJ, Levine M, et al. The relationship between environmental temperature, metabolic rate, sleep state and evaporative water loss in infants from birth to three months. Pediatr Res 1992; 32:417–423.

155. Arkell S, Blair P, Henderson AJ, et al. Is the mattress important in helping babies keep warm? Paradoxical effects of a sleeping surface with negligible thermal resistance. Acta Paediatr 2007; 96(2):199–205.

156. Wigfield RE, Fleming P J, Azaz Y, et al. How much wrapping do babies need at night? Arch Dis Child 1993; 69:181–186.

157. Lodemore MR, Petersen SA, Wailoo MP. Factors affecting the development of night time temperature rhythms. Arch Dis Child 1992; 67(10):1259–1261.

158. Tsogt B, Manaseki-Holland S, Pollock J, et al. The development of thermoregulation in a harsh environment: a prospective controlled study of the effects of swaddling on infants' thermal balance in a Mongolian winter. Early Hum Dev 2006; 82:621.

159. Tsogt B. PhD Thesis. University of the West of England, 2006.

160. Weese-Mayer DE, Berry-Kravis EM, Zhou L, et al. Sudden infant death syndrome: case control frequency differences at genes pertinent to early autonomic nervous system embryologic development. Pediatr Res 2004; 56:391–395.

161. Ackerman MJ, Siu BL, Sturner WQ, et al. Postmortem molecular analysis of SCN5A defects in sudden infant death syndrome. JAMA 2001; 286:2264–2269.

162. Kinney HC, Randall LL, Sleeper LA, et al. Serotonergic brainstem abnormalities in Northern Plains Indians with the sudden infant death syndrome. J Neuropathol Exp Neurol 2003; 62:1178–1191.

163. Paterson DS, Kinney HC. Multiple serotonergic brainstem abnormalities in the sudden infant death syndrome. JAMA 2006; 296:2124–2132.

164. Morris J A. Common bacterial toxins and physiological vulnerability to sudden infant death: the role of deleterious genetic mutations. FEMS Immunology and medical Microbiology 2004; 42:42–47.

165. Blackwell CC, Weir D. The role of infection in sudden infant death syndrome. FEMS Immunol Med Microbiol 1999; 25:1–6.

166. Dashash M, Pravica V, Hutchinson IV, et al. Association of sudden infant death syndrome with VEGF and IL-6 gene polymorphisms. Hum Immunol 2006; 67: 627–633.

167. Vege A, Rognum TO, Scott H, et al. SIDS cases have increased levels of inter-leukin -6 in cerebrospinal fluid. Acta Paediatr 1995; 84:193.

168. Moscovis S, Gordon AE, Hall ST, et al. Interleukin1-β responses to bacterial toxins and sudden infant death stndrome. FEMS Immunology and medical microbiology 2004; 42:139–145.

169. Gunteroth WG, Spiers PS. The triple risk hypotheses in sudden infant death syndrome. Pediatrics 2002; 110:e64. Available at: http://www.pediatrics.org/cgi/content/full/110/5/e64.

13

Sudden Infant Death Syndrome: Genetic Studies in Cardiorespiratory and Autonomic Regulation

DEBRA E. WEESE-MAYER
Northwestern University Feinberg School of Medicine, Chicago, Illinois, U.S.A.

ELIZABETH M. BERRY-KRAVIS
Rush University, Chicago, Illinois, U.S.A.

MICHAEL J. ACKERMAN
Mayo Clinic College of Medicine, Rochester, Minnesota, U.S.A.

MARY L. MARAZITA
University of Pittsburgh, Pittsburgh, Pennsylvania, U.S.A.

I. Introduction

The 1992 "Back to Sleep" campaign identified modifiable environmental risk factors for sudden infant death syndrome (SIDS) and led to a decrease in SIDS incidence from 1.2 per 1000 live births (1) to 0.529 per 1000 live births in 2003 (2). Despite this decline, African-American infants have a 2.7-fold higher SIDS rate than Caucasian infants (2). This ethnic disparity, coupled with SIDS deaths despite improved compliance with modifiable risk factors, led investigators to consider a genetic basis for SIDS. Thus far, all genetic studies have been based on clinical, neuropathological, and epidemiological observations in SIDS victims, with subsequent identification and study of candidate genes. This chapter focuses exclusively on those genes that are pertinent to cardiorespiratory or autonomic regulation.

II. Cardiac Channelopathy Genes in SIDS

These are arrhythmia syndromes due to defective cardiac channels. Congenital long QT syndrome (LQTS), Brugada syndrome (BrS), and catecholaminergic polymorphic ventricular tachycardia (CPVT) are examples of these syndromes.

A. Rationale for Study of Channelopathy Genes

The Schwartz-QT hypothesis proposed a role for abnormal cardiac repolarization with QT prolongation in SIDS (3,4) and was later supported by data indicating prolonged corrected QT (QTc) intervals >440 milliseconds in 50% of electro-cardiograms (ECGs) from 24 SIDS cases versus 2.5% of the entire cohort (34,000 infants, day 3–4 of life ECGs) (5).

B. Molecular Evidence Linking Schwartz-QT Hypothesis and LQTS

Congenital LQTS is characterized by QT interval prolongation and torsades de pointes. Roughly half of the genotype-positive subjects have QT prolongation and symptoms, including syncope, seizures, and sudden death, while the others have nonpenetrant/concealed LQTS with normal or borderline QT intervals at rest. To date, 10 LQTS-susceptibility genes have been discovered (Table 1). Three case reports described sporadic de novo germline mutations in the most common LQTS-susceptibility genes, suggesting that some SIDS cases may have terminal rhythm ventricular fibrillation and/or LQTS-causing cardiac channel mutations (6–8).

Ackerman et al. provided the first genetic epidemiology studies investigating the hypothesis of LQTS-associated cardiac channel mutations in SIDS

Table 1 Summary of LQTS-Susceptibility Genes

LQTS subtype	Locus	Gene	Mode of inheritance	Current	Frequency (%)
LQT1 (JLNS1)	11p15.5	*KCNQ1*	AD (AR in JLNS)	$I_{Ks(\alpha)}$	30–35
LQT2	7q35–36	*KCNH2*	AD	$I_{Kr(\alpha)}$	25–30
LQT3	3p21-p24	*SCN5A*	AD	I_{Na}	5–10
LQT4	4q25-q27	*ANKB*	AD	Na/Ca	<1
LQT5 (JLNS2)	21q22.1	*KCNE1*	AD (AR in JLNS)	$I_{Ks(\beta)}$	~1
LQT6	21q22.1	*KCNE2*	AD	$I_{Kr(\beta)}$	<1
ATS1 (LQT7)	17q23	*KCNJ2*	AD	$I_{K1(\alpha)}$	50 of ATS; <1 of LQTS
TS1 (LQT8)	12p13.3	*CACNA1C*	Sporadic	$I_{Ca.L(\alpha)}$	50 of TS; <1 of LQTS
CAV3-LQTS (LQT9)	3p25	*CAV3*	Sporadic	Caveolin-3 (I_{Na})	<1
SCN4B-LQTS (LQT10)	11q23.3	*SCN4B*	AD	$I_{Na(\beta4)}$	<1

Abbreviations: AD, autosomal dominant; AR, autosomal recessive; ATS, Andersen Tawil syndrome; JLNS, Jervell and Lange-Nielsen syndrome; LQTS, long QT syndrome; TS, Timothy syndrome.

by postmortem mutational analysis of the five major LQTS disease genes (*KCNQ1*, *KCNH2*, *SCN5A*, *KCNE1*, and *KCNE2*) in 93 SIDS cases and 400 controls (9,10). The investigators targeted the *SCN5A*-encoded sodium channel because of known association between LQT3 and sleep events with a high lethality or event rate, and identified 2 of 58 Caucasian SIDS cases (3.4%) (but no African-American SIDS cases) with rare, novel missense mutations that conferred a marked gain of function with accentuation and persistence of late sodium current (9). Subsequently, Tester and Ackerman (10) identified two more cases of probable LQTS-mediated SIDS in their study of the four potassium channel genes. Later, Arnestad et al. validated this observation in a SIDS cohort of 201 Norwegian infants (11), and Crotti et al. reported probable LQTS-causing mutations in ~9% of cases (half in sodium channel, *SCN5A* gene) (12).

Most recently, *CAV3*-encoded caveolin-3 mutations were identified in 3 of 34 African-American infants (13,14). Tester et al. discovered that 2 of the 93 infants harbored gain-of-function mutations in the *RyR2*-encoded cardiac ryanodine receptor and calcium release channel gene (15). Even after excluding the most common channel polymorphisms: K897T-KCNH2, H558R-SCN5A, and G38S-KCNE1, nearly one-third of infants possessed at least one genetic variant noted previously in ethnic-matched reference alleles in one of the five cardiac channel genes (10,16). Whether these channel polymorphisms reduce repolarization reserve and/or facilitate adrenergically mediated cardiac arrhythmias require further investigation. For example, five SIDS victims were positive for R1047L-KCNH2, a polymorphism previously identified as an independent risk factor for drug (dofetilide)-induced torsades (10,17). In addition, the African-American-specific sodium channel common polymorphism, S1103Y-SCN5A, was overrepresented among a cohort of 133 African-American infants and a mexiletine-sensitive increased late sodium current was elicited by cellular acidosis (18).

III. Serotonergic System Genes in SIDS

A. Rationale for Study of Serotonin (*5-HT*) Genes

Panigrahy et al. (19) and later Ozawa and Okado (20) and Kinney et al. (21) reported a decrease in serotonergic receptor binding in medullary regions that contain serotonergic cell bodies. Most recently, Paterson et al. (22) described an increase in the number and density of 5-HT neurons and a lower density of 5-HT$_{1A}$ receptor binding sites in medullary regions of homeostatic control. These neuropathological reports motivated studies focused on genes involved in the serotonergic system.

B. Serotonin Transporter (*5-HTT*) Gene

The 5-HT system is regulated by the action of the serotonin transporter (*5-HTT*) gene. Located at 17q11.1-q12 (23), it controls the duration and strength of interactions between 5-HT and its receptors by regulating membrane reuptake of 5-HT from the extracellular space (24–27).

Two polymorphisms in the 5′ regulatory region of the *5-HTT* gene differentially modulate gene expression: one involves an insertion/deletion in a repeat sequence in the promoter region and the other is a variable number tandem repeat (VNTR) in intron 2. The two most common alleles of the promoter polymorphism include the short allele (S) (corresponds to 14 copies of the 20–23 base pair repeat unit) and the long allele (L) (corresponds to 16 copies). The long allele is a more effective promoter within cell transfection models (25). Subjects with the L/L genotype have an increased availability of raphé serotonin transporters on in vivo neuroimaging studies (28), as well as increased midbrain 5-HTT binding and 5-HTT mRNA levels in the human postmortem brain (29) when compared with individuals carrying at least one S allele. The *5-HTT* promoter allele distribution varies widely by ethnicity (25,30–32). Likewise, SIDS incidence varies widely by ethnicity (2), with rates highest for African-American infants and lowest for Japanese infants (0.248 SIDS deaths per 1000 live births in Japan in 2001) (33).

A polymorphic VNTR containing 9, 10, or 12 copies of a 16 to 17 bp repeat sequence in intron 2 of *5-HTT* (34) also differentially regulates gene expression. Fiskerstrand et al. (24) reported increased expression in promoter-driven reporter gene constructs containing 12 repeats (vs. 10 repeats). The 12-repeat construct was a stronger enhancer in differentiating embryonic stem cells, suggesting that the intron 2 VNTR may affect distribution and rate of transcriptional control (24). MacKenzie and Quinn (27) introduced the VNTR enhancer region coupled to a reporter gene into transgenic mice and noted increased expression levels in the developing rostral hindbrain in mice expressing the 12-repeat construct compared with the 10-repeat construct. Lovejoy et al. (35) identified specific sequence variants within individual repeats in the VNTR that were responsible for high variability in transcriptional efficiency in transfected murine embryonic stem cells and repeat number-dependent variation in VNTR promoter activity in human JAR cells. This suggested that both the repeat copy number and the primary sequence of the repeat units within the intron 2 VNTR may play a role in tissue-specific *5-HTT* expression, leading to variation in *5-HTT* expression in the nervous system and association with disease susceptibility.

Battersby et al. (36) identified a 3′ untranslated region (UTR) single nucleotide polymorphism in *5-HTT*, located within a putative polyadenylation signal for the *5-HTT* mRNA. Although allelic variation at the site does not substantially influence polyadenylation site usage, the 3′ RACE assay used was not quantitative; it remains possible that minor abnormalities in polyadenylation in vivo might affect stability of *5-HTT* mRNA and/or transport into the cytoplasm. A subsequent study (37) did not identify any effect of this 3′ UTR polymorphism on the platelet serotonin transporter expression assayed by [3H] paroxetine binding.

5-HTT Promoter Region Polymorphism in SIDS

Narita et al. (38) examined the role of a functional polymorphism in the promoter region of the *5-HTT* gene in SIDS risk among 27 Japanese SIDS cases and 115 age-matched controls. They genotyped the promoter insertion/deletion polymorphism and demonstrated significant differences in genotype distribution and allele frequency, with an excess of the L/L genotype and L allele in the SIDS group relative to controls [7.4% vs. 1.7% for L/L genotype, 22.2% vs. 13.5% for L allele]. Additionally, they found three extra-long (XL, 18 repeats) alleles in SIDS cases (5.6%) versus one in controls (0.4%). This study provided the first highly significant evidence for the role of a specific gene in SIDS risk.

Weese-Mayer et al. (39) replicated the finding of an increase in frequency of the L allele of the *5-HTT* promoter insertion/deletion polymorphism in SIDS cases in an independent sample of 87 SIDS cases (43 African-American, 44 Caucasian) and 87 gender/ethnicity-matched controls from the United States. They found significant differences in both genotype distribution and allele frequency in the combined (African-American and Caucasian) dataset and for allele frequency in the Caucasian dataset. Specifically, there was an excess of the L/L genotype and the L allele in the SIDS group relative to controls (54.0% vs. 39.1% for L/L genotype; 73.0% vs. 58.6% for L allele). Further, significantly fewer SIDS cases versus controls with no L allele (S/S genotype) were reported in the entire cohort (8.0% vs. 21.8%) and within the Caucasian subgroup (13.6% vs. 34.1%). While the results were not statistically significant within the African-American subgroup (small sample size) there was a trend toward increased frequency of the long allele in the African-American SIDS cases.

In addition to the case-control results, Weese-Mayer et al. (39) examined allele and genotype frequency differences by ethnicity in an additional set of 334 control subjects. The frequency of the long allele was increased in the African-Americans (73.9%) versus Caucasians (53%). Weese-Mayer et al. concluded that the promoter polymorphism in *5-HTT* may play an important role in SIDS risk and may explain, in part, the ethnic differences in SIDS risk. Specifically, SIDS rates are high among African-Americans and low among Japanese, and the *5-HTT* L allele frequency is high among African-Americans (see above) and low among Japanese controls [13.5% in Narita et al. study (38)].

5-HTT Intron 2 VNTR and SIDS

Weese-Mayer et al. (40) subsequently studied the *5-HTT* intron 2 VNTR genotype in a cohort of 90 pairs of SIDS cases and gender/ethnicity-matched controls (46 Caucasians, 44 African-Americans). Genotype distribution, allele frequency for the 12-repeat allele, and frequency of the 12/12 genotype differed significantly between African-American SIDS cases and controls, but not in the overall dataset or the Caucasian subgroup. The association of the 12-allele with SIDS in the African-American group was driven predominantly by a significant increase in 12-alleles in African-American male SIDS cases, which was not observed in females. Similar to the promoter variant, allele frequencies and genotype distribution also varied across ethnic groups, with a higher frequency of the 12-allele in the African-American population, in both cases and controls.

Examination of both promoter polymorphism genotype and intron 2 VNTR genotype in the cohort revealed significant associations between SIDS and the combined "L/L or L/S and 12/12" genotype in the total dataset and the African-American subgroup, but not the Caucasian subgroup. Further, haplotype analysis demonstrated a significant difference in the overall haplotype frequencies between SIDS cases and controls in the entire cohort as well as each ethnic subgroup Finally, the "L-12" haplotype ("long" allele present at the promoter and "12" allele present at intron 2 on the same chromosome) was significantly more frequent in SIDS cases than controls, and also in the African-American SIDS cases versus controls, but not in Caucasian SIDS cases versus controls. These studies established an association between SIDS and the 12-repeat allele of the intron 2 VNTR and the L-12 haplotype in the African-American subgroup.

5-HTT 3' UTR and SIDS

Despite the association of two functional polymorphisms in *5-HTT* with SIDS, a polymorphism in a putative polyadenylation site in the 3' UTR of *5-HTT* (36) was not found to be associated with SIDS (41) in 92 pairs of gender/ethnicity-matched SIDS cases and controls. Specifically, genotype distribution did not differ between the SIDS and control groups in the overall dataset or the Caucasian or African-American subgroups. Analyses performed for haplotypes spanning the *5-HTT* gene (promoter, intron 2 and 3' UTR variants) revealed no significant differences in haplotype frequency distribution either in the total dataset or in the Caucasian or African-American subgroups.

IV. Autonomic Nervous System Genes in SIDS

A. Rationale for Studying ANS Genes, Including *PHOX2B*

5-HT influences a broad range of physiological systems regulated by the autonomic nervous system (ANS), including the regulation of breathing, the cardiovascular system, the temperature, and the sleep-wake cycle (42). Symptoms compatible with ANS dysregulation (ANSD) have been reported in SIDS, including profuse sweating, elevated body temperature, tachycardia then bradycardia preceding the terminal event, reduced heart rate variability, drenching sweats and facial pallor, and decreased responses to obstructive sleep events (43–50). Accordingly, genes pertinent to the early embryology of the ANS were considered to potentially confer SIDS risk. This approach has been successful in clarifying the genetic basis of congenital central hypoventilation syndrome (CCHS), also known to be associated with ANSD (51–53) and thought to be related to SIDS (54). Paired-like homeobox protein (*PHOX2B*) is the disease-defining gene for CCHS such that virtually all individuals with the CCHS phenotype are heterozygous for polyalanine expansion mutations in *PHOX2B* or have a nonpolyalanine expansion mutation in the *PHOX2B* gene (55–60).

PHOX2B encodes a highly conserved homeobox domain transcription factor with two stable polyalanine repeats of 9 and 20 residues and is a key gene in ANS development with a role in early embryologic development as a transcriptional activator in promotion of pan-neuronal differentiation, including upregulation of proneural genes, mammalian achaete-scute homolog-1 (*MASH1*) expression, and motoneural differentiation (61). *PHOX2B* has a separate role by a different pathway wherein it represses expression of inhibitors of neurogenesis (62). Further, *PHOX2B* is required to express tyrosine hydroxylase, dopamine beta hydroxylase (63), and *RET*, and to maintain *MASH1*, thereby regulating noradrenergic neuronal specification in vertebrates (64). Finally, *PHOX2B* knock-out mice (−/−) do not survive as ANS circuits do not form or degenerate (64). Moreover, recent studies indicate that *PHOX2B* plays a regulatory role in the selection between motor neuron or serotonergic neuronal fate in the development of the central nervous system (65,66). Loss of function experiments in mice have shown that for the transition from motor neuron production to 5-HT neuron production to commence downregulation of *PHOX2B* is required (65). Recognizing the identified importance of the 5-HT system in SIDS, as described above, these loss of function experiments identify a role for *PHOX2B* in the development of the 5-HT system and potentially a relationship between the 5-HT system development and *PHOX2B* in SIDS risk.

B. ANS Genes

Weese-Mayer et al. (67) examined several genes thought to play a role in ANS development, including bone morphogenic protein-2(*BMP2*), *MASH1*, *PHOX2A*, rearranged during transfection factor (*RET*), endothelin converting enzyme-1 (*ECE1*), endothelin-1 (*EDN1*), T-cell leukemia homeobox protein (*TLX3*), and engrailed-1 (*EN1*). DNA from 92 SIDS cases and from 26 of the 92 matched controls was sequenced for exon and splice site mutations in *BMP2*, *MASH1*, *PHOX2A*, *RET*, *ECE1*, *EDN1*, *TLX3*, and *EN1*. Any base change expected to affect a splice site or result in modification of the protein sequence that was identified in the SIDS subjects or controls was further screened in all 92 controls (Table 2). Sequence data from *PHOX2A*, *RET*, *ECE1*, *TLX3*, and *EN1* revealed 11 rare protein-changing polymorphisms in 14 SIDS cases (15.2% of SIDS cases) and subsequent genotyping for these polymorphisms in controls identified one polymorphism in two controls (2.2% of controls). Each mutation occurred in one SIDS case with the exception of the *TLX3* base change that occurred in four SIDS cases and two controls. The African-American infants accounted for 10 of the SIDS cases and the two controls with protein-changing mutations. No protein-changing alterations were identified for *MASH1* or *EDN1*.

Four common protein-changing polymorphisms were identified in *BMP2*, *RET*, *ECE1*, and *EDN1*, though allele frequencies did not differ between

Table 2 Protein-Changing Variants in Genes Pertinent to the Early Embryologic Origin of the ANS for 92 SIDS and 92 Control Subjects

			Rare polymorphisms						Common polymorphisms					
			Number of cases with variant						Allele frequency of variant					
			SIDS			Controls			SIDS			Controls		
Gene	Genotype	Amino acid effect	Cauc.	Afr. Amer.	Total	Cauc.	Afr. Amer.	Total	Cauc.	Afr. Amer.	Total	Cauc.	Afr. Amer.	Total
BMP2	T570A	S190R							0.32	0.07	0.19	0.38	0.06	0.22
PHOX2A	C287A	T96K	1	0	1	0	0	0						
RET	G35A	R12H	1	0	1	0	0	0						
	C166A	L56M	1	0	1	0	0	0						
	C1157T	A386V	0	1	1	0	0	0						
	G1253A	R418Q	1	0	1	0	0	0						
	G2071A	G691S							0.07	0.05	0.06	0.11	0.12	0.12
	A2147C	K716T	0	1	1	0	0	0						
ECE1	C1022T	T341I							0.04	0.01	0.02	0.09	0.01	0.05
	A1060G	T354A	0	1	1	0	0	0						
EDN1	G594T	K198N							0.27	0.28	0.26	0.22	0.16	0.19
TLX3	C196T	P66S	0	4	4	0	2	2						
	G152A	R51H	0	1	1	0	0	0						
ENI	C719T	T240I	0	1	1	0	0	0						
	C986A	T329K	0	1	1	0	0	0						

Abbreviations: ANS, autonomic nervous system; SIDS, sudden infant death syndrome; Cauc., Caucasian; Afr. Amer., African-American; BMP 2, bone morphogenic protein-2; PHOX2A, paired-like homeobox gene 2A; RET, rearranged during transfection factor; ECE1, endothelin converting enzyme-1; EDN1, endothelin-1; TLX3, T-cell leukemia homeobox protein; EN1, engrailed-1.

Source: From Ref. 67.

SIDS cases and controls. However, allele frequencies for the *BMP2* common polymorphism differed significantly between Caucasian and African-American infants. Among controls, the allele frequencies for the *BMP2* and *ECE1* polymorphisms differed significantly between Caucasian and African-American infants.

On the basis of the established relationship between SIDS, *5-HTT*, and ANSD coupled with the recognized role of *PHOX2B* in ANS and 5-HT system development, Weese-Mayer et al. (67) studied a cohort of 91 SIDS cases and 91 matched controls for the *PHOX2B* polyalanine expansion mutation characteristic of CCHS. None of the study subjects demonstrated the *PHOX2B* polyalanine mutation characteristic of CCHS.

Subsequently, Rand et al. (68) sequenced the coding regions and intron-exon boundaries of *PHOX2B* in the same SIDS cohort along with 91 gender/ethnicity-matched control subjects, and identified a single common polymorphism (IVS2+101A>G; g.1364A>G) in intron 2 of the *PHOX2B* gene located 100 base pairs downstream of the exon 2 splice site. The frequency of subjects carrying the variant G allele (genotype GG or GA) of this polymorphism was significantly higher in the SIDS group than in the matched control group and also higher in the Caucasian SIDS cases than in the matched control subjects, but did not reach significance in the the African-American SIDS versus control comparison. Likely, the result is nonsignificant in the African-American group because of the high baseline frequency of this polymorphism in the African-American population, which significantly exceeds the frequency of the variant in the Caucasian population as seen in the control groups. The allele frequency of the variant G allele for the intron 2 polymorphism was not significantly increased in the SIDS group relative to controls, although there was a strong trend toward higher G allele frequency in the entire SIDS cohort and Caucasian SIDS group compared with controls that was not seen in the African-American SIDS cases and controls. The difference in allele frequency did not reach significance because the homozygous GG genotype was more frequent in the control group, suggesting that the effect of this polymorphism on SIDS risk is relevant to presence or absence of the G allele and thus is similar in the homozygous and heterozygous state.

Eight polymorphisms located in the third exon of the *PHOX2B* gene (Table 3) occurred significantly more frequently among SIDS cases (34 occurrences observed in 27/91 cases) than controls (19 occurrences observed in 16/91 controls). Likewise, the number of occurrences among SIDS cases in the Caucasian and African-American subgroups was nearly double the number among their respective controls. Among SIDS cases containing a polymorphism in exon 3, 6 of 27 (22%) contained two or more polymorphisms compared to 2 of 16 (12%) controls (Table 3). Each of the eight samples with two or more polymorphisms in exon 3 were African-American. Two of the eight polymorphisms identified were protein-altering missense mutations (F153L and S176T), occurring in nine SIDS cases and four controls (10% and 4%, respectively) (Table 3).

Table 3 PHOX2B Exon 3 Polymorphisms in 91 SIDS Cases and 91 Matched Control Subjects

| | | | Number of patients with rare polymorphism | | | | | |
| | | | SIDS | | | Control | | |
Location	Genotype	Amino acid effect	Caucasian	African-American	Total	Caucasian	African-American	Total
Exon 3	c.459T>G	F153L	0	1	1	2	0	2
Exon 3	c.526T>A	S176T	6	2	8	2	0	2
Exon 3	c.552C>T	silent	1	2	3	0	2	2
Exon 3	c.642C>T	silent	0	2	2	0	0	0
Exon 3	c.726A>G	silent	0	2	2	0	1	1
Exon 3	c.750G>A	silent	1	3	4	0	2	2
Exon 3	c.762A>C	silent	1	7	8	1	5	6
Exon 3	c.870C>A	silent	2	4	6	1	3	4
Total occurrences of polymorphisms[a]			11	23	34	6	13	19

[a]These polymorphisms were identified 34 times in the SIDS group compared with 19 times in the control group ($p = 0.01$) and in 27/91 SIDS cases compared with 16/91 controls ($p = 0.05$).

Abbreviations: PHOX2B, paired-like homeobox gene 2B; SIDS, sudden infant death syndrome.

Source: From Ref. 68.

Gene-gene interaction between the *PHOX2B* exon 3 polymorphisms and the *5-HTT* promoter L/L genotype or the L allele, or the *5-HTT* intron 2 polymorphisms, was not found for SIDS risk, in comparisons of SIDS cases with controls or when the cohort was divided into ethnicity-specific subgroups. Gene interaction analysis revealed that of the 27 SIDS cases containing a *PHOX2B* exon 3 polymorphism(s), three also contained a *RET* mutation compared with 1 of 61 SIDS cases that contained no exon 3 polymorphism and were also tested for *RET* mutations. Significantly, more Caucasian SIDS cases (3/11) with a *PHOX2B* exon 3 polymorphism had an additional *RET* mutation compared with zero of 34 Caucasian SIDS cases containing no exon 3 polymorphism.

Kijima et al. (69) also sequenced the *PHOX2B* gene in 23 Japanese SIDS cases and 50 controls and identified one polymorphism in exon 2 of *PHOX2B* and two intron 2 polymorphisms, none of which were identified in the Rand et al. (68) study. These polymorphisms were identified in 1%, 1% and 9% of subjects, respectively, but the authors do not clarify if these were identified in SIDS cases or controls. Conversely, none of the *PHOX2B* exon 3 polymorphisms that Rand et al. (68) described in the Caucasian and African-Americans were reported in the Japanese cases.

V. Nicotine Metabolizing Genes in SIDS

A. Rationale for Study of Nicotine Metabolizing Genes

Exposure to tobacco, both prenatal as well as postnatal, has been identified as a key risk factor in the etiology of SIDS (70–74). A relationship between tobacco exposure and altered ANS function has long been recognized for adults with both chronic (75–78) and acute (79) exposure and more recently for infants exposed to smoke prenatally (80). On the basis of these relationships between SIDS, tobacco exposure, and ANSD, genes involved in nicotine metabolism were identified as possible candidate genes for further study of the genetic basis for SIDS.

The ability to convert toxic metabolites in cigarette smoke to less harmful compounds is the key to minimize the adverse health effects of tobacco exposure. Polycyclic aromatic hydrocarbons (PAHs), some of the most important carcinogens in cigarette smoke, are metabolized through a two-stage process. In phase 1 inhaled PAHs are activated by converting the hydrophobic compounds into hydrophilic compounds, which are reactive and have electrophilic intermediates capable of binding DNA. Cytochrome P450 1A1 (*CYP1A1*) encodes aryl hydrocarbon hydroxylase, a major enzyme responsible for phase 1 metabolism of PAHs. During the second phase of the metabolism of PAHs detoxification occurs through enzymes, such as glutathione S-transferases (GSTs) or uridine diphosphate (UDP)-glucuronosyltransferase, through transformation into compounds that can be excreted from the body. GSTT1 is encoded by the *GSTT1* gene, and is a major enzyme in phase 2 of cigarette smoke metabolism (81–83). Polymorphisms in both the *CYP1A1* and *GSTT1* genes (81,84) have been reported to impact the metabolic detoxification process of cigarette smoke. Thus, expression of polymorphisms in these genes have been associated with low birth weight (85), and may account for the varying susceptibility to other adverse health consequences of cigarette smoke exposure, including SIDS.

B. Nicotine Metabolizing Genes

Rand et al. (86) reported on frequency of known *CYP1A1* and *GSTT1* polymorphisms in 106 SIDS cases and 106 control subjects matched for gender and ethnicity. The frequency of the *GSTT1* homozygous deletion genotype did not differ between SIDS cases (22/106; 20%) and matched controls (32/106; 30%) in either the complete sample or the Caucasian or African-American subgroups. Likewise, no association with SIDS was observed for genotype distribution or allele frequencies at any of the three *CYP1A1* polymorphisms. When multiple alleles were considered in combination, no association was found between cases containing one or more of the *CYP1A1* rare polymorphic alleles and the SIDS phenotype. Further, no association was observed between cases containing both the *GSTT1* deletion genotype and a *CYP1A1* polymorphism with the SIDS phenotype. Higher frequencies of variant allele combinations were observed in the African-American subgroups compared with Caucasian subgroups likely due to the higher genetic heterogeneity in that population.

VI. Summary and Clinical Significance

A. Significance of Cardiac Channelopathies in SIDS

A primary cardiac channelopathy is estimated to cause 5–15% of SIDS. Even after excluding the most common channel polymorphisms (K897T-*KCNH2*, H558R-*SCN5A*, and G38S-*KCNE1*), nearly one-third of infants possessed at least one genetic variant noted previously in ethnic-matched reference alleles in one of the five cardiac channel genes (10,16,87). Whether these cardiac channel polymorphisms reduce repolarization reserve and/or facilitate adrenergically mediated cardiac arrhythmias requires further investigation.

Routine newborn LQTS genetic screening has not been implemented despite an incidence of 1:2500. Further studies are needed to determine whether polymorphism-specific genotyping for S1103Y should be performed routinely in African-American infants. However, strategies to detect the presence of LQTS preemptively must continue to be sought. To this end, Schwartz et al. continue to investigate the utility and cost-effectiveness of universal ECG screening of Italian infants at 3 to 4 weeks of age (88–90).

B. Significance of *5-HTT* Studies in SIDS

The promoter variant long alleles and VNTR 12-repeat alleles are associated with SIDS. As these alleles are more effective promoters (24,25) of and associated with increased expression of *5-HTT* transporters in various brain regions, synaptic serotonin levels would be expected to be lower in those infants with a long or 12-repeat allele, and perhaps lowest in those with both variants. Increased prevalence of the more effective promoter alleles in SIDS cases would suggest that lower synaptic serotonin levels are associated with SIDS risk, and decreased serotonergic receptor binding may thus occur through downregulation of presynaptic autoreceptors. Alternatively, the long allele, 12-repeat allele, or the combination may relate to SIDS through a developmental effect on raphé neurons. The serotonin transporter is expressed early in ontogenesis in the mouse and the rat (91), and may influence serotonin synapse formation and serotonin-dependent patterning of neuronal networks (92). Moisewitsch et al. (93) have shown that 5-HT, acting through 5-HT1A receptors, stimulates migration of cranial neural crest cells in a dose-dependent fashion in the mouse embryo and in cultured cranial explants. Thus, lower 5-HT levels due to higher *5-HTT* expression during development might lead to alterations in medullary serotonergic neuronal numbers and synaptic connections, with resultant lower serotonin binding in SIDS medullae. Recognizing that the *5-HTT* short allele has been associated with anxiety, phobias, and an increased fear response (26,30,94–96), one might also postulate that SIDS would be less likely in infants with the S/S genotype due to an exaggerated fear response and increased arousability. Differences in risk alleles and haplotypes between Caucasian and African-American populations would likely result from racial differences in modifier genes or other interacting factors that influence 5-HT levels. Alternatively, the risk conferred by the L-12 haplotype may not have directly to do with regulation of *5-HTT* expression by the combined effect of these loci, but could relate to another yet undefined functional polymorphism in linkage disequilibrium with the L-12 haplotype.

Despite localization to a polydenylation signal, the *3' UTR* SNP polymorphism has not been found to have any effect on expression of the 5-HTT transporter protein. Likewise, no association was detected between this polymorphism and SIDS. These data suggest that the *3' UTR* may not really be a functional polymorphism, although it is still expected to be a useful tool for assessment of the contribution of genetic variation in the serotonin transporter gene to disease. Similar to the findings with the SIDS cohort presented here, the *5-HTT* promoter polymorphism was recently shown to be associated with attention-deficit/hyperactivity disorder, while the 3' UTR was not associated (97). Findings in both studies likely relate to the difference in functional effects of the promoter polymorphism and the 3' UTR SNP, such that SIDS risk is specifically related to functional variants that result in increased expression of 5-HT transporter protein. Thus, future investigations on the influence of *5-HTT* on SIDS risk should focus on polymorphisms that directly impact regulation of transporter protein expression or function.

C. Significance of ANS Genes in SIDS

The finding of specific protein-changing mutations in conserved residues (67) of *PHOX2A*, *RET*, *ECE1*, *TLX3*, and *EN1* among 15.2% of SIDS cases versus 2.2%

of controls suggests that specific polymorphisms in these genes may confer some SIDS risk. The observation that 71% of the SIDS cases with these mutations were African-Americans may be consistent with the observed ethnic disparity in SIDS, although African populations tend to exhibit higher levels of genetic variation. The greatest number of rare mutations was identified in the *RET* gene. This is of particular interest because of the relationship of *RET* to Hirschsprung disease and to CCHS (both diseases of neural crest origin), and because of the *RET* knockout model with a depressed ventilatory response to inhaled carbon dioxide with decreased frequency and tidal volume (98). The knockout models for *ECE1* (99) and *TLX3* (100) also include impaired breathing and/or early death in the mouse phenotype, with the suggestion of a central respiratory deficit. On the basis of these findings, further research is necessary to better understand the role of these and other genes in the SIDS phenotype and in explaining the ethnic disparity in SIDS.

The observation that none of the SIDS cases demonstrated the *PHOX2B* polyalanine expansion mutation previously identified in CCHS indicates less specific overlap between the two diseases than previously considered. However, as families of CCHS probands have a higher incidence of SIDS history in a family member (54), and as the anticipated incidence of this *PHOX2B* mutation is low in the general population, our sample size may not have been adequate to detect a case. Therefore, it may still be appropriate to evaluate infants with SIDS for the CCHS *PHOX2B* mutation to ascertain that CCHS was not the cause of death. However, specific (non-CCHS) polymorphisms in *PHOX2B* are more common in SIDS cases (68) and may confer SIDS risk independently or when present in combination with other mutations of ANS genes. Particularly, the *MASH1-PHOX-RET* pathway, in which *PHOX2B* is needed for the expression of *RET*, has been shown to be an integral part of the development of both the sympathetic and enteric nervous systems (64,101). The interaction of *PHOX2B* and *RET* in this pathway is consistent with the finding of a possible interaction between polymorphisms in *PHOX2B* and *RET* in mediating SIDS risk, suggesting that genetic changes at multiple points in the pathway could combine to amplify risk. Although *PHOX2B* plays a key role in the differentiation of central 5-HT neurons (65,66), the absence of significant interactions between *PHOX2B* and *5-HTT* polymorphisms suggests that the two genes exert independent effects on SIDS risk, potentially by acting on different aspects of 5-HT system function.

Although the *PHOX2B* intron 2 polymorphism (IVS2+101A>G; g.1364 A>G) identified is a silent transition in the noncoding region of *PHOX2B*, it was recently linked with Hirschsprung disease (HSCR) (102), another disease of ANSD. The Garcia-Barcelo report of a decreased frequency of the intron 2 polymorphism among 91 ethnic Chinese HSCR cases (19%) compared to 71 unmatched ethnic Chinese controls (36%) strengthens the conclusion that this intron 2 polymorphism is related to ANSD. Although not directly involved in splicing, the *PHOX2B* intron 2 polymorphism could have other regulatory effects and may act in combination with mutations in genes involved in the *RET* and/or *EDNRB* signaling pathway to produce ANSD.

The identification of polymorphisms in genes pertinent to the embryologic origin of the ANS in SIDS cases lends support to the overriding hypothesis that infants who succumb to SIDS have an underlying genetic predisposition. The low rate of occurrence of mutations in ANS genes studied suggests that there are yet unidentified genes that are responsible for the SIDS phenotype, either directly or in conjunction with the polymorphisms identified in *PHOX2B, RET, 5-HTT,* and/or other genes involved in ANS or 5-HT system development. Sequencing of additional genes involved in ANS or 5-HT development in a larger group of SIDS cases will be expected to yield insight into the relationship between *PHOX2B,* additional candidate genes, and SIDS.

D. Significance of Nicotine Metabolizing Genes in SIDS

Genetic traits that alter the metabolic efficiency of toxins encountered through tobacco exposure may also increase susceptibility to damage from these toxins. Further, they could serve as important risk factors for SIDS. However, no defined genetic link was demonstrable in the one study of variations of the *GSTT1* and *CYP1A1* genes carried out thus far. Lack of information and objective testing for tobacco exposure in the SIDS cohort limited the study by Rand et al (86). The SIDS cohort is expected to represent a combination of cases with exposure and without exposure, so the presence of the no exposure cases will be expected to limit significance. Thus, it is possible that an association could be found in a larger group of cases or a group containing only those cases with cigarette smoke exposure. The recognized relationship between tobacco exposure and SIDS risk indicates that examination of these and additional genes involved in tobacco metabolism in a prospective SIDS cohort known to have a history and/or testing of confirmed smoke exposure may shed light on genetic factors that mediate the role that tobacco exposure plays in susceptibility to SIDS.

VII. Future Directions

A number of genetically controlled pathways appear to be involved in at least some cases of SIDS. Given the diversity of results to date, genetic studies support the clinical impression that SIDS is heterogeneous with more than one possible genetic etiology. Future studies should consider expanded dataset size and phenotypic features that might help clarify the heterogeneity and improve the predictive value of the identified genetic factors. Such features should be evaluated to the extent possible in both SIDS victims and their family members. With 2162 infants dying from SIDS in 2003 in the United States alone (2), and improved but still imperfect parent and caretaker compliance with known modifiable risk factors for SIDS, it behooves the scientific community to join in a collaborative multicenter study of candidate genes and genomics to expedite the discovery of the genetic profile of the infant at risk for SIDS.

References

1. Kochanek KD, Hudson BL. Advance Report of Final Mortality Statistics, 1992. Hyattsville, MD: National Center for Health Statistics, 1995.
2. Hoyert DL, Heron MP, Murphy SL, et al. Deaths: final data for 2003. Natl Vital Stat Rep 2006; 54:1–120.
3. Schwartz PJ. Cardiac sympathetic innervation and the sudden infant death syndrome. A possible pathogenetic link. Am J Med 1976; 60:167–172.
4. Maron BJ, Clark CE, Goldstein RE, et al. Potential role of QT interval prolongation in sudden infant death syndrome. Circulation 1976; 54:423–430.
5. Schwartz PJ, Stramba-Badiale M, Segantini A, et al. Prolongation of the QT interval and the sudden infant death syndrome. N Engl J Med 1998; 338:1709–1714.
6. Schwartz PJ, Priori SG, Dumaine R, et al. A molecular link between the sudden infant death syndrome and the long-QT syndrome. N Engl J Med 2000; 343:262–267.
7. Schwartz PJ, Priori SG, Bloise R, et al. Molecular diagnosis in a child with sudden infant death syndrome. Lancet 2001; 358:1342–1343.
8. Christiansen M, Tonder N, Larsen LA, et al. Mutations in the HERG K+-ion channel: a novel link between long QT syndrome and sudden infant death syndrome. Am J Cardiol 2005; 95:433–434.
9. Ackerman MJ, Siu BL, Sturner WQ, et al. Postmortem molecular analysis of SCN5A defects in sudden infant death syndrome. JAMA 2001; 286:2264–2269.
10. Tester DJ, Ackerman MJ. Sudden infant death syndrome: how significant are the cardiac channelopathies? Cardiovasc Res 2005; 67:388–396.
11. Arnestad M, Crotti L, Rognum TO, et al. Prevalence of long-QT syndrome gene variants in sudden infant death syndrome. Circulation 2007; 23:115(3):361–367.
12. Wang DW, Desai RR, Crotti L, et al. Cardiac sodium channel dysfunction in sudden infant death syndrome. Circulation 2007; 115(3):368–376.
13. Vatta M, Ackerman MJ, Ye B, et al. Mutant Caveolin-3 induces persistent late sodium current and is associated with Long QT Syndrome. Circulation 2006; 114 (20):2104–2112.
14. Cronk LB, Ye B, Kaku T, et al. A novel mechanism for sudden infant death syndrome (SIDS): persistent late sodium current secondary to mutations in caveolin-3. Heart Rhythm 2007; 4:161–166.
15. Tester DJ, Dura M, Carturan E, et al. A mechanism for sudden infant death syndrome (SIDS): stress-induced leak via ryanodine receptors. Circulation 2007; 4:733–739.
16. Ackerman MJ, Tester DJ, Jones GS, et al. Ethnic differences in cardiac potassium channel variants: implications for genetic susceptibility to sudden cardiac death and genetic testing for congenital long QT syndrome. Mayo Clin Proc 2003; 78: 1479–1487.
17. Sun Z, Milos PM, Thompson JF, et al. Role of a KCNH2 polymorphism (R1047 L) in dofetilide-induced Torsades de Pointes. J Mol Cell Cardiol 2004; 37:1031–1039.
18. Plant LD, Bowers PN, Liu Q, et al. A common cardiac sodium channel variant associated with sudden infant death in African Americans, SCN5A S1103Y. J Clin Invest 2006; 116:430–435.

19. Panigrahy A, Filiano J, Sleeper LA, et al. Decreased serotonergic receptor binding in rhombic lip-derived regions of the medulla oblongata in the sudden infant death syndrome. J Neuropathol Exp Neurol 2000; 59:377–384.

20. Ozawa Y, Okado N. Alteration of serotonergic receptors in the brainstems of human patients with respiratory disorders. Neuropediatrics 2002; 33:142–149.

21. Kinney HC, Randall LL, Sleeper LA, et al. Serotonergic brainstem abnormalities in Northern Plains Indians with the sudden infant death syndrome. J Neuropathol Exp Neurol 2003; 62:1178–1191.

22. Paterson DS, Trachtenbert FL, Thompson EG, et al. Multiple serotonergic brainstem abnormalities in the sudden infant death syndrome. JAMA 2006; 296:2124–2132.

23. Ramamoorthy S, Bauman AL, Moore KR, et al. Antidepressant- and cocaine-sensitive human serotonin transporter: molecular cloning, expression, and chromosomal localization. Proc Natl Acad Sci U S A 1993; 90:2542–2546.

24. Fiskerstrand CE, Lovejoy EA, Quinn JP. An intronic polymorphic domain often associated with susceptibility to affective disorders has allele dependent differential enhancer activity in embryonic stem cells. FEBS Lett 1999; 458:171–174.

25. Heils A, Teufel A, Petri S, et al. Allelic variation of human serotonin transporter gene expression. J Neurochem 1996; 66:2621–2624.

26. Lesch KP, Bengel D, Heils A, et al. Association of anxiety-related traits with a polymorphism in the serotonin transporter gene regulatory region [see comment]. Science 1996; 274:1527–1531.

27. MacKenzie A, Quinn J. A serotonin transporter gene intron 2 polymorphic region, correlated with affective disorders, has allele-dependent differential enhancer-like properties in the mouse embryo. Proc Natl Acad Sci U S A 1999; 96:15251–15255.

28. Heinz A, Jones DW, Mazzanti C, et al. A relationship between serotonin transporter genotype and in vivo protein expression and alcohol neurotoxicity. Biol Psychiatry 2000; 47:643–649.

29. Little KY, McLaughlin DP, Zhang L, et al. Cocaine, ethanol, and genotype effects on human midbrain serotonin transporter binding sites and mRNA levels. Am J Psychiatr 1998; 155:207–213.

30. Du L, Bakish D, Hrdina PD. Gender differences in association between serotonin transporter gene polymorphism and personality traits. Psychiatr Genet 2000; 10:159–164.

31. Gelernter J, Kranzler H, Coccaro EF, et al. Serotonin transporter protein gene polymorphism and personality measures in African American and European American subjects. Am J Psychiatry 1998; 155:1332–1338.

32. Gelernter J, Cubells JF, Kidd JR, et al. Population studies of polymorphisms of the serotonin transporter protein gene. Am J Med Genet 1999; 88:61–66.

33. Kai B. Maternal and child health statistics of Japan. 2003.

34. Ogilvie AD, Battersby S, Bubb VJ, et al. Polymorphism in serotonin transporter gene associated with susceptibility to major depression. Lancet 1996; 347:731–733.

35. Lovejoy EA, Scott AC, Fiskerstrand CE, et al. The serotonin transporter intronic VNTR enhancer correlated with a predisposition to affective disorders has distinct regulatory elements within the domain based on the primary DNA sequence of the repeat unit. Eur J Neurosci 2003; 17:417–420.

36. Battersby S, Ogilvie AD, Blackwood DH, et al. Presence of multiple functional polyadenylation signals and a single nucleotide polymorphism in the 3′ untranslated region of the human serotonin transporter gene. J Neurochem 1999; 72:1384–1388.

37. Melke J, Westberg L, Landen M, et al. Serotonin transporter gene polymorphisms and platelet [3H] paroxetine binding in premenstrual dysphoria. Psychoneuroendocrinology 2003; 28:446–458.

38. Narita N, Narita M, Takashima S, et al. Serotonin transporter gene variation is a risk factor for sudden infant death syndrome in the Japanese population. Pediatrics 2001; 107:690–692.

39. Weese-Mayer DE, Berry-Kravis EM, Maher BS, et al. Sudden infant death syndrome: association with a promoter polymorphism of the serotonin transporter gene. Am J Med Genet A 2003; 117:268–274.

40. Weese-Mayer DE, Zhou L, Berry-Kravis EM, et al. Association of the serotonin transporter gene with sudden infant death syndrome: a haplotype analysis. Am J Med Genet A 2003; 122:238–245.

41. Maher BS, Marazita ML, Rand C, et al. 3′ UTR polymorphism of the serotonin transporter gene and sudden infant death syndrome: haplotype analysis. Am J Med Genet A 2006; 140:1453–1457.

42. Jacobs BL, Azmitia EC. Structure and function of the brain serotonin system. Physiol Rev 1992; 72:165–229.

43. Kahn A, Groswasser J, Rebuffat E, et al. Sleep and cardiorespiratory characteristics of infant victims of sudden death: a prospective case-control study. Sleep 1992; 15:287–292.

44. Fleming PJ, Gilbert R, Azaz Y, et al. Interaction between bedding and sleeping position in the sudden infant death syndrome: a population based case-control study. BMJ 1990; 301:85–89.

45. Ponsonby AL, Dwyer T, Gibbons LE, et al. Thermal environment and sudden infant death syndrome: case-control study. BMJ 1992; 304:277–282.

46. Meny RG, Carroll JL, Carbone MT, et al. Cardiorespiratory recordings from infants dying suddenly and unexpectedly at home. Pediatrics 1994; 93:44–49.

47. Schechtman VL, Harper RM, Kluge KA, et al. Cardiac and respiratory patterns in normal infants and victims of the sudden infant death syndrome. Sleep 1988; 11: 413–424.

48. Ledwidge M, Fox G, Matthews T. Neurocardiogenic syncope: a model for SIDS. Arch Dis Child 1998; 78:481–483.

49. Taylor BJ, Williams SM, Mitchell EA, et al. Symptoms, sweating and reactivity of infants who die of SIDS compared with community controls. New Zealand National Cot Death Study Group. J Paediatr Child Health 1996; 32:316–322.

50. Franco P, Szliwowski H, Dramaix M, et al. Decreased autonomic responses to obstructive sleep events in future victims of sudden infant death syndrome. Pediatr Res 1999; 46:33–39.

51. Weese-Mayer DE, Shannon DC, Keens TG, et al. Idiopathic congenital central hypoventilation syndrome: diagnosis and management. American Thoracic Society. Am J Respir Crit Care Med 1999; 160:368–373.

52. Weese-Mayer DE, Silvestri JM, Huffman AD, et al. Case/control family study of autonomic nervous system dysfunction in idiopathic congenital central hypoventilation syndrome. Am J Med Genet A 2001; 100:237–245.

53. Marazita ML, Maher BS, Cooper ME, et al. Genetic segregation analysis of autonomic nervous system dysfunction in families of probands with idiopathic congenital central hypoventilation syndrome. Am J Med Genet A 2001; 100: 229–236.

54. Weese-Mayer DE, Silvestri JM, Marazita ML, et al. Congenital central hypoventilation syndrome: inheritance and relation to sudden infant death syndrome. Am J Med Genet A 1993; 47:360–367.
55. Amiel J, Laudier B, Attie-Bitach T, et al. Polyalanine expansion and frameshift mutations of the paired-like homeobox gene PHOX2B in congenital central hypoventilation syndrome. Nat Genet 2003; 33:459–461.
56. Weese-Mayer DE, Berry-Kravis EM, Zhou L, et al. Idiopathic congenital central hypoventilation syndrome: analysis of genes pertinent to early autonomic nervous system embryologic development and identification of mutations in PHOX2B. Am J Med Genet A 2003; 123:267–278.
57. Sasaki A, Kanai M, Kijima K, et al. Molecular analysis of congenital central hypoventilation syndrome. Hum Genet 2003; 114:22–26.
58. Matera I, Bachetti T, Puppo F, et al. PHOX2B mutations and polyalanine expansions correlate with the severity of the respiratory phenotype and associated symptoms in both congenital and late onset central hypoventilation syndrome. J Med Genet 2004; 41(5):373–380.
59. Berry-Kravis EM, Zhou L, Rand CM, et al. Congenital central hypoventilation syndrome: PHOX2B mutations and phenotype. Am J Respir Crit Care Med 2006; 174:1139–1144.
60. Trochet D, O'Brien LM, Gozal D, et al. PHOX2B genotype allows for prediction of tumor risk in congenital central hypoventilation syndrome. Am J Hum Genet 2005; 76(3):421–426.
61. Lo L, Tiveron MC, Anderson DJ. MASH1 activates expression of the paired homeodomain transcription factor Phox2a, and couples pan-neuronal and subtype-specific components of autonomic neuronal identity. Development 1998; 125(4):609–620.
62. Lo L, Morin X, Brunet JF, et al. Specification of neurotransmitter identity by Phox2 proteins in neural crest stem cells. Neuron 1999; 22:693–705.
63. Hirsch MR, Tiveron MC, Guillemot F, et al. Control of noradrenergic differentiation and Phox2a expression by MASH1 in the central and peripheral nervous system. Development 1998; 125:599–608.
64. Pattyn A, Morin X, Cremer H, et al. The homeobox gene Phox2b is essential for the development of autonomic neural crest derivatives. Nature 1999; 399:366–370.
65. Pattyn A, Vallstedt A, Dias JM, et al. Coordinated temporal and spatial control of motor neuron and serotonergic neuron generation from a common pool of CNS progenitors. Genes Dev 2003; 17:729–737.
66. Pattyn A, Simplicio N, van Doorninck JH, et al. Ascl1/Mash1 is required for the development of central serotonergic neurons. Nat Neurosci 2004; 7:589–595.
67. Weese-Mayer DE, Berry-Kravis EM, Zhou L, et al. Sudden infant death syndrome: case-control frequency differences at genes pertinent to early autonomic nervous system embryologic development. Pediatr Res 2004; 56:391–395.
68. Rand CM, Weese-Mayer DE, Maher BS, et al. Sudden infant death syndrome: case-control frequency differences in paired like homeobox (PHOX) 2B gene. Am J Med Genet A 2006; 140A:1687–1691.
69. Kijima K, Sasaki A, Niki T, et al. Sudden infant death syndrome is not associated with the mutation of PHOX2B gene, a major causative gene of congenital central hypoventilation syndrome. Tohoku J Exp Med 2004; 203:65–68.
70. Anderson HR, Cook DG. Passive smoking and sudden infant death syndrome: Review of the epidemiological evidence. Thorax 1997; 52(11):1003–1009.

71. Blair PS, Fleming PJ, Bensley D, et al. Smoking and the sudden infant death syndrome: results from 1993-5 case-control study for confidential inquiry into stillbirths and deaths in infancy. Confidential Enquiry into Stillbirths and Deaths Regional Coordinators and Researchers. BMJ 1996; 313(7051):195–198.
72. Brooke H, Gibson A, Tappin D, et al. Case-control study of sudden infant death syndrome in Scotland, 1992-5. BMJ 1997; 314(7093):1516–1520.
73. MacDorman MF, Cnattingius S, Hoffman HJ, et al. Sudden infant death syndrome and smoking in the United States and Sweden. Am J Epidemiol 1997; 146(3):249–257.
74. Mitchell EA, Tuohy PG, Brunt JM, et al. Risk factors for sudden infant death syndrome following the prevention campaign in New Zealand: a prospective study. Pediatrics 1997; 100(5):835–840.
75. Kotamaki M. Smoking induced differences in autonomic responses in military pilot candidates. Clin Auton Res 1995; 5(1):31–36.
76. Lucini D, Bertocchi F, Malliani A, et al. A controlled study of the autonomic changes produced by habitual cigarette smoking in healthy subjects. Cardiovasc Res 1996; 31(4):633–639.
77. Niedermaier ON, Smith ML, Beightol LA, et al. Influence of cigarette smoking on human autonomic function. Circulation 1993; 88(2):562–571.
78. Piha SJ. Cardiovascular autonomic reflexes in heavy smokers. J Auton Nerv Syst 1994; 48(1):73–77.
79. Pope CA III, Eatough DJ, Gold DR, et al. Acute exposure to environmental tobacco smoke and heart rate variability. Environ Health Perspect 2001; 109(7):711–716.
80. Franco P, Chabanski S, Szliwowski H, et al. Influence of maternal smoking on autonomic nervous system in healthy infants. Pediatr Res 2000; 47(2):215–220.
81. Bartsch H, Nair U, Risch A, et al. Genetic polymorphism of CYP genes, alone or in combination, as a risk modifier of tobacco-related cancers. Cancer Epidemiol Biomarkers Prev 2000; 9(1):3–28.
82. Hayashi S, Watanabe J, Kawajiri K. High susceptibility to lung cancer analyzed in terms of combined genotypes of P450IA1 and Mu-class glutathione S-transferase genes. Jpn J Cancer Res 1992; 83(8):866–870.
83. Nakachi K, Imai K, Hayashi S, et al. Polymorphisms of the CYP1A1 and glutathione S-transferase genes associated with susceptibility to lung cancer in relation to cigarette dose in a Japanese population. Cancer Res 1993; 53(13):2994–2999.
84. Ishibe N, Wiencke JK, Zuo ZF, et al. Susceptibility to lung cancer in light smokers associated with CYP1A1 polymorphisms in Mexican- and African-American. Cancer Epidemiol Biomarkers Prev 1997; 6(12):1075–1080.
85. Wang X, Zuckerman B, Pearson C, et al. Maternal cigarette smoking, metabolic gene polymorphism, and infant birth weight. JAMA 2002; 287(2):195–202.
86. Rand CM, Weese-Mayer DE, Maher BS, et al. Nicotine metabolizing genes GSTT1 and CYP1A1 in sudden infant death syndrome. Am J Med Genet A 2006; 140: 1447–1452.
87. Ackerman MJ, Splawski I, Makielski JC, et al. Spectrum and prevalence of cardiac sodium channel variants among black, white, Asian, and Hispanic individuals: implications for arrhythmogenic susceptibility and Brugada/long QT syndrome genetic testing. Heart Rhythm 2004; 1:600–607.
88. Crotti L, Stramba-Badiale M, Pedrazzini M, et al. Prevalence of the Long QT syndrome. Circulation 2005; 112(suppl 2):660.

89. Goulene K, Stramba-Badiale M, Crotti L, Priori SG, et al. Neonatal electrocardiographic screening of genetic arrhythmogenic disorders and congenital cardiovascular diseases: prospective data from 31,000 infants. Eur Heart J 2005; 26 (abstr suppl):214.

90. Quaglini S, Rognoni C, Spazzolini C, et al. Cost-effectiveness of neonatal ECG screening for the long QT syndrome. Eur Heart J 2006; 27:1824–1832.

91. Zhou FC, Sari Y, Zhang JK. Expression of serotonin transporter protein in developing rat brain. Brain Res Dev Brain Res 2000; 119:33–45.

92. Brüning G, Liangos O, Baumgarten HG. Prenatal development of the serotonin transporter in mouse brain. Cell Tissue Res 1997; 289:211–221.

93. Moiseiwitsch JR, Lauder JM. Serotonin regulates mouse cranial neural crest migration. Proc Natl Acad Sci U S A 1995; 92:7182–7186.

94. Hariri AR, Mattay VS, Tessitore A, et al. Serotonin transporter genetic variation and the response of the human amygdala. Science 2002; 297:400–403.

95. Hu S, Brody CL, Fisher C, et al. Interaction between the serotonin transporter gene and neuroticism in cigarette smoking behavior. Mol Psychiatry 2000; 5:181–188.

96. Katsuragi S, Kunugi H, Sano A, et al. Association between serotonin transporter gene polymorphism and anxiety-related traits. Biol Psychiatry 1999; 45:368–370.

97. Curran S, Purcell S, Craig I, et al. The serotonin transporter gene as a QTL for ADHD. Am J Med Genet B Neuropsychiatr Genet 2005; 134(1):42–47.

98. Burton MD, Kawashima A, Brayer JA, et al. RET proto-oncogene is important for the development of respiratory CO_2 sensitivity. J Auton Nerv Syst 1997; 63:137–143.

99. Renolleau S, Dauger S, Vardon G, et al. Impaired ventilatory responses to hypoxia in mice deficient in endothelin-converting-enzyme-1. Pediatr Res 2001; 49:705–712.

100. Shirasawa S, Arata A, Onimaru H, et al. Rnx deficiency results in congenital central hypoventilation. Nat Genet 2000; 24:287–290.

101. Pattyn A, Morin X, Cremer H, et al. Expression and interactions of the two closely related homeobox genes Phox2a and Phox2b during neurogenesis. Development 1997; 124:4065–4075.

102. Garcia-Barcelo M, Sham MH, Lui VC, et al. Association study of PHOX2B as a candidate gene for Hirschsprung's disease. Gut 2003; 52:563–567.

14

Effects of Intermittent Hypoxia on the Developing Organism

KAREN A. WATERS
University of Sydney and The Children's Hospital at Westmead,
Sydney, Australia

I. Background and Introduction

Intermittent hypoxia is observed in many clinical situations. During early development, hypoxia is frequently externally imposed in an intermittent pattern. Environmental, rather than endogenous, factors during early life including the "in utero" environment may have great consequences during later life. During both the pre- and postnatal periods the supply of oxygen is an important component of overall energy balance. Hypoxia may also be compounded by environmental toxins such as nicotine in cigarette smoke. Cigarette smoke is an important environmental toxin and significant health effects have been demonstrated in infants exposed to cigarette smoke during the pre- and/or the postnatal period. In the postnatal period, new environmental factors such as sleeping in the prone sleep position become relevant. Throughout life, the most common example of a disease resulting in intermittent hypoxia is obstructive sleep apnea (OSA), which in children is most commonly associated with adenotonsillar enlargement.

Regardless of the cause, exposure to hypoxia leads to an array of respiratory, central nervous system (CNS), and systemic responses. The onset of hypoxia activates respiratory activity and stimulates arousal from sleep. With ongoing hypoxia there is a cascade of subsequent neurological and metabolic responses, including changes at the cellular level. Hypoxia is a form of cellular energy deprivation, and as hypoxia continues, adaptive mechanisms progressively shift all systems toward energy conservation. Understanding and recognizing these adaptive responses to hypoxia is the first step to understanding how intermittent, or repeated onsets of, hypoxia can modify those responses.

Recovery refers to the period that follows cessation of hypoxia and during which the animal or human system is exposed to normal or high levels of oxygen. An important characteristic of recovery periods is the time course taken for the energy conservation strategies to return to normal. Energy conservation strategies generally persist after the restoration of normal energy supplies. In the presence of a normal energy supply, energy-conserving adaptive strategies become maladaptive. During the time taken to return from an energy conserving state, even normoxia can produce a state of energy excess. The sequelae of this energy excess provide a plausible explanation for some of the disease links associated with intermittent hypoxic exposures.

Intermittent hypoxia adds new dimensions to the study of energy saving strategies that occur during hypoxia because some pathology only occurs in the presence of such fluctuating levels of oxygen. The pathology of retinopathy of prematurity is only produced under circumstances that produce both oxygen excess and oxygen deprivation (1). Intermittent hypoxic exposure induces repeated onsets of hypoxia, and some energy-conserving strategies recur or persist from cycle to cycle while others are interrupted. The periods between hypoxia are frequently referred to as "recovery periods," but it is important to recognize that they are associated with reoxygenation and therefore that they may be associated with energy excess, particularly when oxygen supplementation is provided. The resulting hyperoxia may be detrimental because it increases the range of partial pressure of O_2 in the arterial blood (PaO_2) over which the oscillation in energy occurs.

This chapter deals with intermittent exposures to whole-body and/or cellular hypoxia. Different combinations of hypoxia and recovery can result in a variety of patterns of pathology and vulnerability. A framework to understand these differences is to evaluate the strategies within a single, prolonged exposure to determine those that are likely to be favored during a particular cyclic pattern of exposure. Responses to repeated onset of hypoxia vary from mimicking repeated acute onsets with minimal chronic adaptation or adaptation equivalent to a single, prolonged period of hypoxia.

Plasticity is another important concept for understanding responses to intermittent hypoxia. During early development, there is potential for systems that are still growing and maturing to become permanently altered when they participate in adaptation to hypoxia. Such changes appear to increase the risk that maladaptive strategies will persist after the insult ceases. The nervous system exhibits considerable plasticity, whereby exposure to intermittent hypoxia can result in changes that persist into adulthood. Therefore, while plasticity enhances the short-term adaptation to hypoxia, it also translates into the more severe sequelae of intermittent hypoxia because the individual previously experienced and adapted to (was "primed by") chronic energy deprivation during early development. These priming events result in poorer tolerance to subsequent periods of energy excess. Some evidence suggests that plasticity is enhanced by intermittent exposures.

II. Clinical Context (Diseases Producing Intermittent Hypoxia)

In pediatrics, the availability of oxygen saturation monitors has led to the identification of varying degrees of repetitive hypoxia in many clinical conditions. Although the clinical value of the oximetry is sometimes debated, it has allowed the documentation that severe but brief episodes of hypoxia are a relatively frequent occurrence particularly during sleep periods (2) (Fig. 3). The addition of oxygen supplementation, on the basis of oximetry values that may be clinically undetectable, has been shown to improve clinical outcomes for infants (3). The fetus and infants have considerable tolerance to both low and high extremes of oxygen levels, although both may result in long-term tissue or end organ toxicity (4,5).

OSA is a common disease that causes repetitive or intermittent hypoxia. It has been identified from the newborn period through to adulthood. The medical importance of OSA, particularly in children, was not appreciated until the 1970s and 1980s, when Guilleminault authored several papers on the topic (6,7) and other investigators began to describe the pathological sequelae of the disease (8,9). The disease is most commonly attributed to adenotonsillar hypertrophy in toddlers and children up to the teenage years (10). Snoring is common during infancy affecting up to 26% of infants up to the age of one year (11). However, reports of clinically significant OSA in infants are most frequently associated with anatomical abnormalities, particularly craniofacial ones such as micrognathia (Pierre-Robin), or with neuromuscular disease or dysfunction (12,13).

During early development, infants also frequently experience central apnea. Infants, especially those born prematurely, frequently suffer brief episodes of hypoxia in association with spontaneous central apneic events with desaturations to <80% (14). But inhibitory reflexes are also dominant during infancy, so other stimuli can frequently precipitate reflex apnea (15). The frequency and severity of both spontaneous and reflex apneas increase with the degree of prematurity (16). Although these episodes of apnea were described in detail when infants began being monitored in intensive care settings (17), interventions to prevent or abort the events became more common as the sequelae of these perturbations in ventilation, including compromised development, became better recognized (18,19).

Factors in the antenatal or intrauterine environment can impact on postnatal function predominantly through plasticity of the fetal systems (20,21). Intrauterine growth is a strong indicator of antenatal energy supplies, and intrauterine growth retardation signals antenatal energy deprivation (22,23). Maternal nutrition is not the major determinant of fetal energy supplies. A research model for intermittent hypoxia during fetal life is intermittent umbilical cord occlusion (24). It is estimated that a 50% reduction in oxygen supply is required for permanent brain damage to occur in the fetus (4). A study of brief hypoxia in rats showed that a brief period of hypoxia per day induced intrauterine growth retardation without affecting maternal intake, whereas twice the duration of hypoxia reduced maternal intake and produced similar levels of growth retardation in the fetus (25). A simple paradigm relates the major change to a model of glucose utilization (26). Growth-retarded fetuses may be exposed to both hypoxic and hypoglycemic energy deprivation (27). Recent studies of gene expression of placental tissue suggest that several genes may be upregulated by hypoxia (28). Among these are leptin, soluble vascular endothelial growth factor receptor (sFlt-1), hypoxia inducible factor (HIF2), and human chorionic gonadotrophin (HCG) (28).

Exposure to cigarette smoke may affect the fetus as well as the infant and young child (29). During pregnancy, maternal smoking results in significant exposure of the fetus to a number of chemicals and toxins, including nicotine and carbon monoxide. Nicotine causes vasoconstriction in the placenta and less efficient delivery of oxygen to the fetus (30). Carbon monoxide binds with greater affinity to fetal than maternal hemoglobin and results in chronic hypoxia in the fetus. Therefore, the fetus exposed to cigarette smoke experiences chronic hypoxia, but may well experience additional intermittent hypoxic insults. In the postnatal environment, cigarette smoke exposure continues to be an important environmental toxin. Cigarette smoking creates significant oxidative stress that has been demonstrated in infants exposed to passive smoking (31,32).

III. Risk Factors for Sudden Infant Death Syndrome

Other important clinical situations where infants and children may be exposed to hypoxia have been identified through epidemiological studies identifying risk factors for sudden infant death syndrome (SIDS) (33). Sleeping in the facedown position (prone) is a major risk for sudden infant death (34). Prone sleeping can result in acute and chronic changes in ventilatory responses (35). The sequelae of sleeping prone include rebreathing of exhaled gases leading to suffocation, changes in sleep architecture, depressed arousal, and altered cardiorespiratory responses (36–38). Other respiratory disorders may also be associated with nocturnal hypoventilation. An important inherited disorder is congenital central hypoventilation syndrome (CCHS), a rare condition that results in hypoventilation, which is most severe in slow-wave sleep. Research into the effects of the genetic abnormality underlying this condition will be very informative regarding mechanisms of respiratory control and arousal from sleep in response to blood gas disturbances (39). Other conditions include chronic lung disease or neuromuscular disorders where the infant or child is unable to achieve adequate gas exchange.

The sequelae of diseases that cause intermittent hypoxia during development cover a variety of body systems. These include the nervous system, control of ventilation, control of glucose and its metabolism (particularly liver function), sleep architecture, and brain development. One of the major concerns is the effect on behavior and cognition in children. As with many clinical areas of medicine, the level of evidence is not ideal and more controlled studies need to be undertaken; however, there are a number of studies indicating that hypoxia does have significant effects on cognition in children (40,41). One of the major sequelae of blunted ventilatory responses is reduced arousability from sleep (42,43). Brain development can be significantly affected by hypoxia in the fetus and the infant (44). Interventions and treatments have included closer monitoring of oxygenation and treatment with supplementary drugs, oxygen, continuous positive airway pressure, or ventilation (45–47). Some of these produce secondary injury, such as bronchopulmonary dysplasia, which requires treatment strategies of its own (48).

IV. Responses to Hypoxia

Regardless of the cause, exposure to hypoxia leads to an extensively studied array of responses. The onset of hypoxia activates the peripheral chemoreceptors that lead to increased respiration and to arousal (43,49) (Fig. 1). With ongoing hypoxia, an array of neurological and metabolic responses are then stimulated, including changes at the cellular level (50). Metabolic responses include a decrease in oxygen utilization and hypometabolism (51) (Fig. 1). As hypoxia is a form of cellular energy deprivation, adaptive mechanisms initiated throughout the body, including at cellular level, during hypoxia are geared toward energy conservation (52). Understanding and recognizing these adaptive responses to hypoxia is the first step to understanding how intermittent, or repeated onsets of, hypoxia can modify those responses.

Exposure to continuous hypoxia during early development is associated with a series of sequential responses. These include an initial increase in ventilation and heart rate. If hypoxia continues, there is a secondary falloff in ventilation, which is the result of several contributing factors. These include decreased chemoreceptor responsiveness, decreased carotid body input, increased levels of inhibitory

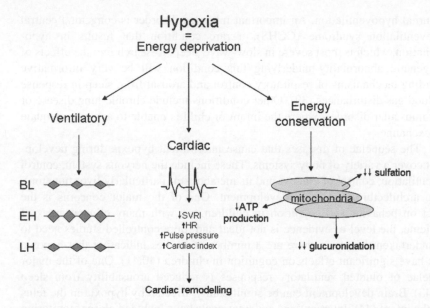

Figure 1 The responses to hypoxia include early stimulation of ventilation (represented here as a schematic of phrenic nerve activity). The early increase in ventilation is predominantly due to an increased respiratory rate but later ventilatory depression, which may be to levels at, or below baseline. In mitochondria, energy cardiac effects, including changes in vascular resistance and heart rate are detailed in the text. Changes in mitochondria primarily serve to reduce oxidative metabolism. *Abbreviations*: BL, baseline; EH, early hypoxia; LH, late hypoxia; SVRI, systemic vascular resistance index (incorporating pressure differential and cardiac output); HR, heart rate.

transmitters within the CNS, reduced metabolic rate, reduced efficiency of the respiratory pump (chest and diaphragm muscles), and decreased levels of carbon dioxide (50). At a cellular level, HIF1 is a key regulator of cellular processes that induce many of the responses to hypoxia, whether the exposure is intermittent or continuous (53,54).

Hypoxic insults result in physiological adjustments to increase oxygen delivery to the tissues. Minute ventilation increases through increased tidal volume and respiratory rate. During early infancy, the response is characterized by an early increase in ventilation followed by a secondary falloff in minute ventilation to levels that may reach below the baseline (55). This pattern is observed in human infants as well as a number of other species, and there has been extensive investigation of the contributory mechanisms for this response (55–57).The direct effect of hypoxia on the cardiovascular system is bradycardia and peripheral vasoconstriction, but because hypoxia also causes arousal (''the alerting response''), there is tachycardia with vasoconstriction in renal, splanchnic, and cutaneous circulations along with vasodilation of the skeletal muscle circulation (58,59) (Fig. 1). Local effects in the CNS serve to maintain circulation (and therefore oxygen and energy supplies) to the brain (60).

The receptors, transmitters, and pathways that are stimulated to produce these responses include stimulation of the carotid bodies, which depolarize neurons of the nucleus tractus solitarius (NTS) via glutamate-sensitive N-methyl-D-aspartate (NMDA) receptors (61). This excitation results in increased tidal volume and respiratory rate. The NTS also receives input from the sympathetic nervous system, which activates cardiac activity (62). Cardiac activity mediated from the NTS is predominantly excitatory and also mediated by glutamatergic pathways, and serotoninergic pathways appear to facilitate the excitatory responses (63,64).

Longer-term hypoxia results in a depression of ventilation and is attributable to reduced activity of the carotid body inputs at the NTS as well as the accumulation of inhibitory transmitters within the brain stem areas controlling ventilation. Adenosine plays a significant role in the central depression of ventilation (and cardiac activity) (65). Modeling suggests that the secondary decline may be entirely attributable to central depression (66). Among the neurotransmitters that are associated with central depression are GABA, adenosine, serotonin, opioids and platelet-derived growth factor (PDGF)-β (67). Clinical situations vary regarding carbon dioxide (CO_2) levels; thus, whereas experimental exposure to hypocarbic hypoxia is not associated with CO_2 retention secondary to hypoventilation, CO_2 tends to fall as ventilation becomes more effective, and this reduces the normal CO_2 stimulus, which maintains ventilation and predisposes to cycles of further apnea as well as contributes to neurological damage (68). Simultaneously, intracellular pathways including those within cytochromes and mitochondria are sensitive to the availability of oxygen and will regulate glycolytic enzymes involved in anaerobic production of ATP and other survival pathways such as phosphatidylinositol 3-kinase (PL3K/Akt) and NF-$\kappa\beta$, as well as producing free radicals that participate in the production of HIF1α (69,70). There may be some preference for suppression of nonessential mitochondrial processes where possible (52). The precise mechanism by which mitochondria detect the hypoxic environment is still debated (71). The decrease in metabolic rate that is observed during hypoxia is most marked in younger and smaller animals, resulting in decreased demand for O_2 and reduced CO_2 output (51).

V. Responses to Reoxygenation

As more information becomes available about the processes that take place during reoxygenation, it is clear that there is a similar cascade of effects, which produces both early and late changes, during early development and in

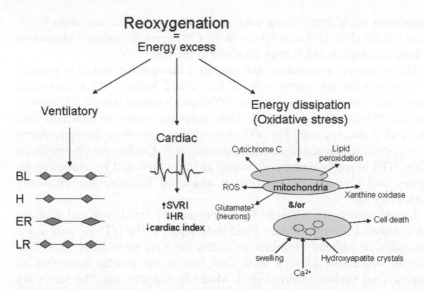

Figure 2 The responses to reoxygenation, including ventilatory, cardiac, and cellular (within mitochondria) reoxygenation. The ventilatory patterns depicted here specifically relate to the production and recovery from gasping, where Akay et al. detailed that the differences in phrenic response during early and late reoxygenation and recovery of ventilation (119). Stimulation of ventilation is represented as a schematic of phrenic nerve activity. The cardiac responses depicted here were measured in response to hyperoxia rather than to reoxygenation (59). Viable mitochondrial responses include energy dissipation by production of ROS, but mitochondria may also demonstrate calcium influx, swelling, and deposition of hydroxyapatite crystals with progression onto cell death (predominantly apoptosis). *Abbreviations*: BL, baseline; H, hypoxia; ER, early reoxygenation; LR, late reoxygenation; SVRI, systemic vascular resistance index (incorporating pressure differential and cardiac output), HR, heart rate; ROS, reactive oxygen species.

adulthood (72,73) (Fig. 2). A state of "energy excess" is induced when oxygen is delivered including the production of free radicals and oxidative stress. Restoration of normoxia in an environment adapted to energy deprivation can result in the increased production of free radicals and thus lead to cellular oxidative stress (74). The provision of oxygen during recovery periods can exacerbate the climate of energy excess, and if the internal environment has adapted to oxygen deprivation, the energy excess this produces can increase free radical production (75,76).

Energy restoration after hypoxia, or after other forms of energy deprivation, is associated with an oxidative stress at the cellular level. Processes induced by oxidative stress, such as brain damage secondary to lipid peroxidation, can be initiated during hypoxia but may continue in the recovery phase (77). This is consistent with evidence that some biochemical substances, such as xanthine oxidase that increase during hypoxia, can produce free radicals in the presence of oxygen (74,78). These cellular effects may be modified by the timing at which the hyperoxia occurs, as well as by the developmental stage of the subject (76,79).

Pre-exposure can, in some circumstances, cause sensitization to greater injury (80). The developing organisms is vulnerable to particular patterns of injury, particularly highlighted with regard to brain injury, can induce sensitization to reoxygenation injury, and these would very likely be exacerbated in intermittent hypoxic exposures (78,81). Obesity is a form of energy excess that is exacerbated by prior energy deprivation because adipose-specific suppression of thermogenesis occurs along with reduced metabolic rate of muscle, predisposing to insulin resistance (82). Large weight fluctuations increase the risk for future cardiac morbidity and mortality more than obesity per se (82).

In cells, the main effecter of the production of free radicals is the mitochondria where pathways shift to allow uncoupling of the oxidative pathways (83,84). Free radical production is a specific mechanism by which injury is produced during reoxygenation. Energy excess during recovery encourages further production of free radicals and superoxides by mitochondria, which increases with the level of oxygen, up to a saturation of 100% (76). Clinical studies now suggest that neonates recover better if they are resuscitated in room air rather than supplemental oxygen (85). However, reactive oxygen species (ROS) production is not always harmful and can enhance recovery of cardiac function (73). Free radical production is also activated in studies that utilize prior exposure to hypoxia or pharmacological agents to precondition and therefore protect against hypoxia-reperfusion injury (86). Preconditioning by exposure to hypoxia or by nutritional deprivation can lead to relative protection (tolerance) against subsequent injury by induction of protective molecules, including HIF1 (87,88).

Other cellular effects include increased adhesiveness of epithelium for T-lymphocyte (89) and increased expression and function of the GLUT 3 glucose transporter (90,91). In muscle, reoxygenation is associated with increased production of growth hormone (GH) and testosterone (92). The pro-inflammatory cytokines ↑ IL-6, IL-1b, and TNF-α, which contribute to cellular damage in the brain, are increased during reoxygenation (83). In addition, there is an almost immediate reduction in sympathetic activity mediated by nitric oxide in the brain stem (93) (Table 1).

Chronic energy excess is also associated with chronic oxidative stress. There has been considerable recent attention to oxidative stress as a mechanism for metabolic and cardiovascular complications in conditions of repetitive hypoxia and reoxygenation such as OSA (94,95). These principles can be applied to an organism that has adapted to energy deprivation and is subsequently exposed to normoxia, resulting in alterations to the glucose transport pathways (96).

Table 1 Summary of Documented Responses During Hypoxia and During
Reoxygenation

	Cellular	Serological	Whole body
Hypoxia	↓ Aerobic processes	↑ Acute glucose uptake	↓ Energy
	↓ Biosynthesis	↑ Sympathetic activity	expenditure
	↑ Anaerobic processes	↓ GH and IGF-1	↓ Metabolism
	↑ HIF1α	↑ Insulin resistance	↓ Growth
	NF-κβ	↑ Inflammatory markers	
		↑ Free fatty acids	
Reoxygenation	↑ ROS [superoxide	↑ T-lymphocyte adhesion	Obesity
	(O)] and H_2O_2	↑ GLUT 3	Chronic
	↑ RNS	↑ GH, testosterone	inflammation
	↑ xanthine oxidase	↑ IL-6, IL-1b, and TNF-α	Metabolic
		↓ Sympathetic activity	syndrome
		(BS NO)	

Not all of these relate specifically to models of intermittent hypoxia, for example, some of the responses
were measured after a single episode of ischemic hypoxia and reoxygenation. *Abbreviations*: ROS,
reactive oxygen species, RNS, Reactive nitrogen species; Metabolic syndrome, hypertension (↑BP),
Type 2 diabetes, obesity; GLUT3, glucose transporter; TNF-α, tumor necrosis factor alpha (TNF-alpha);
GH, growth hormone; BS NO, brain stem nitric oxide.

VI. Effects of Intermittent Hypoxia and Reoxygenation

In contrast to continuous hypoxia, intermittent hypoxia is characterized by
the repeated onset of hypoxia interspersed with periods of recovery. One of the
important physiological impacts of intermittent hypoxia is disruption of the
orderly cascade of adaptive processes that are initiated during a single, prolonged
exposure to hypoxia (50). This process may be beneficial or harmful depending
on the nature of the intermittent stimulus (97,98).

With regard to the hypoxic responses, the effect of the repeated onset and
cessation of hypoxia is to initiate but then disrupt the usual sequence of adaptive
responses. Some of the sensitizing effects of hypoxia, such as increased sympathetic activity or activation of inflammatory markers, are particularly harmful in the
long term (98,99). Changes in sympathetic responses have only been studied in
adults. They are thought to occur in the NTS, persistent activation of sympathetic
output and reorganization of the adrenal medulla to dampen chronic, but enhance
the acute release of catecholamines in response to hypoxia, with these changes
mediated at a cellular level by ROS and hypoxia inducible factor (100). The nature
of this sensitization also depends on the stage of development when the insult
occurs. After "chronic" intermittent hypoxia, adult rats demonstrate reversible,
long-term facilitation (increased baseline response) of the sensory response of the
carotid body. In contrast, neonates exposed to intermittent hypoxia for even a few

hours show a rapid, nonreversible induction and enhancement of the sensory response of the carotid body to hypoxia without a change in the baseline response (long-term facilitation is absent) (99). Upregulation of inflammatory markers has been demonstrated in cell lines in newborn animals and in adults after exposure to various patterns of intermittent hypoxia (98,101–103).

Prior exposure to hypoxia alters ventilatory responses to a further insult in a number of research paradigms (104). Differences attributable to intermittent compared with continuous hypoxic exposure are seen during the second and subsequent periods of hypoxia or recovery. For example, during early development, the fall in ventilation that would otherwise be observed may be attenuated, or follow a longer time course, because the repeated cycles of hypoxia and recovery interrupt or stop the adaptive processes that normally contribute to a falloff in ventilation (105). Whether ventilation is depressed or enhanced is determined by whether the exposure and recovery (cycle) times for the intermittent hypoxia are shorter or longer than the time course of the adaptive processes to enhance or depress ventilation (50). As greater chronicity of intermittent hypoxia is studied, the target of adaptation moves from carotid body to CNS to the end organs of the lungs and musculature of breathing (106,107).

At the brain stem level, postnatal exposures to intermittent hypoxia can effect changes in cardiorespiratory control areas, with effects in the dorsal motor nucleus of the vagus (DMNV) and the NTS (108,109). Infants experience episodes of intermittent hypoxia when they sleep prone or are exposed to cigarette smoke exposure, both of which are risk factors for SIDS. Prone sleeping causes hypoxia when it leads to rebreathing, and cigarette smoke causes exposure to carbon monoxide and exacerbates other respiratory illnesses. Such exposures can be modeled in animals, and changes in the brain stem of piglets after exposure to intermittent hypoxia are similar to those found in infants who died from SIDS (109,110). It appears that during early development, the longer the time course of the exposure to hypoxia (intermittent or sustained), the greater the pattern moves toward recovery of functionally normal ventilation, regardless of the abnormalities that are demonstrable.

VII. Specific Effects of Intermittent Hypoxia and Reoxygenation Cycle During Early Development

A. Ventilation and Ventilatory Responses

Among the responses to hypoxia, a number of processes have been shown to exhibit plasticity. These include serotoninergic, adrenergic, and NMDA pathways with downstream molecules such as nitric oxide and protein kinase C (27,111). During early development, compensatory mechanisms at both vascular and cellular levels work to minimize the impact of both hypoxia and hyperoxia in organs such as the brain and kidney (75,79).

In the newborn, evidence for adaptive responses that show less activation during succeeding cycles is stronger for arousal than for ventilation (43,112). Prolonged hypoxic or hyperoxic exposure results in depression of ventilatory responses in adulthood by depressing development of the carotid body chemoreflex response (113–115). After intermittent hypoxia, serotonin-dependent long-term facilitation is now a well-described response (116,117). Some studies demonstrate subsequent depression of ventilation, and others show enhancement of the ventilatory response to subsequent hypoxia (118). These variations may be attributable to species differences, differences in the developmental stage, and/or differences in the pattern of exposure (107). After hypoxia severe enough to induce gasping, there is no initial increase in the rate of phrenic discharge although there is an increase in the duration of the bursts with full recovery to baseline after 30 minutes in piglets (119). Cardiac output initially increases, then decreases during hypoxia with recovery to baseline during reoxygenation, with the main mechanisms for changes in the cardiac system being tachycardia throughout all phases, including the reoxygenation phase (120).

B. Metabolism During Early Development

During an acute exposure to hypoxia, a relatively unique feature of early development is the ability to drop the metabolic rate by reducing whole-body oxygen consumption per unit time (VO_2). The characteristics of such hypometabolism have been extensively investigated by Mortola and colleagues (121,122). The main contributing process is a drop in body temperature, with reduced production of CO_2, and as hypoxia continues, there is reduced tissue growth and reduced tissue differentiation. In the long term, this may lead to changes such as persisting alterations in mechanical properties of the respiratory system or changes in ventilatory control responses that persist into adulthood, but metabolic rate apparently returns rapidly to normal after return to normoxia (123).

Glucose metabolism, particularly hepatic glucose metabolism, is affected by hypoxia, but exposure to hypoxia by sleep apnea also has implications for metabolic syndrome. The results of hypoxic exposure may also differ depending on whether or not this occurs on a background of obesity. Hyperinsulinemic euglycemic clamp studies report that intermittent hypercapnic hypoxia in genetically normal, lean mice reduces whole-body insulin sensitivity (increase insulin resistance) (124). In a study comparing lean mice with and without exposure to intermittent hypoxia, lean mice showed an upregulation of leptin but no change in insulin resistance, whereas leptin-deficient obese mice developed significant insulin resistance (125). The fact that obesity constitutes chronic oxidative stress is also seen as a possible mechanism for long-term morbidity associated with obesity per se (126,127).

C. Sleep (Arousal and Clarification of Arousal Frequency in Early Development)

Sleep itself is susceptible to intermittent hypoxia. During sleep, the onset of hypoxia is associated with arousal (128). Given the vulnerabilities to hypoxia that are associated with sleep, arousal is an important protective response to the onset of hypoxia that, in the short term, does not habituate (129). However, younger infants and children do not always arouse in response to hypoxia (104).

Although arousal seems to predominate in rapid eye movement (REM) sleep in response to hypoxia for infants (128), sleep deprivation has been associated with an increase in the number of obstructive apneas (130). Snoring, whether associated with desaturation or frequent arousals that have been linked to snoring without hypoxia, has been associated with lower scores on neurocognitive testing for young infants and children (131,132).

Sleep deprivation has been demonstrated to precipitate abnormalities of glucose metabolism, dysregulation of appetite, and decreased energy expenditure, all of which predispose to diabetes and obesity (133,134). In addition to these effects, there is thought to be an increased stress-associated change, including increased appetite associated with an increase in the grehlin/leptin ratio, increased levels of pro-inflammatory cytokines, decreased parasympathetic and increased sympathetic tone, increased blood pressure, increased evening cortisol, and elevated insulin and glucose levels (135). Some of these stress responses can be precipitated by hypoxia (as a stressor), including changes in insulin and glucose, metabolism, and blood pressure, as detailed above.

Some of these dysregulatory processes may be through common stress pathways, particularly HIFs (2 and 3, not 1α, which is responsible for downstream effects of hypoxia) and corticosteroids, which can be activated by other forms of energy disturbance, particularly hypoglycemia (53,136) (137). The common associations among obesity, sleep disorders, and other forms of stress such as depression and other mental disorders are being increasingly recognized. Whether this is due to a single common denominator is still much debated (138,139). Repeated stress is associated with structural remodeling in brain regions associated with memory and emotions, including the hippocampus, amygdala, and prefrontal cortex (140). Memory is impaired and anxiety and aggression are increased (141). Extrapolating from other studies, functional brain activity (especially in these regions) is also impaired when exposed to hyperinsulinemia and hyperglycemia. Extrapolating from animal studies, depletion of glycogen stores, increased oxidative stress, and free radical production are contributors to such brain dysfunction (135,142).

The effect of reoxygenation likely depends on the severity and duration of the preceding anoxia or hypoxia, and free radical production may occur during moderate hypoxia, but is not present in severe hypoxia (143). Where hypoxic injury is limited, reoxygenation in the young animal can be associated with increased energy expenditure as in the newborn experiencing catch-up growth (121). If the cells have been irreversibly damaged, then the replenishment of oxygen cannot recover function. In studies of neurological damage after hypoxia, a penumbral zone is defined as a region where cells show unstable but potentially recoverable function (144). However, the finding of potentially recoverable cells after such an insult also extends to other tissues, and these cells are a target for various therapeutic options (145).

D. Brain Pathology with Changes in Learning and Daytime Behavior

It is well known that brain injury occurs in response to severe or prolonged hypoxia. However, the spectrum of disorders arising from brief, less severe, or repeated episodes of hypoxia is still being defined. A specific impetus for evaluating these latter responses is clinical research suggesting that neuro psychological abnormalities may occur secondary to OSA during early development with debate on the relative contributions of sleep deprivation and hypoxia as contributing mechanisms (146,147). The clinical imperative is to determine the threshold of sleep disturbance and/or hypoxic exposure that would cause subsequent (and/or irreversible) neurological dysfunction, especially now that brain changes have been demonstrated on magnetic resonance spectroscopy (MRS) imaging (148). There is some evidence in pediatric studies that memory dysfunction in children is more closely associated with sleep disruption than with hypoxia (131). Children whose oxygen saturation levels remain within normal limits and whose apnea indices are not different from control children showed neurocognitive (memory) dysfunction in proportion to their respiratory arousals (sleep disturbance) (147). Thus, consideration of non–respiratory sleep disorders will also be important in the future (131).

A number of studies have assessed the relative recovery of brain function or neurons depending on whether recovery from hypoxia is undertaken in hyperoxia or normoxia (i.e., 21% oxygen) (85). Control of tissue oxygenation limits the magnitude of subsequent neurological injury, suggesting that energy excess in this tissue is damaging during recovery, whether due to hyperoxia or hyperglycemia, although apparently by different pathways (136,149). The time course of these changes is important, so a biphasic change may mean that early studies suggest limited damage, whereas prolonged observation reveals a second wave of damage during recovery such as in apoptosis within the brain (72). The recovery of responses may also differ depending on the nature of the preceding hypoxia. Paradoxically, one study demonstrated that recovery of nonessential aerobic pathways in mitochondria of hepatocytes was slower after "acute" compared with "chronic" exposure to hypoxia (52). The stage of development at which exposure occurs can influence which pathways respond preferentially to the different stimuli. Finally, and specifically with regard to intermittent hypoxia, the number and duration of cycles required to produce the particular effect can differ. For example, protection of the myocardium against arrhythmias during subsequent hypoventilation required at least three prior cycles of five-minute hypercapnic hypoxia (pO_2 49.9 ± 13.5 mmHg, and pCO_2 61.6 ± 8.6 mmHg, pH 7.093 ± 0.097) and five-minute recovery, raising the possibility of thresholds for the effect (150).

In clinical situations, another factor that may contribute to brain injury is the intermittent disturbances in CO_2 that almost always accompany intermittent hypoxia. Exposure to hypoxia is the focus of most studies because of the correlations between hypoxic exposure and clinical sequelae. Clinically, hypoxia is most often associated with hypercapnia, which exacerbates any tendency toward acidosis, reduces the autoregulation of cerebral blood flow, and is at least partly responsible for ventilatory responses of the whole organism during the exposure (68,151) (Fig. 3). Evidence of brain injury has been demonstrated in animal studies of both hyper- and hypocapnia, suggesting that any perturbations of CO_2 that accompany hypoxia may exacerbate the injury observed (68).

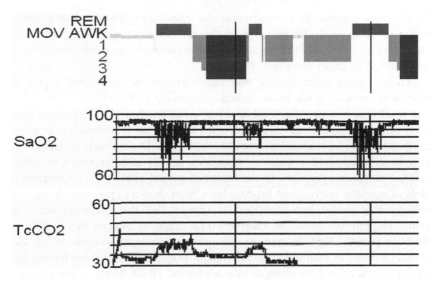

Figure 3 Changes in oxygen (saturation) and carbon dioxide (transcutaneous) observed during sleep. Intermittent hypoxia in this disease is generally associated with hypercapnia. There are also three time cycles over which the hypoxia is repeated: (1) Repetitive hypoxia occurs at rapidly recurring (frequent) intervals almost exclusively during REM sleep (2). These bouts of hypoxia also recur at the intervals that separate REM sleep periods (3). Finally, those two time cycles recur with sleep and are not generally present during wakefulness. *Abbreviations*: REM, rapid eye movement (sleep); NREM, non–rapid eye movement (sleep); MOV, movement; AWK, awake, sleep states are represented as awake, and stages 1, 2, 3, and 4 NREM sleep, as well as, REM sleep; $SaO_2(\%)$, arterial oxygen saturation measured by oximeter; $TcPCO_2$ (mmHg), transcutaneous carbon dioxide tension.

VIII. Plasticity

The major importance of the underlying changes in maturation is that during early development, many systems are plastic, meaning that they can still change and adapt. Plasticity refers to persistence of changes after removal of the stimulus that induced those changes (152). During early development, the maturation of these systems is not only incomplete but the pattern of ongoing development is clearly under the ongoing influence of external or environmental factors (153).

Breathing control exhibits plasticity throughout life in response to (1) hypoxia or chemoafferent neuron activation, (2) abnormal O_2 levels or stress during development, (3) exercise, (4) hypercapnia, (5) sensory denervation, (6) neural injury, and (7) conditioning. Neuroplasticity in the respiratory system helps to maintain regulatory function in the face of normal development and aging, altered environmental conditions, and cardiopulmonary or brain injury or disease (116). The long developmental period (in utero until several months after birth) provides opportunity for environmental interactions that can lead to long-standing or permanent changes in how the system develops. The points and mechanisms by which such plasticity can occur during early development have been reviewed in detail elsewhere (154).

These studies make it clear that plasticity can be considered a part of normal development. It has been studied extensively in the visual system, also giving rise to the concept of critical developmental windows (155). Critical time periods reflect a stage of development when the system is vulnerable to influences that may not have great influence at other times. During early development long-term depression of ventilatory responses occurs after exposure to either hyperoxia or chronic hypoxia in the neonatal period (154,156). Experimental models of neonatal intermittent hypoxia have been shown to produce changes in ventilation that persist into adulthood. It appears that these changes occur in response to perturbation of the relatively low range of oxygen that is normal during that period (156). In contrast, intermittent exposure to hypoxia has the potential to result in facilitation of subsequent responses, while also having the potential to maintain these changes into adulthood (105). Many of the changes that occur in the respiratory network are mediated by the serotoninergic system (107,116). Exposure to CO_2 has a limited duration of effect, which is not unique to early development and does not persist into adulthood (157). Antenatal exposure to hypoxia appears to produce enhancement of the postnatal responses to an acute hypoxic stimulus (156). The areas that are most affected appear to be the carotid body, chemoafferent neurons, diaphragm, and possibly other aspects of pulmonary mechanics (156).

The "Barker hypothesis" is now a well-known clinical context for plasticity in response to prolonged energy deprivation affecting metabolic function in a lifelong manner. Barker first described an association between low birth weight and cardiac disease in adulthood (158); however, subsequent studies have demonstrated association with other diseases and the term "Barker hypothesis" has come to describe the fetal origins of adult disease (159). The original pathology associated with the Barker hypothesis is that a compromised in utero environment, illustrated by infants who were born growth retarded, increases an individual's risk for ischemic heart disease (IHD) in adulthood (158). The risk for IHD is amplified as the amount of energy excess during the immediate postnatal recovery period increases, so the risk for adult IHD is greater with more rapid postnatal weight gain or even weight gain after a period of considerable weight loss in later life (21,82). In either case, this weight gain is particularly pertinent to factors underlying risk for cardiac disease such as obesity, hypertension, insulin resistance, and type 2 diabetes (82).

Infants who are small for their gestational age are vulnerable to disease later in life. The mechanisms underlying this vulnerability include a reduced number of cells in some organs such as the kidneys (160). A second mechanism is the "thrifty hypothesis"; their system is geared to efficient use of substrates so hormonal and cellular responses are altered to maintain blood glucose levels for the brain, at the expense of transporting glucose into the muscles for activity or growth. The third mechanism is apparent poor tolerance to environmental perturbations with excessive (or increased) stress responses that translate into increased blood pressure and increased blood glucose. Regardless of the mechanism, the increase in cardiovascular disease also relates to the rate of increased weight gain or growth that occurs after the initial growth retardation, and those infants with higher rates of weight gain show increased risk for disease (160).

IX. Models of Intermittent Hypoxia

Investigators who model intermittent hypoxia during early development use different durations of hypoxia and recovery. Different components of the "cascade" of responses to (hypercapnic) hypoxia show different time courses of response, and stimulus intervals will potentially disrupt either the induction or the cessation of these responses. Patterns of rapidly repeated intermittent hypoxia may cause repeated onset of the acute adaptive response with complete failure to transition chronic adaptation. Alternatively, slower cycles of intermittent hypoxia may induce disrupted transition to chronic adaptation so that some, but not other aspects of the chronic adaptation response occur. This can result in a variety of patterns of vulnerability and pathology.

The patterns of intermittent hypoxia that are seen clinically do not follow well-ordered intervals with specific cycle times, so it is likely that more complex modeling would be required to predict the final outcome of intermittent hypoxia in association with illness (Fig. 3). Nonetheless, the studies that utilize prolonged or discrete cycle times of exposure provide information about the time course of various responses, which is vital information for complex modeling as well as for developing relevant therapeutic interventions (119,161,162). A framework to understand these differences is to evaluate the energy-saving strategies that are favored during any particular pattern of exposures. A shift among strategies appears to be dependent on patterns of exposure, so that the repeated onset of hypoxia may vary from acute responses without chronic adaptation or adaptation equivalent to a single, prolonged period of hypoxia.

X. Implications of Current Research and Future Directions

The study of intermittent hypoxia is an exciting area that requires an understanding of processes that are elicited during hypoxia, but also during reoxygenation. Repeated episodes of hypoxia and reoxygenation create a dynamic interplay between these contrasting insults. Factors that influence the outcome include the rapidity of onset and offset, severity of the stimulus (energy deprivation and energy excess), developmental stage of the subject, and the cycle duration and frequency, as well as the duration and refractory period of various responses that are being interrupted. The developmental stage of the subject, cycle duration, and cycle frequency tend to affect which systems exhibit plasticity. Screening for sequelae assists the search for treatments that will limit the negative impact of these responses in clinical situations.

References

1. Tasman W, Patz A, McNamara JA, et al. Retinopathy of prematurity: the life of a lifetime disease. Am J Ophthalmol 2006; 141(1):167–174.
2. Salyer JW. Neonatal and pediatric pulse oximetry. Respir Care 2003; 48(4): 386–396; discussion 97–98.
3. Poets CF. When do infants need additional inspired oxygen? A review of the current literature. Pediatr Pulmonol 1998; 26(6):424–428.
4. Parer JT. Effects of fetal asphyxia on brain cell structure and function: limits of tolerance. Comp Biochem Physiol A Mol Integr Physiol 1998; 119(3):711–716.
5. Bhandari V, Elias JA. Cytokines in tolerance to hyperoxia-induced injury in the developing and adult lung. Free Radic Biol Med 2006; 41(1):4–18.
6. Guilleminault C, Korobkin R, Winkle R. A review of 50 children with obstructive sleep apnea syndrome. Lung 1981; 159(5):275–287.
7. Guilleminault C, Eldridge FL, Simmons FB, et al. Sleep apnea in eight children. Pediatrics 1976; 58(1):23–30.
8. Brouillette RT, Fernbach SK, Hunt CE. Obstructive sleep apnea in infants and children. J Pediatr 1982; 100(1):31–40.
9. Hunt CE, Brouillette RT. Abnormalities of breathing control and airway maintenance in infants and children as a cause of cor pulmonale. Pediatr Cardiol 1982; 3(3): 249–256.
10. Rosen CL. Clinical features of obstructive sleep apnea hypoventilation syndrome in otherwise healthy children. Pediatr Pulmonol 1999; 27(6):403–409.
11. Mitchell EA, Thompson JM. Snoring in the first year of life. Acta Paediatr 2003; 92(4): 425–429.
12. Goldberg S, Shatz A, Picard E, et al. Endoscopic findings in children with obstructive sleep apnea: effects of age and hypotonia. Pediatr Pulmonol 2005; 40(3): 205–210.
13. Lin SY, Halbower AC, Tunkel DE, et al. Relief of upper airway obstruction with mandibular distraction surgery: long-term quantitative results in young children. Arch Otolaryngol Head Neck Surg 2006; 132(4):437–441.
14. Richard D, Poets CF, Neale S, et al. Arterial oxygen saturation in preterm neonates without respiratory failure. J Pediatr 1993; 123(6):963–968.
15. Martin RJ, Abu-Shaweesh JM. Control of breathing and neonatal apnea. Biol Neonate 2005; 87(4):288–295.
16. Theobald K, Botwinski C, Albanna S, et al. Apnea of prematurity: diagnosis, implications for care, and pharmacologic management. Neonatal Netw 2000; 19(6): 17–24.
17. Roberton NR. Effect of acute hypoxia on blood pressure and electroencephalogram of newborn babies. Arch Dis Child 1969; 44(238):719–725.
18. Finer NN, Higgins R, Kattwinkel J, et al. Summary proceedings from the apnea-of-prematurity group. Pediatrics 2006; 117(3 pt 2):S47–S51.
19. Janvier A, Khairy M, Kokkotis A, et al. Apnea is associated with neurodevelopmental impairment in very low birth weight infants. J Perinatol 2004; 24(12): 763–768.
20. Gluckman PD, Cutfield W, Hofman P, et al. The fetal, neonatal, and infant environments-the long-term consequences for disease risk. Early Hum Dev 2005; 81(1): 51–59.

21. Barker DJ. The developmental origins of adult disease. J Am Coll Nutr 2004; 23 (6 suppl):588S–595S.
22. Luther JS, Redmer DA, Reynolds LP, et al. Nutritional paradigms of ovine fetal growth restriction: implications for human pregnancy. Hum Fertil (Camb) 2005; 8(3):179–187.
23. Schroder HJ. Models of fetal growth restriction. Eur J Obstet Gynecol Reprod Biol 2003; 110(suppl 1):S29–S39.
24. Bennet L, Roelfsema V, George S, et al. The effect of cerebral hypothermia on white and grey matter injury induced by severe hypoxia in preterm fetal sheep. J Physiol 2007; 578(pt 2):491–506.
25. Schwartz JE, Kovach A, Meyer J, et al. Brief, intermittent hypoxia restricts fetal growth in Sprague-Dawley rats. Biol Neonate 1998; 73(5):313–319.
26. Hay WW Jr. Recent observations on the regulation of fetal metabolism by glucose. J Physiol 2006; 572(pt 1):17–24.
27. Wallace JM, Regnault TR, Limesand SW, et al. Investigating the causes of low birth weight in contrasting ovine paradigms. J Physiol 2005; 565(pt 1):19–26.
28. McCarthy C, Cotter FE, McElwaine S, et al. Altered gene expression patterns in intrauterine growth restriction: potential role of hypoxia. Am J Obstet Gynecol 2007; 196(1):70.e1–70.e6.
29. Cook DG, Strachan DP. Health effects of passive smoking-10: summary of effects of parental smoking on the respiratory health of children and implications for research. Thorax 1999; 54(4):357–366.
30. Dempsey DA, Benowitz NL. Risks and benefits of nicotine to aid smoking cessation in pregnancy. Drug Saf 2001; 24(4):277–322.
31. Morrow JD, Frei B, Longmire AW, et al. Increase in circulating products of lipid peroxidation (F2-isoprostanes) in smokers. Smoking as a cause of oxidative damage. N Engl J Med 1995; 332(18):1198–1203.
32. Noakes PS, Thomas R, Lane C, et al. Association of maternal smoking with increased infant oxidative stress at 3 months of age. Thorax 2007; 62(8):714–117.
33. Kleemann WJ, Schlaud M, Fieguth A, et al. Body and head position, covering of the head by bedding and risk of sudden infant death (SID). Int J Legal Med 1999; 112(1):22–26.
34. Mitchell EA. Recommendations for sudden infant death syndrome prevention: a discussion document. Arch Dis Child 2007; 92(2):155–159.
35. Galland BC, Bolton DP, Taylor BJ, et al. Ventilatory sensitivity to mild asphyxia: prone versus supine sleep position. Arch Dis Child 2000; 83(5):423–428.
36. Guntheroth WG, Spiers PS. Are bedding and rebreathing suffocation a cause of SIDS? Pediatr Pulmonol 1996; 22(6):335–341.
37. Horne RS, Parslow PM, Ferens D, et al. Arousal responses and risk factors for sudden infant death syndrome. Sleep Med 2002; 3(suppl 2):S61–S65.
38. Horne RS, Franco P, Adamson TM, et al. Effects of body position on sleep and arousal characteristics in infants. Early Hum Dev 2002; 69(1–2):25–33.
39. Gaultier C, Amiel J, Dauger S, et al. Genetics and early disturbances of breathing control. Pediatr Res 2004; 55(5):729–733.
40. Ebert CS Jr., Drake AF. The impact of sleep-disordered breathing on cognition and behavior in children: a review and meta-synthesis of the literature. Otolaryngol Head Neck Surg 2004; 131(6):814–826.

41. Bass JL, Corwin M, Gozal D, et al. The effect of chronic or intermittent hypoxia on cognition in childhood: a review of the evidence. Pediatrics 2004; 114(3):805–816.

42. Hunt CE. Impaired arousal from sleep: relationship to sudden infant death syndrome. J Perinatol 1989; 9(2):184–187.

43. Waters KA, Tinworth KD. Habituation of arousal responses after intermittent hypercapnic hypoxia in piglets. Am J Respir Crit Care Med 2005; 171(11): 1305–1311.

44. Billiards SS, Pierson CR, Haynes RL, et al. Is the late preterm infant more vulnerable to gray matter injury than the term infant? Clin Perinatol 2006; 33(4): 915–933.

45. McNamara HM, Dildy GA III. Continuous intrapartum pH, pO_2, pCO_2, and SpO_2 monitoring. Obstet Gynecol Clin North Am 1999; 26(4):671–693.

46. Perlman JM. Intervention strategies for neonatal hypoxic-ischemic cerebral injury. Clin Ther 2006; 28(9):1353–1365.

47. Kennedy JD, Waters KA. 8. Investigation and treatment of upper-airway obstruction: childhood sleep disorders I. Med J Aust 2005; 182(8):419–423.

48. Ambalavanan N, Carlo WA. Ventilatory strategies in the prevention and management of bronchopulmonary dysplasia. Semin Perinatol 2006; 30(4):192–199.

49. Carroll JL, Bureau MA. Peripheral chemoreceptor $CO2$ response during hyperoxia in the 14-day-old awake lamb. Respir Physiol 1988; 73(3):339–349.

50. Waters KA, Gozal D. Responses to hypoxia during early development. Respir Physiol Neurobiol 2003; 136(2–3):115–29.

51. Mortola JP. How newborn mammals cope with hypoxia. Respir Physiol 1999; 116 (2–3):95–103.

52. Subramanian RM, Chandel N, Budinger GR, et al. Hypoxic conformance of metabolism in primary rat hepatocytes: a model of hepatic hibernation. Hepatology 2007; 45(2):455–464.

53. Semenza GL. Regulation of physiological responses to continuous and intermittent hypoxia by hypoxia-inducible factor 1. Exp Physiol 2006; 91(5):803–806.

54. Semenza GL, Shimoda LA, Prabhakar NR. Regulation of gene expression by HIF-1. Novartis Found Symp 2006; 272:2–8; discussion, 14, 33–36.

55. Rigatto H. Ventilatory response to hypoxia. Semin Perinatol 1977; 1(4):357–362.

56. Mortola JP, Rezzonico R. Metabolic and ventilatory rates in newborn kittens during acute hypoxia. Respir Physiol 1988; 73(1):55–67.

57. Cohen G, Malcolm G, Henderson-Smart D. Ventilatory response of the newborn infant to mild hypoxia. Pediatr Pulmonol 1997; 24(3):163–172.

58. Marshall JM. The Joan Mott Prize Lecture. The integrated response to hypoxia: from circulation to cells. Exp Physiol 1999; 84(3):449–470.

59. Thomson AJ, Drummond GB, Waring WS, et al. Effects of short-term isocapnic hyperoxia and hypoxia on cardiovascular function. J Appl Physiol 2006; 101(3): 809–816.

60. Acker T, Acker H. Cellular oxygen sensing need in CNS function: physiological and pathological implications. J Exp Biol 2004; 207(pt 18):3171–3188.

61. Sapru HN. Carotid chemoreflex. Neural pathways and transmitters. Adv Exp Med Biol 1996; 410:357–364.

62. Milner TA, Pickel VM. Receptor targeting in medullary nuclei mediating baroreceptor reflexes. Cell Mol Neurobiol 2003; 23(4–5):751–760.

63. Lawrence AJ, Jarrott B. Neurochemical modulation of cardiovascular control in the nucleus tractus solitarius. Prog Neurobiol 1996; 48(1):21–53.

64. Raul L. Serotonin2 receptors in the nucleus tractus solitarius: characterization and role in the baroreceptor reflex arc. Cell Mol Neurobiol 2003; 23(4–5):709–726.

65. Phillis JW, Scislo TJ, O'Leary DS. Purines and the nucleus tractus solitarius: effects on cardiovascular and respiratory function. Clin Exp Pharmacol Physiol 1997; 24(9–10):738–742.

66. Zhou H, Saidel GM, Cabrera ME. Multi-organ system model of O_2 and CO_2 transport during isocapnic and poikilocapnic hypoxia. Respir Physiol Neurobiol 2007; 156(3):320–330.

67. Simakajornboon N, Kuptanon T. Maturational changes in neuromodulation of central pathways underlying hypoxic ventilatory response. Respir Physiol Neurobiol 2005; 149(1–3):273–286.

68. Fritz KI, Delivoria-Papadopoulos M. Mechanisms of injury to the newborn brain. Clin Perinatol 2006; 33(3):573–591, v.

69. Tamatani M, Mitsuda N, Matsuzaki H, et al. A pathway of neuronal apoptosis induced by hypoxia/reoxygenation: roles of nuclear factor-kappaB and Bcl-2. J Neurochem 2000; 75(2):683–693.

70. Chandel NS, Budinger GR. The cellular basis for diverse responses to oxygen. Free Radic Biol Med 2007; 42(2):165–174.

71. Lahiri S, Roy A, Baby SM, et al. Oxygen sensing in the body. Prog Biophys Mol Biol 2006; 91(3):249–286.

72. Parker J, Ashraf QM, Akhter W, et al. Effect of post-hypoxic reoxygenation on DNA fragmentation in cortical neuronal nuclei of newborn piglets. Neurosci Lett 2007; 412(3):273–277.

73. Sarre A, Lange N, Kucera P, et al. mitoKATP channel activation in the postanoxic developing heart protects E-C coupling via NO-, ROS-, and PKC-dependent pathways. Am J Physiol Heart Circ Physiol 2005; 288(4):H1611–H1619.

74. Saugstad OD. Oxidative stress in the newborn–a 30-year perspective. Biol Neonate 2005; 88(3):228–236.

75. Richards JG, Todd KG, Emara M, et al. A dose-response study of graded reoxygenation on the carotid haemodynamics, matrix metalloproteinase-2 activities and amino acid concentrations in the brain of asphyxiated newborn piglets. Resuscitation 2006; 69(2):319–327.

76. Vereczki V, Martin E, Rosenthal RE, et al. Normoxic resuscitation after cardiac arrest protects against hippocampal oxidative stress, metabolic dysfunction, and neuronal death. J Cereb Blood Flow Metab 2006; 26(6):821–835.

77. Mishra OP, Delivoria-Papadopoulos M. Cellular mechanisms of hypoxic injury in the developing brain. Brain Res Bull 1999; 48(3):233–238.

78. Buonocore G, Perrone S, Bracci R. Free radicals and brain damage in the newborn. Biol Neonate 2001; 79(3–4):180–186.

79. Adachi S, Zelenin S, Matsuo Y, et al. Cellular response to renal hypoxia is different in adolescent and infant rats. Pediatr Res 2004; 55(3):485–491.

80. Hagberg H, Dammann O, Mallard C, et al. Preconditioning and the developing brain. Semin Perinatol 2004; 28(6):389–395.

81. Painter MJ. Animal models of perinatal asphyxia: contributions, contradictions, clinical relevance. Semin Pediatr Neurol 1995; 2(1):37–56.

82. Dulloo AG, Jacquet J, Seydoux J, et al. The thrifty 'catch-up fat' phenotype: its impact on insulin sensitivity during growth trajectories to obesity and metabolic syndrome. Int J Obes (Lond) 2006; 30(suppl 4):S23–S35.

83. Feng Y, LeBlanc MH. Effect of agmatine on the time course of brain inflammatory cytokines after injury in rat pups. Ann N Y Acad Sci 2003; 1009:152–156.

84. Arsenijevic D, Onuma H, Pecqueur C, et al. Disruption of the uncoupling protein-2 gene in mice reveals a role in immunity and reactive oxygen species production. Nat Genet 2000; 26(4):435–439.

85. Saugstad OD. Room air resuscitation-two decades of neonatal research. Early Hum Dev 2005; 81(1):111–116.

86. Ljubkovic M, Mio Y, Marinovic J, et al. Isoflurane preconditioning uncouples mitochondria and protects against hypoxia-reoxygenation. Am J Physiol Cell Physiol 2007; 292(5):C1583–C1590.

87. Trescher WH, Lehman RA, Vannucci RC. The influence of growth retardation on perinatal hypoxic-ischemic brain damage. Early Hum Dev 1990; 21(3):165–173.

88. Sharp FR, Ran R, Lu A, et al. Hypoxic preconditioning protects against ischemic brain injury. NeuroRx 2004; 1(1):26–35.

89. Kokura S, Wolf RE, Yoshikawa T, et al. Endothelial cells exposed to anoxia/reoxygenation are hyperadhesive to T-lymphocytes: kinetics and molecular mechanisms. Microcirculation 2000; 7(1):13–23.

90. Devaskar SU, Rajakumar PA, Mink RB, et al. Effect of development and hypoxic-ischemia upon rabbit brain glucose transporter expression. Brain Res 1999; 823 (1–2):113–128.

91. Zovein A, Flowers-Ziegler J, Thamotharan S, et al. Postnatal hypoxic-ischemic brain injury alters mechanisms mediating neuronal glucose transport. Am J Physiol Regul Integr Comp Physiol 2004; 286(2):R273–R282.

92. Hoffman JR, Im J, Rundell KW, et al. Effect of muscle oxygenation during resistance exercise on anabolic hormone response. Med Sci Sports Exerc 2003; 35(11): 1929–1934.

93. Zanzinger J, Czachurski J, Seller H. Nitric oxide in the ventrolateral medulla regulates sympathetic responses to systemic hypoxia in pigs. Am J Physiol 1998; 275(1 Pt 2):R33–R39.

94. Lavie L. Obstructive sleep apnoea syndrome–an oxidative stress disorder. Sleep Med Rev 2003; 7(1):35–51.

95. Prabhakar NR. Sleep apneas: an oxidative stress? Am J Respir Crit Care Med 2002; 165(7):859–860.

96. Bruckner BA, Ammini CV, Otal MP, et al. Regulation of brain glucose transporters by glucose and oxygen deprivation. Metabolism 1999; 48(4):422–431.

97. Manukhina EB, Downey HF, Mallet RT. Role of nitric oxide in cardiovascular adaptation to intermittent hypoxia. Exp Biol Med (Maywood) 2006; 231(4): 343–365.

98. Ryan S, McNicholas WT, Taylor CT. A critical role for p38 map kinase in NF-kappaB signaling during intermittent hypoxia/reoxygenation. Biochem Biophys Res Commun 2007; 355(3):728–733.

99. Prabhakar NR, Dick TE, Nanduri J, et al. Systemic, cellular and molecular analysis of chemoreflex-mediated sympathoexcitation by chronic intermittent hypoxia. Exp Physiol 2007; 92(1):39–44.

100. Prabhakar NR, Peng YJ, Kumar GK, et al. Altered carotid body function by intermittent hypoxia in neonates and adults: relevance to recurrent apneas. Respir Physiol Neurobiol 2007; 157(1):148–153.

101. Altay T, Gonzales ER, Park TS, et al. Cerebrovascular inflammation after brief episodic hypoxia: modulation by neuronal and endothelial nitric oxide synthase. J Appl Physiol discussion 196 2004; 96(3):1223–1230.

102. Tam C, Wong M, Tam K, et al. The effect of acute intermittent hypercapnic hypoxia treatment on IL-6, TNF-alpha, and CRP levels in piglets. Sleep 2007; 30 (6):723–727.

103. Ryan S, Taylor CT, McNicholas WT. Selective activation of inflammatory pathways by intermittent hypoxia in obstructive sleep apnea syndrome. Circulation 2005; 112(17):2660–2667.

104. Fewell JE. Protective responses of the newborn to hypoxia. Respir Physiol Neurobiol 2005; 149(1–3):243–255.

105. Reeves SR, Gozal D. Developmental plasticity of respiratory control following intermittent hypoxia. Respir Physiol Neurobiol 2005; 149(1–3):301–311.

106. Peng Y, Yuan G, Overholt JL, et al. Systemic and cellular responses to intermittent hypoxia: evidence for oxidative stress and mitochondrial dysfunction. Adv Exp Med Biol 2003; 536:559–564.

107. Mahamed S, Mitchell GS. Is there a link between intermittent hypoxia-induced respiratory plasticity and obstructive sleep apnoea? Exp Physiol 2007; 92(1):27–37.

108. Machaalani R, Waters KA. NMDA receptor 1 expression in the brainstem of human infants and its relevance to the sudden infant death syndrome (SIDS). J Neuropathol Exp Neurol 2003; 62(10):1076–1085.

109. Say M, Machaalani R, Waters KA. Changes in serotoninergic receptors 1A and 2A in the piglet brainstem after intermittent hypercapnic hypoxia (IHH) and nicotine. Brain Res 2007; 1152:17–26.

110. Kinney HC. Abnormalities of the brainstem serotonergic system in the sudden infant death syndrome: a review. Pediatr Dev Pathol 2005; 8(5):507–524.

111. Herlenius E, Lagercrantz H. Development of neurotransmitter systems during critical periods. Exp Neurol 2004; 190(suppl 1):S8–S21.

112. Johnston RV, Grant DA, Wilkinson MH, et al. Repetitive hypoxia rapidly depresses cardio-respiratory responses during active sleep but not quiet sleep in the newborn lamb. J Physiol 1999; 519(pt 2):571–579.

113. Hanson MA, Kumar P, Williams BA. The effect of chronic hypoxia upon the development of respiratory chemoreflexes in the newborn kitten. J Physiol 1989; 411:563–574.

114. Ling L, Olson EB Jr., Vidruk EH, et al. Attenuation of the hypoxic ventilatory response in adult rats following one month of perinatal hyperoxia. J Physiol 1996; 495(pt 2):561–571.

115. Tatsumi K, Pickett CK, Weil JV. Attenuated carotid body hypoxic sensitivity after prolonged hypoxic exposure. J Appl Physiol 1991; 70(2):748–755.

116. Feldman JL, Mitchell GS, Nattie EE. Breathing: rhythmicity, plasticity, chemosensitivity. Annu Rev Neurosci 2003; 26:239–266.

117. Cao KY, Zwillich CW, Berthon-Jones M, et al. Increased normoxic ventilation induced by repetitive hypoxia in conscious dogs. J Appl Physiol 1992; 73(5): 2083–2088.

118. Prabhakar NR, Kline DD. Ventilatory changes during intermittent hypoxia: importance of pattern and duration. High Alt Med Biol 2002; 3(2):195–204.
119. Akay M, Sekine N. Investigating the complexity of respiratory patterns during recovery from severe hypoxia. J Neural Eng 2004; 1(1):16–20.
120. Fugelseth D, Borke WB, Lenes K, et al. Restoration of cardiopulmonary function with 21% versus 100% oxygen after hypoxaemia in newborn pigs. Arch Dis Child Fetal Neonatal Ed 2005; 90(3):F229–F234.
121. Mortola JP. Implications of hypoxic hypometabolism during mammalian onto-genesis. Respir Physiol Neurobiol 2004; 141(3):345–356.
122. Mortola JP, Besterman AD. Gaseous metabolism of the chicken embryo and hatchling during post-hypoxic recovery. Respir Physiol Neurobiol 2007; 156(2): 212–219.
123. Frappell P, Lanthier C, Baudinette RV, et al. Metabolism and ventilation in acute hypoxia: a comparative analysis in small mammalian species. Am J Physiol 1992; 262(6 pt 2):R1040–R1046.
124. Iiyori N, Alonso LC, Li J, et al. Intermittent hypoxia causes insulin resistance in lean mice independent of autonomic activity. Am J Respir Crit Care Med 2007; 175(8): 851–857.
125. Polotsky VY, Li J, Punjabi NM, et al. Intermittent hypoxia increases insulin resistance in genetically obese mice. J Physiol 2003; 552(pt 1):253–264.
126. Semenkovich CF. Insulin resistance and atherosclerosis. J Clin Invest 2006; 116(7): 1813–1822.
127. Trayhurn P, Wood IS. Adipokines: inflammation and the pleiotropic role of white adipose tissue. Br J Nutr 2004; 92(3):347–355.
128. Richardson HL, Parslow PM, Walker AM, et al. Maturation of the initial ven-tilatory response to hypoxia in sleeping infants. J Sleep Res 2007; 16(1):117–127.
129. Richardson HL, Parslow PM, Walker AM, et al. Variability of the initial phase of the ventilatory response to hypoxia in sleeping infants. Pediatr Res 2006; 59(5): 700–704.
130. Gaultier C. Apnea and sleep state in newborns and infants. Biol Neonate 1994; 65 (3–4):231–234.
131. Kennedy JD, Blunden S, Hirte C, et al. Reduced neurocognition in children who snore. Pediatr Pulmonol 2004; 37(4):330–337.
132. Montgomery-Downs HE, Gozal D. Snore-associated sleep fragmentation in infancy: mental development effects and contribution of secondhand cigarette smoke exposure. Pediatrics 2006; 117(3):e496–e502.
133. Knutson KL, Spiegel K, Penev P, et al. The metabolic consequences of sleep deprivation. Sleep Med Rev 2007; 11(3):163–178.
134. Van Cauter E, Holmback U, Knutson K, et al. Impact of sleep and sleep loss on neuroendocrine and metabolic function. Horm Res 2007; 67(suppl 1):2–9.
135. McEwen BS. Sleep deprivation as a neurobiologic and physiologic stressor: allo-stasis and allostatic load. Metabolism 2006; 55(10 suppl 2):S20–S23.
136. Schurr A. Bench-to-bedside review: a possible resolution of the glucose paradox of cerebral ischemia. Crit Care 2002; 6(4):330–334.
137. Heidbreder M, Qadri F, Johren O, et al. Non-hypoxic induction of HIF-3alpha by 2-deoxy-D-glucose and insulin. Biochem Biophys Res Commun 2007; 352(2): 437–443.

138. Alam I, Lewis K, Stephens JW, et al. Obesity, metabolic syndrome and sleep apnoea: all pro-inflammatory states. Obes Rev 2007; 8(2):119–127.

139. Vogelzangs N, Suthers K, Ferrucci L, et al. Hypercortisolemic depression is associated with the metabolic syndrome in late-life. Psychoneuroendocrinology 2007; 32(2):151–159.

140. McEwen BS. The neurobiology of stress: from serendipity to clinical relevance. Brain Res 2000; 886(1–2):172–189.

141. McEwen BS. Glucocorticoids, depression, and mood disorders: structural remodeling in the brain. Metabolism 2005; 54(5 suppl 1):20–23.

142. Copinschi G. Metabolic and endocrine effects of sleep deprivation. Essent Psychopharmacol 2005; 6(6):341–347.

143. Grune T, Muller K, Zollner S, et al. Evaluation of purine nucleotide loss, lipid peroxidation and ultrastructural alterations in post-hypoxic hepatocytes. J Physiol 1997; 498(Pt 2):511–522.

144. Back T. Pathophysiology of the ischemic penumbra–revision of a concept. Cell Mol Neurobiol 1998; 18(6):621–638.

145. Hara Y, Fujino M, Adachi K, et al. The reduction of hypoxia-induced and reoxygenation-induced apoptosis in rat islets by epigallocatechin gallate. Transplant Proc 2006; 38(8):2722–2725.

146. Beebe DW. Neurobehavioral morbidity associated with disordered breathing during sleep in children: a comprehensive review. Sleep 2006; 29(9):1115–1134.

147. Blunden SL, Beebe DW. The contribution of intermittent hypoxia, sleep debt and sleep disruption to daytime performance deficits in children: consideration of respiratory and non-respiratory sleep disorders. Sleep Med Rev 2006; 10(2):109–118.

148. Halbower AC, Degaonkar M, Barker PB, et al. Childhood obstructive sleep apnea associates with neuropsychological deficits and neuronal brain injury. PLoS Med 2006; 3(8):E301.

149. Balan IS, Fiskum G, Hazelton J, et al. Oximetry-guided reoxygenation improves neurological outcome after experimental cardiac arrest. Stroke 2006; 37(12): 3008–3013.

150. Svorc P, Bracokova I. Preconditioning by hypoventilation increases ventricular arrhythmia threshold in Wistar rats. Physiol Res 2003; 52(4):409–416.

151. Kaiser Jr., Gauss CH, Williams DK. The effects of hypercapnia on cerebral autoregulation in ventilated very low birth weight infants. Pediatr Res 2005; 58(5): 931–935.

152. Morris KF, Baekey DM, Nuding SC, et al. Invited review: neural network plasticity in respiratory control. J Appl Physiol 2003; 94(3):1242–1252.

153. Nathanielsz PW. Animal models that elucidate basic principles of the developmental origins of adult diseases. ILAR J 2006; 47(1):73–82.

154. Carroll JL. Developmental plasticity in respiratory control. J Appl Physiol 2003; 94(1): 375–389.

155. Maurer D, Mondloch CJ, Lewis TL. Sleeper effects. Dev Sci 2007; 10(1):40–47.

156. Bavis RW. Developmental plasticity of the hypoxic ventilatory response after perinatal hyperoxia and hypoxia. Respir Physiol Neurobiol 2005; 149(1–3): 287–299.

157. Bavis RW, Johnson RA, Ording KM, et al. Respiratory plasticity after perinatal hypercapnia in rats. Respir Physiol Neurobiol 2006; 153(1):78–91.

158. Barker DJ, Osmond C. Infant mortality, childhood nutrition, and ischaemic heart disease in England and Wales. Lancet 1986; 1(8489):1077–1081.

159. Gluckman PD, Hanson MA, Morton SM, et al. Life-long echoes–a critical analysis of the developmental origins of adult disease model. Biol Neonate 2005; 87(2): 127–139.

160. Barker DJ. The developmental origins of chronic adult disease. Acta Paediatr 2004; 93(suppl 446):26–33.

161. Sun TB, Yang CC, Lai CJ, et al. Time course of cardiovascular neural regulation during programmed 20-sec apnea in rats. Crit Care Med 2006; 34(3):765–770.

162. Cleave JP, Levine MR, Fleming PJ, et al. Hopf bifurcations and the stability of the respiratory control system. J Theor Biol 1986; 119(3):299–318.

15

Influence of Prenatal Nicotine Exposure on Development of Neurotransmission in Central Respiratory Neurons

RALPH F. FREGOSI
The University of Arizona, Tucson, Arizona, U.S.A.

I. Introduction

This chapter considers the influence of prenatal nicotine exposure on the development of neurotransmission in central respiratory neurons. Neonatal mammals that are nicotine exposed in utero show abnormalities in central ventilatory control, such as reduced ventilatory output (1,2), altered breathing pattern (2–4), increased apnea frequency (2,4) and duration (5), delayed arousal in response to hypoxia (6,7), decreased sensitivity to hypoxia (1,4,5,8–11), and diminished capacity for autoresuscitation following severe hypoxic exposure (12,13). Although these findings provide substantial evidence that development of central ventilatory control is altered by prenatal nicotine exposure, the mechanism of nicotine's action on respiratory-related neurons has not been identified. Identifying these mechanisms is important clinically, as epidemiological findings show that exposure to tobacco smoke is now the number one risk factor for the sudden infant death syndrome (SIDS), accounting for approximately one-third of all SIDS deaths (14,15). The major hypothesis addressed in this chapter is that prenatal nicotine exposure enhances inhibitory neurotransmission, and may also depress excitatory neurotransmission. It is envisaged that these alterations make the neonate more vulnerable to exogenous stressors, such as hypoxia, hypercapnia, asphyxia, and laryngeal irritation. The increased vulnerability is likely manifest as a diminution of protective reflex responses to these stressors, leading to life-threatening events.

The task of critiquing and synthesizing data on the influence of prenatal nicotine exposure on neurotransmission in central, respiration-related neurons is complicated by the diversity of animal models and model systems that have been used to address this issue. These range from in vitro brain stem slices to the postmortem analysis of brain tissue from SIDS victims. To avoid confusion, I have attempted, where possible, to organize each section of the chapter according to the complexity of the experimental model, starting with the most reduced preparations and ending with the most intricate. The majority of the work in this area is based on studies where nicotine is infused into a pregnant animal throughout gestation, using an osmotic minipump that is implanted subdermally. Although this model is not an exact representation of smoking, Slotkin and others have elegantly demonstrated that it is the best model, largely on the basis of data showing that nicotine is the major neuroteratogen in smoke-exposed neonates (16–20), and that this method avoids serious confounds associated with other models, such as daily nicotine injection or exposure to cigarette smoke (16).

With this qualification in mind, the chapter evaluates available data on the influence of prenatal nicotine exposure on cholinergic neurotransmission, fast inhibitory and excitatory neurotransmission, and modulatory neurotransmission in central respiratory neurons. When relevant and available, information on neurons involved in central cardiovascular control is also included. Because Hafstrom et al. (11) have recently contributed an excellent summary of the influence of prenatal nicotine exposure on protective reflexes in neonates, this topic will not be covered here, unless such coverage is needed for clarity.

II. Prenatal Nicotine Exposure and Cholinergic Neurotransmission

Nicotine is a potent neuroteratogen that crosses the mammalian blood brain barrier, leading to alterations in neuronal differentiation (16,21) and a striking increase in the density of nicotinic cholinergic receptors (nAChRs) throughout the brain (18,22,23). Mothers who smoke during and after pregnancy expose their progeny to nicotine in utero, as well as postnatally owing to "second hand" smoke exposure (14,17). This scenario is thought to influence one-quarter of all pregnancies in the United States, and children thus exposed are more likely to have learning, attention, and breathing abnormalities (14,24,25). In the early developmental period, neurotransmitters play trophic roles in nervous system development by activating neurotransmitter receptors and promoting neuronal replication and differentiation, synaptogenesis, apoptosis, and neuronal migration. That nAChRs are expressed in the neural tube stage suggests that nicotine can evoke developmental alterations early in embryogenesis. This is consistent with data showing significant correlations between maternal smoke exposure and SIDS (14,26).

It is clear from the above that any discussion of how nicotine exposure alters development of central ventilatory control begins with its effects on nAChRs. Mammalian neurons express many subtypes of nAChRs, each composed of a variety of identified subunits. Most of the nAChRs in the mammalian brain are made from pentameric combinations of α and β subunits ($\alpha2$–$\alpha6$, and $\beta2$–$\beta4$), although there are also homomeric nAChRs composed of the $\alpha7$–$\alpha9$ subunits (27–31). It appears that only the $\alpha4\beta2$ and $\alpha7$ subunit combinations are widely expressed in the mammalian brain. The $\alpha7$ subunits have high Ca^{2+} permeability and rapid activation and desensitization and are inhibited by α-bungarotoxin, while the $\alpha4\beta2$ receptors have a lower calcium permeability and a relatively slower response to agonist application and are not sensitive to α-bungarotoxin (32–37). The majority of nAChRs expressed on respiratory neurons are the $\alpha7$ and $\alpha4$ homomeric receptors and $\alpha4\beta2$ heteroreceptors (38–40).

The acute effects of nicotine applied to the brain stem or through the bloodstream have been studied in a variety of experimental preparations, and the results suggest an overall excitation of central ventilatory output. Thus, bath application of nicotine to brain stem slices enhances an excitatory, tetrodotoxin-insensitive inward current in hypoglossal motoneurons (41–43). Similarly, nicotine increased the frequency of inspiratory bursts in brain stem/spinal cord or slice preparations from neonatal mice (44) and rats (39,42,43). Brain stem neurons involved in respiratory rhythm generation are also subject to cholinergic influences. For example, bath application of antagonists of both $\alpha4\beta2$ and $\alpha7$ nAChRs produced dose-dependent reductions in the frequency of C4 ventral root nerve bursts (presumed inspiratory bursts) in the brain stem/spinal cord preparation of the neonatal rat, and this effect was accompanied by hyperpolarization of inspiratory and pre-inspiratory neurons in the medulla (45). In contrast, the frequency (and also the amplitude) of phrenic motor nerve bursts was decreased by injection of carbachol into the medial pontine reticular formation in decerebrate neonatal rats (46), suggesting heterogeneity of cholinergic responses in the various regions that are importantly involved in respiratory rhythm generation.

Phrenic motoneurons and bulbospinal neurons projecting to the phrenic motor nucleus in the adult rat express $\alpha7$ nAChRs, documenting that inspiratory pumping muscles, and thus ventilatory output, are also subject to cholinergic control (47). Similarly, in vivo studies in anesthetized adult rats show that microdialysis of nicotinic agonists into the hypoglossal motor nucleus increased genioglossus muscle activity (48). Genetic manipulations that knock out specific nAChR subunits can also provide some insight into the role of nAChRs on breathing. For example, two-day-old mutant mice lacking the $\beta2$ subunit of the nAChR had greater rates of pulmonary ventilation, a reduced ventilatory decline during acute exposure to hypoxia and a shorter arousal latency than wild-type littermates (49). These data suggest that nicotinic receptors containing the $\beta2$ subunit are normally inhibitory.

Thus, if chronic nicotine exposure alters the density of these receptors then inhibitory pathways may be reinforced. However, the differences reported above were abolished on the eighth day of life suggesting that the system is plastic and can adapt with time (49). Moreover, the nicotinic receptor knockout is presumably widespread in these animals, affecting both brain stem and spinal neurons, which complicates interpretation of the knockout studies. Thus, we know surprisingly little about the cholinergic control of medullary respiratory neurons or the motoneurons of the inspiratory and expiratory pumping muscles. Nevertheless, the results outlined above show that motoneurons controlling the respiratory pump and upper airway muscles express nAChRs, suggesting that they are subject to plastic changes accompanying chronic nicotine exposure. However, it is important to keep two caveats in mind: First, the reported quantitative and qualitative effects of cholinergic stimulation on phrenic nerve burst amplitude or pulmonary ventilation in anesthetized, decerebrate or awake animal preparations vary greatly, owing largely to the difficulty in applying nicotine to identified respiratory neurons, and to the wide constellation of receptor subtypes that may or may not be present on each neuron type (50). Second, the direct excitatory effects of nicotine on these cells are minor compared to those mediated by glutamate, as the magnitude of the hypoglossal motoneuron inward current evoked by nicotinic receptor activation is responsible for only 5–10% of the total excitatory current, with glutamate accounting for 60–70% of the total, via non-methyl-D-aspartate (NMDA) receptors (51).

There are limited data on the influence of chronic nicotine exposure on the density, structure, or functional state of nAChRs. nAChRs composed of $\alpha4\beta2$ subunits were upregulated in cultured human cells that were exposed to nicotine as they developed (52). Similarly, nicotine-induced release of ACh in rats was abolished in hippocampal synaptosomes following chronic nicotine treatment, with additional experiments showing that these effects were due to desensitization of the nAChRs (53). Thus, although several studies show that chronic nicotine exposure leads to an increase in the density of nAChRs in animal and human brains (54–59), this may be secondary to desensitization, resulting in a "functional downregulation" of the receptors (see below). Interestingly, SIDS victims born to smoking mothers did not show the expected increase in nicotine binding, suggesting a complex alteration in nicotine receptor development in smoke-exposed human neonates (60).

In summary, acute nicotine application increases the excitability of hypoglossal motoneurons and accelerates the respiratory rhythm, but has more variable effects on the drive to respiratory pump and upper airway muscles. In contrast, chronic nicotine exposure upregulates but also desensitizes nAChRs, resulting in an overall inhibition of ventilatory output (1,2,42,61). This paradox between the acute and chronic effects of nicotine on central neurons has been recognized and discussed previously (18,23) and has lead to the idea that the effects of chronic nicotine exposure are mediated largely by alterations in non-cholinergic receptors, and that it is these secondary effects that lead to the coexisting breathing instability. For example, the release of excitatory and inhibitory neurotransmitters evoked by activation of presynaptic nAChRs on the dendrites and terminals of GABAergic, glycinergic, glutamatergic, serotonergic, and catecholaminergic central neurons is increased following prenatal nicotine exposure (37,62,63). Just how the increased transmitter release influences the structure and function of the post-synaptic neuron is poorly understood. However, a growing body of evidence showing that chronic nicotine exposure, as well as exposure to other neuroteratogens (e.g., alcohol), results in an upregulation of inhibitory neurotransmitter receptors and a downregulation of glutamatergic receptors in neurons found throughout the brain. Accordingly, the remainder of this chapter deals with the issue of nicotine exposure–induced alterations in inhibitory and excitatory neurotransmission among respiration-related neurons.

III. Prenatal Nicotine Exposure and Fast Inhibitory Neurotransmission

The influence of prenatal nicotine exposure on inhibitory neurotransmitter systems is now well established. Prenatal nicotine exposure leads to an upregulation of presynaptic nicotinic receptors on GABAergic (64–69) and glycinergic (70) neurons. Persistent stimulation of these receptors increases the release of γ-aminobutyric acid (GABA) and glycine onto cerebellar, midbrain, and brain stem neurons, with complex changes in receptor density or function (18,64,71–73), as explained below.

There is some evidence that chronic nicotine exposure alters inhibitory pathways in neurons involved in cardiorespiratory control in the neonate. For example, Neff et al. (68) showed that the frequency of GABAergic and glycinergic synaptic events increased during the inspiratory phase in rodent cardiac vagal neurons (Fig. 1). The respiratory-modulated increase in GABAergic (but not glycinergic) firing frequency was blocked by antagonism of nAChRs (specifically, the α4β2 subunit of the receptor), consistent with nicotinic modulation of GABAergic inputs to respiration-related neurons. Interestingly, prenatal nicotine exposure enhanced the respiratory-modulated increase in GABAergic synaptic events in these cardioinhibitory neurons (68), suggesting that prenatal nicotine exposure may cause exaggerated respiratory sinus arrhythmia and may be responsible for the abnormal cardiac rhythm observed in some SIDS victims (74). Moreover, whereas hypoxia is normally associated with an initial increase followed by a decrease in the frequency of GABAergic inhibitory postsynaptic currents in these cells, prenatal nicotine exposure was associated with only a large reduction in GABAergic currents (75). This would be expected to release these cells from inhibition, leading to marked slowing of the heart rate during hypoxia, as observed in rats exposed to nicotine in utero (76). Moreover, although respiration-related excitatory (glutamatergic) inputs to cardiac vagal neurons were not observed in eupnea or hypoxia in control animals, prenatal nicotine exposure was associated with excitatory currents in eupnea, and an

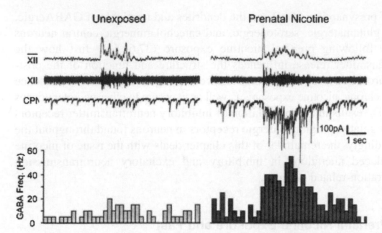

Figure 1   Inhibitory inward currents in cardiac vagal neurons studied in vitro increase during inspiration. From top down, the traces represent the moving time average of hypoglossal nerve activity (XII) in a brain stem slice preparation containing the core neural elements to generate a neural respiratory pattern; the unprocessed hypoglossal nerve activity; GABAergic currents obtained from voltage-clamped cardiac vagal neurons. Hypoglossal nerve discharge is typically associated with the inspiratory phase of the respiratory cycle, and in this preparation serves as an index of inspiratory discharge. The bar graphs show the frequency of inhibitory postsynaptic currents at different epochs throughout the respiratory cycle. Note that the frequency of GABAergic postsynaptic potentials increases during inspiration, and that the increase is significantly greater in animals that were exposed to nicotine in utero. *Abbreviations*: GABA, γ-aminobutyric acid. *Source*: From Ref. 68.

increase in these currents in hypoxia (77). These studies suggest that prenatal nicotine exposure makes the neonate vulnerable to bradycardia and/or arrhythmia during hypoxia by reducing inhibitory inputs and increasing excitatory inputs to cardiac vagal neurons.

These observations are supported by recent studies showing that the slowing of the respiratory rhythm by GABA-A receptor agonists in the in vitro brain stem spinal cord preparation of the neonatal rat was significantly greater in rats that were exposed to nicotine in the prenatal period, compared with saline-exposed control animals (73) (Fig. 2). More recent data suggest that prenatal nicotine exposure enhances glycinergic inhibition of the respiratory rhythm as well (78); when glycine was microinjected into the pre-Botzinger complex, transient apnea ensued, but the duration of the apneic period was significantly greater in animals that were exposed to nicotine in utero (79,80) (Fig. 3). Thus, there is ample evidence that prenatal nicotine exposure enhances synaptic inhibition in brain stem neurons, including those involved in the central control of breathing and cardiovascular function. These data are consistent with recent immunocytochemical studies showing an upregulation of the α3 subunit of the

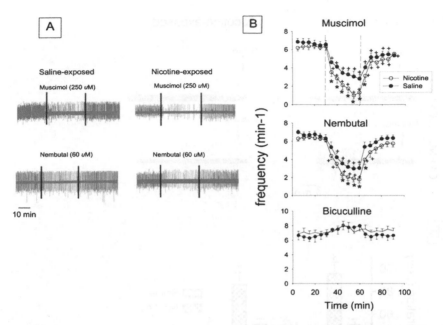

Figure 2 An enhanced response to muscimol and Nembutal in respiratory activity from control mice and mice exposed to prenatal nicotine. (**A**) Change in the discharge of C4 ventral root nerve activity (the C4 ENG) before, during, and after bath application of muscimol (250 μM) or Nembutal (60 μM) to the medulla of a neonatal brain stem–spinal cord preparation in representative saline-exposed or nicotine-exposed neonates. (**B**) Average changes in the frequency of C4 ENG bursts obtained from 12 saline-exposed and 12 nicotine-exposed neonates. Responses to the GABA-A receptor antagonist bicuculline methiodide are also shown. Values are means and SEM. Asterisks (*) indicate a significant difference ($p < 0.05$) between saline-exposed and nicotine-exposed neonates at a given time point. *Abbreviations*: ENG, electroneurogram; GABA, γ-aminobutyric acid; SEM, standard error of measurement. *Source*: From Ref. 73.

GABA-A receptor in the pre-Botzinger complex of nicotine-exposed animals, as illustrated in Figure 4 (Luo, McMullen, and Fregosi, unpublished observations).

The above observations are incorporated into a simple working model that was designed to help us understand these complex changes, and to develop testable hypotheses for further study. The model is shown in Figure 5. On the basis of the above discussion, prenatal nicotine exposure leads to an upregulation of nAChRs on GABAergic (and possibly glycinergic) neurons that are pre-synaptic to respiratory neurons in the pre-Botzinger complex region, and perhaps at other sites known to participate in ventilatory neurogenesis. But subsequent desensitization of the nAChRs leads to a diminution of GABA release, as has been demonstrated in synaptosomes from rat hippocampal neurons (53). The

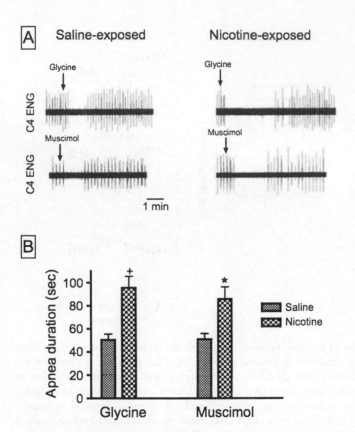

Figure 3 (**A**) Representative records showing the influence of microinjecting glycine (*top panels*) or muscimol (*bottom panels*) into the pre-Botzinger complex in saline-exposed (*left panels*) and nicotine-exposed (*right panels*) neonates. Drugs were injected at the downward facing arrows, with the duration of injection 250 milliseconds. Note that both drugs evoked abrupt, transient apnea in all animals, but that apnea duration is longer in the nicotine-exposed animals with either glycine or muscimol injection. (**B**) The average apnea duration evoked by glycine and muscimol in saline-exposed and nicotine-exposed neonates. Microinjection of glycine was done in 12 saline-exposed and 12 nicotine-exposed neonates, and muscimol was injected into 10 saline-exposed and 12 nicotine-exposed neonates. $^+p < 0.001$ versus saline; $^*p < 0.05$ versus saline. From Ref. 79.

prolonged reduction in GABA release then leads to an upregulation of GABA-A receptors on the postsynaptic neuron, consistent with data shown in Figure 4. As a consequence, application of GABA or GABA-A receptor agonists to cardiorespiratory neurons in nicotine-exposed brains evokes enhanced functional responses, as shown in Figures 1–3, and as discussed above (73,79,80). This scenario is functionally significant in the context of this chapter (see section VII), because it is now well known that, contrary to some data in mouse brain stem

Saline-exposed   Nicotine-exposed

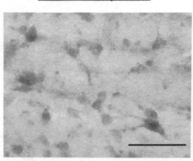

Figure 4 (*See color insert.*) Photomicrographs from the pre-Botzinger complex region in a saline-exposed and nicotine-exposed neonatal rat; both animals studied on the second day of life. Sections were stained immunocytochemically with antibodies against the α-3 subunit of the GABA-A receptor complex. Brain stem sections (40-μm thick) from saline-exposed and nicotine-exposed animals were assayed together to control for exposure time. Note darker staining in the nicotine-exposed neonate, suggesting that prenatal nicotine exposure increases the density of GABA-A receptors in the pre-Botzinger complex region. Calibration bar 50 μm. $N = 3$ nicotine-exposed and 3 saline-exposed neonates. *Abbreviation*: GABA, γ-aminobutyric acid. *Source*: From Luo, McMullen, and Fregosi, unpublished observations.

slices (81,82), GABA is inhibitory in mice and rats, not only in the early neonatal period (83–86) but also in the late embryonic period (85). Moreover, this holds true not only in reduced in vitro preparations but also in awake neonatal rats (85).

Finally, it is important to point out that, in contrast to information on the GABA-A and glycine receptor, there are only limited data on the influence of prenatal nicotine exposure on the density and/or function of the GABA-B receptor. Information on the influence of prenatal nicotine exposure on GABA-B receptor function and development is needed because inhibitory synaptic depression of CNS neurons is mediated by both receptor subtypes (123).

IV. Prenatal Nicotine Exposure and Fast Excitatory Neurotransmission

Although the data on excitatory neurotransmitter systems are sparse compared with those for the GABAergic and glycinergic inhibitory systems, prenatal nicotine exposure has been shown to change the density and/or function of glutamate receptors. For example, Hsieh et al. (87) reported reduced NMDA receptor binding in the rat thalamus following chronic nicotine exposure, and Aramakis et al. (88) have recently reported significant disruption of NMDA receptor development in the auditory cortex of neonatal rats that were nicotine

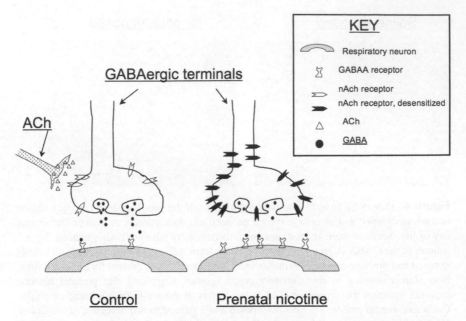

Figure 5 Schematic diagram summarizing physiologic and anatomic findings on the influence of prenatal nicotine exposure on inhibitory synaptic transmission in brain stem respiratory neurons. Prenatal nicotine exposure results in an upregulation of nicotinic acetylcholine receptors, but these are subsequently desensitized leading to a diminution of GABA release. The reduction in GABA release leads to an upregulation of GABA-A receptors on the postsynaptic neuron. As a result, any endogenous stressor associated with an increase in GABA release (e.g., hypoxia) would be associated with an exaggerated postsynaptic response. *Abbreviation*: GABA, γ-aminobutyric acid. *Source*: From Ref. 79.

exposed in utero. Similarly, repeated exposure to rewarding stimulation of the medial forebrain bundle (a model for repetitive nicotine, alcohol, or cocaine use) selectively decreases expression of an AMPA receptor subunit in the ventral tegmentum of the rat (89). Abnormalities of the NMDA receptor or the mRNA expression in various brain regions (90), as well as a reduction in the binding of tritiated kainate in the arcuate nucleus (124), have been observed in SIDS victims. Glutamatergic neurons are the major neuron subtype in the arcuate nucleus in human infants (91), and this nucleus is believed to be the homologue of the retrotrapezoid nucleus in the rat, a region with neurons that are sensitive to high CO_2/low pH (92). It is certainly possible that chemosensitive glutamatergic neurons in the ventral-lateral medulla (93,94) play a role in the association of prenatal nicotine exposure with the reduced chemosensitivity and arousal responses observed shortly after birth. Unfortunately, there have been no detailed studies of the interconnection between prenatal nicotine exposure and glutamatergic control of breathing in the neonate.

V. Prenatal Nicotine Exposure and Modulatory Neurotransmission: Serotonin

To the best of my knowledge, there are no published data on the influence of prenatal nicotine exposure on the serotonergic control of breathing. This may be due in part to the fact that the mechanism by which serotonin modulates central ventilatory control is profoundly complex and poorly understood, even in reduced preparations (95). For example, in the brain stem–spinal cord preparation of the neonatal rat, serotonin increases the frequency of respiratory motor nerve bursts if the pons is intact, but reduces frequency if the pons is removed (see Fig. 16 in Ref. 95). Some of the variability reported in these studies may indeed be the result of how much pontine tissue is attached to the preparation. Under conditions where the entire pons is removed, we consistently find that brain stem application of the 5-HT1A receptor agonist 8-OH-DPAT slows the frequency of C4 ventral root nerve bursts (Fig. 6), whereas the 5-HT2 receptor agonist 1-(2,5-dimethoxy-4-iodophenyl)-2-aminopropane (DOI) has no consistent effects (78). However, the key observation in the context of this chapter is that the responses evoked by either drug were not altered by prenatal nicotine exposure (Fig. 6). These findings were initially surprising to us, but are in fact consistent with other data showing that prenatal nicotine exposure alters the density of 5-HT1A receptors and the binding of paroxetine (a marker for serotonin transporter activity) in the cortex of neonatal rats and monkeys, but not in more caudal brain regions, including the midbrain, pons, or medulla (96,97).

Results in more intact preparations suggest that exogenously applied serotonergic agonists modulate the ventilatory response to CO_2 (98,99). And, as with glutamatergic neurons, there is also evidence that some serotonergic neurons are intrinsically chemosensitive (100–102). Thus, in addition to modulating the ventilatory response by synaptically modifying the excitability of respiration-related neurons, some serotonergic neurons appear to play a direct role in the sensory response to elevated CO_2. These data suggest that any insult that alters the 5-HT system may also alter CO_2 chemosensitivity, which may be impaired in SIDS victims (see above). However, the influence of prenatal nicotine exposure on the interaction between the serotonergic system and CO_2 chemosensitivity is unknown.

Studies of the serotonergic control of breathing in human subjects also yield complex and conflicting results. For example, tryptophan depletion does not alter breathing in normal human subjects (103), and subjects with either Joubert syndrome, the congenital central hypoventilation syndrome, or apneustic breathing of unknown etiology showed no significant alterations in the density of 5-HT1A receptors in the brain stem (104). In contrast to these observations in adults, the groundbreaking observations of Kinney and colleagues clearly demonstrate that brain stem serotonergic systems are abnormal in 50% of SIDS cases (26). They used autoradiography to demonstrate that the binding of [3H]-lysergic acid diethylamide was reduced in the brains of SIDS victims relative

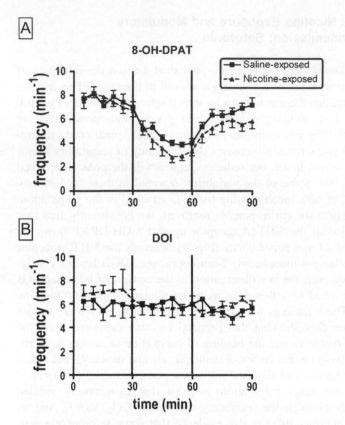

Figure 6 Change in the discharge frequency of C4 ventral root nerve bursts (the C4 ENG) before, during, and after bath application of serotonin receptor agonists to the brain stem compartment in saline-exposed and nicotine-exposed neonatal rat brain stem–spinal cord preparations. (**A**) The response to the 5-HT1A receptor agonist 8-OH-DPAT. Although 8-OH-DPAT (100 μM) slowed the frequency significantly at all time points, the extent of the slowing was the same in both saline ($N = 8$) and nicotine-exposed ($N = 8$) preparations. (**B**) The response to the 5-HT2A receptor agonist DOI. Note that DOI (120 μM) had no discernible influence on frequency in either group. $N = 6$ animals in each group. Values are means and SEM. *Abbreviations*: ENG, electroneurogram; DOI, 1-(2,5-dimethoxy-4-iodophenyl)-2-aminopropane; 8-OH-DPAT, 8-hydroxy-2-di-*n*-propylamino-tetralin; SEM, standard error of measurement. *Source*: From Ref. 78.

to the binding observed in brain tissue obtained from control infants that died of non-SIDS causes (105–107). Specific brain regions affected included the arcuate nucleus, raphe obscurus, raphé pallidus, nucleus gigantocellularis and para-gigantocellularis, parapyramidal nucleus, retrotrapezoid nucleus, the intermediate reticular zone, and the inferior olivary nucleus; all of these regions play at least some role in cardiorespiratory reflex responses. The most recent study from

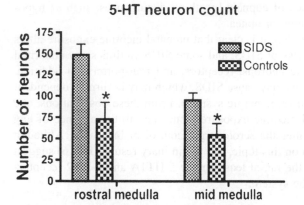

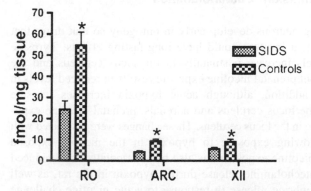

Figure 7 This figure summarizes the results of serotonin (5-HT) neuron count and serotonin receptor–binding density in 16 infants who die of SIDS, and 7 control cases who die of other causes. The data are taken from Table 2 in Ref. 108. Serotonin neuron count is reduced significantly (*) in rostral and mid medulla, and serotonin-binding density is significantly reduced in RO, the ARC, and the hypoglossal nucleus (**XII**), among other regions described in their paper. *Abbreviations*: RO, raphe obscurus; ARC, arcuate nucleus; SIDS, Sudden Infant Death Syndrome. *Source*: Adapted from Ref. 108.

this group (108) showed an increase in the number of serotonergic neurons, coupled to a decrease in the relative density of the 5-HT1A receptor subtype and the 5-HT-transporter protein, in various brain stem regions in SIDS victims as compared to the controls (Fig. 7). These anatomic changes would presumably influence the release and clearance of 5-HT, and would also have as yet unde-fined influences on the behavior of neurons with 5-HT receptors. Indeed, as the authors acknowledge, we have no data on brain 5-HT levels in SIDS, how the serotonergic modulation of cardiorespiratory protective reflexes might be altered, or if there is an association between serotonin neuron and receptor pathology, and the incidence of eupneic breathing disturbances, such as hypoventilation, periodic breathing, or apnea.

To summarize this section, it is clear that prenatal nicotine exposure alters protective reflexes and the risk of SIDS, and some SIDS victims show abnormal development of serotonergic neurons, receptors, and transporters. In addition, inadequate protective reflexes may cause SIDS, which may in turn be dependent on the integrity of the brain serotonergic systems. From these observations, one might predict that prenatal nicotine exposure alone (i.e., in the absence of any other risk factors) would alter the serotonergic control of breathing. Although there are no published data on this topic, our preliminary results (Fig. 6) suggest that this is not the case in the rat, at least for the 5-HT1A and 5-HT2 receptor-mediated components of the system.

VI. Prenatal Nicotine Exposure and Modulatory Neurotransmission: Catecholamines

Catecholamine-containing neurons develop early in ontogeny so that drugs that influence their development in utero could have long-lasting effects. Tyrosine hydroxylase mRNA levels increase postnatally in the locus ceruleus and the adrenal glands of mice, but prenatal nicotine exposure results in reduced levels in the adrenals (109). In addition, although acute hypoxia increases tyrosine hydroxylase mRNA in the locus ceruleus and adrenals, prenatal nicotine exposure eliminates the increase in the locus ceruleus. These changes were associated with increased mortality following exposure to hypoxia in the nicotine-exposed animals (109). Prenatal nicotine exposure has also been associated with reduced adrenal and forebrain catecholamine release during hypoxia in the rat, as well as a diminished norepinephrine release in response to acute nicotine challenge (110). Additionally, prenatal nicotine exposure is associated with reduced dopamine content in the cortex, midbrain, pons, and medulla of 15- to 18-day-old neonates (96), and the alteration persists into adulthood in both male and female rats (96,111,112). Receptor binding studies show that the density of cardiac β-adrenergic receptors is reduced in rats exposed to nicotine in utero. These changes were associated with diminished excitatory responses to isoproterenol (113), and with increased mortality in response to severe hypoxic challenge.

VII. Translational Physiology

Available evidence on the effects of chronic nicotine exposure on inhibitory and excitatory neurotransmitter receptors suggest that synaptic inhibition is enhanced, while synaptic excitation is reduced. This idea is entirely consistent with recent data showing that behavioral deficits induced by abuse of ethanol, inhaled toxins, and volatile anesthetics are the result of enhanced glycinergic and GABAergic neurotransmission and reduced glutamatergic transmission (114–118). I believe that this general model may also play a role in neonatal breathing instability following prenatal nicotine exposure. Although there is at present much more information on inhibitory than excitatory or modulatory neurotransmission, the working model presented in Figure 5 can be expanded as more information is gained.

An interesting question is how such changes could help explain why infants born to smoking mothers have a greater incidence of ventilatory control abnormalities. One of the most widely accepted models of SIDS is the "triple risk model," which involves the following factors: a vulnerable infant; a critical developmental period in homeostatic control, and an exogenous stressor, or stressors (119). In our model, prenatal nicotine exposure would make an infant vulnerable by evoking an abnormal increase in GABA (and perhaps glycine) receptors, and a decrease in excitatory or modulatory receptors on neurons involved in respiratory and cardiovascular control. Any exogenous stressor that is associated with increased GABA release could then enhance GABAergic and/ or glycinergic inhibition of ventilatory control, and the weakened excitatory pathways would be unable to adequately compensate. For example, both hypoxia (120,121) and hypercapnia (122) increase GABA release in various brain stem regions. Thus, one might imagine a vulnerable, nicotine-exposed infant within a critical developmental window becoming hypoxic and hypercapnic due to partial suffocation by bedding, for example. The increased GABA release evoked by the ensuing hypoxic or hypercapnic insult would enhance GABA-mediated inhibition of the ventilatory response, which in turn could lead to hypoventilation and apnea, followed by even more severe hypoxia or hypercapnia, and subsequent cardiorespiratory failure.

References

1. St-John WM, Leiter JC. Maternal nicotine depresses eupneic ventilation of neonatal rats. Neurosci Lett 1999; 267(3):206–208.
2. Huang YH, Brown AR, Costy-Bennett S, et al. Influence of prenatal nicotine exposure on postnatal development of breathing pattern. Respir Physiol Neurobiol 2004; 143(1):1–8.
3. Hafstrom O, Milerad J, Sundell HW. Altered breathing pattern after prenatal nicotine exposure in the young lamb. Am J Respir Crit Care Med 2002; 166(1):92–97.
4. Fewell JE, Smith FG, Ng VK. Prenatal exposure to nicotine impairs protective responses of rat pups to hypoxia in an age-dependent manner. Respir Physiol 2001; 127(1):61–73.
5. Froen JF, Akre H, Stray-Pedersen B, et al. Prolonged apneas and hypoxia mediated by nicotine and endotoxin in piglets. Biol Neonate 2002; 81(2):119–125.
6. Lewis KW, Bosque EM. Deficient hypoxia awakening response in infants of smoking mothers: possible relationship to sudden infant death syndrome. J Pediatr 1995; 127(5):691–699.
7. Hafstrom O, Milerad J, Asokan N, et al. Nicotine delays arousal during hypoxemia in lambs. Pediatr Res 2000; 47(5):646–652.

8. Bamford OS, Carroll JL. Dynamic ventilatory responses in rats: normal development and effects of prenatal nicotine exposure. Respir Physiol 1999; 117(1):29–40.
9. Bamford OS, Schuen JN, Carroll JL. Effect of nicotine exposure on postnatal ventilatory responses to hypoxia and hypercapnia. Respir Physiol 1996; 106(1): 1–11.
10. Fewell JE, Smith FG, Ng VK. Threshold levels of maternal nicotine impairing protective responses of newborn rats to intermittent hypoxia. J Appl Physiol 2001; 90(5):1968–1976.
11. Hafstrom O, Milerad J, Sandberg KL, et al. Cardiorespiratory effects of nicotine exposure during development. Respir Physiol Neurobiol 2005; 149(1–3):325–341.
12. Fewell JE, Smith FG. Perinatal nicotine exposure impairs ability of newborn rats to autoresuscitate from apnea during hypoxia. J Appl Physiol 1998; 85(6):2066–2074.
13. Froen JF, Akre H, Stray-Pedersen B, et al. Adverse effects of nicotine and interleukin-1beta on autoresuscitation after apnea in piglets: implications for sudden infant death syndrome. Pediatrics 2000; 105(4):E52.
14. Mitchell EA, Milerad J. Smoking and the sudden infant death syndrome. Rev Environ Health 2006; 21(2):81–103.
15. Anderson ME, Johnson DC, Batal HA. Sudden Infant Death Syndrome and prenatal maternal smoking: rising attributed risk in the Back to Sleep era. BMC Med 2005; 3:4.
16. Slotkin TA. Fetal nicotine or cocaine exposure: which one is worse? J Pharmacol Exp Ther 1998; 285(3):931–945.
17. Slotkin TA. Cholinergic systems in brain development and disruption by neurotoxicants: nicotine, environmental tobacco smoke, organophosphates. Toxicol Appl Pharmacol 2004; 198(2):132–151.
18. Slotkin TA, Pinkerton KE, Auman JT, et al. Perinatal exposure to environmental tobacco smoke upregulates nicotinic cholinergic receptors in monkey brain. Brain Res Dev Brain Res 2002; 133(2):175–179.
19. Slotkin TA, Lappi SE, Seidler FJ. Impact of fetal nicotine exposure on development of rat brain regions: critical sensitive periods or effects of withdrawal? Brain Res Bull 1993; 31(3–4):319–328.
20. Sugiyama H, Hagino N, Moore G, et al. [3H]Nicotine binding sites in developing fetal brains in rats. Neurosci Res 1985; 2(5):387–392.
21. Slikker W Jr., Xu ZA, Levin ED, et al. Mode of action: disruption of brain cell replication, second messenger, and neurotransmitter systems during development leading to cognitive dysfunction—developmental neurotoxicity of nicotine. Crit Rev Toxicol 2005; 35(8–9):703–711.
22. Yates SL, Bencherif M, Fluhler EN, et al. Up-regulation of nicotinic acetylcholine receptors following chronic exposure of rats to mainstream cigarette smoke or alpha 4 beta 2 receptors to nicotine. Biochem Pharmacol 1995; 50(12):2001–2008.
23. Wonnacott S. The paradox of nicotinic acetylcholine receptor upregulation by nicotine. Trends Pharmacol Sci 1990; 11(6):216–219.
24. DiFranza JR, Lew RA. Effect of maternal cigarette smoking on pregnancy complications and sudden infant death syndrome. J Fam Pract 1995; 40(4):385–394.
25. Bardy AH, Seppala T, Lillsunde P, et al. Objectively measured tobacco exposure during pregnancy: neonatal effects and relation to maternal smoking. Br J Obstet Gynaecol 1993;100(8):721–726.

26. Kinney HC. Abnormalities of the brainstem serotonergic system in the sudden infant death syndrome: a review. Pediatr Dev Pathol 2005; 8(5):507–524.
27. Dani JA, Mayer ML. Structure and function of glutamate and nicotinic acetylcholine receptors. Curr Opin Neurobiol 1995; 5(3):310–317.
28. Dani JA. Overview of nicotinic receptors and their roles in the central nervous system. Biol Psychiatry 2001; 49(3):166–174.
29. Le Novere N, Changeux JP. Molecular evolution of the nicotinic acetylcholine receptor: an example of multigene family in excitable cells. J Mol Evol 1995; 40(2): 155–172.
30. Colquhoun LM, Patrick JW. Alpha3, beta2, and beta4 form heterotrimeric neuronal nicotinic acetylcholine receptors in Xenopus oocytes. J Neurochem 1997; 69(6): 2355–2362.
31. Patrick J, Sequela P, Vernino S, et al. Functional diversity of neuronal nicotinic acetylcholine receptors. Prog Brain Res 1993; 98:113–120.
32. Gerzanich V, Wang F, Kuryatov A, et al. alpha 5 Subunit alters desensitization, pharmacology, Ca++ permeability and Ca++ modulation of human neuronal alpha 3 nicotinic receptors. J Pharmacol Exp Ther 1998; 286(1):311–320.
33. Lindstrom J, Peng X, Kuryatov A, et al. Molecular and antigenic structure of nicotinic acetylcholine receptors. Ann N Y Acad Sci 1998; 841:71–86.
34. Alkondon M, Pereira EF, Wonnacott S, et al. Blockade of nicotinic currents in hippocampal neurons defines methyllycaconitine as a potent and specific receptor antagonist. Mol Pharmacol 1992; 41(4):802–808.
35. Albuquerque EX, Pereira EF, Castro NG, et al. Nicotinic receptor function in the mammalian central nervous system. Ann N Y Acad Sci 1995; 757:48–72.
36. Gray R, Rajan AS, Radcliffe KA, et al. Hippocampal synaptic transmission enhanced by low concentrations of nicotine. Nature 1996; 383(6602):713–716.
37. Dajas-Bailador F, Wonnacott S. Nicotinic acetylcholine receptors and the regulation of neuronal signalling. Trends Pharmacol Sci 2004; 25(6):317–324.
38. Dehkordi O, Millis RM, Dennis GC, et al. Alpha-7 and alpha-4 nicotinic receptor subunit immunoreactivity in genioglossus muscle motoneurons. Respir Physiol Neurobiol 2005; 145(2–3):153–161.
39. Shao XM, Feldman JL. Pharmacology of nicotinic receptors in preBotzinger complex that mediate modulation of respiratory pattern. J Neurophysiol 2002; 88(4): 1851–1858.
40. Quitadamo C, Fabbretti E, Lamanauskas N, et al. Activation and desensitization of neuronal nicotinic receptors modulate glutamatergic transmission on neonatal rat hypoglossal motoneurons. Eur J Neurosci 2005; 22(11):2723–2734.
41. Chamberlin NL, Bocchiaro CM, Greene RW, et al. Nicotinic excitation of rat hypoglossal motoneurons. Neuroscience 2002; 115(3):861–870.
42. Robinson DM, Peebles KC, Kwok H, et al. Prenatal nicotine exposure increases apnoea and reduces nicotinic potentiation of hypoglossal inspiratory output in mice. J Physiol 2002;538(pt 3):957–973.
43. Shao XM, Feldman JL. Mechanisms underlying regulation of respiratory pattern by nicotine in preBotzinger complex. J Neurophysiol 2001; 85(6):2461–2467.
44. Chatonnet F, Boudinot E, Chatonnet A, et al. Respiratory survival mechanisms in acetylcholinesterase knockout mouse. Eur J Neurosci 2003; 18(6):1419–1427.

45. Hatori E, Sakuraba S, Kashiwagi M, et al. Association of nicotinic acetylcholine receptors with central respiratory control in isolated brainstem-spinal cord preparation of neonatal rats. Biol Res 2006; 39(2):321–330.
46. Fung ML, St John WM. Pontine cholinergic respiratory depression in neonatal and young rats. Life Sci 1998; 62(24):2249–2256.
47. Dehkordi O, Haxhiu MA, Millis RM, et al. Expression of alpha-7 nAChRs on spinal cord-brainstem neurons controlling inspiratory drive to the diaphragm. Respir Physiol Neurobiol 2004;141(1):21–34.
48. Liu X, Sood S, Liu H, et al. Opposing muscarinic and nicotinic modulation of hypoglossal motor output to genioglossus muscle in rats in vivo. J Physiol 2005; 565(pt 3):965–980.
49. Dauger S, Durand E, Cohen G, et al. Control of breathing in newborn mice lacking the beta-2 nAChR subunit. Acta Physiol Scand 2004; 182(2):205–212.
50. Kubin L, Fenik V. Pontine cholinergic mechanisms and their impact on respiratory regulation. Respir Physiol Neurobiol 2004; 143(2–3):235–249.
51. Wang J, Irnaten M, Venkatesan P, et al. Synaptic activation of hypoglossal respiratory motorneurons during inspiration in rats. Neurosci Lett 2002; 332(3): 195–199.
52. Darsow T, Booker TK, Pina-Crespo JC, et al. Exocytic trafficking is required for nicotine-induced up-regulation of alpha 4 beta 2 nicotinic acetylcholine receptors. J Biol Chem 2005;280(18):18311–18320.
53. Grilli M, Parodi M, Raiteri M, et al. Chronic nicotine differentially affects the function of nicotinic receptor subtypes regulating neurotransmitter release. J Neurochem 2005; 93(5):1353–1360.
54. Mueller RA, Lundberg DB, Breese GR, et al. The neuropharmacology of respiratory control. Pharmacol Rev 1982; 34(3):255–285.
55. Marks MJ, Stitzel JA, Collins AC. Time course study of the effects of chronic nicotine infusion on drug response and brain receptors. J Pharmacol Exp Ther 1985; 235(3):619–628.
56. Schwartz RD, Kellar KJ. Nicotinic cholinergic receptor binding sites in the brain: regulation in vivo. Science 1983; 220(4593):214–216.
57. Peng X, Gerzanich V, Anand R, et al. Nicotine-induced increase in neuronal nicotinic receptors results from a decrease in the rate of receptor turnover. Mol Pharmacol 1994; 46(3):523–530.
58. Buisson B, Bertrand D. Nicotine addiction: the possible role of functional upregulation. Trends Pharmacol Sci 2002; 23(3):130–136.
59. Flores CM, Davila-Garcia MI, Ulrich YM, et al. Differential regulation of neuronal nicotinic receptor binding sites following chronic nicotine administration. J Neurochem 1997; 69(5):2216–2219.
60. Nachmanoff DB, Panigrahy A, Filiano JJ, et al. Brainstem 3H-nicotine receptor binding in the sudden infant death syndrome. J Neuropathol Exp Neurol 1998; 57 (11):1018–1025.
61. Hafstrom O, Milerad J, Sundell HW. Prenatal nicotine exposure blunts the cardiorespiratory response to hypoxia in lambs. Am J Respir Crit Care Med 2002; 166 (12 pt 1):1544–1549.
62. Barazangi N, Role LW. Nicotine-induced enhancement of glutamatergic and GABAergic synaptic transmission in the mouse amygdala. J Neurophysiol 2001; 86(1): 463–474.

63. Vizi ES, Lendvai B. Modulatory role of presynaptic nicotinic receptors in synaptic and non-synaptic chemical communication in the central nervous system. Brain Res Brain Res Rev 1999; 30(3):219–235.

64. Zhu PJ, Chiappinelli VA. Nicotine modulates evoked GABAergic transmission in the brain. J Neurophysiol 1999; 82(6):3041–3045.

65. Zhu PJ, Chiappinelli VA. Nicotinic receptors mediate increased GABA release in brain through a tetrodotoxin-insensitive mechanism during prolonged exposure to nicotine. Neuroscience 2002; 115(1):137–144.

66. Neal MJ, Cunningham JR, Matthews KL. Activation of nicotinic receptors on GABAergic amacrine cells in the rabbit retina indirectly stimulates dopamine release. Vis Neurosci 2001; 18(1):55–64.

67. Fisher JL, Pidoplichko VI, Dani JA. Nicotine modifies the activity of ventral tegmental area dopaminergic neurons and hippocampal GABAergic neurons. J Physiol Paris 1998; 92(3–4):209–213.

68. Neff RA, Wang J, Baxi S, et al. Respiratory sinus arrhythmia: endogenous activation of nicotinic receptors mediates respiratory modulation of brainstem cardioinhibitory parasympathetic neurons. Circ Res 2003; 93(6):565–572.

69. Covernton PO, Lester RA. Prolonged stimulation of presynaptic nicotinic ace-tylcholine receptors in the rat interpeduncular nucleus has differential effects on transmitter release. Int J Dev Neurosci 2002; 20(3–5):247–258.

70. Lim DK, Park SH, Choi WJ. Subacute nicotine exposure in cultured cerebellar cells increased the release and uptake of glutamate. Arch Pharm Res 2000; 23(5): 488–494.

71. Magata Y, Kitano H, Shiozaki T, et al. Effect of chronic (-)-nicotine treatment on rat cerebral benzodiazepine receptors. Nucl Med Biol 2000; 27(1):57–60.

72. Meier E, Drejer J, Schousboe A. GABA induces functionally active low-affinity GABA receptors on cultured cerebellar granule cells. J Neurochem 1984; 43(6): 1737–1744.

73. Luo Z, Costy-Bennett S, Fregosi RF. Prenatal nicotine exposure increases the strength of GABA(A) receptor-mediated inhibition of respiratory rhythm in neonatal rats. J Physiol 2004; 561(pt 2):387–393.

74. Ottaviani G, Matturri L, Rossi L, et al. Crib death: further support for the concept of fatal cardiac electrical instability as the final common pathway. Int J Cardiol 2003; 92(1):17–26.

75. Neff RA, Simmens SJ, Evans C, et al. Prenatal nicotine exposure alters central cardiorespiratory responses to hypoxia in rats: implications for sudden infant death syndrome. J Neurosci 2004; 24(42):9261–9268.

76. Slotkin TA, Saleh JL, McCook EC, et al. Impaired cardiac function during post-natal hypoxia in rats exposed to nicotine prenatally: implications for perinatal morbidity and mortality, and for sudden infant death syndrome. Teratology 1997; 55(3):177–184.

77. Evans C, Wang J, Neff R, et al. Hypoxia recruits a respiratory-related excitatory pathway to brainstem premotor cardiac vagal neurons in animals exposed to prenatal nicotine. Neuroscience 2005; 133(4):1073–1079.

78. Luo Z, Costy-Bennett S, Fregosi RF. Prenatal nicotine exposure does not alter the central ventilatory response to serotonin receptor agonists. FASEB J 2006; 20:A1214.

79. Luo Z, McMullen NT, Costy-Bennett S, Fregosi RF. Prenatal nicotine exposure alters glycinergic and GABAergic control of respiratory frequency in the neonatal rat brainstem-spinal cord preparation. Respir Physiol Neurobiol 2007; 157(2–3): 226–234.

80. Luo Z, Rometo A, Costy-Bennett S, Fregosi RF. Microinjection of muscimol and glycine into the ventrolateral medulla in neonatal rat brainstem spinal cord preparations exposed to nicotine or saline in the prenatal period. FASEB J 2004; 18:A335.

81. Ritter B, Zhang W. Early postnatal maturation of GABAA-mediated inhibition in the brainstem respiratory rhythm-generating network of the mouse. Eur J Neurosci 2000; 12(8):2975–2984.

82. Zhang W, Barnbrock A, Gajic S, et al. Differential ontogeny of GABA (B)-receptor-mediated pre- and postsynaptic modulation of GABA and glycine transmission in respiratory rhythm-generating network in mouse. J Physiol 2002; 540(pt 2):435–446.

83. Murakoshi T, Otsuka M. Respiratory reflexes in an isolated brainstem-lung preparation of the newborn rat: possible involvement of gamma-aminobutyric acid and glycine. Neurosci Lett 1985; 62(1):63–68.

84. Fregosi RF, Luo Z, Iizuka M. GABA(A) receptors mediate postnatal depression of respiratory frequency by barbiturates. Respir Physiol Neurobiol 2004; 140(3): 219–230.

85. Ren J, Greer JJ. Modulation of respiratory rhythmogenesis by chloride-mediated conductances during the perinatal period. J Neurosci 2006; 26(14):3721–3730.

86. Onimaru H, Arata A, Homma I. Inhibitory synaptic inputs to the respiratory rhythm generator in the medulla isolated from newborn rats. Pflugers Arch 1990; 417(4): 425–432.

87. Hsieh CY, Leslie FM, Metherate R. Nicotine exposure during a postnatal critical period alters NR2A and NR2B mRNA expression in rat auditory forebrain. Brain Res Dev Brain Res 2002; 133(1):19–25.

88. Aramakis VB, Hsieh CY, Leslie FM, et al. A critical period for nicotine-induced disruption of synaptic development in rat auditory cortex. J Neurosci 2000; 20(16): 6106–6116.

89. Carlezon WA Jr., Todtenkopf MS, McPhie DL, et al. Repeated exposure to rewarding brain stimulation downregulates GluR1 expression in the ventral tegmental area. Neuropsychopharmacology 2001; 25(2):234–241.

90. Waters KA, Machaalani R. NMDA receptors in the developing brain and effects of noxious insults. Neurosignals 2004; 13(4):162–174.

91. Paterson DS, Thompson EG, Kinney HC. Serotonergic and glutamatergic neurons at the ventral medullary surface of the human infant: observations relevant to central chemosensitivity in early human life. Auton Neurosci 2006; 124(1–2): 112–124.

92. Nattie EE, Li A. Substance P-saporin lesion of neurons with NK1 receptors in one chemoreceptor site in rats decreases ventilation and chemosensitivity. J Physiol 2002; 544(pt 2):603–616.

93. Mulkey DK, Stornetta RL, Weston MC, et al. Respiratory control by ventral surface chemoreceptor neurons in rats. Nat Neurosci 2004; 7(12):1360–1369.

94. Richerson GB, Wang W, Hodges MR, et al. Homing in on the specific phenotype(s) of central respiratory chemoreceptors. Exp Physiol 2005; 90(3):259–266; discussion 66–69.

95. Ballanyi K, Onimaru H, Homma I. Respiratory network function in the isolated brainstem-spinal cord of newborn rats. Prog Neurobiol 1999; 59(6):583–634.

96. Muneoka K, Ogawa T, Kamei K, et al. Nicotine exposure during pregnancy is a factor which influences serotonin transporter density in the rat brain. Eur J Pharmacol 2001; 411(3):279–282.

97. Slotkin TA, Pinkerton KE, Tate CA, et al. Alterations of serotonin synaptic proteins in brain regions of neonatal Rhesus monkeys exposed to perinatal environmental tobacco smoke. Brain Res 2006; 1111(1):30–35.

98. Taylor NC, Li A, Nattie EE. Medullary serotonergic neurones modulate the ventilatory response to hypercapnia, but not hypoxia in conscious rats. J Physiol 2005; 566(pt 2):543–557.

99. Messier ML, Li A, Nattie EE. Inhibition of medullary raphe serotonergic neurons has age-dependent effects on the CO2 response in newborn piglets. J Appl Physiol 2004; 96(5):1909–1919.

100. Richerson GB, Wang W, Tiwari J, et al. Chemosensitivity of serotonergic neurons in the rostral ventral medulla. Respir Physiol 2001; 129(1–2):175–189.

101. Severson CA, Wang W, Pieribone VA, et al. Midbrain serotonergic neurons are central pH chemoreceptors. Nat Neurosci 2003; 6(11):1139–1140.

102. Nattie EE, Li A, Richerson G, et al. Medullary serotonergic neurones and adjacent neurones that express neurokinin-1 receptors are both involved in chemoreception in vivo. J Physiol 2004; 556(pt 1):235–253.

103. Kent JM, Coplan JD, Martinez J, et al. Ventilatory effects of tryptophan depletion in panic disorder: a preliminary report. Psychiatry Res 1996; 64(2):83–90.

104. Saito Y, Ito M, Ozawa Y, et al. Changes of neurotransmitters in the brainstem of patients with respiratory-pattern disorders during childhood. Neuropediatrics 1999; 30(3):133–140.

105. Panigrahy A, Filiano J, Sleeper LA, et al. Decreased serotonergic receptor binding in rhombic lip-derived regions of the medulla oblongata in the sudden infant death syndrome. J Neuropathol Exp Neurol 2000; 59(5):377–384.

106. Kinney HC, Filiano JJ, White WF. Medullary serotonergic network deficiency in the sudden infant death syndrome: review of a 15-year study of a single dataset. J Neuropathol Exp Neurol 2001; 60(3):228–247.

107. Panigrahy A, Rosenberg PA, Assmann S, et al. Differential expression of glutamate receptor subtypes in human brainstem sites involved in perinatal hypoxia-ischemia. J Comp Neurol 2000; 427(2):196–208.

108. Paterson DS, Trachtenberg FL, Thompson EG, et al. Multiple serotonergic brainstem abnormalities in sudden infant death syndrome. JAMA 2006; 296(17): 2124–2132.

109. Wickstrom HR, Mas C, Simonneau M, et al. Perinatal nicotine attenuates the hypoxia-induced up-regulation of tyrosine hydroxylase and galanin mRNA in locus ceruleus of the newborn mouse. Pediatr Res 2002; 52(5):763–769.

110. Seidler FJ, Levin ED, Lappi SE, et al. Fetal nicotine exposure ablates the ability of postnatal nicotine challenge to release norepinephrine from rat brain regions. Brain Res Dev Brain Res 1992; 69(2):288–291.

111. Ribary U, Lichtensteiger W. Effects of acute and chronic prenatal nicotine treatment on central catecholamine systems of male and female rat fetuses and offspring. J Pharmacol Exp Ther 1989; 248(2):786–792.

112. Herrenkohl LR, Ribary U, Schlumpf M, et al. Maternal stress alters monoamine metabolites in fetal and neonatal rat brain. Experientia 1988; 44(5):457–459.

113. Slotkin TA, Epps TA, Stenger ML, et al. Cholinergic receptors in heart and brainstem of rats exposed to nicotine during development: implications for hypoxia tolerance and perinatal mortality. Brain Res Dev Brain Res 1999; 113(1–2):1–12.

114. Downie DL, Hall AC, Lieb WR, et al. Effects of inhalational general anaesthetics on native glycine receptors in rat medullary neurones and recombinant glycine receptors in Xenopus oocytes. Br J Pharmacol 1996; 118(3):493–502.

115. Franks NP, Lieb WR. Molecular and cellular mechanisms of general anaesthesia. Nature 1994; 367(6464):607–614.

116. Lovinger DM. Alcohols and neurotransmitter gated ion channels: past, present and future. Naunyn Schmiedebergs Arch Pharmacol 1997; 356(3):267–282.

117. Mihic SJ. Acute effects of ethanol on GABAA and glycine receptor function. Neurochem Int 1999; 35(2):115–123.

118. Beckstead MJ, Weiner JL, Eger EI, et al. Glycine and gamma-aminobutyric acid(A) receptor function is enhanced by inhaled drugs of abuse. Mol Pharmacol 2000; 57 (6):1199–1205.

119. Filiano JJ, Kinney HC. A perspective on neuropathologic findings in victims of the sudden infant death syndrome: the triple-risk model. Biol Neonate 1994; 65(3–4): 194–197.

120. Huang J, Suguihara C, Hehre D, et al. Effects of GABA receptor blockage on the respiratory response to hypoxia in sedated newborn piglets. J Appl Physiol 1994; 77(2):1006–1010.

121. Xiao Q, Suguihara C, Hehre D, et al. Effects of GABA receptor blockade on the ventilatory response to hypoxia in hypothermic newborn piglets. Pediatr Res 2000; 47(5):663–668.

122. Zhang L, Wilson CG, Liu S, et al. Hypercapnia-induced activation of brainstem GABAergic neurons during early development. Respir Physiol Neurobiol 2003; 136(1):25–37.

123. Mitoma H, Ishida K, Shizuka-Ikeda M, and Mizusawa H. Dual impairment of GABAA- and GABAB-receptor-mediated synaptic responses by autoantibodies to glutamic acid decarboxylase. J Neurol Sci 2003; 208:51–56.

124. Panigrahy A, Filiano JJ, Sleeper LA, Mandell F, Valdes-Dapena M, Krous HF, Rava LA, White WF, and Kinney HC. Decreased kainate receptor binding in the arcuate nucleus of the sudden infant death syndrome. J Neuropathol Exp Neurol 1997; 56:1253–1261.

16

Central Hypoventilation Syndromes

THOMAS G. KEENS and SALLY L. DAVIDSON WARD
University of Southern California, Los Angeles, California, U.S.A.

I. Introduction

In 1962, Severinghaus first used the term "Ondine's curse" to describe three adults who lacked ventilatory responsivity to CO_2 following surgery to the brain stem (1). This term has been most frequently used to describe a rare disorder where infants appear to breathe reasonably well while awake, but severely hypoventilate and/or become apneic during sleep. Central hypoventilation syndromes, although uncommon, are now more frequently diagnosed. They range in frequency, severity, and clinical presentation, but advances in our knowledge and technology now permit prompt diagnosis and comprehensive treatment. Thus, many of these patients survive with a good quality of life. This chapter will describe some of the disorders in infants and children known to cause hypoventilation during sleep.

II. Congenital Central Hypoventilation Syndrome

Congenital central hypoventilation syndrome (CCHS), or Ondine's curse, is defined as the failure of automatic control of breathing, present from birth, now known to be due to a mutation in the *PHOX2B* gene (2–10) (see chap. 19). In this disorder, ventilation is severely affected during quiet sleep and is abnormal during active sleep and wakefulness, though usually to a milder degree (3–5,8). Disordered ventilatory control may range in severity from hypoventilation during quiet sleep with adequate ventilation during wakefulness to complete apnea during sleep and severe hypoventilation during wakefulness. Other signs of brain stem dysfunction may be present (1–5,7,8). The incidence of CCHS is not known, but it is generally considered to be rare.

A. Etiology

The cause of CCHS is a mutation in the *PHOX2B* gene, which is an important gene in the development of the autonomic nervous system (9,10). CCHS is a generalized disorder of the autonomic nervous system, which affects more than just control of breathing (11–13). Hirschsprung's disease is associated with CCHS in about 15–20% of cases (4,14). Multiple mediastinal and adrenal ganglioneuromas (12), and other tumors of neural crest origin, have been described. Ophthalmologic abnormalities, especially those of neural control of eye movement, pupillary response, etc., are frequently seen in CCHS (15). These abnormalities all suggest that CCHS is a generalized neurologic disorder, possibly due to abnormal embryonic development and/or nerve cell migration during development of the central nervous system.

B. Physiologic Pattern of Respiratory Control Abnormality

Paton et al. found that children with CCHS have absent chemoreceptor responses to both hypercapnia and hypoxia, even while awake, when tested by the rebreathing technique (3). Because chemoreceptors are in two anatomically distinct sites, postulating one abnormality in the brain stem respiratory center, which receives input from both chemoreceptors, is more likely (3). Humans also have an arousal response to CO_2 and hypoxia. If children with CCHS have a disorder of chemoreceptor input integration for ventilation, they may still arouse to respiratory stimuli, because ventilatory and arousal responses to respiratory stimuli use different neural pathways. Marcus showed that most children with CCHS arouse to hypercapnia under very controlled circumstances, indicating intact central chemoreceptor input (16). Thus, CCHS is most likely due to brain stem dysfunction in the area where input from chemoreceptors is integrated for ventilation (16).

Harper and colleagues compared functional MRI (fMRI) scans during hypercapnia and hypoxia among children with CCHS and controls (17–19). Because children with CCHS have absent ventilatory responses to both hypercapnia and hypoxia, areas of neural activation present in controls, but not in CCHS, should indicate brain regions responsible for neurologic control of breathing. Children with CCHS had a notable absence of neural activation in the cerebellum in response to hypercapnia and hypoxia, as well as midbrain regions (17–19). These findings suggest that children with CCHS have neural dysfunction in many brain areas, not just in the brain stem, and that many brain regions participate in neurologic control of breathing. In addition, Kumar and colleagues showed that there were neural deficits in the same brain regions (20). It is not clear whether these neural deficits are a primary abnormality in CCHS or secondary to chronic hypoxia.

Chemoreceptors are thought to be important controllers of ventilation during exercise. Thus, one would predict that CCHS patients may have trouble with exercise. In fact, Silvestri and associates showed severe gas exchange abnormalities in full-time ventilatory-dependent CCHS patients during moderate exercise (21). However, Paton et al. showed that exercise-induced hyperpnea does occur in CCHS patients who require ventilatory assistance only during sleep (22). These patients showed only mild gas exchange abnormalities (decrease in oxygenation and increase in P_{CO_2}), though not enough to limit exercise. These CCHS patients increased the minute ventilation and tidal volume with increasing exercise, but not as much as normal subjects. Paton et al. found that body movement during exercise entrained ventilation in the absence of chemoreceptor function (22). Gozal et al. showed that passive leg motion also increased alveolar ventilation in CCHS (23). Therefore, the rhythmic entrainment of respiration plays a significant role in the modulation of breathing in CCHS children, and thus some may tolerate exercise well (23). This finding also suggests that CCHS patients may be at a higher risk for hypoventilation when they are inactive, as when watching television, reading, or studying (22,23).

C. Diagnosis and Clinical Course

The clinical presentation of CCHS may vary, depending on the severity of the disorder (4). Most patients with CCHS present with symptoms in the newborn period. Many will not breathe at birth and will require assisted ventilation in the newborn nursery. Many do not breathe at all during the first few months of life but may mature to a pattern of adequate breathing during wakefulness, while apnea or hypoventilation persists only during sleep. This apparent improvement is due to normal maturation of the respiratory system and does not represent a change in the basic disorder (3). Other infants may present at a later age with cyanosis, edema, and signs of right heart failure as the first indications of CCHS (4). These infants have often been mistaken for patients with cyanotic congenital heart disease. However, cardiac catheterization reveals only pulmonary hypertension. Other infants may present with severe apnea or an apparent life-threatening event (4). All patients with CCHS have abnormal ventilation both awake and asleep, but spontaneous breathing is always worse while asleep. Approximately one-third of patients with CCHS have such severe spontaneous hypoventilation while awake that they require full-time ventilatory support. The remainder of patients with CCHS, though not normal while awake, breathe well enough that sleeping ventilatory support is all that is required to avoid pulmonary hypertension and central nervous system complications.

The diagnosis of CCHS is confirmed by testing for mutations in the *PHOX2B* gene (9,10). While waiting for this test result, which is run in only a few laboratories, other causes of hypoventilation should be ruled out to facilitate proper treatment. Primary lung disease, ventilatory muscle weakness, and cardiac disease should be ruled out. MRI and/or CT scans of the brain and brain stem should be performed to rule out gross anatomic lesions, which are absent in CCHS (24). A variety of inborn errors of metabolism may cause apnea or hypoventilation. Thus, a metabolic screen should be performed. Similarly, patients should have a neurologic evaluation to rule out known neurologic conditions that may cause these symptoms.

CCHS is characterized by abnormal ventilatory control in the absence of obvious brain stem anatomic lesions (3,16,24). However, patients with CCHS have other abnormalities in autonomic nervous system function. Woo and coworkers found that all patients with CCHS showed decreased beat-to-beat heart rate variability, indicating a dysfunction in autonomic nervous system control of the heart (11). Patients with CCHS frequently exhibit ophthalmologic abnormalities reflecting neural control of eye function (15). There are anecdotal reports that children with CCHS have poor heat tolerance. Some of our patients sweat on only one side of their bodies. Bradycardia is not uncommon in CCHS, especially during sleep, though it rarely necessitates implantation of cardiac pacemakers (5). Two studies have reported poor school performance and/or decreased intellectual function in patients with CCHS (4,13). It is unclear whether these symptoms are due to hypoxia or a direct result of CCHS.

D. Clinical Management

The treatment of CCHS is to ensure adequate ventilation when the patient is unable to achieve adequate gas exchange by spontaneous breathing (4–7). This requires mechanically assisted ventilation, as no pharmacologic respiratory stimulants have been shown to be effective (2,4,6). CCHS does not resolve spontaneously, therefore, chronic ventilatory support at home is necessary for these patients to leave the hospital (3). Positive pressure ventilators (PPV) via tracheostomy, bi-level positive airway pressure (4,25,26), negative-pressure ventilators (27), and diaphragm pacing (28,29) are options for these patients. Although oxygen administration improves the Pao_2 and relieves cyanosis, this treatment is inadequate as hypoventilation persists and pulmonary hypertension ensues (13).

CCHS patients lack a very essential protective physiologic response, the ventilatory response to hypoxia and CO_2. Trying to compensate for this in a child at all times is not easy. During the first years of life, CCHS infants may be very unstable. Even minor respiratory infections may cause complete apnea during both sleep and wakefulness. As they mature, the neurologic condition does not change, but the other parts of the respiratory system (lungs, ventilatory muscles, chest wall) mature. Older children and adolescents are usually more stable.

Respiratory infections usually do not cause the degree of ventilatory depression that was seen in the first few years of life. However, CCHS patients do not regain their ventilatory responses to hypoxia or CO_2 at any age.

It cannot be overemphasized that CCHS patients may suffer complete respiratory arrest or severe hypoventilation at sleep onset. Thus, they require continuous observation and/or monitoring so that ventilatory support can be initiated with each sleep episode. Apnea/bradycardia monitoring alone is not sufficient, as many patients hypoventilate but are not apneic. An impressive finding in CCHS is the complete absence of subjective or objective responses to hypoxia or hypercapnia while awake or asleep (3). Clinicians usually recognize hypoxia or respiratory failure in a child by manifestations of intact ventilatory control. Hypoxia and hypercapnia ordinarily stimulate respiratory drive, which increases ventilation, retractions, nasal flaring, a sense of dyspnea, etc. However, in CCHS, respiratory drive is absent. Thus, hypoxia is detected only much later, when it has already caused central nervous system depression (lethargy), cyanosis, or other complications. Therefore, these children need to be monitored continually by trained observers to prevent significant and sustained hypoxia and its sequelae.

Progressive pulmonary hypertension and cor pulmonale may occur in these patients and must be assumed to be due to inadequate ventilation until proven otherwise. Some infants will have progressive pulmonary hypertension even when ventilation during sleep is controlled. This symptom is usually due to hypoventilation during wakefulness. These patients require ventilatory support during wakefulness as well (4). For such patients, diaphragm pacing is an optimal form of ventilatory support during wakefulness, because it is portable and permits these children to participate in normal activities while receiving "assisted ventilation" (28,29).

E. Medical Complications and Outcome

In patients with CCHS, the most common problem is inadequate ventilation, which occurs both during sleep and wakefulness. Thus, if these patients have any unexplained problem (seizure, lethargy, etc.), they should be stabilized by hyperventilation with 100% oxygen until the source of the problem can be identified. In children with CCHS, the etiology of any such problem is likely to be hypoventilation until proven otherwise. A brief period of hyperventilation will not be harmful, but may be lifesaving if the child has inadequate ventilation.

Frequent and severe hypoxemic episodes may be associated with permanent neurologic sequelae. Children with CCHS are generally in the slow learner range of mental processing abilities, compounded by significant learning disabilities. Neuropsychological function appears to correlate with the severity of CCHS. Children with the mildest form of CCHS may function in the above average range. Children who function in the mentally retarded range often have severe forms of CCHS and may require ventilatory support during wakefulness as well as during sleep (4,13).

There is no known cure for CCHS. The disorder appears to be lifelong (3,4). With modern techniques for home ventilation, most children with CCHS survive with a good quality of life (4), although they are at risk of having offspring with CCHS (see chap. 19).

III. Myelomeningocele with Arnold-Chiari Malformation

The Arnold-Chiari malformation (ACM) of the brain stem is a complex deformity of the central nervous system, bone, and soft tissues (30). There is herniation of the medulla and cerebellum, giving rise to obstruction of the cerebrospinal fluid flow at the fourth ventricular outlet. Thus, hydrocephalus is common. Type II ACM, commonly associated with myelomeningocele, is characterized by displacement of the cerebellar vermis, caudal brainstem, and fourth ventricle through the foramen magnum. It can be predicted that the ACM of the brain stem should affect the brain stem respiratory centers and thus affect the neurologic control of breathing.

A. Etiology

There are two basic theories about the etiology of ACM in the myelomeningocele. One group of theories suggests that the actual brain in ACM is normal but was deformed by mechanical processes: (*i*) traction from the myelomeningocele, which tethers the spinal cord to the skin opening, pulling the brain stem down through the foramen magnum with growth; and (*ii*) hydrocephalus and increased intracranial pressure, which causes reopening of the previously closed neural tube, pushing the brain stem down through the foramen magnum (30,31). The second theory suggests that ACM represents a primary, unidentified insult to central nervous system tissue and that it is not secondary to other mechanical actions (30). This latter view is supported by the high incidence of brain stem nuclear hypoplasia noted in one study (30). Elements of both theories are probably correct, and ACM is associated with abnormal formation and/or destruction of brain stem nuclei.

B. Ventilatory Control Abnormalities

Abnormal vocal cord motility and the resultant obstructive apnea in infants with myelomeningocele are a major manifestation of abnormal ventilation (31–36). It has been suggested that this is due to increased intracranial pressure and is often successfully treated when this pressure is reduced. Infants have also been noted to have clinically significant sleep hypoventilation, obstructive apneas, and breath-holding spells (37). In some cases, these symptoms resolve following posterior fossa decompression surgery (37).

Infants with myelomeningocele, hydrocephalus, and ACM have abnormalities in their ventilatory pattern during sleep, even if they do not have obvious clinical apneas (37,38).

Swaminathan and coworkers found that hypercapnic ventilatory responses were significantly lower in adolescents with ACM compared with controls (39). These results suggest that the ACM interferes with central chemosensitivity (39,40). Although the exact anatomic location of the central chemoreceptors has not been defined, it is believed to be in the ventrolateral medulla. This is compatible with the anatomic defect in ACM. Swaminathan and Gozal also demonstrated depressed hypoxic ventilatory responses in some subjects with ACM, though as a group they were not significantly different from control values (39,40). This fact could indicate involvement of central integrating pathways and/or respiratory neurons in some patients with ACM.

C. Clinical Management

Hays and coworkers reported the outcome of 616 infants and children with ACM (41). Thirty-five children, or 5.7%, had evidence of central ventilatory dysfunction, which included apnea, bradycardia, aspiration, vocal cord paralysis, and stridor. Twenty-four of these 35 patients died (69%) (41). Apnea, stridor, and/or aspiration were the primary causes of death in 14 of the 24 patients. Two had sudden, unexplained deaths during sleep without previous clinical respiratory problems (3.2/1000 ACM). Six additional children died from acute apnea (9.7/1000 ACM). Three died from increased intracranial pressure (4,9/1000 ACM). Thus, infants and children with ACM have an increased incidence of sudden death, presumably due to apnea (41). Others have documented a high incidence of acute respiratory arrest in children with ACM, presumably due to increased intracranial pressure (42).

It cannot be distinguished whether these signs of abnormal ventilatory control are due to abnormal brain stem nuclei or to mechanical compression of the brain stem. Little can be done for abnormally developed nuclei. However, mechanical compression can be relieved. Therefore, infants with ACM should be evaluated for hydrocephalus, which is present in nearly all patients. This abnormality should be corrected as soon as possible with a ventriculoperitoneal shunt. If symptoms persist after correction of the hydrocephalus, then a posterior fossa decompression of the brain stem should be seriously considered (37,43). Kirk and coworkers reviewed treatment of sleep-disordered breathing in ACM from six centers and found that posterior fossa decompression was only effective in four of 13 patients (31%) (43). If performed, posterior fossa decompression must be performed as soon as possible to prevent progressive brain stem damage. It is possible that once significant respiratory symptoms are clinically evident, irreversible brain stem damage has already occurred. On the other hand, having a high clinical suspicion for sleep-disordered breathing in infants with ACM, early investigation, and early treatment may improve the clinical outcome of these, and other, therapeutic interventions (43).

Patients with ACM commonly develop upper airway obstruction during wakefulness and/or sleep, as a result of vocal cord paralysis. Signs of obstruction should be investigated by laryngoscopy. If vocal cord paralysis is present, a tracheostomy is usually required.

Some infants and children with ACM develop inadequate ventilation during sleep or during both sleep and wakefulness. This central hypoventilation syndrome requires chronic ventilatory support (43). Some of those who require only sleeping ventilatory support may be able to attend school and have a reasonable quality of life while off the ventilator during wakefulness. However, progressive neurologic problems, such as syrinx formation and hydrocephalus, may occur. On the other hand, infants and children with myelomeningocele and severe neurologic damage, who also require assisted ventilation, have a poor prognosis due to progressive neurologic deterioration, and many die despite mechanically assisted ventilation (44). Therefore, the benefits and burdens of home mechanical ventilation should be weighed individually for each child, considering the current neurologic condition, overall function, and expected benefits (44).

IV. Prader-Willi Syndrome

Prader-Willi syndrome is characterized by obesity, hyperphagia, hypogonadism, mental retardation, hypotonia, and behavioral and sleep disorders. One of the most remarkable features is an apparently insatiable appetite, resulting in obesity. Reduced life expectancy is probably related to complications of morbid obesity. Prader-Willi syndrome is associated with a deletion of the long arm of the paternally derived chromosome 15 (15q11–q13) in approximately 50–70% of the patients. It is believed that a primary hypothalamic dysfunction leads to the typical clinical and behavioral manifestations of Prader-Willi syndrome.

A. Respiratory Control Abnormalities

Patients with Prader-Willi syndrome often exhibit sleep-disordered breathing. This syndrome is characterized by snoring, obstructive sleep apnea, restless movements during sleep, hypoventilation, hypoxia, excessive daytime sleepiness, and abnormalities of sleep architecture (45). However, it is unclear how much of this is related to obesity alone versus an intrinsic disorder of ventilatory control.

Arens and coworkers found that ventilatory responses to hypercapnia were normal in non-obese Prader-Willi patients but blunted in obese patients (46). Thus, abnormalities in response to CO_2 are probably explained by obesity, rather than a primary disorder of ventilatory control (46). It is also possible that obesity could be a marker for severity of the ventilatory control disturbance in these patients. Conversely, rebreathing ventilatory responses to hypoxia were completely absent in about one-third of patients, and blunted in the remainder (46). This finding was consistent in all Prader-Willi subjects, whether or not they were obese. Thus, hypoxic ventilatory responses were decreased in both obese and non-obese Prader-Willi patients, suggesting a primary ventilatory control abnormality in peripheral chemoreceptor function (46). Gozal et al. studied peripheral chemoreceptor function specifically with hyperoxia, and acute hypoxic and hypercapnic challenges, and found absent or depressed peripheral chemoreceptor function in all patients with Prader-Willi syndrome (47).

Arens and coworkers found that patients with Prader-Willi syndrome rarely aroused from quiet sleep in response to hypoxia, compared to control subjects (48). Similarly, the increase in heart rate stimulated by hypoxia was blunted in Prader-Willi syndrome compared with controls (48). Since peripheral chemoreceptor function is required for intact hypoxic arousal, this finding supports the hypothesis that patients with Prader-Willi syndrome have absent peripheral chemoreceptor function (48). Livingston and coworkers found that all patients and controls aroused from quiet sleep in response to a hypercapnic challenge. However, the level of Pco_2 at which arousal occurred was significantly higher in Prader-Willi syndrome than in controls (49). Since ventilatory responses to hypercapnia appear to be intact, this increased CO_2 arousal threshold may also reflect abnormal peripheral chemoreceptor function (decreased tonic stimulation). Brain stem dysfunction in areas of integration and/or reticular activating system may also be present.

Prader-Willi syndrome is thought to represent a primary hypothalamic dysfunction. Altered hypothalamic function may lead to abnormal ventilatory responses (50). The hypothalamus may modulate both hypercapnic and hypoxic ventilatory responses (50,51). Thus, the hypothalamic dysfunction in Prader-Willi syndrome may contribute to the ventilatory control abnormality seen in these patients.

B. Clinical Management

In patients with Prader-Willi syndrome, the main clinical problem related to ventilatory control appears to be sleep-disordered breathing. One can reduce the severity of this problem by avoiding obesity. Unfortunately, this is difficult in Prader-Willi syndrome, because patients have an insatiable appetite on the one hand and mental retardation on the other. The mental retardation makes it difficult to motivate these patients to decrease caloric intake. Obstructive sleep apnea should be treated as in other patients and may require nasal continuous positive airway pressure (CPAP), bi-level positive airway pressure, or upper airway surgery. In our experience, it is uncommon for patients with Prader-Willi syndrome to require home mechanical ventilation. Since the primary defect is peripheral chemoreceptor dysfunction, one should be especially concerned about situations where the patient's inadequate response to hypoxia may be life-threatening.

Growth hormone therapy has been proposed as a useful intervention for children with Prader-Willi syndrome in order to increase lean tissue mass and growth velocity. There are also reports that this therapy enhances behavior, physical activity, and respiratory function (52). However, there have been a number of reports of death shortly after the initiation of growth hormone therapy, raising concerns about the safety of this therapy. Deaths have been attributed to obstructive sleep apnea, respiratory infection, and pulmonary aspiration. Many, but not all, of the deaths occurred in obese children with Prader-Willi syndrome (52,53). It is not entirely clear, if deaths were caused by unrecognized preexisting conditions or were triggered by the use of growth hormone therapy. A case report of respiratory difficulty during growth hormone therapy resolving after it was discontinued supports the latter possibility (54). A prospective study of 25 children with Prader-Willi syndrome found that all patients had some degree of sleep-disordered breathing prior to growth hormone therapy and that the majority (19 of 25) had an improvement in their breathing pattern after six weeks of growth hormone therapy. However, six patients had a worsening of obstructive sleep apnea. The authors attributed the worsening to intercurrent upper respiratory tract infections and an increase in tonsillar size. All of these patients had adenotonsillectomy with clinical resolution of the obstructive sleep apnea syndrome (OSAS) (55). Thus, it is recommended that children with Prader-Willi syndrome, especially those with history of snoring, sleep-disordered breathing, or obesity, should have an examination of the upper airway and an overnight polysomnogram prior to commencing growth hormone therapy. If sleep-disordered breathing is identified, appropriate therapy should be initiated before administering growth hormone. All patients should be followed for any change in sleep- or breathing-related symptoms, and some would recommend a repeat polysomnogram for all patients after six weeks of therapy (52,55).

V. Achondroplasia and Other Skeletal Dysplasias

Achondroplasia is an autosomal dominant disorder characterized by inhibition of endochondral bone formation. Affected individuals have disproportionate shortening of the proximal limbs, a small thoracic cage, and a large head with a depressed nasal bridge. It is caused by mutations in the fibroblast growth factor receptor 3 gene. The base of the skull is involved and there is midfacial hypoplasia. Thus, obstructive sleep apnea is common and may be severe. However, the membranous bones of the skull grow normally, which results in a large skull resting on a small base with spinal stenosis. Therefore, compression of the medullary and cervical cord and hydrocephalus are common. These abnormalities lead to a high risk for abnormalities of central respiratory control, such as hypoventilation, apnea, and sudden death.

Mogayzel and colleagues found that nearly half of 88 infants and children with achondroplasia had abnormalities documented by overnight polysomnography (56). The most common abnormality was hypoxemia. The majority did not have significant obstructive or central apnea or hypoventilation, but a small number of subjects were severely affected (56).

Treatment options include ventriculoperitoneal shunt for hydrocephalus, cervicomedullary decompression for central respiratory control abnormalities and other neurologic dysfunctions, oxygen for hypoxemia, adenotonsillectomy for OSAS, or bi-level positive airway pressure for hypoventilation and/or OSAS. Some infants and children with achondroplasia will require tracheostomy for severe OSAS, and a few will need positive pressure ventilation via tracheostomy for central hypoventilation. Despite these difficulties, children with achondroplasia have normal intelligence and do well with appropriate therapy (57–59).

Other skeletal dysplasias may also affect the brain stem area and/or thoracic restriction. The thoracic restriction in skeletal dysplasias may occur prior to birth, restricting growth of the rapidly developing lungs and causing structural hypoplasia of the lungs. Even with subsequent growth of the thoracic cage, or attempted surgical reconstruction, the hypoplastic lungs may not be reversible. Thus, the presence of hypoplastic lungs is an important prognosticator for these patients.

VI. Leigh's Disease

Leigh's disease, also called subacute necrotizing encephalomyelopathy, is a group of inherited disorders in infancy and childhood characterized by a progressive clinical course of deterioration in brain stem dysfunction (60–63). Patients may appear normal during infancy but develop progressive neurologic symptoms later. Clinical symptoms include poor feeding, vomiting, apnea, alveolar hypoventilation, and regression of development. Occasionally, hypoventilation can precede other neurologic symptoms. Brain stem symptoms may include nystagmus, bizarre eye movements, pupillary changes, hypotonia, seizures, and sleep/wakefulness disturbances. Brain stem lesions are bilateral, but not necessarily symmetrical. There is preferential gray matter involvement with vascular proliferation, endothelial swelling, and progressive neuronal destruction. There is also loss of myelin. Changes are predominantly seen in the midbrain, pons, periaqueductal gray matter, posterior colliculi, medulla, floor of the fourth ventricle, and posterior olive. CT or MRI of the brain stem often shows changes suggesting this diagnosis. Leigh's disease was once thought to be an autosomal recessive disorder. It is now clear that Leigh's disease is a syndrome with many etiologies; presumably all are due to inborn errors of metabolism (62,63).

There is no specific treatment for Leigh's disease. Chronic ventilatory support is the only treatment for chronic respiratory failure, but it is not offered to some of these patients because of their poor prognosis due to neurologic deterioration (61).

VII. Joubert Syndrome

Joubert syndrome is due to agenesis of the cerebellar vermis, with associated episodes of tachypnea (as high as 100–200 breaths/min) alternating with prolonged apneas (64,65). Patients also exhibit abnormal eye movements, hypotonia, and severe psychomotor retardation. Tachypnea and apnea may occur during sleep or wakefulness. The tachypnea spontaneously resolves after infancy. We provided medical care to one patient who had moderate hypoventilation in addition to the apneas (Pco_2 50–55 Torr). The child also had significant obstructive apnea and vocal cord paralysis, which are presumed to be nonspecific signs of brain stem involvement. However, her symptoms progressed to requiring full-time mechanical ventilation, accompanied by deteriorating mental function. The disorder is often progressive and the ventilatory pattern abnormalities can cause death.

VIII. Acquired Central Hypoventilation Syndromes

Abnormalities in neurologic control of breathing can be acquired, usually because of damage to relevant areas of the brain stem. When sufficient damage occurs, it can result in a central hypoventilation syndrome, with attendant hypoxia and hypercapnia. In less severe cases, intermittent apnea may occur with adequate baseline ventilation. Causes of acquired central hypoventilation syndrome can include brain tumors (66), infections (encephalitis) (61,67), trauma, congenital vascular malformations (such as rupture of aneurysms), neurologic surgery, central nervous system radiation, and cerebrovascular accidents (61). In our experience, these conditions are uncommon and are often associated with other severe neurologic damages. While damage to the brain stem can cause a disorder in neurologic control of breathing, there is no characteristic pattern of the abnormality, as it will depend on the specific area of injury and extent of damage. However, because peripheral chemoreceptors are anatomically distinct from the brain stem, one is not likely to see a primary peripheral chemoreceptor dysfunction. Rather, these patients usually have a combination of central chemoreceptor and central integration (ventilatory controller) dysfunction. In addition to a true disorder of neurologic control of breathing, brain stem injury may also disrupt motor tracts leading to the ventilatory muscles. Thus, respiratory control dysfunction in these children is usually accompanied by ventilatory muscle weakness or paralysis from damage to motor tracts.

We have experience providing medical care to brain stem tumor patients with acquired central hypoventilation syndrome severe enough to require chronic ventilatory support. These children usually have signs of generalized severe neurologic damage in addition to hypoventilation. In general, these patients require full-time ventilatory support. We have also seen a number of children with acquired central hypoventilation following resection of craniopharyngioma. In addition to multiple endocrine problems from panhypopituitarism, many of these children are obese and have OSAS, which may also have elements of central hypoventilation syndrome. We have treated some of these patients with bi-level positive airway pressure using a back-up rate.

IX. Management of Respiratory Failure in Children with Respiratory Control Disorders

In children with respiratory control disorders, usually there is little that can be done to augment central respiratory drive. However, central respiratory drive can be further inhibited by metabolic imbalance, such as chronic metabolic alkalosis. Thus, serum chloride concentrations should be maintained greater than 95 mEq/dL, and alkalosis avoided. Pharmacologic respiratory stimulants are not helpful (3,4). Sedative medications and central nervous system depressants should be avoided.

Children with respiratory control disorders are generally good candidates for chronic home mechanical ventilation (25). Any coexisting pulmonary disease must be sufficiently stable so that the child does not require frequent adjustments in ventilator settings to maintain adequate gas exchange. In general, children with chronically elevated P_{CO_2} greater than ~60 Torr, due to decreased central respiratory drive, will develop progressive pulmonary hypertension. Although oxygen administration improves the Pa_{O_2} and relieves cyanosis, this treatment alone is inadequate, as hypoventilation persists with resulting pulmonary hypertension. Thus, these children require home mechanical ventilation.

A. Philosophy of Chronic Ventilatory Support

For most children going home with chronic ventilatory support, weaning from the ventilator is not a realistic goal. In order to optimize quality of life, these children must have energy available for other physical activities. Thus, ventilators are adjusted to completely meet the ventilatory demands of these children, leaving much of their energy available for other activities. For children with respiratory control disorders, ventilators are adjusted to provide end-tidal CO_2 pressure (PET_{CO_2}) of 30–35 mmHg and arterial oxygen saturation of hemoglobin (SpO_2) greater than 95% (25). Optimal ventilation also avoids atelectasis and the development of coexisting lung disease. Children who are hyperventilated at night have better spontaneous ventilation while awake than those who are ventilated to higher Pco_2 levels (68). It has also been our experience that children with respiratory control disorders have fewer complications, and generally do better clinically, with hyperventilation during assisted ventilation.

B. Modalities of Chronic Ventilatory Support

The ideal ventilators for home use are different from those used in hospitals for the treatment of acute respiratory failure (25). Because children with respiratory control disorders usually do not have severe lung disease, they have the greatest number of options for different techniques to provide chronic ventilatory support at home. These include (*i*) portable positive pressure ventilator via tracheostomy (25,26); (*ii*) bi-level positive airway pressure via nasal or face mask (25,26); (*iii*) negative-pressure chest shell (cuirass) (27), wrap, or portable tank ventilator; and (*iv*) diaphragm pacing (28,29). Details of management of patients requiring home mechanical ventilation prior to discharge and in the home are beyond the scope of this chapter, and they have been described elsewhere (6,7,25). The different modalities of home mechanical ventilation relevant to central hypoventilation syndromes will be briefly reviewed.

PPV Through Tracheostomy

The PPV is the most common method of providing home mechanical ventilation for infants and children (4,25). Commercially available electronic PPVs are capable of battery operation and are relatively portable and thus maximize mobility. A tracheostomy is required for positive-pressure ventilator access. We prefer to maintain a small tracheostomy in ventilator-assisted children for two reasons: (*i*) the small tracheostomy is less likely to cause tracheomalacia, and (*ii*) the small tracheostomy allows a large expiratory leak so that the child may speak. While use of the small tracheostomy necessitates a large leak around the tracheostomy, using the home ventilator in a pressure plateau mode allows us to compensate for this leak (69)

Bi-Level Positive Airway Pressure Ventilation by Mask or Nasal Prongs

Noninvasive intermittent positive pressure ventilation is delivered via a nasal mask, nasal prongs, or face mask using a bi-level positive airway pressure ventilator (7,70–73). This technique is commonly used in older children, but has also been used successfully in infants and small children. When bi-level ventilators are used for ventilatory assistance rather than for obstructive sleep apnea, a large inspiratory positive airway pressure (IPAP) to expiratory positive airway pressure (EPAP) difference is desirable. The lowest EPAP that can be used without CO_2 accumulation at the interface is 4 cmH_2O. The highest IPAP that can be used is generally 20 cmH_2O. However, most children need to begin with lower IPAP in the range of 10 to 14 cmH_2O and increase slowly as tolerated and as necessary (70).

Only the spontaneous/timed and timed modes of ventilation guarantee breath delivery. These modes should be used in children with respiratory control disorders because these patients cannot be trusted to generate their own adequate respirations. Noninvasive bi-level ventilation is not as powerful as PPV via tracheostomy. Thus, children may require intubation and more sophisticated ventilatory support during acute exacerbations. The major benefit of bi-level ventilation is that a tracheostomy is not required.

Negative-Pressure Ventilation

Negative-pressure ventilators apply a negative pressure outside the chest and abdomen during inspiration to generate ventilation. A chest shell ventilator uses a dome-shaped shell that is fitted over the anterior chest and abdomen (27). The negative-pressure wrap ventilator is a "jump suit" that fits snugly around the neck, wrists, and ankles to minimize leaks. A metal "cage" inside the jump suit creates a space where negative pressure can be generated during inspiration. A portable tank is a negative-pressure ventilator, and an infant or child may fit inside. Negative inspiratory pressure is generated inside the chest shell, wrap, or portable tank, which expands the chest and upper abdomen. The ventilator rate and the negative pressure developed inside the chest shell, wrap, or portable tank can be selected. The negative pressure is proportional to the tidal volume, but may be limited by leaks around the chest shell or wrap. These ventilators can provide effective ventilation in children and adolescents, sometimes without a tracheostomy (27). However, with negative-pressure ventilation there is no synchronous activation of the upper airway muscles as normally occurs during spontaneous breathing. Thus, airway occlusion can occur when breaths are generated by a negative-pressure ventilator during sleep.

Negative-pressure ventilation may permit decannulation of a tracheostomy. We have successfully transitioned children with CCHS from positive pressure ventilation via tracheostomy to negative-pressure ventilation in order to allow them to be decannulated after five to six years of age. Upper airway obstruction can be minimized by tonsillectomy and adenoidectomy, which optimizes the size of the upper airway. However, these ventilators are not portable, and most of our patients utilizing this technique have changed to bi-level positive airway pressure ventilation via mask.

Diaphragm Pacing

Diaphragm pacing generates breathing using the child's own diaphragm as the respiratory pump (28,29). Commercially available diaphragm pacing systems have battery-operated external transmitters. An antenna is taped on the skin over subcutaneously implanted receivers. The transmitter generates a train of pulses for each breath, which is transmitted through the antenna to the receiver under the skin, similar to radio transmission. The receiver converts this energy to standard electrical current, which is directed to a phrenic nerve electrode by lead wires. The electrical stimulation of the phrenic nerve causes a diaphragmatic contraction, which generates the breath. The amount of electrical voltage is proportional to the diaphragmatic contraction, which generates tidal volume. In children, simultaneous bilateral diaphragm pacing is generally required to achieve optimal ventilation. In older children or adolescents who have stable chest walls, adequate ventilation may be achieved by pacing only one side.

Use of pacers requires that the phrenic nerves and the diaphragm function appropriately to enable effective ventilation. Therefore, ventilatory muscle myopathy and phrenic neuropathy are contraindications to pacer use. Obstructive apnea can be a complication of diaphragm pacing during sleep because synchronous upper airway skeletal muscle contraction does not occur with inspiration. However, this complication can often be overcome by adjusting settings on the pacers to lengthen inspiratory time and/or decrease the force of inspiration. In general, diaphragm pacers can only be used up to approximately 14 hours a day and cannot be used for 24 hours continuously. Thus, patients who require ventilatory support 24 hours a day should have an alternate form of ventilation for part of the day if pacers are used. Pacers can be used for daytime support of ambulatory children who require full-time ventilatory support, in combination with PPV at night (28,29).

X. Summary

There are no generally effective pharmacologic treatments for true disorders of neurologic control of breathing. Thus, therapeutic management usually requires mechanically assisted ventilation or close monitoring of less severe clinical problems (apnea). The prognosis for children with syndromes affecting respiratory control during sleep depends primarily on associated neurologic problems, the extent of central nervous system injury or involvement, whether the disorder is progressive, and the severity of hypoventilation. Some children with central hypoventilation syndromes, such as CCHS, can have prolonged survival, associated with a good quality of life for them and their families, using mechanically assisted ventilation. For other children with progressive or severe neurologic disorders, the prognosis is poor, and mechanically assisted ventilation may not be indicated. Complications in these children may result from delayed diagnosis and intermittent hypoxemia. We believe that early diagnosis of central hypoventilation and treatment of occult hypoxemia or hypoventilation will result in the best outcome. The level of treatment ultimately instituted must be individually tailored to the child and specific respiratory control disorder.

References

1. Severinghaus J, Mitchell RA. Ondine's curse—failure of respiratory center automaticity while awake. Clin Res 1962; 10:122.
2. Mellins RB, Balfour HH Jr., Turino GM, et al. Failure of automatic control of ventilation (Ondine's curse). Medicine 1970; 49:487–504.
3. Paton JY, Swaminathan S, Sargent CW, et al. Hypoxic and hypercapneic ventilatory responses in awake children with congenital central hypoventilation syndrome. Am Rev Respir Dis 1989; 140:368–372.

4. Marcus CL, Jansen MT, Poulsen MK, et al. Medical and psychosocial outcome of children with congenital central hypoventilation syndrome. J Pediatr 1991; 119: 888–895.

5. Weese-Mayer DE, Silvestri JM, Menzies LJ, et al. Congenital central hypoventilation syndrome: diagnosis, management, and long-term outcome in thirty-two children. J Pediatr 1992; 120:381–387.

6. Weese-Mayer DE, Shannon DC, Keens TG, et al. Idiopathic congenital central hypoventilation syndrome: diagnosis and management. Am J Respir Crit Care Med 1999; 160:368–373.

7. Chen ML, Keens TG. Congenital central hypoventilation syndrome: not just another rare disorder. Paediatr Respir Rev 2004; 5(3):182–189.

8. Gozal D. Congenital central hypoventilation syndrome: an update. Pediatr Pulmonol 1998; 26:273–282.

9. Amiel J, Laudier B, Attie-Bitach T, et al. Polyalanine expansion and frameshift mutations of the paired-like homeobox gene PHOX2B in congenital central hypoventilation syndrome. Nat Genet, 2003; 33:459–461.

10. Weese-Mayer DE, Berry-Kravis EM, Zhou L, et al. Idiopathic congenital central hypoventilation syndrome: analysis of genes pertinent to early autonomic nervous system embryonic development and identification of mutations in PHOX2B. Am J Med Genet 2003; 123A:267–278.

11. Woo MS, Woo MA, Gozal D, et al. Heart rate variability in congenital central hypoventilation syndrome. Pediatr Res 1992;31:291–296.

12. Swaminathan S, Gilsanz V, Atkinson J, et al. Congenital central hypoventilation syndrome associated with multiple ganglioneuromas. Chest 1989; 96:423–424.

13. Silvestri JM, Weese-Mayer DE, Nelson MN. Neuropsychologic abnormalities in children with congenital central hypoventilation syndrome. J Pediatr 1992; 120: 388–393.

14. Haddad GG, Mazza NM, Defendini R, et al. Congenital failure of automatic control of ventilation, gastrointestinal motility and heart rate. Medicine (Baltimore) 1978; 57:517–526.

15. Goldberg DS, Ludwig IH. Ocular signs in children with congenital central hypoventilation syndrome. Pediatr Pulmonol 1997; 23:150–151.

16. Marcus CL, Bautista DB, Amihyia A, et al. Hypercapneic arousal responses in children with congenital central hypoventilation syndrome. Pediatrics 1991; 88: 993–998.

17. Macey PM, Valderama C, Kim AH, et al. Temporal trends of cardiac and respiratory responses to ventilatory challenges in congenital central hypoventilation syndrome. Pediatr Res 2004; 55:953–959.

18. Macey PM, Woo MA, Macey KE, et al. Hypoxia reveals posterior thalamic, cerebellar, midbrain and limbic deficits in congenital central hypoventilation syndrome. J Appl Physiol 2005; 98:958–969.

19. Harper RM, Macey PM, Woo MA, et al. Hypercapnic exposure in congenital hypoventilation syndrome reveals central respiratory control mechanisms. J Neurophysiol 2005; 93:1647–1658.

20. Kumar R, Macey PM, Woo MA, et al. Neuroanatomic deficits in congenital central hypoventilation syndrome. J Comp Neurol 2005; 487:361–371.

21. Silvestri JM, Weese-Mayer DE, Flanagan EA. Congenital central hypoventilation syndrome: cardiorespiratory responses to moderate exercise simulating daily activity. Pediatr Pulmonol 1995; 20:89–93.
22. Paton JY, Swaminathan S, Sargent CW, et al. Ventilatory response to exercise in children with congenital central hypoventilation syndrome. Am Rev Respir Dis 1993; 147:1185–1191.
23. Gozal D, Marcus CL, Davidson Ward SL, et al. Ventilatory responses to passive leg motion in children with congenital central hypoventilation syndrome. Am J Respir Crit Care Med 1996; 153:761–768.
24. Weese-Mayer DE, Brouillette RT, Naidich TP, et al. Magnetic resonance imaging and computerized tomography in central hypoventilation. Am Rev Respir Dis 1988; 137:393–398.
25. Witmans MB, Chen ML, Davidson Ward SW, et al. Congenital syndromes affecting respiratory control during sleep. In: Lee-Chiong T, ed. Sleep: A Comprehensive Handbook. Hoboken, New Jersey: John Wiley and Sons, 2006:517–527.
26. Beckerman RC. Home positive pressure ventilation in congenital central hypoventilation syndrome: more than twenty years of experience. Pediatr Pulmonol 1997; 23:154–155.
27. Hartman H, Samuels MP, Noyes JP, et al. Negative extrathoracic pressure ventilation in infants and young children with central hypoventilation syndrome. Pediatr Pulmonol 1997; 23155–157.
28. Weese-Mayer DE, Hunt CE, Brouillette RT. Diaphragm pacing in infants and children. J Pediatr 1992; 120(1):1–8.
29. Chen ML, Tablizo MA, Kun S, et al. Diaphragm pacers as a treatment for congenital central hypoventilation syndrome. Expert Rev Med Dev 2005; 2:577–585.
30. Gilbert JN, Jones KL, Rorke LB, et al. Central nervous anomalies associated with meningomyelocele, hydrocephalus, and Arnold-Chiari malformation: reappraisal of theories regarding the pathogenesis of posterior neural tube closure defects. Neurosurgery 1986; 18:559–564.
31. Ruff ME, Oakes WJ, Fisher SR, et al. Sleep apnea and vocal cord paralysis secondary to type I Arnold-Chiari malformation. Pediatrics 1987; 80:231–234.
32. Morley AR. Laryngeal stridor, Arnold-Chiari malformation and medullary hemorrhages. Dev Med Child Neurol 1969; 11:471–474.
33. Bluestone CD, Delevine AN, Samuelson GH. Airway obstruction due to vocal cord paralysis in infants with hydrocephalus and meningomyelocele. Ann Otol Rhinol 1972; 81:778–783.
34. Krieger AJ, Detwiler JS, Trooskin SZ. Respiratory function in infants with Arnold-Chiari malformation. Laryngoscope 1976; 86:718–723.
35. Hollinger PC, Hollinger LD, Reichert TJ, et al. Respiratory obstruction and apnea in infants with bilateral abductor vocal cord paralysis, meningomyelocele, hydrocephalus and Arnold-Chiari malformation. J Pediatr 1978; 92:368–373.
36. Badr AI, McLone D, Seleny FL. Intraoperative autonomic dysfunction associated with Arnold-Chiari malformation. Childs Brain 1980; 7:146–149.
37. Oren J, Kelly DH, Todres ID, et al. Respiratory complications in patients with myelodysplasia and Arnold-Chiari malformation. Am J Dis Child 1986; 140:221–224.
38. Davidson Ward SL, Jacobs RA, Gates EP, et al. Abnormal ventilatory patterns during sleep in infants with myelomeningocele. J Pediatr 1986; 109:631–634.

39. Swaminathan S, Paton JY, Ward SLD, et al. Abnormal control of ventilation in adolescents with myelomeningocele. J Pediatr 1989; 115:898–903.

40. Gozal D, Arens R, Omlin KJ, et al. Peripheral chemoreceptor function in children with myelomeningocele and Arnold Chiari malformation type 2. Chest 1995; 108: 425–431.

41. Hays RM, Jordan RA, McLaughlin JF, et al. Central ventilatory dysfunction in myelodysplasia: an independent determinant of survival. Dev Med Child Neurol 1989; 31:366–370.

42. Tomita T, McLone DG. Acute respiratory arrest: a complication of malformation of the shunt in children with myelomeningocele and Arnold-Chiari malformation. Am J Dis Child 1983;137:142–144.

43. Kirk VG, D'Andrea L, Marcus CL, et al. Efficacy of treatments for sleep-disordered breathing (SDB) in patients with spina bifida/myelomeningocele (SB/MM). Am J Respir Crit Care Med 1998; 157(3):A534.

44. Woo MS, Jansen MT, Jacobs RA, et al. Home mechanical ventilation for children with Arnold-Chiari malformation. Am J Respir Crit Care Med 1994; 149(4):A376.

45. Cassidy SB, McKillop J, Morgan W. Sleep disorders in Prader-Willi syndrome. Dysmorphol Clin Genet 1990; 4:13–17.

46. Arens R, Gozal D, Omlin KJ, et al. Hypoxic and hypercapnic ventilatory responses in Prader-Willi syndrome. J Appl Physiol 1994; 77:2224–2230.

47. Gozal D, Arens R, Omlin KJ, et al. Absent peripheral chemosensitivity in the Prader-Willi syndrome. J Appl Physiol 1994; 77:2231–2236.

48. Arens R, Gozal D, Burrell BC, et al. Arousal and cardiorespiratory responses to hypoxia in Prader-Willi syndrome. Am J Respir Crit Care Med 1996; 153:283–287.

49. Livingston FR, Arens R, Bailey SL, et al. Hypercapnic arousal responses in Prader-Willi syndrome. Chest 1995; 108:1627–1631.

50. Dillon GH, Waldrop TG. Electrophysiological and morphologic properties of caudal hypothalamic hypoxic- and hypercapneic-sensitive neurons in vitro. Soc Neurosci Abstr 1992; 492:10A.

51. Waldrop TG. Posterior hypothalamic modulation of the respiratory response to CO_2. Pflugers Arch 1992; 418:7–13.

52. Craig ME, Cowell CT, Larssons P, et al. Growth hormone treatment and adverse events in Prader-Willi syndrome: data from the KIGS. Clin Endocrinol 2006; 65: 178–185.

53. Wilson SS, Cotterill AM, Harris MA. Growth hormone and respiratory compromise in Prader-Willi syndrome. Arch Dis Child 2006; 91:349–350.

54. Miller J, Silverstein J, Shuster J, et al. Short-term effects of growth hormone on sleep abnormalities in Prader-Willi syndrome. J Clin Endocrinol Metab 2006; 91: 413–417.

55. Grugni G, Livicri C, Corrias A, et al. Death during growth hormone therapy in children with Prader-Willi syndrome: description of two new cases. J Endocrinol Invest 2005; 28:554–557.

56. Mogayzel PJ, Carroll JK, Loughlin GM, et al. Sleep disordered breathing in children with achondroplasia. J Pediatr 1998; 13:667–671.

57. Pauli RM, Scott CI, Wassman ER, Gilbert EF, et al. Apnea and sudden death in infants with achondroplasia. J Pediatr 1984; 104:342–348.

58. Reid CS, Pyeritz RE, Kopits SE, et al. Cervicomedullary compression in young patients with achondroplasia: value of comprehensive neurologic and respiratory evaluation. J Pediatr 1987; 110:522–530.

59. Stokes DC, Phillips JA, Leonard CO, et al. Respiratory complications of achondroplasia. J Pediatr 1983; 102:534–541.

60. Koch TK, Lo WD, Berg BO. Variability of serial CT scans in subacute necrotizing encephalomyelopathy (Leigh's disease). Pediatr Neurol 1985; 1:48–51.

61. Beckerman RC, Hunt CE. Neuromuscular diseases. In: Beckerman RC, Brouillette RT, Hunt CE, eds. Respiratory Control Disorders in Infants and Children. Baltimore, Maryland: Williams and Wilkins, Baltimore, 1992:251–270.

62. Devivo DC, Hammond MW, Obert KA, et al. Defective activation of the pyruvate dehydrogenase complex in subacute necrotizing encephalomyelopathy (Leigh's disease). Ann Neurol 1979; 6:483–494.

63. Willem JL, Monnens LAH, Trijbels JMF, et al. Leigh's encephalomyelopathy in a patient with cytochrome c oxidase deficiency in muscle tissue. Pediatrics 1977; 60:850–857.

64. Joubert M, Eisenring JJ, Robb JP, et al. Familial dysgenesis of the cerebellar vermis. Neurology 1969; 19:813–825.

65. Harmant van Rijckervorsel G, Aubert-Tulkens G, Moulin D, et al. Le syndrome de Joubert. Etude clinique et anatomopathologique. Rev Neurol 1983; 139:715–724.

66. Kuna ST, Smickley JS, Murchison LC. Hypercarbic periodic breathing during sleep in a child with a central nervous system tumor. Am Rev Respir Dis 1990; 142: 880–883.

67. Brouillette RT, Hunt CE, Gallemore GE. Respiratory dysrhythmia: a new cause of central alveolar hypoventilation (case report). Am Rev Respir Dis 1986; 134: 609–611.

68. Gozal D, Keens TG. Passive nighttime hypocapnic hyperventilation improves daytime eucapnia in mechanically ventilated children. Am J Respir Crit Care Med 1998; 157(3):A779.

69. Gilgoff IS, Peng R-C, Keens TG. Hypoventilation and apnea in children during mechanical assisted ventilation. Chest 1992; 101:1500–1506.

70. Kerbl R, Litscher H, Grubbauer HM, et al. Congenital central hypoventilation syndrome (Ondine's curse syndrome) in two siblings: delayed diagnosis and successful noninvasive treatment. Eur J Pediatr 1996; 155:977–980.

71. Marcus CL. Ventilator management of abnormal breathing during sleep: continuous positive airway pressure and nocturnal noninvasive intermittent positive pressure ventilation. In: Loughlin GM, Marcus CL, Carroll JL, eds. Sleep and Breathing in Children: A Developmental Approach. Lung Biology in Health and Disease series. New York: Marcel Dekker, Inc., 2000:797–811.

72. Simonds AK, Ward S, Heather S, et al. Outcome of paediatric domiciliary mask ventilation in neuromuscular and skeletal disease. Eur Respir J 2000; 16:476–481.

73. Teague WG. Non-invasive positive pressure ventilation: current status in paediatric patients. Paediatr Respir Rev 2005; 6:52–60.

17

Genetic Basis for Congenital Central Hypoventilation Syndrome

CLAUDE GAULTIER
Hospital Robert Debré and University Paris 7 Denis Diderot,
Paris, France

I. Introduction

Congenital central hypoventilation syndrome (CCHS) was first described by Mellins in 1970 (1). Now, more than 30 years later, approximately 300 to 350 patients with CCHS have been reported (2–28). Moreover, late-onset central hypoventilation syndrome (LO-CHS) has been recognized as a respiratory control disorder that manifests only in late infancy or childhood (20,29), or even in adulthood (30,31).

Early clinical observations in patients with CCHS supported a genetic basis for the condition. A few familial cases were reported (3,8,9,12,13,19,23). Some patients with CCHS also had inherited conditions, such as Hirschsprung disease (HSCR) and/or neuroblastoma (10,14,16,21,22,25,32). Finally, transmission of CCHS from parents to their offspring was reported recently (33,34).

Studies in mutant newborn mice unveiled the molecular mechanisms underlying the genetic basis for CCHS. In 2003, Amiel et al. discovered that *PHOX2B* was the major disease-causing gene (17). Moreover, *PHOX2B* gene mutations were reported in children and adults with LO-CHS (20,23,29–31).

This chapter reviews tentative mutant newborn mouse models for CCHS, genetic data from CCHS and LO-CHC patients, phenotype-genotype relationships, and the molecular consequences of *PHOX2B* gene mutations.

II. Tentative Mutant Newborn Mouse Models of CCHS

Recent studies described the respiratory phenotype of mutant newborn mice with targeted deletions of genes involved in respiratory control development (35). The first mutant newborn mouse model for CCHS was the null mutant for the rearranged during transfection (*Ret*) gene (36). This mutant has blunted ventilatory responses to hypercapnia and dies from respiratory failure soon after birth. Intestinal aganglionosis is another feature. However, few CCHS patients carry *RET* gene mutations (37–40). Another model of CCHS was the neonatal mouse invalidated for the mammalian homologue of the *Drosophila* archaete scute gene complex (*Mash1*), involved in the *Ret* signaling pathway (41). *Mash1* male mutant newborn mice exhibited mild impairments in the hypercapnic ventilatory response, which were not present in adulthood (41). Only few CCHS patients were found to carry mutations of the *HASH1* gene, the human *Mash1* homologue (18,42). Null mutant mice lacking the respiratory neuron homeobox (*Rnx*) gene exhibit numerous apneas and respiratory failure leading to death soon after birth (43). However, two studies ruled out a major role for *RNX* in the pathogenesis of CCHS (44,45).

Studies of mouse embryos lacking the gene for the transcription factor paired-like homeobox *Phox2b* proved more rewarding. Pattyn et al. described the $Phox2b^{-/-}$ phenotype in mice (46) and demonstrated that *Phox2b* was crucial to autonomic nervous system development. $Phox2b^{-/-}$ mouse embryos died shortly after mid-gestation because they had no noradrenergic neurons in the central nervous system, including the locus coeruleus. $Phox2b^{-/-}$ embryos were rescued up to birth by the administration of noradrenergic agonists to the mothers (47). Furthermore, the transcription factor Phox2b was necessary for the development of other neural crest derivatives: $Phox2b^{-/-}$ embryos lacked sympathetic, parasympathetic, and enteric ganglia (46). *Phox2b* dependency extended to the three-relay visceral reflex pathway comprising the carotid bodies, cranial ganglia, and nucleus tractus solitarius (nTS) (48). $Phox2b^{-/-}$ mouse embryos exhibited degeneration of the neural crest–derived carotid body and the three epibranchial placode–derived visceral sensory ganglia whereas the nTS (the site of integration of all visceral input) failed to develop (48).

Studies of *Phox2b* null mutant mouse embryos established a key role for *Phox2b* in the development of neural crest derivatives in mice. Neural crest stem cells in the developing nervous system can give rise to a variety of distinct neural subtypes. Considerable progress has been made in identifying the molecular signals that control neuronal specification and differentiation. For example, the generation of autonomic neurons from neural crest cells is induced by an extrinsic signal (bone morphogenic proteins) that elicits the expression of a network of transcription factors, which in turn control autonomic differentiation (49). This network includes the transcription factors *Mash1* and *Phox2b*. *Phox2b* and its paralogue, the paired-like homeobox *Phox2a*, bind to the promoter of the subtype-specific noradrenergic marker genes tyrosine hydroxylase and dopamine-β-hydroxylase, thus activating their transcription. *Mash1* and *Phox2b* can induce the differentiation of noradrenergic neurons from neural crest precursor cells (50–54) and are essential determinants of the noradrenergic phenotype, both central and peripheral (46,47,50,54,55). Depending on the subtype of noradrenergic neuron, *Mash1* and *Phox2b* can act in different epistatic orders and interact with distinct transcription factors in various noradrenergic cell types (49,55).

Heterozygous *Phox2b*-deficient newborn mice develop normally after birth. The respiratory phenotype of these mutant newborn mice has been investigated by our colleagues. It partly models the respiratory phenotype of CCHS patients (56). Abnormally long apneas and decreased ventilation during sleep compared with littermates are present on postnatal day 5 (57). The significant decrease in ventilatory responses to hypercapnia compared with wild-type pups on postnatal day 2 (48) also resembles CCHS (58). However, ventilatory responses to hypercapnia return to normal between postnatal days 2 and 10 (48) whereas 6-day-old pups exhibit a phenotype intermediate between those of 2- and 10-day-old pups (56). This functional recovery of the neonatal impairment in hypercapnia-induced ventilatory responses contrasts with the life-long impairment seen in CCHS patients (58). *Phox2b* is expressed in brainstem neuron groups believed to be involved in central chemosensitivity, such as the nTS (48) and retrotrapezoid nucleus (59). No data are available on the level of *Phox2b* expression in brainstem structures involved in central chemosensitivity in $Phox2b^{+/-}$ pups. Thus, the compensatory mechanisms underlying the functional recovery of central chemosensitivity in $Phox2b^{+/-}$ pups are unknown.

Two-day-old $Phox2b^{+/-}$ pups exhibit the biphasic ventilatory response to sustained hypoxia that is typical of newborn mammals. The hyperpneic response to hypoxia is normal, but the hypoxic ventilatory decline is markedly increased in the $Phox2b^{+/-}$ pups (48). The characteristics of the ventilatory response of $Phox2b^{+/-}$ pups to hyperoxia suggest strong tonic activity of oxygen-sensitive peripheral chemoreceptors (60). Interestingly, normal function of peripheral chemoreceptors has been documented in a group of CCHS patients who are able to breathe spontaneously while awake (61). Finally, a preliminary study in $Phox2b^{+/-}$ pups suggests thermoregulatory and respiratory abnormalities reminiscent of the thermoregulatory abnormalities seen in CCHS patients (56).

The key role for the transcription factor Phox2b in autonomic nervous system development and the similarities between the respiratory phenotype of $Phox2b^{+/-}$ newborn mice and CCHS prompted us to look for *PHOX2B* gene mutations in our CCHS patients. We found that *PHOX2B* was the major disease-causing gene of CCHS (17).

III. *PHOX2B* Gene Mutations in CCHS and LO-CHS Patients

The human *PHOX2B* gene is located on chromosome 4p12 and encodes a highly conserved homeobox domain transcription factor (314 amino acids) containing two short, stable polyalanine repeats of nine and 20 residues, respectively (62). *PHOX2B* mutations were first identified in a study of 27 CCHS patients (17). Further data were then generated by three single-center studies in Japan, the United States, and Italy (18–20) and by two large multicenter studies in Europe and the United States. One multicenter study was conducted by us (23) in France, other European countries, and the United States in 2005 and the other was done by Berry-Kravis et al. in CCHS patients from the United States and Europe in 2006 (27). Approximately 300 patients with CCHS have been screened for *PHOX2B* gene mutations around the world (17–20,23–28). However, an international registry for CCHS remains to be established. Therefore, an unknown number of patients may have been included in several reports, resulting in errors in prevalence estimates of the various *PHOX2B* mutation types. Accurate estimates require that an international registry be created.

The percentage of CCHS patients carrying *PHOX2B* mutations ranged across studies from 92.5% (23) to 100% (27). Of note, most of the CCHS patients carrying *PHOX2B* gene mutations are heterozygous for a polyalanine repeat expansion mutation involving the second polyalanine repeat sequence in exon 3 of the *PHOX2B* gene. Expansions range from 15 to 39 alanine insertions and result in expansion of the normal 20-repeat polyalanine tract by 5 to 13 additional alanine repeats. Importantly, unsuccessful amplification by DNA polymerase has been reported in individuals who are heterozygous for length variants of the polyalanine segment of the *PHOX2B* exon 3. The largest allele is prone to unsuccessful amplification, indicating a need for specific gene-analysis methods (20,23,26,27).

Figure 1 shows the distribution of *PHOX2B* alanine expansion mutations in our series of 179 patients with CCHS from France, other European countries, and the United States (23). *PHOX2B* expansion mutations with no more than 7 additional alanine repeats were more common than larger numbers of repeats in this series, the +7 alanine mutation being the most prevalent.

A small percentage of CCHS patients [7% in our multicenter study (23) and in the study by Berry-Kravis et al. (27)] carry nonpolyalanine *PHOX2B* mutations, all located within exon 3 or at the end of exon 2. These mutations include frameshift, missense, and nonsense mutations, as well as a missense mutation with a stop codon alteration (17,20,23–25,27,28,63).

Results of *PHOX2B* gene mutation testing have been reported for 14 children with LO-CHS (20,23,29,30,31). Nine of these patients carried a *PHOX2B* gene mutation, which was consistently a polyalanine expansion mutation with the shortest reported alanine repeat, i.e., 5 additional alanines. The respiratory disorders were less severe in the LO-CHS patients than in CCHS patients, and none of the LO-CHS patients had HSCR or symptoms of hypothalamic dysfunction (29; H. Trang, unpublished data; I. Ceccherini, unpublished data). This last point is of particular interest because late occurrence of central alveolar hypoventilation was associated with hypothalamic symptoms in some patients (64). In our experience with a few patients exhibiting central alveolar hypoventilation and hypothalamic symptoms (H. Trang, unpublished data), *PHOX2B* gene mutations were not found, suggesting different pathogenic mechanisms to those found in CCHS. Importantly, *Phox2b* is not expressed in the hypothalamus in mice (C. Goridis, unpublished data).

Finally, a recent and very important report described LO-CHS in five adults, three of whom have offspring with CCHS or LO-CHS (30,31). These adults experienced symptoms of chronic and/or acute hypoventilation that started after 21 years of age and were not associated with primary lung disease, heart disease, or neuromuscular disorders. In one of them, the ventilatory response to CO_2 was examined and found to be attenuated. These five adults carried the shortest alanine expansion mutation of the *PHOX2B* gene, i.e., +5 alanines. Very interestingly, careful examination of the history of these patients revealed abnormal symptoms such as cyanotic apnea spells or unexplained "epilepsy" during childhood (31). The pathogenic mechanisms underlying the onset of central alveolar hypoventilation in late infancy, childhood, or adulthood are unknown. They may include compensatory mechanisms involving redundant respiratory control systems that counteract, at least partly, the consequences of the genetic defect during a specific period of life. The role for interactions between genetic abnormalities and environmental factors triggering the occurrence of central alveolar hypoventilation remains to be elucidated.

IV. Mode of Inheritance

The mode of inheritance is autosomal dominant. Vertical transmission of a stable alanine expansion *PHOX2B* gene mutation has been observed in offspring born to CCHS probands (19,20,23,27). Therefore, an infant born to a parent with CCHS has a 50% risk of being affected. Most of the mutations found so far in affected probands with unaffected parents occurred de novo (17,19,20,27). However, somatic mosaicism was detected in 4.5% of 105 pairs of parents in our multicenter study (23) and 10% of 43 pairs of parents in another study (19,27). These findings have implications for genetic counseling: the risk of CCHS cannot be predicted accurately, as the percentage of germline mosaicism is unknown. Nevertheless, in parents with mosaicism and a child with CCHS, the risk of CCHS in future children should be up to 50%. Finally, penetrance can be incomplete, as two parents of CCHS probands carried *PHOX2B* gene mutations but had no detectable symptoms (20).

Vertical transmission has been also reported in patients with LO-CHS. A stable +5 alanine expansion mutation was found in two children with LO-CHS each of whom had one parent who carried the mutation and developed central hypoventilation during adulthood (30,31).

V. Phenotype-Genotype Relationships

Several groups have investigated phenotype-genotype relationships, especially regarding the severity of respiratory impairments and the diversity of autonomic nervous system abnormalities (19,20,23,27). Phenotype-genotype relationships were influenced by the type of *PHOX2B* gene mutation. The length of the alanine expansion correlated with the severity of the respiratory phenotype (19,23,27), the extent of ventilatory dependence (19,23,27), and the severity of symptoms related to autonomic dysfunction (19,27).

Alanine repeats in LO-CHS patients involved the addition of only 5 alanines (20,23,29–31). However, this short repeat was found also in several patients with neonatal onset of central alveolar hypoventilation (23) (Fig. 1). Therefore, the type of *PHOX2B* gene mutation does not determine the age of

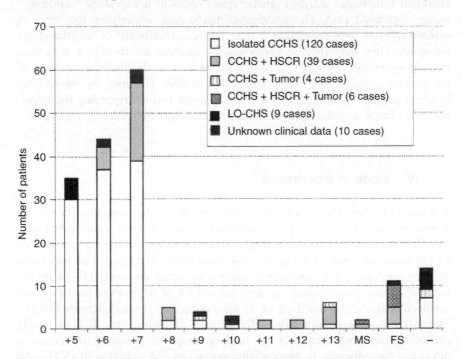

Figure 1 *PHOX2B* mutations among subgroups of patients with CCHS or LO-CHS. The mutation types are reported on the x-axis. Alanine expansions are symbolized by a plus sign (+) followed by the number of extra alanines. The minus sign (−) represents the groups of patients with no *PHOX2B* mutation identified. Clinical groups are listed in the graph key. *Abbreviations*: MS, missense mutations; FS, frameshift mutations. Reprinted with permission from Trochet et al. Am J Hum Genet, 2005; 76:421–426.

onset of central alveolar hypoventilation, a fact that suggests a role for mutations at other sites and/or interactions with environmental factors.

In our multicenter studies, the type of *PHOX2B* mutation was not correlated with the occurrence of HSCR in addition to CCHS (23) (Fig. 1). Furthermore, among patients with the same type of *PHOX2B* mutation (e.g., +7 alanine repeats), some did and some did not have HSCR. HSCR was common in CCHS patients who had non–polyalanine expansion *PHOX2B* gene mutations, both in our multicenter study (23) and in a recent study conducted on a large series (27). Molecular mechanisms involving the *RET* gene have been investigated in an attempt to explain the association of HSCR with CCHS. Because *RET* is the main gene involved in the complex genetics of HSCR, patients with CCHS have been investigated for *RET* gene mutations. Three patients with CCHS have been found to carry *RET* mutations, and among them only two have HSCR (38–41). Recent studies have shown that the weak *RET* predisposing haplotype is carried by most patients with sporadic HSCR (65). De Pontual et al. investigated whether this HSCR-predisposing haplotype was involved in the association between CCHS and HSCR in patients carrying *PHOX2B* mutations (66,67). The haplotype was significantly more common in CCHS patients with than without HSCR. Thus, *RET* may act as a modifier gene for the HSCR phenotype to occur in CCHS patients. Nevertheless, a strict digenic model does not account for all cases, indicating that one or more modifier genes—with or without interactions with environmental factors—are involved in the pathogenesis of HSCR associated with CCHS.

We reported an association between non–polyalanine expansion *PHOX2B* mutations and the occurrence of neural crest tumors (Fig. 1) (23). This association was also found in a recent report (27). Therefore, molecular testing can identify a subset of CCHS children at very high risk for developing malignant tumors, who need to be carefully monitored.

VI. Molecular Consequences of *PHOX2B* Gene Mutations

The molecular basis for the impaired function of the mutant PHOX2B protein was investigated recently (63,68–70). Bachetti et al. (68) and Trochet et al. (69) used transfection experiments to test the transcriptional activity of wild-type and mutant *PHOX2B* expression constructs on the regulatory regions of the target gene dopamine-β-hydroxylase. They observed that both expansion and frameshift mutations reduced transcriptional activity. The length of the alanine expansion correlated with the severity of the transcriptional activity reduction, indicating that the size of the alanine tract influenced the level of transactivation. Trochet et al. (69) tested whether reduced transactivation was due to decreased DNA binding to the dopamine-β-hydroxylase promoter. They found impaired DNA binding with both frameshift mutations and +9 alanine or greater expansion mutations. The same group established that the mutant PHOX2B protein associated with the alanine expansion mutation formed cytoplasmic aggregates in transfected cells. Cytoplasmic aggregation was influenced by the length of the alanine repeat: proteins encoded by short expansions remained nuclear, whereas those encoded by +9 alanine or greater expansions formed cytoplasmic aggregates. One way cells handle misfolded and aggregate-prone proteins is by attempting to refold them using molecular chaperones such as heat-shock proteins (HSP) (71). Trochet et al. (69) found that HSP70 colocalized with the aggregates formed by the +13 alanine PHOX2B mutant protein. Boosting HSP70 expression via exposure to the antibiotic geldamycine reduced the cytoplasmic aggregates. Thus, with short expansions, chaperone proteins may promote either refolding or degradation of the expanded protein at a rate that is sufficient to prevent the accumulation of intracellular aggregates. With long expansions, in contrast, failure of chaperone-mediated refolding and of the proteasome system to cope with the misfolding proteins may lead to aggregation. Finally, recent experiments by Bachetti et al. (70) suggest that PHOX2B aggregates may impair cell viability and that geldamycine may prevent cell death.

These new findings indicating a role for the chaperone system in correcting the molecular consequences of impaired function of long-expansion mutant PHOX2B proteins raises the issue of gene-environment interactions. Environmental factors such as stress induction or temperature elevation influence the level of expression of HSP. Such epigenetic effects probably contribute to the marked interindividual and intraindividual variability of the clinical phenotype. These findings may lead to new treatments involving manipulation of chaperone activity.

VII. Does the *PHOX2B* Gene Defect Fully Account for the Pathogenesis of CCHS?

This question is legitimate, for at least two reasons. First, the recently described functional and neuroanatomical abnormalities reported in CCHS patients extend beyond the brainstem areas where *PHOX2B* is expressed. Second, mutations in genes other than *PHOX2B* were found in several CCHS patients.

Noninvasive functional magnetic imaging provides functional maps of brain responses to specific challenges, such as hypercapnia, hypoxia, and loaded breathing (72–74). This investigation was used in a group of CCHS patients who were able to breathe independently when awake. The results showed functional impairments extending far beyond the areas of *PHOX2B* expression during development, as observed in mice, for instance in the limbic and cerebellar structures. Neuroanatomical defects have been recently identified in CCHS patients (75,76). Defects were found in the periventricular white matter and in the cortical, cerebellar, and diencephalic structures involved in autonomic patterning, coordination of sympathetic and parasympathetic outflows, and coordination of muscles (including respiratory muscles). These defects provide an anatomic basis for several components of the CCHS phenotype. The presence of functional and neuroanatomic abnormalities in CCHS patients outside the brainstem areas of *PHOX2B* gene expression casts doubt on whether *PHOX2B* mutations can fully explain CCHS. Nevertheless, Kumar et al. and Harper et al. (75–77) hypothesized that impaired function of the *PHOX2B* gene, which targets autonomic ganglia, exerts a direct effect on blood flow by controlling the cerebral vasculature, the consequence being abnormal development of cerebral structures involved in respiratory and cardiovascular functions.

Other gene mutations associated with *PHOX2B* mutations have been found in 11 of about 100 tested patients with CCHS (17–19,42,78). These patients with CCHS had heterozygous mutations affecting genes involved in neural crest cell development [*RET*; genes encoding the glial cell line–derived neurotrophic (GDNF) factor and the GDNF family receptor α 1, respectively; *HASH1*; and *PHOX2A*] and one gene encoding the brain-derived neurotrophic factor (BDNF) (17,18,42,78). The number of CCHS patients carrying mutations of one of the six genes listed above was too small for an investigation of phenotype-genotype relationships. Nevertheless, the existence of these mutations suggests that modifier genes may be involved in the variability of the CCHS phenotype and that further investigations for mutations in genes other than *PHOX2B* may be in order. So far, no studies have looked for other gene mutations in children or adults with LO-CHS.

VIII. Conclusion and Perspectives

Combined studies in humans and newborn mouse models have supplied new insights into the molecular mechanisms underlying the pathogenesis of CCHS. *PHOX2B* is the major disease-causing gene of CCHS. The identification of this gene allows familial counseling and prenatal diagnosis. The phenotype-genotype relationships reported for the various *PHOX2B* gene mutations have opened the way to outcome prediction. However, clinicians should be aware that clinical experience in individual CCHS patients does not consistently match predictions based on statistical analyses of CCHS patient populations. International databases of phenotypes and genotypes of CCHS patients are urgently needed to enable accurate analyses of phenotype-genotype relationships with the goal of elucidating the mechanisms of phenotypic variability in CCHS patients.

CCHS may be less uncommon than previously thought. The identification of the shortest +5 alanine expansion mutation of the *PHOX2B* gene in a few adults with LO-CHS indicates a need for genetic studies in adults, or even children, who have hypoventilation, unexplained by abnormal respiratory system effectors. Such patients may carry *PHOX2B* gene mutations.

The heterozygous $Phox2b^{+/-}$ newborn mouse model has helped us to understand the pathogenesis of CCHS. The persistence of a single functional allele, which may ensure adequate protein function, is associated with a less severe phenotype than that of CCHS patients. Nevertheless, investigations into the mechanisms that lead to functional recovery of central chemosensitivity found in *Phox2b*$^{+/-}$ newborn mice would produce valuable information.

A knock-in newborn mouse model with a *Phox2b* +7 alanine expansion has been generated recently. The mutation in this new strain replicates the most common mutation found in CCHS patients. Preliminary data indicate that severity of the respiratory phenotype is similar to that in CCHS patients (79). These knock-in models will serve to investigate means of correcting the respiratory deficits in mutant models, with the goal of designing new treatments for CCHS patients.

Recent findings indicate a pressing need for all researchers—neonatologists, pediatricians, adult pulmonologists, geneticists, neurobiologists, and respiratory physiologists—to work jointly to elucidate the molecular mechanisms of central alveolar hypoventilation occurring in the neonatal period or later on in humans.

References

1. Mellins RB, Balfour HH, Turino GM, et al. Failure of autonomic control of ventilation (Ondine's curse): report of an infant born with this syndrome and review of the literature. Medicine 1970; 49:487–504.
2. Shannon DC, Marsland DW, Gould JB, et al. Central hypoventilation during quiet sleep in two infants. Pediatrics 1976; 57:342–346.
3. Haddad GG, Mazza NM, Defendini R, et al. Congenital failure of autonomic control of ventilation, gastrointestinal motility and heart rate. Medicine 1978; 57:517–526.
4. Fleming PJ, Cade D, Bryan MH, et al. Congenital central hypoventilation and sleep state. Pediatrics 1980; 66:425–428.
5. Bower RJ, Adkins JC. Ondine's curse and neurocristopathy. Clin Pediatr 1980; 19: 665–668.
6. Guilleminault C, McQuitty J, Ariagno RL, et al. Congenital central alveolar hypoventilation in six infants. Pediatrics 1982; 70:684–694.
7. Oren J, Kelly DH, Shannon DC. Long-term follow-up of children with congenital central hypoventilation syndrome. Pediatrics 1987; 80:375–380.
8. Khalifa MM, Flavin MA, Wherrett BA. Congenital central hypoventilation syndrome in monozygous twins. J Pediatr 1988; 113:853–855.
9. Hamilton J, Bodurtha JN. Congenital central hypoventilation syndrome and Hirschsprung's disease in half sibs. J Med Genet 1989; 26:272–274.
10. Swaminathan S, Gilsanz V, Atkinson J, et al. Congenital central hypoventilation associated with multiple ganglioneuromas. Chest 1989; 96:423–424.
11. Marcus CL, Jansen MT, Poulsen MK, et al. Medical and psychosocial outcome of children with congenital central hypoventilation syndrome. J Pediatr 1991; 119: 888–895.
12. Weese-Mayer DE, Silvestri JM, Menzies LJ, et al. Congenital central hypoventilation syndrome: diagnosis, management, and long-term outcome in thirty-two children. J Pediatr 1992; 120:381–387.
13. Kerbl R, Litscher H, Grubbauer HM, et al. Congenital central hypoventilation syndrome (Ondine's curse syndrome) in two siblings: delayed diagnosis and successful noninvasive treatment. Eur J Pediatr 1996; 155:977–980.

14. Croaker GDH, Shi E, Simpson E, et al. Congenital central hypoventilation syndrome and Hirschsprung's disease. Arch Dis Child 1998; 78:316–322.
15. Devriendt K, Fryns JP, Naulaers G, et al. Neuroblastomas in a mother and congenital central hypoventilation in her daughter: variable expression of the same genetic disorder? Am J Med Genet 2000; 90:430–431.
16. Rohrer T, Trachsel D, Engelcke G, et al. Congenital central hypoventilation syndrome associated with Hirschsprung's disease and neuroblastomas: case of multiple neurocristopathies. Pediatr Pulmonol 2002; 33:71–76.
17. Amiel J, Laudier B, Attié-Bitach T, et al. Polyalanine expansion and frameshift mutations of the paired-like homeobox gene *PHOX2B* in congenital central hypoventilation syndrome. Nat Genet 2003; 33:459–461.
18. Sasaki A, Kanai M, Kijima K, et al. Molecular analysis of congenital central hypoventilation syndrome. Hum Genet 2003; 114:22–26.
19. Weese-Mayer DE, Berry-Kravis EM, Zhou L, et al. Idiopathic congenital central hypoventilation syndrome: analysis of genes pertinent to early autonomic nervous system embryologic development and identification of mutations of *PHOX2B*. Am J Med Genet 2003; 123:267–278.
20. Matera I, Bachetti T, Puppo F, et al. *PHOX2B* mutations and polyalanine expansions correlate with the severity of the respiratory phenotype and associated symptoms in both congenital and late-onset central hypoventilation syndrome. J Med Genet 2004; 41:373–380.
21. Vanderlaan M, Holbrook CR, Wang M, et al. Epidemiologic survey of 196 patients with congenital central hypoventilation syndrome. Pediatr Pulmonol 2004; 37: 217–229.
22. Trang H, Dehan M, Beaufils F, et al. The French congenital central hypoventilation syndrome registry: general data, phenotype, genotype. Chest 2005; 127:72–79.
23. Trochet D, O'Brien LM, Gozal D, et al. *PHOX2B* genotype allows for prediction of tumour risk in congenital central hypoventilation syndrome. Am Hum Genet 2005; 76:421–426.
24. Bajaj R, Smith J, Trochet D, et al. Congenital central hypoventilation syndrome and Hirschsprung's disease in an extremely preterm infant. Pediatrics 2005; 115: e737–e738.
25. Holzinger A, Mittal RA, Kachel W, et al. A novel 17 bp deletion in the *PHOX2B* gene causes congenital central hypoventilation syndrome with total aganglionosis of the small and large intestine. Am J Med Genet A 2005; 139:50–51.
26. Horiuchi H, Sasaki A, Osawa M, et al. Sensitive detection of polyalanine expansion in *PHOX2B* by polymerase chain reaction using bisulfite converted DNA. J Mol Diagn 2005; 7:638–640.
27. Berry-Kravis EM, Zhou L, Rand CM, et al. Congenital central hypoventilation syndrome. *PHOX2B* mutations and phenotype. Am J Respir Crit Care Med 2006; 174:1139–1144.
28. Or SF, Tong MF, Lo FM, et al. *PHOX2B* mutations in three Chinese patients with congenital central hypoventilation syndrome. Chin Med J 2006; 119:1749–1752.
29. Trang H, Laudier B, Trochet D, et al. *PHOX2B* gene mutation in a patient with late-onset central hypoventilation. Pediatr Pulmonol 2004; 38:349–351.
30. Weese-Mayer DE, Berry-Kravis EM, Zhou L. Adult identified with congenital central hypoventilation syndrome-mutation in *PHOX2B* gene and late-onset CHS. Am J Respir Crit Care Med 2005; 171:88.

31. Antic NA, Malow BA, Lange N, et al. *PHOX2B* mutation-confirmed congenital central hypoventilation syndrome. Presentation in adulthood. Am J Respir Crit Care Med 2006; 174:923–927.

32. Gaultier C, Trang H, Dauger S, et al. Pediatric disorders with autonomic dysfunction: what role for *PHOX2B*? Pediatr Res 2005; 58:1–6.

33. Sritippayawan S, Hamutcu R, Run SS, et al. Mother-daughter transmission of congenital central hypoventilation syndrome. Am J Respir Crit Care Med 2002; 166: 367–369.

34. Silvestri JM, Chen ML, Weese-Mayer DE, et al. Idiopathic congenital central hypoventilation syndrome: the next generation. Am J Med Genet 2002; 112:46–50.

35. Gaultier C, Matrot B, Gallego J. Transgenic models to study disorders of respiratory control in newborn mice. ILAR J 2005; 47:15–21.

36. Burton MD, Kawashima A, Brayer JA, et al. RET proto-oncogene is important for the development of respiratory CO_2 sensitivity. J Auton Nerv Syst 1997; 63: 137–143.

37. Bolk S, Angrist M, Schwartz S, et al. Congenital central hypoventilation syndrome: mutation analysis of the receptor tyrosine kinase RET. Am J Med Gen 1996; 63:603–609.

38. Amiel J, Salomon R, Attié T, et al. Mutations of the *RET-GDNF* pathway in Ondine's curse. Am J Hum Genet 1998; 62:715–717.

39. Sakai T, Wakizaka A, Matsuda H, et al. Point mutation in exon 12 of the receptor tyrosine kinase proto-oncogene RET in Ondine-Hirschsprung syndrome. Pediatrics 1998; 101:924–926.

40. Kanai M, Namakura C, Sasaki A, et al. Congenital central hypoventilation syndrome: a novel mutation of the RET gene in an isolated case. Tohoku J Exp Med 2002; 196:241–246.

41. Dauger S, Renolleau S, Vardon G, et al. Ventilatory responses to hypercapnia and hypoxia in Mash-1 heterozygous newborn and adult mice. Pediatr Res 1999; 46: 535–542.

42. De Pontual L, Nepote V, Attie-Bitach T, et al. Noradrenergic neural development is impaired by mutation of the proneural HASH-1 gene in congenital central hypoventilation syndrome (Ondine's curse). Hum Mol Genet 2003; 12:3173–3180.

43. Shirasawa S, Arata A, Onimaru H, et al. Rnx deficiency results in congenital central hypoventilation. Nat Genet 2000; 24:287–290.

44. Matera I, Bachetti T, Cinti R, et al. Mutational analysis of the RNX gene in congenital central hypoventilation syndrome. Am J Med Genet 2003; 113:178–182.

45. Amiel J, Pelet A, Trang H, et al. Exclusion of Rnx as a major gene in congenital central hypoventilation syndrome. Am J Med Genet 2003; 117:18–20.

46. Pattyn A, Morin X, Cremer H, et al. The homeobox gene Phox2b is essential for the development of autonomic neural crest derivatives. Nature 1999; 399:366–370.

47. Pattyn A, Goridis C, Brunet JF. Specification of the central noradrenergic phenotype by the homeobox gene Phox2b. Mol Cell Neurosci 2000; 15:235–243.

48. Dauger S, Pattyn A, Lofaso F, et al. Phox2b controls the development of peripheral chemoreceptors and afferent visceral pathways. Development 2003; 130: 6635–6642.

49. Goridis C, Rohrer H. Specification of catecholaminergic and serotonergic neurons. Nat Rev Neurosci 2002; 3:531–541.

50. Guillemot F, Lo LC, Johnson JE, et al. Mammalian achaete-scute homolog 1 is required for the early development of olfactory and autonomic neurons. Cell 1993; 75:463–476.

51. Stanke M, Junghans D, Geissen M, et al. The Phox2b homeodomain proteins are sufficient to promote the development of sympathetic neurons. Development 1999; 126:4087–4094.

52. Stanke M, Stubbusch J, Rohrer H. Interactions of Mash1 and Phox2b in sympathetic neuron development. Mol Cell Neurosci 2004; 25:374–382.

53. Lo L, Morin X, Brunet JF, et al. Specification of neurotransmitter identify by Phox2b proteins in neural crest stem cells. Neuron 1999; 22:693–705.

54. Lo L, Tiveron MC, Anderson DJ. MASH1 activated expression of the paired homeodomain transcription factor Phox2a and couples pan-neural and subtype-specific components of autonomic neuronal activity. Development 1998; 125:609–620.

55. Brunet JF. Phox2b and the homeostatic brain. In: Gaultier C, ed. Genetic Basis for Respiratory Control Disorders. New York: Springer, 2007; 25–44.

56. Gallego J, Ramanantsoa N, Vaubourg V. Tentative mouse model for the congenital central hypoventilation syndrome: heterozygous mutant newborn mice. In: Gaultier C, ed. Genetic Basis for Respiratory Control Disorders. New York: Springer, 2007; 243–257.

57. Durand E, Dauger S, Pattyn A, et al. Sleep-disordered breathing in newborn mice heterozygous for the transcription factor Phox2b. Am J Respir Crit Care Med 2005; 172:238–243.

58. Gozal D. Congenital central hypoventilation syndrome: an update. Pediatr Pulmonol 1998; 26:273–282.

59. Stornetta RL, Moreira TS, Takakura AC, et al. Expression of Phox2b by brainstem neurons involved in chemosensory integration in the adult rat. J Neurosci 2006; 26: 10305–10314.

60. Ramanantsoa N, Vaubourg V, Dauger S, et al. Ventilatory responses to hyperoxia in newborn mice heterozygous for the transcription factor Phox2b. Am J Physiol Regul Integr Comp Physiol 2006; 290:R1691–R1696.

61. Gozal D, Marcus CL, Shoyov D, et al. Peripheral chemoreceptor function in children with the congenital central hypoventilation syndrome. J Appl Physiol 1993; 74: 379–387.

62. Yokoyama M, Watanabe H, Nakamura M. Genomic structure and functional characterization of NBPhox (PMX2B), a homeodomain protein specific to catecholaminergic cells that is involved in second messenger-mediated transcriptional activation. Genomics 1999; 59:40–50.

63. Bachetti T, Ceccherini I. *In vitro* studies of *PHOX2B* gene mutations in congenital central hypoventilation syndrome. In: Gaultier C, ed. Genetic Basis for Respiratory Control Disorders. New York: Springer, 2007; 71–83.

64. Katz ES, McGrath S, Marcus CL. Late-onset central hypoventilation with hypothalamic dysfunction: a distinct clinical syndrome. Pediatr Pulmonol 2000; 29: 62–68.

65. Emison ES, McCallion AS, Kashuk CS, et al. A common sex-dependent mutation in a RET enhancer underlies Hirschsprung disease risk. Nature 2005; 434:857–863.

66. De Pontual L, Pelet A, Trochet D, et al. Mutations of the ret gene in isolated and syndromic Hirschsprung disease disclose major and modifier alleles at a single locus. J Med Genet 2006; 43:419–423.

67. De Pontual L, Pelet A, Clement-Ziza M, et al. Epistatic interactions with a common hypomorphic Ret allele in syndromic Hirschsprung disease. Hum Mutat 2007; 28:790–796.
68. Bachetti T, Matera I, Borghini S, et al. Distinct pathogenic mechanisms for *PHOX2B* associated polyalanine expansions and frameshift mutations in congenital central hypoventilation syndrome. Hum Mol Genet 2005; 14:1815–1824.
69. Trochet D, Hong SJ, Brunet JF, et al. Molecular consequences of *PHOX2B* missense, frameshift and alanine expansion mutations leading to autonomic dysfunction. Hum Mol Genet 2005; 14:3697–3708.
70. Bachetti T, Bocca P, Borghini S, et al. Geldanamycine promotes nuclear localization and clearance of PHOX2B misfolded proteins containing polyalanine expansions. Int J Biochem Cell Biol 2006; 39:327–339.
71. Albrecht A, Mundlos S. The other trinucleotide repeat: polyalanine expansion disorders. Curr Opin Genet Dev 2005; 15:285–293.
72. Macey KE, Macey PM, Woo MA, et al. fMRI signal changes in response to forced expiratory loading in congenital central hypoventilation syndrome. J Appl Physiol 2004; 97:1897–1907.
73. Macey PM, Woo MA, Macey KE, et al. Hypoxia reveals posterior thalamic, cerebellar, midbrain and limbic deficit in congenital central hypoventilation syndrome. J Appl Physiol 2005; 98:958–969.
74. Harper RM, Macey PM, Woo MA, et al. Hypercapnic exposure in congenital central hypoventilation syndrome reveals CNS respiratory control mechanisms. J Neurophysiol 2005; 93:1647–1658.
75. Kumar R, Macey PM, Woo MA, et al. Neuroanatomic deficits in congenital central hypoventilation syndrome. J Comp Neurol 2005; 487:361–371.
76. Kumar R, Macey PM, Woo MA, et al. Elevated mean diffusivity in widespread brain regions in congenital central hypoventilation syndrome. J Magn Reson Imaging 2006; 24:1252–1258.
77. Harper RM, Woo MA, Macey PM, et al. Structural and functional abnormalities in congenital central alveolar hypoventilation. In: Gaultier C, ed. Genetic Basis for Respiratory Control Disorders. New York: Springer, 2007; 57–70.
78. Weese-Mayer DE, Bolk S, Silvestri JM, et al. Idiopathic congenital central hypoventilation syndrome: evaluation of brain-derived neurotrophic factor genomic DNA sequence variation. Am J Med Genet 2002; 107:306–310.
79. Dubreuil V, Ramanantsoa N, Trochet D, et al. A mutation of the transcription factor *Phox2b* causes look of CO_2 chemosensitivity, fatal apnea and specific loss of parafacial neurons. Third international meeting on Congenital central hypoventilation syndrome, Sestri Levante, Italy, 7–9 November 2007.

18

Epidemiology of Pediatric Obstructive Sleep Apnea

JAMES C. SPILSBURY and SUSAN REDLINE
Case Western Reserve University, Cleveland, Ohio, U.S.A.

I. Introduction

Despite increased experience in diagnosing and treating the pediatric obstructive sleep apnea syndrome (OSAS), data are limited regarding its overall prevalence, risk, and protective factors, natural course, and consequences. This chapter focuses on the epidemiology of OSAS among children and adolescents (2–18 years of age). The chapter sections will cover current knowledge pertaining to its overall prevalence, distribution in various population subgroups, identified risk factors and comorbidities associated with the disorder and, briefly, health outcomes related to OSAS. The chapter closes with recommendations for future research on the epidemiology of OSAS.

II. Prevalence

One of the major challenges of obtaining accurate estimates of OSAS prevalence is deciding on a suitable definition for the disorder. OSAS is defined by the American Thoracic Society as a "disorder of breathing during sleep characterized

397

by prolonged partial upper airway obstruction and/or intermittent complete obstruction (obstructive apnea) that disrupts normal ventilation during sleep and normal sleep patterns'' (1). OSAS is considered the severe end of a spectrum of related clinical conditions grouped together as ''sleep-disordered breathing'': primary snoring, upper airway resistance syndrome, obstructive hypoventilation, hypopneas, and OSAS (2). For ease of presentation, we will refer to data from all studies in which objective nocturnal monitoring data were used to identify abnormalities as OSAS. In the scientific literature, definitions of OSAS are varied and have been based on (*i*) presence of symptoms, such as habitual snoring; (*ii*) physiological measures based on overnight polysomnography, such as obstructive events with corroborative oxygen desaturation levels; and (*iii*) presence of the syndrome, which is presence of both symptoms and physiological perturbation on polysomnography. The definition selected is critical in assessment of prevalence and in quantifying risk associations: prevalence estimates may vary as much as 20-fold depending on how liberal (e.g., central or obstructive apneas and hypopneas with no requirement for associated desaturation) or restrictive (obstructive apnea only or obstructive apnea and hypopnea with a 5% associated desaturation) is the OSAS definition (3).

Besides definitional issues related to OSAS, prevalence estimates may vary due to other factors. Prevalence assumes a threshold level that identifies (*i*) the tail of a distribution or (*ii*) individuals at increased risk of negative outcomes or those who would benefit from treatment. However, there is limited research with large population-based samples necessary to identify such threshold levels for OSAS. In general, OSAS prevalence estimates have been based on small samples of normal children and have not applied threshold definitions that have been shown to discriminate clinical abnormalities or treatment responders from other groups.

Tables 1 and 2 summarize prevalence studies grouped by OSAS definition. Table 1 includes studies that have estimated OSAS prevalence largely from questionnaire surveys of habitual snoring and sleep habits (4–14). Table 1 also includes studies using objective measures of OSAS (see below), but which also reported estimates of habitual snoring (15–23). In the studies shown in Table 1, habitual snoring has been defined in various ways, such as snoring ''always,'' ''on most nights,'' or ''at least three nights per week.'' Habitual snoring has been reported for 3–35% of young children (<13 years) from the United States, European, and Asian population-based surveys (Table 1) (4–23). One study found OSAS symptoms, defined as an aggregate of responses to loud snoring, stopping breathing, or snorts/gasps, present in 4% of U.S. school-age children (24).

Eight studies—five in Europe (15,18–20,23), two in Asia (16,17), and one in the United States(25)—have employed ''two-staged'' sampling estimates to derive OSAS prevalence (Table 2). These approaches first identified "symptomatic" children from broad community surveys (e.g., parent report of habitual snoring) and then followed up by measuring overnight breathing patterns or oximetry in the "high-level snorers" subsample. Five of these studies reported prevalence estimates ranging from 0.7% to 2.9% (15,17,18,20,23). However, two studies have reported much higher estimates. Castronovo et al. (19) reported an OSAS estimate of 13%, which they attributed to (*i*) high sensitivity of the snoring "screening question" in stage 1 of the sampling procedure, which therefore generated a larger sample of children to follow-up with the more objective oximetry measure and (*ii*) the cultural practice of children and parents sleeping in the same room, which likely made parents more aware of snoring and other sounds during sleep.

The second study reporting a higher prevalence estimate is the U.S.-based Tucson Children's Assessment of Sleep Apnea (TuCASA), which is a prospective cohort study of a population-based sample of 1219 Hispanic and White children (12,25). TuCASA has utilized a two-staged sampling strategy similar to the European and Asian studies described above, but with a less restricted definition of OSAS: >1 apnea and hypopnea per hour, with an event having >3% oxygen desaturation. TuCASA investigators have reported an OSAS prevalence of 24% (25). Two studies have taken a different methodological approach by foregoing the initial screening stage and instead using objective measures on the entire study sample of children. The Cleveland Children's Sleep and Health Study is an urban U.S. population-based cohort study created via stratified random sampling of full-term and preterm children born between 1988 and 1993 and identified from the birth records of Cleveland's three major hospitals (3,21,26). The study includes 907 children (50% female; 40% minority, mostly African-American) studied at 8 to 11 years of age with in-home sleep studies (117 also with in-lab polysomnography and collection of data on symptoms, behavior and cognition, physiology, and anthropometry. The Cleveland Children's Sleep and Health Study, using objective measures obtained from children without "prescreening," revealed a sleep-disordered breathing prevalence of 2.2% (95% CI, 1.2, 3.2) using a definition based on >1 apnea or >5 apneas and hypopneas per hour (21). Similarly, another large prospective cohort study involves a population-based sample of 966 German schoolchildren (mean age, 9.6 years; 95% White) (22). This investigation utilized pulse oximetry data and reported a prevalence of 3.8% (95% CI, 2.7, 4.9) using their most inclusive definition: (*i*) three events with a fall in arterial oxygen saturation (SaO_2) to $\leq 90\%$ and three clusters of ≥ 5 desaturations within a 30-minute period over the course of one night ($3D_{90}$ and $3D_C$); (*ii*) if the number of desaturations to $\leq 90\%$ exceeded 0.6/hr ($DI_{90} > 0.6$); or (*iii*) if the number of desaturations with >4% fall in saturation exceeded 3.9/hr, with at least 0.4 desaturation clusters per hour ($DI_4 > 3.9$ and $DI_C > 0.4$).

Table 1 Prevalence of OSAS Based on Measure of Habitual Snoring

First author (reference)	Date	Sample size	Age (yr)	Sample type	Country	Definition	Finding
Corbo (4)	1989	1615	6–13	Population based, school	Italy	Snores "often"	7.3%
Teculescu (5)	1992	190	5–6	Population based, school	France	Snores "often"	10%
Ali (15)	1993	782	4–5	Clinic based, visitor register	U.K.	Snores "most nights"	12.1%
Ali (6)	1994	507	6–7	Clinic based, visitor register	U.K.	Snores "most nights"	11.4%
Gislason (20)	1995	454	0.5–6	All children in town	Iceland	Snores "often" or "very often"	3.2%
Hultcrantz (7)	1995	325	4	Clinic based, 4 year checkup	Sweden	Snores "every night"	6.2%
Owen (8)	1995	222	1–10	Clinic based, general register	U.K.	Snores "often"	11%
Ferreira (9)	2000	976	6–11	Population based, school	Portugal	Snores loudly "frequently" or "always"	8.6%
Anuntaseree (16)	2001	1008	6–13	Population based, school	Thailand	Snores "on most nights"	8.5%
Brunetti (18)	2001	895	3–11	Population based, school	Italy	Snores "always"	4.9%
Corbo (10)	2001	2209	10–15	Population based, school	Italy	Snores "often"	5.6%
Stein (11)	2001	472	4–12	Clinic based, pediatric practices	U.S.A	Snoring "every night"	12.0%
Castronovo (19)	2003	595	3–6	Cross sectional, population based, school	Italy	Snoring "always" or "often"	34.5%

	Year	N	Age	Study type	Country	Definition	Prevalence
Goodwin (12)	2003	1494	6-11	Community-based cohort, school	U.S.A	Snoring "frequently" or "almost always"	10.5%
Rosen (21)	2003	850	8-11	Population-based cohort, birth hospital	U.S.A	"Loud" snoring at least 1-2 times per week	17%
Shin (13)	2003	3871	15-18	Cross sectional, population based, school	Korea	Snoring $\geq$ 3 days per week	11.2%
Schlaud (22)	2004	1129	9.6 (0.66)[a]	Population based, school	Germany	Snores "frequently" or "always"	10.1% (95% CI, 8.3, 11.9)
Anuntaseree (17)	2005	755	9-12	Population based, school	Thailand	Snores "on most nights"	6.9%
Liu (14)	2005	5979	2-12	Population based, school	China	"frequent" snoring	5.6%
Sogut (23)	2005	1198	3-11	Population based, school	Turkey	Snores "always": $\geq$3 times per week	3.3%

[a]Mean age and standard deviation.

Table 2 Prevalence of OSAS Based on Polysomnography/Oximetry

First author (reference)	Date	Overall sample size	Subsample objectively measured	Child age (yr)	Sample type	Country	OSAS Threshold	Prevalence[a]
Ali (15)	1993	782	132	4–5	Clinic based, general register	U.K.	$\geq$5 events per hour with $\geq$4% decrease in SaO_2	0.7%
Gislason (20)	1995	454	11	0.5–6	All children in one town	Iceland	$\geq$3 events per hour with $\geq$4% decrease in SaO_2	2.9% (SE = 0.5%)
Redline (52)	1999	126	126	126	Children of probands with and without sleep apnea	U.S.A.	AHI > 10 AHI > 5	1.6% 10.3%
Anuntaseree (16)	2001	1008	8	6–13	Population-based cohort, school	Thailand	AHI > 1	0.69%
Brunetti (18)	2001	895	14	3–11	Population based, school	Italy	AHI > 3	1.8% (95% CI, 1.6, 2.0)[b]
Castronovo (19)	2003	595	204	3–6	Cross sectional, population based, school	Italy	$\geq$5 events per hour with SaO_2 decrease $\geq$ 4%	13.0% (95% CI, 8.7, 17.3)
Rosen (21)	2003	850	850	8–11	Population-based cohort, birth hospital	U.S.A.	AHI > 5 OAI > 1 Either of the above	0.9% (95% CI, 0.4, 1.3) 1.9% (95% CI, 1.0, 2.9) 2.2% (95% CI, 1.2, 3.2)

Study	Year	N		Age	Design	Country	Definition[c]	Prevalence
Schlaud (22)	2004	996	996	9.6 (0.66)	Population-based cohort, school	Germany	$3D_{90}$ and $3D_C$	2.4% (95% CI, 1.5, 3.4)
							$DI_{90} > 0.6$	1.0% (95% CI, 0.4, 1.6)
							$DL_4 > 3.9$ and $DI_C > 0.4$	3.3% (95% CI, 2.2, 4.4)
							Any definition above[c]	3.8% (95% CI, 2.7, 4.9)
Anuntaseree (17)	2005	755		10	Population-based cohort, school	Thailand	AHI > 1	1.3%
Goodwin (25)	2005	1219	480	6–11	Population-based cohort, school	U.S.A.	RDI ≥ 1 (with ≥3% decrease in SaO_2)	24%
Sogut (23)	2005	1215	39	3–11	Population based, school	Turkey	AHI > 3	1.3% (95% CI, 0.8, 1.8)[a]

[a]Estimate is extrapolated to overall sample in studies utilizing a two-staged sampling procedure.

[b]Included children who underwent adenotonsillectomy because of worsening clinical condition and/or oxygen desaturation index >2 events with desaturation cf 4% or more, but who refused follow-up polysomnography.

[c]$3D_{90}$ and $3D_C$ = three events with a fall in arterial oxygen saturation to ≤90% and three clusters of ≥5 desaturations within a 30-minute period over the course of one night; $DI_{90} > 0.6$ = the number of desaturations to ≤90% exceeded 0.6 per hour; $DL_4 > 3.9$ and $DI_C > 0.4$ = the number of desaturations with >4% fall in saturation exceeded 3.9/hr, with at least 0.4 desaturation clusters per hour.

Abbreviations: OSAS, obstructive sleep apnea syndrome; AHI, apnea-hypopnea index; RDI = respiratory disturbance index.

III. Distribution of OSAS Among Population Subgroups

Evidence suggests that OSAS varies among age, gender, and ethnicity subgroups of the population. First, OSAS prevalence tends to peak at two ages. The first peak occurs in children from two to six years of age and coincides with the peak age of adenotonsillar hypertrophy (see below) (2). A second peak occurs during adolescence and appears related to an increase in prevalence of overweight children (2). Gender differences have been observed among adolescents, with greater OSAS prevalence among boys (27). In contrast, most studies have found approximately equal distribution of OSAS among preadolescent boys and girls, though a few have reported greater prevalence of OSAS-related symptoms in boys. (12) A greater prevalence of OSAS or OSAS-related symptoms has been reported among African-American (21) and Hispanic children (12) compared with White children.

IV. OSAS Risk Factors

OSAS is a complex, chronic disease that may be expressed after a given threshold level of susceptibility is exceeded. Susceptibility relates to the propensity for repetitive upper airway collapse. In any individual, propensity for such airway collapse is determined by anatomic and neuromuscular factors that influence upper airway size and/or function. In adults, the strongest risk factors for OSAS are obesity and male sex (28,29). In children, there is less information regarding OSAS risk factors besides those associated with adenotonsillar hypertrophy, specific congenital anomalies, or neurological disorders. The latter two likely impact susceptibility to OSAS because of their associations with craniofacial morphology that reduces nasopharyngeal area (30) or because of associated abnormalities in ventilatory control (31,32). Specific risk factors for childhood OSAS are described below. In this section, we expand our focus to sleep-disordered breathing in general to provide a more comprehensive examination of factors that might be implicated in the development of OSAS.

A. Lymphoid Hypertrophy

Adenotonsillar hypertrophy is the most commonly recognized risk factor for childhood OSAS, especially in younger children. Increased risk is likely due to reduced upper airway volume (discussed in chap. 21). Several studies, however, suggest that sleep-disordered breathing may persist in 9–30% of children post-adenotonsillectomy (33–35). Paradoxically, a history of adenotonsillectomy increases the risk of snoring two- to threefold (4,5,20). Recent data suggest that sleep-disordered breathing post adenotonsillectomy is especially common among African-American children (36). Thus, sleep-disordered breathing may often present because of several factors that interact to increase susceptibility. A history of adenotonsillectomy may be a marker of disease severe enough to warrant intervention, and having had an adenotonsillectomy may identify children with a propensity for more severe disease, which may or may not have been resolved with a reduction in lymphoid tissue. It may be inappropriate to assume that sleep-disordered breathing is uncommon in children whose tonsils have regressed or been removed.

B. Developmental Risk Factors

Premature birth (<36 weeks' gestational age) has been identified as a significant risk factor for sleep-disordered breathing, with children aged 8 to 11 years who were born premature three to five times more likely to have sleep-disordered breathing after controlling for obesity and child ethnicity (21). This observed association could be due to several reasons. For example, delayed linear craniofacial growth and mandibular retrognathia have been reported for children born small for gestational age (37). Ventilatory chemosensitivity and load compensation are other traits relevant to sleep-disordered breathing that may be shaped both by genetic factors and developmental influences. Experimental data indicate substantial plasticity of the neural control systems in infancy (38). Maturation of respiratory chemoafferents occurs in the first few days of life (39–42). Animal studies show that exposure to hypoxia during this time, but not later, results in blunted ventilatory responses later in life (43,44). These observations may be explained by experimental work demonstrating that exposure to hypoxia or hyperoxia after birth can fundamentally alter the development of the chemoafferent pathway through changes in neuronal growth factor expression (45). In humans, blunted chemosensitivity has been observed in infants who receive supplemental oxygen after birth (46); the magnitude of the ventilatory response appears to be inversely correlated with the time spent by the infant on a ventilator (47).

Preterm infants are also more likely to have medical problems ranging from neurological injuries to chronic respiratory disease, which could influence sleep-disordered breathing later in childhood. Much research has focused on the relationships of prematurity with sudden infant death syndrome and acute life-threatening events in infancy. Preterm infants are predisposed to apnea in infancy partly because of neuronal immaturity leading to cardiorespiratory system instability. Although risk of apnea appears to decrease with increasing postgestational age, some data suggest that apneas may persist beyond 40 weeks' gestational age in subgroups of infants, such as those born prematurely (48,49). Persistent apneas have been observed beyond one year of life in a subgroup of children followed after an acute life-threatening event (50). These children have been described as initially being noisy breathers with a family history of snoring.

C. Obesity

Obesity is an epidemic in the developed world: >50% of the U.S. population is now estimated to be overweight and 20% is considered obese (51). Childhood obesity in the United States has increased as well. National surveys indicate that from 1980 to 2000, the prevalence of overweight tripled among 12- to 19-year-olds and doubled among 2- to 11-year-olds (52). The obesity risk appears to be particularly high for minority children, with proportions among non-Hispanic Black and Mexican-American children aged 6 to 19 years being twice that of similarly aged non-Hispanic White children (52).

Obesity may precipitate or exacerbate sleep-disordered breathing by influences related to abdominal mass loading, with effects on breathing pattern and responsiveness to respiratory drive, or via upper airway fat deposition, compromising airway patency. Obesity is prevalent among older children and adolescents referred to sleep laboratories who are subsequently found to have sleep-disordered breathing. However, the relative importance of obesity as a risk factor for childhood OSAS may vary across the pediatric age. Data from the Cleveland Family Study, which included children aged 4 to 18 years, indicate that children who are overweight are at a 4.6-fold increased risk for sleep-disordered breathing compared with normal weight children (53). In contrast, in a Cleveland cohort of 8 to 11 years of age (the Cleveland Children's Sleep and Health Study), the odds ratio (OR) for adjusted obesity was only 1.3 (95% CI, 0.5, 3.1) (21). However, a follow-up study of this cohort, assessed at ages 13 to 16 years, showed an OR greater than 6.0 (unpublished). These studies thus demonstrate marked differences in estimates of the influence of obesity depending on the age of the sample, with evidence of weak associations in prepubertal children and strong associations, similar to what has been described in adults, in adolescents. This pattern is consistent with several reports of snoring, which provide evidence of stronger associations between snoring and obesity in older rather than younger children, in whom ORs have been generally >2.0 (10,16,19,23). One exception to this is a study of 90 Chinese children aged 7 to 11 years that reported OSAS in 32.6% of the children who were overweight compared with 4.5% of their normal weight peers (54). In this study, obesity was associated both with adenoid hypertrophy and velopharyngeal narrowing, suggesting that obesity may increase susceptibility to OSAS through several different pathways. Other data have demonstrated that Asian individuals are at an increased risk for OSAS at lower levels of body mass index (BMI) than individuals of European descent (55), possibly due to differences in body fat composition or to craniofacial features (56). Thus, young Chinese children may be more susceptible to the effects of overweight than children in other ethnic groups.

Central obesity, as measured by the waist circumference or by visceral fat detected by specialized imaging of the abdomen, appears to be particularly important among adults as a risk factor both for sleep-disordered breathing and for cardiovascular disease-associated comorbidities. In children, the role of body fat distribution as a risk factor for sleep-disordered breathing has not been established. However, gender-specific patterns of body fat distribution begin to establish during adolescence, and these patterns may be useful for identifying high-risk subgroups.

D. Congenital Factors

Over 20 common syndromes or disorders, several of them resulting in craniofacial anomalies (e.g., Down syndrome, Marfan syndrome, Apert Syndrome), that affect the size of the upper airway are associated with OSAS (57). OSAS is present in 30–60% of persons with Down syndrome, the most common genetic disorder affecting craniofacial structure (57). Other studies have revealed OSAS prevalence rates ranging from 12% in Pierre Robin syndrome (58) to nearly 90% in mucopolysaccharidosis (59).

E. Upper and Lower Respiratory Disease

Upper and lower respiratory problems may influence the expression of childhood OSAS. For example, nasal obstruction caused by allergic or inflammatory conditions, by increasing nasopharyngeal resistance, may cause an increased subatmospheric airway pressure and thereby enhance collapsibility of the upper airway. Increased nasal resistance may also favor mouth breathing, which chronically may result in changes in craniofacial form that restricts airway patency. Questionnaire surveys have suggested significant relationships of snoring with asthma, cough and wheeze symptoms (4,5), and allergic rhinitis in children (5). ORs relating symptoms of cough, wheeze, or a history of asthma for snorers versus nonsnorers range from 1.3 to 8.7 (4). Passive smoking also may be more prevalent in snorers, with one study showing a significantly increased OR of 1.9 (4). According to the "unified airway theory," (60) sleep-disordered breathing and asthma may share common risk factors: generalized abnormalities of the nasopharynx and lower airway may coexist either because of common airway responses to inflammatory or atopic stimuli, or because other developmental factors similarly affect the upper and lower airways (61).

We have examined the association of respiratory symptoms with objectively measured sleep-disordered breathing in the Cleveland Family Study, which is a genetic epidemiology and natural history study of sleep-disordered breathing. Over 2500 members from 375 families have been enrolled; many reevaluated at six- and nine-year follow-up. In this sample, a history of persistent wheeze increased the risk of sleep-disordered breathing ≈ fivefold (OR 4.7), and a history of cough was associated with an OR of 10.5 (53). Independent of lower respiratory symptoms, a history of sinus problems had an OR of 3.5. Thus, it appears likely that exposures or physiological processes promoting nasal or pharyngeal inflammation influence susceptibility to sleep-disordered breathing. Other research also indicates that asthma and obesity are associated (62). Further work is needed to assess the extent to which any relationship between sleep-disordered breathing and asthma or allergies reflects causal associations.

F. Ethnic or Racial Variation

African-American children are four- to sixfold more likely to have sleep-disordered breathing than White children, independent of other factors such as obesity, premature birth, and maternal smoking (21). Other research has reported increased frequency of parent-witnessed apneas among Hispanic children compared with White non-Hispanic children (12). Although part of this association may be due to factors related to socioeconomic status (see below), there are also likely genetically based differences in craniofacial structure. In adults, we found that sleep-disordered breathing is associated with different craniofacial characteristics specific to race: in Whites, sleep-disordered breathing is associated with a brachycephalic head form and reduced bony dimensions (63), and in African-Americans, sleep-disordered breathing is related to soft tissue dimensions, such as tongue mass. Our genetic studies demonstrate different allele frequencies for African-Americans compared with Whites (64), and different linkages for sleep-disordered breathing (65,66). Further work is needed to understand the basis for the apparent increased susceptibility of African-American children to sleep-disordered breathing as well as its consequences.

G. Familial Risk Factors

Many of the established risk factors for sleep-disordered breathing (e.g., obesity, fat distribution, craniofacial morphology) have a known or suspected genetic basis. Sleep-disordered breathing aggregates significantly within families (67–69). Family studies suggest that the risk of sleep-disordered breathing may be two- to fourfold greater in relatives of patients with sleep-disordered breathing compared with controls and that nearly 40% of the variance in the apnea hypopnea index (AHI) may be explained by familial factors (67). Segregation analysis of >2000 members of the Cleveland Family Study showed evidence of a major gene explaining 20–30% of the variance in the AHI. After BMI adjustment, evidence for a major gene effect was stronger in African-Americans than in Whites, and was consistent with codominant segregation. In a preliminary linkage analysis using genome scan data on 636 members of the Cleveland Family Study (70), several suggestive areas of linkage were demonstrated for the AHI, including loci on chromosomes 2,8, and 12 (65,66). These findings were based on pedigrees (of children and adults) in which age-adjusted values for the AHI were determined using similar methodology in children and adults. In follow-up work, we recalculated estimates of the AHI in pedigrees with and without inclusion of children. Results showed no substantive change in estimates (Larkin E, personal communication). The intergenerational transmission patterns suggest that adults and children share common genetic risk factors for OSAS.

H. Environmental and Socioeconomic Factors

Using data from the Cleveland Children's Sleep and Health Study, we have recently established an association between OSAS and residence in severely disadvantaged or "distressed" neighborhoods (i.e., neighborhoods characterized by high levels of poverty, single-female-headed families with children, high-school dropouts, and noninstitutionalized, civilian, working-age males who are disengaged from the labor force) (71). After controlling for obesity, ethnicity, prematurity, and individual or household measures of socioeconomic status and health characteristics (i.e., maternal smoking, enlarged tonsils, asthma) children residing in a distressed neighborhood had over three times the odds of OSAS (95% CI, 1.53, 7.75) than children not residing in a distressed neighborhood.

The reasons for this observed association are speculative; the association could be due to greater exposure to allergens or irritants (passive cigarette smoke) (72–75). Chronic exposure to these factors might increase inflammation of the upper airway, increase nasal resistance, and perhaps trigger lymphoid hypertrophy or pharyngeal obstruction (76,77). Alternatively, children face increased exposure to environmental toxins such as lead in poor neighborhoods (73,78), and perhaps early life exposure to an environmental neurotoxin could adversely affect the upper airway's neuromuscular function. Children living in distressed neighborhoods also face increased exposure to community violence and environmental noise, which may increase stress (79,80). Noise, stress, or both may decrease sleep quality or quantity, and sleep deprivation or fragmentation may increase the propensity for OSAS (81). This underscores the need to further assess the role of environmental factors—specifically, characteristics of severely disadvantaged neighborhoods—as those shaping children's sleep because the nature of interventions to improve sleep may greatly differ depending on the actual etiological mechanisms involved.

I. Age-Specific Variation in Sleep-Disordered Breathing Risk Factors

As described above, the relative impact of any given group of risk factors on the expression of sleep-disordered breathing may vary across age. Any set of risk factors may have variable effects depending on the prevalence of that risk factor at given ages and may be influenced by age-related changes in airway size and collapsibility, hormonal changes, and maturation of breathing control systems. Figure 1 shows hypothesized changes in the likelihood of OSAS over time, and the contributions of obesity and lymphoid hyperplasia as risk factors for OSAS. Two peaks are hypothesized. The first occurs from the ages two to six years, in which lymphoid hyperplasia constitutes the most significant risk factor. However, as children enter puberty the likelihood of OSAS decreases as airway size increases, and in girls, hormonal influences alter ventilation.

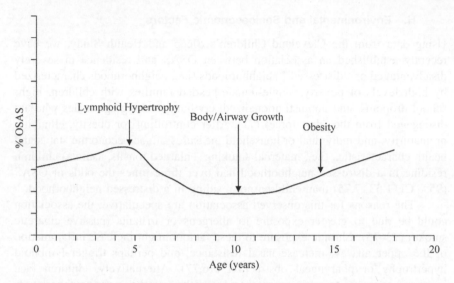

Figure 1 Change in relative contribution of different risk factors to OSAS likelihood across childhood. *Abbreviation*: OSAS, obstructive sleep apnea syndrome.

V. Natural History of OSAS

Data pertaining to the longitudinal study of pediatric sleep-disordered breathing are very limited but seem to generally support the long-held assumption that sleep-disordered breathing occurring in children without underlying neurological or congenital disorders often resolves with either growth or maturation. Moreover, sleep-disordered breathing often resolves after adenotonsillectomy, although this is not always the case (see above).

Four studies have followed samples of preadolescents and adolescents for one to three years to assess the natural course of primary snoring or OSAS (6,17,82,83). Collectively, the results of these studies indicate that only 8–10% of children with primary snoring progress to OSAS (17,82,83). However, although most children with primary snoring did not progress to OSAS, one study found that children with OSAS at baseline generally had developed more severe OSAS (i.e., >AHI) at follow-up (17). Urschitz et al. (84) conducted a one-year follow-up of 80 habitual snorers (average age approximately 10 years) and found that approximately half (49%) still snored habitually, whereas 51% no longer snored habitually. Moreover, in the studies with larger sample sizes (n > 700), the majority of children with primary snoring improved or resolved spontaneously, but the overall prevalence of primary snoring at follow-up resembled that at baseline because of new cases among previous nonhabitual snorers (6,17).

The Cleveland Family Study has followed 174 children with sleep studies done on an average of five years apart. Among children initially studied before age 7, the AHI decreased on average by 2.4 events per hour (unpublished). In contrast, in children greater than age 12, the average AHI increased on an average of ≈ 1 event per hour on the second exam. These data are consistent with some improvement in sleep-disordered breathing with growth (and regression of lymphoid tissue) in growing prepubertal children but not with progression of sleep-disordered breathing in adolescents. Collectively, the above studies suggest that sleep-disordered breathing has a different progression if onset is in adolescence versus preadolescence. Two studies suggested that children who present with primary snoring at early ages might be at particular risk for developing OSAS (82,83). However, the sample size of these studies was small (≤ 20).

Although limited follow-up among adolescents suggests persistence of risk factors for OSAS (e.g., narrow upper airway) (85,86), there are no longitudinal data following children through adulthood to assess whether OSAS in childhood leads to OSAS in adulthood.

Some research suggests that tonsillar hypertrophy in childhood may contribute to the development of skeletal features, such as a "longer lower facies" and relative retrognathia, which may increase susceptibility to OSAS across the life span (87).

VI. Health Outcomes Associated with OSAS

Chapters 21 through 24 in this volume cover consequences of OSAS in detail. Briefly, untreated OSAS is associated with a wide range of serious health, behavioral, and physiological disorders in children, including cor pulmonale, hypertension, and failure to thrive (88–91). A growing number of studies has documented links between pediatric OSAS and deficits in behavioral and neurocognitive or neuropsychological domains, many after controlling for potential confounders, including measures of socioeconomic status. For example, investigations have found associations between OSAS and behavior regulation and a wide spectrum of behavior problems, such as externalizing, hyperactive, aggressive, and internalizing (92–95). Other research has revealed decreased attention and executive functioning (92–94) as well as problems in learning and memory (96–99), social functioning (95), and school performance (100,101) in children with OSAS. A few studies have reported associations between OSAS and decreased measures of intelligence or intellectual ability (99,102,103). Given the range of problems associated with OSAS, it is not surprising that OSAS has been linked to poorer child-reported quality of life (e.g., domains of bodily pain, somatic complaints, overall physical health status), even among children with mild OSAS symptoms (104). Recent research has also implicated abnormalities in cardiac and metabolic function in children with even milder forms of OSAS (105,106).

A full understanding of the health outcomes associated with sleep-disordered breathing are limited by the largely cross-sectional design of most of the existing research, limiting assessment of causality, reversibility, and threshold effects. For example, many of the studies of behavioral outcomes have implicated habitual snoring as a key exposure (93,95). In contrast, recent work examining the association of C-reactive protein levels (a marker of inflammation and cardiovascular disease risk) with sleep-disordered breathing identified an AHI of at least 5 as a threshold above which associations were observed (106).

VII. Research Needs

Although significant progress has been made in the last decade to identify risk factors for OSAS, there is a critical need for further epidemiological research to understand the basis for individual susceptibility to the disorder, long-term outcomes, and to identify responsiveness to therapy. Longitudinal studies are needed to define temporal associations between sleep-disordered breathing and outcomes, and to elucidate the interaction among risk and protective factors during specific periods of human development (i.e., prenatal, infancy, adolescence) to shape particular OSAS "trajectories." Greater understanding of the differential contribution of risk factors and underlying etiological mechanisms leading to OSAS is critical because the nature of interventions to improve children and adolescents with OSAS sleep may differ greatly depending on the actual etiological mechanism(s) involved.

One research need is the adoption of a standard, objectively measured definition of OSAS. The large number of definitions currently in use makes comparisons across studies problematic, and the recent demonstration that definitional differences change OSAS prevalence estimates by over 20-fold in the same sample of children underscores the need for a uniform definition (3). Continued use of diverse definitions will only make the task of understanding the etiology and natural course of OSAS slower and more difficult.

A potentially fruitful, yet understudied area lies in identifying social and environmental characteristics that may operate as risk or protective factors for OSAS. For example, on a "community/neighborhood level," residence in an extremely disadvantaged neighborhood is associated with OSAS in a large cohort of Cleveland, Ohio children (71). Why? Moreover, on a "household or family level," specific parenting practices (e.g., vigilance, encouragement of maturity, consistency) have been shown to improve children's sleep outcomes (107–109). Perhaps household or family environmental factors may reduce or exacerbate the development and symptomatology of OSAS. An ecological or biopsychosocial perspective, simultaneously taking into account multiple risk and protective factors on several contextual levels (e.g., genetic, individual, household, neighborhood, or community), may identify unique and potentially modifiable risk factors.

References

1. American Thoracic Society. Standards and indications for cardiopulmonary sleep studies in children. Am J Respir Crit Care Med 1996; 153:866–878.
2. Mindell JA, Owens, JA. A Clinical Guide to Pediatric Sleep. Philadelphia: Lippincott Williams & Wilkins, 2003.

3. Tang J, Rosen C, Larkin E, et al. Identification of sleep-disordered breathing in children: variation with event definition. Sleep 2002; 25:72–79.
4. Corbo GM, Fuciarelli F, Foresi A. Snoring in children: association with respiratory symptoms and passive smoking. BMJ 1989; 299:1491–1494.
5. Teculescu DB, Caillier I, Perrin P, et al. Snoring in French preschool children. Pediatr Pulmonol 1992; 13:239–244.
6. Ali NJ, Pitson D, Stradling JR. Natural history of snoring and related behavior problems between the ages of 4 and 7 years. Arch Dis Child 1994; 71:74–76.
7. Hulcrantz E, Lofstrand-Tidestrom B, Ahlquist-Rastad J. The epidemiology of sleep related breathing disorder in children. Int J Pediatr Otorhinolaryngol 1995; 32 (suppl):S63–S66.
8. Owen GO, Canter RJ, Robinson A. Overnight pulse oximetry in snoring and non-snoring children. Clin Otolaryngol 1995; 20:402–406.
9. Ferreira AM, Clemente V, Gozal D, et al. Snoring in Portuguese primary school children. Pediatr 2000; 106: e64.
10. Corbo GM, Forastiere F, Agabiti N, et al. Snoring in 9- to 15-year-old children: risk factors and clinical relevance. Pediatrics 2001; 108:1149–1154.
11. Stein MA, Mendelsohn J, Obermeyer WH, et al. Sleep and behavior problems in school-aged children. Pediatrics 2001; 107:e60.
12. Goodwin JL, Babar SI, Kaemingk KL, et al. Symptoms related to sleep-disordered breathing in White and Hispanic children: the Tucson Children's Assessment of Sleep Apnea Study. Chest 2003; 124:196–203.
13. Shin C, Joo SJ, Kim JK, et al. Prevalence and correlates of habitual snoring in high school students. Chest 2003; 124:1709–1715.
14. Liu X, Ma Y, Want Y, et al. Brief report: an epidemiogical survey of the prevalence of sleep disorders among children 2 to 12 years old in Beijing, China. Pediatr 2005; 115: 266–268.
15. Ali NJ, Pitson DJ, Stradling JR. Snoring, sleep disturbance, and behaviour in 4–5-year-olds. Arch Dis Child 1993; 68:360–366.
16. Anuntaseree W, Rookkapan K, Kuasirikul S, et al. Snoring and obstructive sleep apnea in Thai school-age children: prevalence and predisposing factors. Pediatr Pulmonol 2001; 32:222–227.
17. Anuntaseree W, Kuasirikul S, Suntornlohanakul S. Natural history of snoring and obstructive sleep apnea in Thai school-age children. Pediatr Pulmonol 2005; 39:415–420.
18. Brunetti L, Rana S, Lospalluti ML, et al. Prevalence of obstructive sleep apnea syndrome in a cohort of 1,207 children of southern Italy. Chest 2001; 120:1930–1935.
19. Castronovo V, Zucconi M, Nosetti L, et al. Prevalence of habitual snoring and sleep-disordered breathing in preschool-aged children in an Italian community. J Pediatr 2003; 142:377–382.
20. Gislason T, Benediktsdottir B. Snoring, apneic episodes, and nocturnal hypoxemia among children 6 months to 6-years-old. An epidemiologic study of lower limit of prevalence. Chest 1995; 107:963–966.
21. Rosen CL, Larkin EK, Kirchner HL, et al. Prevalence and risk factors for sleep-disordered breathing in 8- to 11-year-old children: association with race and prematurity. J Pediatr 2003; 142:383–389.
22. Schlaud M, Urschitz MS, Urschitz-Duprat PM, et al. The German study on sleep-disordered breathing in primary school children: epidemiological approach,

representativeness of study sample, and preliminary screening results. Paediatr Perinat Epidemiol 2004; 18:431–440.

23. Sogut A, Altin R, Uzun L, et al. Prevalence of obstructive sleep apnea syndrome and associated symptoms in 3–11-year-old Turkish children. Pediatr Pulmonol 2005; 39:251–256.

24. Owens JA, Spirito A, McGuinn M, et al. Sleep habits and sleep disturbances in elementary school-aged children. J Dev Behav Pediatr 2000; 21:27–36.

25. Goodwin JL, Kaemingk KL, Mulvaney SA, et al. Clinical screening of school children for polysomnography to detect sleep-disordered breathing—the Tucson Children's Assessment of Sleep Apnea Study (TuCASA). J Clin Sleep Med 2005; 1:247–254.

26. Spilsbury JC, Storfer-Isser A, Drotar D, et al. Sleep behavior of an urban U.S. sample of school-aged children. Arch Pediatr Adolesc Med 2004; 158:988–994.

27. Redline S, Cartar L, Rosen CL, et al. Insulin resistance in adolescents with sleep-disordered breathing. Am J Respir Crit Care Med 2004; 169(abstr suppl):A758.

28. Guilleminault C, Dement WC. Sleep apnea syndromes and related disorders. In: Williams RL, Katacan I, eds. Sleep Disorders: Diagnosis and Treatment. New York: Wiley, 1978:9–28.

29. Redline S, Kump K, Tishler PV, et al. Gender differences in sleep disordered breathing in a community-based sample. Am J Respir Crit Care Med 1994; 149:722–726.

30. Bacon WH, Krieger J, Turlot JC, et al. Craniofacial characteristics in patients with obstructive sleep apneas syndrome. Cleft Palate J 1988; 25:374–378.

31. Redline S, Leitner J, Arnold J, et al. Ventilatory-control abnormalities in familial sleep apnea. Am J Respir Crit Care Med 1997; 156:155–160.

32. Marcus CL, Lutz J, Carroll JL, et al. Arousal and ventilatory responses during sleep in children with obstructive sleep apnea. J Appl Physiol 1998; 84:1926–1936.

33. Suen JS, Arnold JE, Brooks LJ. Adenotonsillectomy for treatment of obstructive sleep apnea in children. Arch Otolaryngol Head Neck Surg 1995; 121:525–530.

34. Nishimura T, Morishima N, Hasegawa S, et al. Effect of surgery on obstructive sleep apnea. Acta Otolaryngol 1996; 523:231–233.

35. Contencin P, Guilleminault C, Manach Y. Long-term follow-up and mechanisms of obstructive sleep apnea (OSAS) and related syndromes through infancy and childhood. Int J Pediatr Otorhinolaryngol 2003; 67(suppl 1):S119–S123.

36. Morton S, Rosen C, Larkin E, et al. Sleep disordered breathing in children post-surgery. Sleep 2001; 24:823–829.

37. Van Erum R, Mulier M, Carels C, et al. Craniofacial growth in short children born small for gestational age: effect of growth hormone treatment. J Dent Res 1997; 76:1579–1586.

38. Ling L, Olson E, Vidruk E, et al. Developmental plasticity of the hypoxic ventilatory response. Respir Physiol 1998; 110:261–268.

39. Barrington KJ, Finer NN. Periodic breathing and apnea in preterm infants. Pediatr Res 1990; 27:118–121.

40. Elnazir B, Marshall JM, Kumar P. Postnatal development of the pattern of respiratory and cardiovascular response to systemic hypoxia in the piglet: the roles of adenosine. J Physiol 1996; 492:573–585.

41. Rigatto H, Brady JP, de la Torre-Verduzco R. Chemoreceptor reflexes in preterm infants: I. The effect of gestational and postnatal age on the ventilatory response to inhalation of 100% and 15% oxygen. Pediatrics 1975; 55:604–613.

42. Bonora M, Marlot D, Gautier H, et al. Effects of hypoxia on ventilation during postnatal development in conscious kittens. J Appl Physiol 1984; 56:1464–1471.
43. Okubo S, Mortola J. Long term respiratory effects of neonatal hypoxia in the rat. J Appl Physiol 1988; 64:952–958.
44. Ling L, Olson E, Vidruk E, et al. Attenuation of the hypoxic ventilatory response in adult rats following one month of perinatal hypoxia. J Physiol 1996; 39:561–571.
45. Wang H, Yuan G, Prabhakar NR, et al. Secretion of brain-derived neurotropic factor from PC12 cells in response to oxidative stress requires autocrine dopamine signaling. J Neurochem 2006; 96:694–705.
46. Calder NA, Williams BA, Smyth J, et al. Absence of ventilatory responses to alternating breaths of mild hypoxia and air in infants who have had broncho-pulmonary dysplasia: implications for the risk of sudden infant death. Pediatr Res 1994; 35:677–681.
47. Katz-Salamon M, Jonsson B, Lagercrantz H. Blunted peripheral chemoreceptor response to hyperoxia in a group of infants with bronchopulmonary dysplasia. Pediatr Pulmonol 1995; 20:101–106.
48. Ramanathan R, Corwin MJ, Hunt CE, et al. Cardiorespiratory events recorded on home monitor: comparison of healthy infants with those at increased risk for SIDS. JAMA 2001; 285:2199–2207.
49. Eichenwald E, Aina A, Stark A. Apnea frequently persists beyond gestation in infants delivered at 24 to 28 weeks. Pediatrics 1997; 100:354–359.
50. Guilleminault C, Stoohs R. From apnea of infancy to obstructive sleep apnea syndrome in the young child. Chest 1992; 102:1065–1071.
51. Visscher TL, Seidell JC. The public health impact of obesity. Annual Rev Pub Health 2001; 22:355–375.
52. Ogden CL, Flegal KM, Carroll MD, et al. Prevalence and trends in overweight among US children and adolescents, 1999–2000. JAMA 2002; 288:1728–1732.
53. Redline S, Tishler PV, Schluchter M, et al. Risk factors for sleep-disordered breathing in children. Associations with obesity, race, and respiratory problems. Am J Respir Crit Care Med 1999; 159(5 pt 1):1527–1532.
54. Wing YK, Hui SH, Pak WM, et al. A controlled study of sleep related disordered breathing in obese children. Arch Dis Child 2003; 88:1043–1047.
55. Ip MSM, Tsang WT, Lam WK, et al. Obstructive sleep apnea syndrome: an experience in Chinese adults in Hong Kong. Chin Med J 1998; 111:257–260.
56. Liu Y, Lowe AA, Zeng X, et al. Cephalometric comparisons between Chinese and Caucasian patients with obstructive sleep apnea. Am J Orthod Dentofacial Orthop 2000; 117:479–485.
57. Arens R, Marcus CL. Pathophysiology of upper airway obstruction: a developmental perspective. Sleep 2004; 27:997–1019.
58. Spier S, Riulin J, Rowe R, et al. Sleep in Pierre Robin syndrome. Chest 1986; 90:711–715.
59. Semenza GL, Pyertz RF. Respiratory complications of mucopolysaccharide storage disorder. Medicine (Baltimore) 1988; 67:209–219.
60. Nayak AS. A common pathway: asthma and allergic rhinitis. Allergy Asthma Proc 2002; 23:359–365.
61. Sulit LG, Storfer-Isser A, Rosen CL, et al. Associations of obesity, sleep-disordered breathing, and wheezing in children. Am J Respir Crit Care Med 2005; 171:659–664.

62. Figueroa-Munoz JI, Chinn S, Rona RJ. Association between obesity and asthma in 4–11 year old children in the UK. Thorax 2001; 56:133–137.

63. Redline S, Tishler PV, Hans MG, et al. Racial differences in sleep-disordered breathing in African-Americans and Caucasians. Am J Respir Crit Care Med 1997; 155:186–192.

64. Sinha M, Larkin EK, Elston RC, et al. Self-reported race and genetic admixture. N Engl J Med 2006; 354:421–422.

65. Palmer LJ, Buxbaum SG, Larkin EK, et al. Whole genome scans for obstructive sleep apnea and obesity in African-American families. Am J Respir Crit Care Med 2004; 169:1314–1321.

66. Palmer LJ, Redline S. Genomic approaches to understanding obstructive sleep apnea. Respir Phys Neurobiol 2003; 135:187–205.

67. Redline S, Tishler PV, Tosteson TD, et al. The familial aggregation of obstructive sleep apnea. Am J Respir Crit Care Med 1995; 151:682–687.

68. Mathur R, Douglas NJ. Family studies in patients with the sleep apnea-hypopnea syndrome. Ann Intern Med 1995; 122:174–178.

69. Guilleminault C, Partinen M, Hollman K, et al. Familial aggregates in obstructive sleep apnea syndrome. Chest 1995; 107:1545–1551.

70. Buxbaum SG, Elston RC, Tishler PV, et al. Linkage analysis of the Respiratory Disturbance Index in African Americans and Caucasians. Genet Epidemiol 2001; 21(2):145 (abstr).

71. Spilsbury JC, Storfer-Isser A, Kirchner HL, et al. Neighborhood disadvantage as a risk factor for pediatric obstructive sleep apnea. J Pediatr 2006; 149:342–347.

72. Evans GW. The environment of childhood poverty. Am Psychol 2004; 59:77–92.

73. Chen E, Matthews KA, Boyce WT. Socioeconomic differences in children's health: how and why do these relationships change with age? Psychol Bull 2002; 128:295–329.

74. Rauh V, Chew G, Garfinkel R. Deteriorated housing contributes to high cockroach allergen levels in inner-city households. Environ Health Perspect 2002; 110: 323–327.

75. Whitlock G, MacMahon S, Vander Hoorn S, et al. Association of environmental tobacco smoke exposure with socioeconomic status in a population of 7725 New Zealanders. Tob Control 1998; 7:276–280.

76. Rizzi M, Onorato J, Andreoli A, et al. Nasal resistances are useful in identifying children with severe obstructive sleep apnea before polysomnography. Int J Pediatr Otorhinolaryngol 2002; 65:7–13.

77. Young T, Finn L, Kim H. Nasal obstruction as a risk factor for sleep-disordered breathing. J Allergy Clin Immunol 1997; 99:S757–S762.

78. Bullard R, Wright B. Environmental justice for all: current perspectives on health and research needs. Toxicol Ind Health 1993; 9:821–841.

79. Attar BK, Guerra NG, Tolan PH. Neighborhood disadvantage, stressful life events, and adjustments in urban elementary-school children. J Clin Child Psychol 1994; 23:391–400.

80. Evans GW, English K. The environment of poverty. Child Dev 2002; 73:1238–1248.

81. Persson HE, Svanborg E. Sleep deprivation worsens obstructive sleep apnea: comparison between diurnal and nocturnal polysomnography. Chest 1996; 109: 645–650.

82. Marcus CL, Hamer A, Loughlin GM. Natural history of primary snoring in children. Pediatr Pulmonol 1998; 26:6–11.
83. Topol HI, Brooks LJ. Followup of primary snoring in children. J Pediatr 2001; 138: 291–293.
84. Urschitz MS, Eitner S, Guenther A, et al. Habitual snoring, intermittent hypoxia, and impaired behavior in primary school children. Pediatrics 2004; 114:1041–1048.
85. Guilleminault C, Partinen M, Praud JP, et al. Morphometric facial changes and obstructive sleep apnea in adolescents. J Pediatr 1989; 114:997–999.
86. Tasker C, Crosby JH, Stradling JR. Evidence for persistence of upper airway narrowing during sleep, 12 years after adenotonsillectomy. Arch Dis Child 2002; 86:34–37.
87. Shintani T, Asakura K, Kataura A. Adenotonsillar hypertrophy and skeletal morphology of children with obstructive sleep apnea syndrome. Acta Otolaryngol 1996; 423(suppl): 222–224.
88. Marcus CL, Chapman D, Davidson-Ward SL, et al. Clinical practice guideline: diagnosis and management of childhood obstructive sleep apnea syndrome. Pediatrics 2002; 109:704–712.
89. Nieto FJ, Young TB, Lind BK, et al. Association of sleep-disordered breathing, sleep apnea, and hypertension in a large community-based study. JAMA 2000; 283:1077–1085.
90. Schechter MS. Technical report: diagnosis and management of childhood obstructive sleep apnea syndrome. Pediatrics 2002; 109:e69.
91. Young T, Peppard P. Sleep-disordered breathing and cardiovascular disease: epidemiologic evidence for a relationship. Sleep 2000; 23(suppl 4):S122–S126.
92. Beebe DW, Wells CT, Jeffries J, et al. Neurophysiological effects of pediatric obstructive sleep apnea. J Int Neuropsychol Soc 2004; 10:962–975.
93. Gottlieb D, Vezina R, Chase C, et al. Symptoms of sleep disordered breathing in 5-year-old children are associated with sleepiness and problem behaviors. Pediatrics 2003; 112:870–877.
94. Lewin DS, Rosen RC, England SJ, et al. Preliminary evidence of behavioral and cognitive sequelae of obstructive sleep apnea in children. Sleep Med 2002; 3:5–13.
95. Rosen CL, Storfer-Isser A, Taylor HG, et al. Increased behavioral morbidity in school-aged children with sleep-disordered breathing. Pediatrics 2004; 114: 1640–1648.
96. Adams N, Strauss M, Schluchter M, et al. Relation of measures of sleep disordered breathing to neuropsychological functioning. Am J Respir Crit Care Med 2001; 163:1626–1631.
97. Blunden S, Lushington K, Kennedy D, et al. Behavior and neurocognitive performance in children aged 5–10 years who snore compared to controls. J Clin Exp Neuropsychol 2000; 22:554–568.
98. Kaemingk KL, Pasvogel AE, Goodwin JL, et al. Learning in children and sleep disordered breathing: findings of the Tucson Children's Assessment of Sleep Apnea (TuCASA) prospective cohort study. J Int Neuropsychol Soc 2003; 9:1016–1026.
99. Kennedy JD, Blunden S, Hirte C, et al. Reduced neurocognition in children who snore. Pediatr Pulmonol 2004; 37:330–337.
100. Gozal D. Sleep-disordered breathing and school performance in children. Pediatrics 1998; 102:616–620.

101. Weissbluth M, Davis A, Poncher J, et al. Signs of airway obstruction during sleep and behavioral, developmental, and academic problems. Dev Behav Pediatr 1983; 4:119–121.

102. Gottleib DJ, Chase C, Vezina RM, et al. Sleep-disordered breathing symptoms are associated with poorer cognitive function in 5-year-old children. J Pediatr 2004; 145:458–464.

103. O'Brien LM, Mervis CB, Holbrook CR, et al. Neurobehavioral correlates of sleep-disordered breathing in children. J Sleep Res 2004; 13:165–172.

104. Rosen CL, Palermo TM, Larkin EK, et al. Health-related quality of life and sleep-disordered breathing in children. Sleep 2002; 25:657–663.

105. Amin R, Kimball TR, Kalra M, et al. Left ventricular function in children with sleep-disordered breathing. Am J Cardiol 2005; 95:801–804.

106. Larkin EK, Rosen CL, Kirchner HL, et al. Variation in C-reactive protein levels in adolescents: associations with sleep disordered breathing and sleep duration. Circulation 2005; 111:1978–1984.

107. Meijer AM, Habekothe RT, Van Den Witenboer GLH. Mental health, parental rules, and sleep in pre-adolescents. J Sleep Res 2001; 10:297–302.

108. Owens-Stively J, Frank N, Smith A, et al. Child temperament, parenting discipline style, and daytime behavior in childhood sleep disorders. J Dev Behav Pediatr 1997; 18:314–321.

109. Spilsbury JC, Storfer-Isser A, Drotar D, et al. Effects of the home environment on school-aged children's sleep. Sleep 2005; 28:1419–1427.

19

Pathophysiology of Childhood OSAS: Structural Factors

RAANAN ARENS
Albert Einstein College of Medicine, Bronx, New York, U.S.A.

I. Introduction

The structure and the neural control of the upper airway have evolved to serve four important physiologic functions: (*i*) respiration, (*ii*) deglutition, (*iii*) speech, and (*iv*) local immunity. The upper airway is collapsible to accommodate these functions. During wakefulness, upper airway collapse can be prevented by an increase in pharyngeal neuromuscular tone (1). However, this mechanism is decreased during sleep, predisposing the upper airway to obstruction (2).

The obstructive sleep apnea syndrome (OSAS) refers to a breathing disorder characterized by recurrent, partial, or complete episodes of upper airway obstruction, commonly associated with intermittent hypoxemia and sleep fragmentation (3). OSAS affects individuals of all ages, from neonates to the elderly. However, it is still not known whether OSAS represents a continuum of a disorder that places pediatric patients at risk for the disease as adults (4), or whether OSAS during different stages of life comprises distinct clinical entities (5–8) (Table 1).

The anatomic factors predisposing to OSAS differ over the lifespan. However, a smaller upper airway is noted in patients with OSAS in all age

Table 1 Developmental Aspects of Obstructive Sleep Apnea Syndrome

	Infancy	Childhood	Adolescence	Adulthood
Demographics				
Estimated prevalence (%)	?	2	2	4–9
Peak age (yr)	<1	2–8	12–18	30–60
Gender	M > F	M = F	?	M > F
Weight	Normal	Normal May be underweight or obese	Obese	Obese
Risk factors	Craniofacial anomalies	Adenotonsillar hypertrophy	Obesity	Obesity
	Prematurity	Obesity	Adenotonsillar hypertrophy	Postmenopause in women
	Gastroesophageal reflux			
	Adenotonsillar hypertrophy			
Level of obstruction	Nasopharyngeal	Nasopharyngeal	?	Retropalatal
	Retropalatal	Retropalatal		Retroglossal
Anatomic findings				
Airway	Small?	Small	Small?	Small
Craniofacial features	May have craniofacial anomalies: - midfacial hypoplasia - micrognathia	Majority normal	?	Retrognathia Micrognathia
Soft tissues	May have adenoidal hypertrophy; usually normal tonsils	Adenotonsillar hypertrophy Large soft palate	Adenotonsillar hypertrophy Other soft tissues?	Large lateral pharyngeal walls, tongue, soft palate, parapharyngeal fat pads
Treatment				
Treatment of choice	Craniofacial surgery CPAP	Adenotonsillectomy	CPAP Weight reduction Adenotonsillectomy	CPAP Weight reduction
Treatment success	High	High	Low	Moderate

Abbreviation: CPAP, continuous positive airway pressure.
Source: From Ref. 8.

groups, and probably predisposes to airway collapse during sleep. Despite the known anatomic factors, such as craniofacial anomalies, obesity, and adenotonsillar hypertrophy, which contribute to OSAS throughout life, a clear anatomic factor cannot always be identified. This suggests that alterations in upper airway neuromotor tone also play an important role in the etiology of OSAS. The present chapter will focus on the known anatomic risk factors leading to OSAS during child development, with emphasis on studies using magnetic resonance imaging (MRI) that provide the most quantitative and reproducible data.

A. Pharyngeal Anatomy

The pharynx is generally divided into three anatomic regions (Fig. 1A):

1. The nasopharynx, located superior to the level of the soft palate and continuous anteriorly, through the choanae, with the nasal cavities. This region contains the pharyngeal tonsil (adenoid).
2. The oropharynx, located between the level of the soft palate and the larynx, communicating anteriorly with the oral cavity and having the posterior one-third of the tongue as its anterior border. On the basis of the midsagittal view, the oropharynx is subdivided into retropalatal (bounded by the level of the hard palate and the caudal margin of the soft palate) and retroglossal (bounded by the caudal margin of the soft palate to the tip of the epiglottis) regions. In infants and young children the oropharynx includes mostly the retropalatal region (Fig. 1A), since the soft palate and the epiglottis are in close proximity. The anterior oropharyngeal wall is formed primarily by the tongue and soft palate, while the posterior wall of the oropharynx is formed by the superior, middle, and inferior constrictor muscles (9,10). The lateral pharyngeal walls are formed by several different soft tissues, including muscles [hyoglossus, styloglossus, stylohyoid, stylopharyngeus, palatoglossus, palatopharyngeus, and the lateral aspects of the superior, middle, and inferior pharyngeal constrictors (11,12)], lymphoid tissue, primarily the palatine tonsils (noted more in children) (Fig. 1B) (13), and adipose tissue (lateral parapharyngeal fat pads).
3. The hypopharynx, located posterolateral to the larynx and communicating with the cavity of the larynx through the auditus. It includes the pyriform recesses and the valleculae.

II. The Role of Anatomic Factors in the Pathophysiology of OSAS

A. Infancy

OSAS has been described in premature infants, newborns, and infants during the first year of life. Criteria and definitions for OSAS in these groups vary among investigators. The exact prevalence of OSAS early in infancy is not well documented. It is a more frequent phenomenon in premature infants than in full-term infants and continues to decrease with postnatal age until 43 weeks postconceptional age (14). Preterm infants may have OSAS secondary to hypotonia and central nervous system immaturity. Neonates with craniofacial anomalies often have OSAS. In some young infants, OSAS may be idiopathic. After the first few months of life, adenoidal hypertrophy, and subsequently tonsillar hypertrophy, may develop and contribute to OSAS.

Premature and newborn infants are predisposed to upper airway obstruction and oxygen desaturation during sleep mainly because of decreased upper airway muscle tone, high nasal resistance, and a highly compliant chest wall. Dransfield et al. studied 76 premature infants presenting clinically with apnea and found that 68% of them had obstructive events whereas 32% had only central events (15). Milner et al. found that half of the apneic events associated with periodic breathing in eight premature infants were the result of upper airway obstruction and glottic closure (16). Spontaneous neck flexion was also found to cause upper airway obstruction in premature infants (17).

Studies on full-term infants show that obstructive events occur mostly during active sleep, are more frequently observed in males, and usually resolve by eight weeks of life (18–20). In full-term infants, Kahn et al. found a median obstructive apnea index of 0.1/hr, compared with zero in older infants (21). In this age group, OSAS is not likely to be attributable to adenotonsillar hypertrophy. Full-term neonates are preferential nasal breathers and may develop upper airway obstruction whenever mild nasal obstruction, such as an upper respiratory infection, is present. In addition, a highly compliant chest wall predisposes newborn infants to gas exchange abnormalities during even brief episodes of obstruction.

Don et al. (22) studied the anatomic site of upper airway obstruction in 19 infants between 1 and 36 weeks of age evaluated for possible OSAS. They used a combination of MRI and airway manometry to evaluate the site of obstruction. Obstruction with clinically significant OSAS [respiratory disturbance index (RDI) > 3/hr] occurred in the retropalatal region 80% of the time and the retroglossal region 20% of the time.

In infants over six months of age, the association of snoring, obstructive apnea, failure to thrive, developmental delay, and adenotonsillar hypertrophy has been established by several investigators (23,24). These studies also demonstrated the efficacy of early adenotonsillectomy in decreasing the morbidity of OSAS in this young age group (23,24).

Several reports describe the association between OSAS and apparent life-threatening event (ALTE) during early infancy. Guilleminault et al. reported a high number of mixed and obstructive apneic events in infants with ALTE (25). Moreover, a report from the same group described five infants with ALTE who subsequently developed severe OSAS. Polysomnography in these infants at the time of the initial ALTE (3 weeks to 6 months) demonstrated a high index of mixed and obstructive events. These infants became progressively more symptomatic by 6 to 10 months and improved only after adenotonsillectomy (26), supporting the role of adenotonsillar hypertrophy as a main cause for OSAS in these infants.

A familial association has been described between adults with OSAS and infants who died of sudden infant death syndrome (SIDS) or had ALTEs. Mathur and Douglas found that SIDS occurred more commonly in families with a history of OSAS (27). Tishler et al. (28) found a significant association between altered cephalometrics, atopy, and decreased hypoxic chemosensitivity in family members with OSAS who had a first-degree relative who died of SIDS or had an ALTE. These findings suggest that genetically determined mechanisms might influence airway size or other mechanisms that could link SIDS, ALTE, and OSAS.

Risk Factors

Three known risk factors contribute to OSAS in infants (Table 2): (*i*) craniofacial anomalies, (*ii*) altered soft tissue size, and (*iii*) neurologic disorders.

Craniofacial Anomalies

The relationship between craniofacial structure and OSAS is most compelling in infants with distinct craniofacial anomalies seen with craniofacial synostosis, such as Crouzon, Pfeiffer, and Apert syndromes (29,30), and with mandibulofacial dysostoses, such as Robin sequence (31–34) and Treacher-Collins syndrome (35). Altered facial skeletal development, especially the association of maxillary and/or mandibular hypoplasia, may lead to airway narrowing due to crowding of adenoid, tonsils, and other soft tissues within the mid- and lower-face skeletal boundaries. Decreased neuromotor tone may further reduce airway size by inducing glossoptosis and hypopharyngeal collapse during sleep. Children with craniofacial anomalies may present with OSAS soon after birth and during the first years of life. In some cases, OSAS does not occur until the child is older and develops adenotonsillar hypertrophy in conjunction with the narrow upper airway. Some craniofacial syndromes, such as Down syndrome, are also associated with hypotonia, which can contribute to upper airway obstruction. Children with associated central nervous system abnormalities may also have central hypoventilation.

Down syndrome is the most common genetic disorder associated with craniofacial anomalies. OSAS is present in 30–60% of these patients (36–39). Anatomic factors related to the Down syndrome phenotype, including midfacial and mandibular hypoplasia, glossoptosis, adenoid, and tonsillar hypertrophy, laryngotracheal anomalies and obesity, are the most common causes of OSAS in this group (40,41). In addition, reduction in neuromuscular tone may also play a role in the development of sleep-disordered breathing in these children.

Altered Soft Tissue Size

The size of the upper airway soft tissues (tonsils, adenoid, fat pads, and musculature) are determined by genetic factors. In addition, the size of these tissues may be affected by inflammation, infection, and infiltration by various metabolic or storage components. Finally, abnormally neuromotor tone may further alter the shape of upper airway musculature, predisposing to airway narrowing and collapse during sleep.

Table 2 Common Pediatric Disorders Affecting Upper Airway Size
and Associated With Obstructive Sleep Apnea Syndrome

I. Craniofacial anomalies
    Apert syndrome
    Crouzon syndrome
    Pfeiffer syndrome
    Treacher-Collins syndrome
    Robin sequence
    Stickler syndrome
    Nager syndrome
    Hallerman-Streiff syndrome
    Goldenhar syndrome
    Rubinstein-Taybi
    Down syndrome
    Beckwith-Wiedemann
    Achondroplasia
    Klippel-Feil syndrome
    Marfan syndrome
    Choanal stenosis
    Mucopolysaccharidoses (Hurler, Hunter)

II. Neurologic Disorders
     Cerebral palsy
     Syringobulbia
     Syringomyelia
     Myasthenia gravis
     Möbius syndrome
     Arnold-Chiari malformation
     Poliomyelitis

III. Miscellaneous Disorders
      Obesity
      Prader-Willi syndrome
      Congenital hypothyroidism
      Sickle cell disease
      Laryngomalacia
      Subglottic stenosis
      Airway papillomatosis
      Face and neck burns
      Gastroesophageal reflux

IV. Postoperative Disorders
     Post-adenotonsillectomy leading to naso- and/or oropharyngeal stenosis
     Post-pharyngeal flap leading to naso- and/or oropharyngeal stenosis

Source: From Ref. 8.

Inflammatory changes leading to adenotonsillar hypertrophy are seen in some infants prior to one year of age, leading to the full clinical spectrum of OSAS (23,24). Macroglossia can significantly reduce upper airway size. It commonly occurs in infants and children with Down syndrome as well as in infants and children with various storage and metabolic disorders, such as mucopolysaccharidosis (42) and Beckwith-Wiedemann syndrome (43). In patients with glossoptosis, the tongue may prolapse posteriorly and occlude the airway. Glossoptosis is commonly seen in patients with a small and retroposed mandible, as in the Robin sequence (31–34), or in conditions associated with poor upper airway muscle tone, such as Down syndrome (36–41). Anomalies of the soft palate, such as cleft palate and velopharyngeal insufficiency, are not usually associated with OSAS. However, the surgical correction of these malformations by palatoplasty and pharyngeal flap, respectively, are associated at times with a moderate degree of OSAS (44,45).

Neurologic Disorders

Various central nervous system disorders have been associated with OSAS in infants. All induce pharyngeal hypotonia and predispose to sleep-disordered breathing and airway obstruction. Common causes include cerebral palsy, increased intracranial pressure, brain stem compression/dysplasia, such as Arnold Chiari malformations, recurrent laryngeal nerve palsy, palsies of the cranial nerves, and syrinx (46–49). Neurologic disorders are discussed in further detail in chapter 22.

B. Childhood

In preschool children, the incidence of OSAS is estimated to be 2% (50,51), whereas primary snoring is more common and is estimated as 6–9% in school-aged children (52). Although the exact mechanism for OSAS in children is not fully understood, important anatomic risk factors have been identified and are linked to the anatomic structures surrounding the airway that affect the size and shape of the airway.

Waldeyer's ring, which is the lymphoid immunocompetent tissue within the upper airway, is comprised of the pharyngeal tonsil or adenoid, the paired palatine tonsils, and the lingual tonsil. These tend to enlarge during childhood in response to somatic growth (13,53,54) and are a potential focus for infection and inflammation (55). Therefore, in this age group, in the absence of obesity and when no apparent craniofacial anomalies or neurologic disorders exist, adenotonsillar hypertrophy is considered the most significant anatomic risk factor for OSAS.

MRI of the Upper Airway

Physical examination of the upper airway of the child is important and should be performed in each child as part of the general assessment. However, in order to more thoroughly evaluate the airway, endoscopy (56) and imaging techniques such as lateral neck radiographs, cephalometrics, fluoroscopy, acoustic reflection, computerized tomography, and MRI are available (57–62). The above modalities have all demonstrated that the upper airway of children with OSAS is smaller on average than that of the normal child.

MRI is a particular powerful tool because (*i*) it provides excellent upper airway and soft tissue resolution (Figs. 1A–D); (*ii*) it provides accurate,

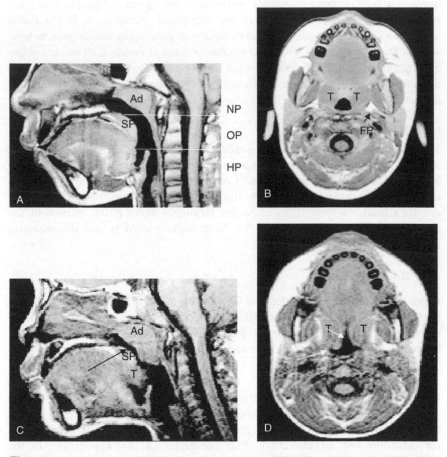

Figure 1 A midsagittal (**A**) and axial retropalatal (**B**) MRI of the upper airway in a control child. The airway is shown in black. Note in (**A**) the three main anatomic regions of the upper airway in the child: nasopharynx, oropharynx adjacent to the retropalatal region, and hypopharynx. Note in (**B**) the lateral pharyngeal walls formed mainly by the palatine tonsils and parapharyngeal fat pad. A midsagittal (**C**) and axial retropalatal (**D**) MRI of the upper airway in a child with OSAS. The airway is shown in black. Note in (**C**) the airway narrowing that occurs in the nasopharyngeal and high oropharyngeal regions, where the adenoid and tonsils overlap (black arrow). Note in (**D**) the narrowing of the airway (white arrow) due to tonsillar hypertrophy. *Abbreviations*: NP, nasopharynx; OP, oropharynx; HP; hypopharynx; SP, soft palate; Ad, adenoid; T, tonsils; FP, fat pad; OSAS, obstructive sleep apnea syndrome; Ad, adenoid; T, tonsils.

reproducible quantification of the upper airway and surrounding soft tissue structure; (*iii*) imaging can be performed in the axial, sagittal, and coronal planes; (*iv*) volumetric data analysis including three-dimensional reconstructions of upper airway soft tissue and craniofacial structures can be performed (63) (Fig. 2); (*v*) dynamic images provide four-dimensional data of the size and shape of the airway during breathing (Fig. 3); and (*vi*) it does not expose subjects to ionized radiation. On the other hand several limitations should be noted: (*i*) young children need to be sedated to avoid motion artifact; (*ii*) studies cannot be performed in sleep conditions in the MRI environment because of noise, arousals, and movement artifact; and (*iii*) MRI is expensive and not always available.

Airway Size

Using MRI, Arens et al. (57) studied the upper airway in 18 children with moderate OSAS (age 4.8 ± 2.1 years) with an apnea/hypopnea index of 11.2 ± 6.8 and compared these findings to 18 matched controls. MRI was performed under sedation, and axial and sagittal T1- and T2-weighted sequences were obtained. The volume of the upper airway was smaller in subjects with OSAS than in controls (1.5 ± 0.8 cm^3 vs. 2.5 ± 1.2 cm^3, $p < 0.005$). This finding was later reproduced by other investigators (64,65) using similar techniques.

Airway Architecture

To determine the anatomic region of maximal narrowing in children with OSAS, Isono et al. performed upper airway endoscopy under general anesthesia, evaluating discrete levels of the upper airway including the adenoid, soft palate, tonsil, and tongue (56) (see chap. 8). The minimum cross-sectional area was found to be at the level of the adenoid and the soft palate. These findings, along with high closing pressures noted at these points in the same study, suggest that the superior upper airway segments are most involved in children with OSAS. These findings are supported by two recent studies evaluating upper airway size with MRI. Arens et al. (66) showed that airway narrowing in children with OSAS occurred along the upper two-third of the airway and was maximal in the region where the adenoid overlapped the tonsils (Fig. 4). Similar findings were noted by Fregosi et al. (65), who described maximal narrowing in the retropalatal region where the soft palate, adenoid, and tonsils overlap.

Airway Dynamics Depicted by MRI

More recently, Arens et al. used respiratory-gated MRI to demonstrate the kinematics of the upper airway during tidal breathing in children with OSAS (67). They showed that the maximum restriction in patients with OSAS occurred in midinspiration (Fig. 3) and that dynamic fluctuations in the airway overlap region were sixfold higher than in controls. They speculated that such changes may have been induced by one of the following: altered upper airway motor tone, increased airway compliance, or excessive inspiratory driving pressures caused by proximal airway narrowing.

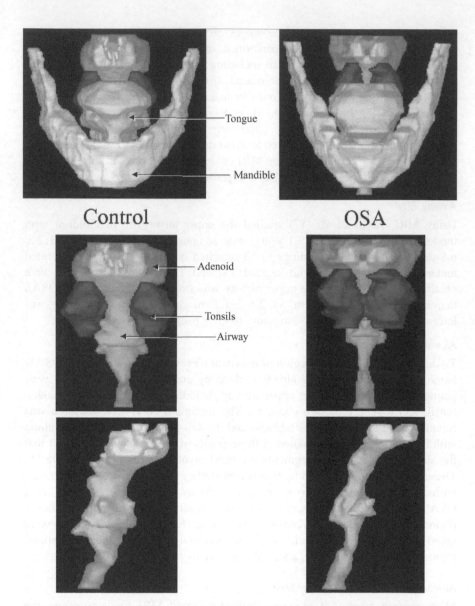

Figure 2 (*See color insert.*) Three-dimensional reconstruction of airway (light blue), adenoid (orange) and tonsils (red), tongue (pink), and mandible (white) in a normal child and a child with obstructive sleep apnea syndrome. Note differences in airway size and shape. *Source*: From Ref. 63.

In the above study, shape analysis demonstrated a different configuration of the airway in children with OSAS in both inspiration and expiration, compared with control subjects. Subjects with OSAS exhibited an airway shape narrowed across the A–P axis. This narrowing could be caused by anatomic features

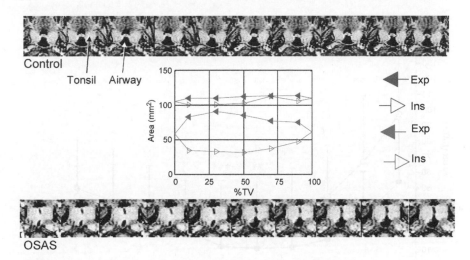

Figure 3 (*See color insert.*) Dynamic changes in cross-sectional area at midtonsillar level during tidal breathing (TV) at 20% increments of tidal volume (5 increments in inspiration [Ins] and 5 expiration [Exp]) in a control child (*top panels*) and a child with obstructive sleep apnea syndrome (*bottom panels*).

influencing the width of the lateral pharyngeal wall and/or by neuromotor factors affecting upper airway dilator muscle activity along this axis (i.e., genioglossal activation). These differences, together with the magnitude of area changes during tidal breathing, may contribute to a more collapsible airway in children with OSAS during sleep, as suggested by functional studies (56,60,68).

Soft Tissues

Adenoid and Tonsils Soft tissues, particularly the tonsils and adenoid, can also narrow the pharynx. These tissues grow progressively during childhood (13,53,54,69) and are maximal in the prepubertal years (54), coinciding with the peak incidence of childhood OSAS (70). In normal children, the airway size grows proportionately with the soft tissues surrounding it (13). However, it is not known how the airway grows in proportion to the surrounding tissues in children with OSAS.

Arens et al. measured the size of the adenoid and tonsils in children with OSAS compared with controls (57). They noted that both were significantly larger in the OSAS group; 9.9 ± 3.9 cm^3 and 9.1 ± 2.9 cm^3 vs. 6.4 ± 2.3 cm^3, and 5.8 ± 2.2 cm^3 ($p < 0.005$; $p < 0.0005$, respectively). In addition, a significant correlation between the combined size of the adenoid and tonsils and the apnea/hypopnea index was found ($p = 0.03$, $r = 0.51$), suggesting that volumetric measurements of these tissues may be useful in predicting the severity of OSA in these children.

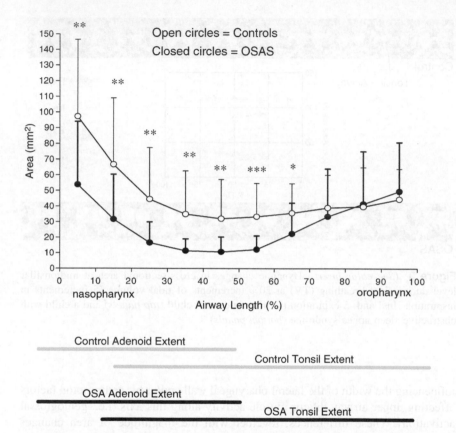

Figure 4 Airway length versus cross-sectional area in 20 control children (*open circles*) and 20 children with OSAS (*closed circles*). Data points are means ± SD. Horizontal bars show the regions of the adenoid and tonsils adjacent to the airway. Gray represents controls; black, OSAS. *$p < 0.5$, **$p < 0.005$; ***$p < 0.0005$. Note that the overlap region of the adenoid and tonsils in both groups corresponds to the minimal airway cross-sectional area. *Source*: Modified from Ref. 66.

In most cases, large tonsils and/or adenoid can explain the clinical symptoms of children with OSAS; surgical removal of these tissues cures or ameliorates the disorder in the majority of cases (23,71–73). However, it is estimated that in 10–15% of otherwise normal children with OSAS, this disorder is not resolved by the simple removal of the tonsils and adenoid (74–76).

Although the importance of adenoidal and tonsillar hypertrophy in the pathogenesis of childhood OSAS is unquestioned, much remains to be learned. It is possible that the three-dimensional orientation of these tissues, and how they overlap in the airway, is a more important factor and may significantly affect flow resistance during sleep. This is suggested by recent reports using three-dimensional MRI techniques, showing that maximal airway narrowing occurred in subjects with OSAS along an airway segment where both the adenoid and tonsils overlap (Fig. 4) (57,65,66).

Tongue Size The tongue is one of the largest structures defining the oropharyngeal airway and bounds its anterior aspect. It is composed of extrinsic muscles (genioglossus, hyoglossus, and styloglossus), which alter its position, and intrinsic muscles, which alter its shape; both can affect airway size and shape. Arens et al. found that the overall volume of the tongue in nonsyndromic children with OSAS did not differ from controls (57).

Soft Palate There are few data on the dimensions of the soft palate in children with OSAS. Using direct measurements, Brodsky et al. (77) did not find a correlation between soft palate length and severity of tonsillar hypertrophy in children with OSAS. Using MRI, Arens et al. (57) noted a 30% increase in the volume of the soft palate of children with mild to moderate OSAS compared with controls. They speculated that the larger palatal volume might have been due to edema and inflammatory changes secondary to chronic snoring, as described in adults (78–80).

Craniofacial Structure

Several studies using cephalometrics support the idea that children without distinct craniofacial anomalies have subtle craniofacial morphometric features associated with OSAS (59,81–84). Kawashima et al. (85) reported that children with OSAS and more pronounced tonsillar hypertrophy had retrognathic mandibles and increased posterior facial height compared with children with OSAS and less pronounced tonsillar hypertrophy. Shintani et al. (81) noted that the relationship of the mandible with respect to the cranial base was retrognathic in children with OSAS than in normal children. Zucconi et al. (86) noted that children with OSAS had increased craniomandibular, intermaxillary, goniac, and mandibular plane angles, indicating a hyperdivergent growth pattern (angle between nasion-sella line and mandibular line > 38°).

In contrast, other investigators suggested that the craniofacial changes found in children with OSAS are mild and reversible following adeno-tonsillectomy (84,87,88). In a recent study evaluating upper airway structure, Arens et al. noted no significant differences in the size of the mandible and maxilla of children with OSAS versus controls (57). Furthermore, in a more comprehensive evaluation of the mandible after three-dimensional reconstruction, these authors found no difference in eight dimensions of the mandible between children with OSAS and controls, suggesting that mandibular size and shape do not play a significant role in the causation of childhood OSAS in nonsyndromic children (89).

Childhood Obesity

Earlier descriptions of childhood OSAS characterized children as being of normal weight, and failure to thrive was a common complication (23,90). However, the dramatic increase in pediatric obesity (91,92) is not reflected in most of literature characterizing risk for OSAS from early infancy to late childhood (51,92–98), although a large epidemiologic study involving 399 children between 2 and 18 years of age found that obesity was the most significant risk factor for OSAS, with an odds ratio of 4.5 (51). Guilleminault et al. and Brouillette et al. reported that ~ 10% of children diagnosed with OSAS were obese (47). The prevalence of OSAS was reported to be 46% by Marcus et al. in unselected obese children undergoing polysomnography (96); Silvestri et al. reported a prevalence of 59% in obese children referred for evaluation of sleep-disordered breathing (95) and Kalra et al. reported a prevalence of 55% in morbidly obese children undergoing bariatric surgery (99). The reason for such a high prevalence of OSAS in obese children compared with the 2% reported in the general pediatric population (51) is unknown. However, it may be related to a different underlying pathophysiology of the disorder distinguishing it from OSAS in nonobese children and/or an augmented effect on regular causative factors resulting from their obesity.

In nonobese children with OSAS the most common treatment is adenotonsillectomy (100). Adenotonsillectomy cures or ameliorates the disorder in the majority of cases (23,71–73). However, as noted earlier, it is estimated that in 10–20% of otherwise normal children, significant residual symptoms exists after surgery (74–76,101). Similarly, several investigators emphasize the role of adenoid and tonsillar hypertrophy in obese children with OSAS (96,102–104). A recent study suggests that 45% of morbidly obese children and adolescents with OSAS have evidence of adenotonsillar hypertrophy (105). However, after adenotonsillectomy in obese children with OSAS, residual OSAS is noted in up to 50% of children (106). This finding suggests that other anatomic and/or functional factors play a significant role in the pathophysiology of OSAS in this group.

Obese children may have excess deposition of adipose tissue within the muscles and tissues surrounding the airway, limiting airway size and increasing airway resistance, as observed in adults (107). Additional factors that may predispose obese children to OSAS include altered chest wall mechanics and reduced lung volumes resulting in decreased oxygen reserves and decreased central ventilatory drive (93,108). However, the exact effects of weight gain or weight loss on upper airway structure and function have not been studied in obese children. Moreover, as mentioned above, other mechanisms affecting upper airway neuromotor tone and increasing upper airway collapsibility could have a compound effect in these children with an anatomically compromised airway.

C. Adolescence

There are few data related to the epidemiology of OSAS in adolescence. Only one study assessed the prevalence of the disorder in this age group and estimated it at 1.9% (109). It is not known whether OSAS appearing in adolescence is an extension of the clinical disorder of childhood, with adenotonsillar hypertrophy as a major risk factor, or whether it represents an early manifestation of the adult form of OSAS, with obesity as a major risk factor.

Several studies have addressed the relationship between childhood OSAS and OSAS during adolescence. In a retrospective study, Morton et al. (110) found that sleep-disordered breathing in adolescence was more common in those who had undergone adenotonsillectomy during early childhood. Tasker et al. (111) noted a significant increase in inspiratory effort and snoring during sleep in adolescents 12 years after adenotonsillectomy, compared with controls. The latter authors speculated that airway narrowing could have originated in childhood and predisposed to OSAS during adolescence. Guilleminault et al. noted alterations in craniofacial morphology in three adolescents with OSAS and a history of upper airway obstruction in childhood. They hypothesized that both genetic factors altering craniofacial growth and secondary modification of craniofacial growth secondary to adenotonsillar hypertrophy predisposed these patients to OSAS (112,113).

Another possibility is that OSAS during adolescence represents an early manifestation of the adult form of OSAS, especially when associated with obesity. It is well established that the antecedents of adult obesity begin during childhood and adolescence (91). Childhood obesity in all age groups is currently on the rise and the highest prevalence (15.5%) is seen in adolescent children between 12 and 19 years of age (114). Recent studies have revealed the presence of all components of the metabolic syndrome in this age group (115–117). Finally, a fivefold rise in the prevalence of OSAS in obese children admitted for hospital care has been observed in recent years (92). The above observation supports an association between the increased prevalence of obesity seen in recent years in children and adolescence and the consequences of the disorder, including OSAS.

III. Summary

Various anatomic and functional mechanisms may lead to OSAS in children. However, a smaller upper airway is noted in all age groups and probably predisposes to airway narrowing and collapse during sleep. OSAS is uncommon during infancy. However, children born with craniofacial anomalies are at increased risk for the development of a severe form of the disorder. The most common type of childhood OSAS occurs in children between two and eight years of age and is associated with adenotonsillar hypertrophy in most cases. Surgical removal of the adenoid and tonsils ameliorates the disorder in most but not all children, suggesting that other anatomic factors or mechanisms such as those leading to altered upper airway neuromotor tone during sleep may contribute to OSAS in these children.

Recent data suggest that obesity may be a leading cause for OSAS during adolescent years. This form of OSAS shares much with the adult form of OSAS. Additional factors that may cause restriction of the upper airway in adolescents include adenotonsillar hypertrophy and altered craniofacial morphology.

References

1. Mezzanotte WS, Tangel DJ, White DP. Waking genioglossal electromyogram in sleep apnea patients versus normal controls (a neuromuscular compensatory mechanism). J Clin Invest 1992; 89(5):1571–1579.
2. Mezzanotte WS, Tangel DJ, White DP. Influence of sleep onset on upper-airway muscle activity in apnea patients versus normal controls. Am J Respir Crit Care Med 1996; 153(6 pt 1):1880–1887.
3. Cardiorespiratory sleep studies in children. Establishment of normative data and polysomnographic predictors of morbidity. American Thoracic Society. Am J Respir Crit Care Med 1999; 160(4):1381–1387.
4. McNamara F, Sullivan CE. Pediatric origins of adult lung diseases 3: the genesis of adult sleep apnoea in childhood. Thorax 2000; 55(11):964–969.
5. Rosen CL, D'Andrea L, Haddad GG. Adult criteria for obstructive sleep apnea do not identify children with serious obstruction. Am Rev Respir Dis 1992; 146(5 pt 1): 1231–1234.
6. Carroll JL, Loughlin GM. Diagnostic criteria for obstructive sleep apnea syndrome in children. Pediatr Pulmonol 1992; 14(2):71–74.
7. Standards and indications for cardiopulmonary sleep studies in children. American Thoracic Society. Am J Respir Crit Care Med 1996; 153(2):866–878.
8. Arens R, Marcus CL. Pathophysiology of upper airway obstruction: a developmental perspective. Sleep 2004; 27(5):997–1019.
9. van Lunteren E. Muscles of the pharynx: structural and contractile properties. Ear Nose Throat J 1993; 72(1):27–29, 33.
10. van Lunteren E, Strohl KP. The muscles of the upper airways. Clin Chest Med 1986; 7(2):171–188.
11. Kuna ST, Smickley JS, Vanoye CR. Respiratory-related pharyngeal constrictor muscle activity in normal human adults. Am J Respir Crit Care Med 1997; 155 (6):1991–1999.
12. Schwab RJ, Gupta KB, Gefter WB, et al. Upper airway and soft tissue anatomy in normal subjects and patients with sleep-disordered breathing. Significance of the lateral pharyngeal walls. Am J Respir Crit Care Med 1995; 152(5 pt 1):1673–1689.
13. Arens R, McDonough JM, Corbin AM, et al. Linear dimensions of the upper airway structure during development: assessment by magnetic resonance imaging. Am J Respir Crit Care Med 2002; 165:117–122.
14. Ramanathan R, Corwin MJ, Hunt CE, et al. Cardiorespiratory events recorded on home monitors: comparison of healthy infants with those at increased risk for SIDS. JAMA 2001; 285(17):2199–2207.
15. Dransfield DA, Spitzer AR, Fox WW. Episodic airway obstruction in premature infants. Am J Dis Child 1983; 137(5):441–443.

16. Milner AD, Boon AW, Saunders RA, et al. Upper airways obstruction and apnoea in preterm babies. Arch Dis Child 1980; 55(1):22–25.
17. Thach BT, Stark AR. Spontaneous neck flexion and airway obstruction during apneic spells in preterm infants. J Pediatr 1979; 94(2):275–281.
18. Flores-Guevara R, Plouin P, Curzi-Dascalova L, et al. Sleep apneas in normal neonates and infants during the first 3 months of life. Neuropediatrics 1982; 13 (suppl):21–28.
19. Kahn A, Groswasser J, Rebuffat E, et al. Sleep and cardiorespiratory characteristics of infant victims of sudden death: a prospective case-control study. Sleep 1992; 15 (4):287–292.
20. Guilleminault C, Ariagno RL, Forno LS, et al. Obstructive sleep apnea and near miss for SIDS: I. Report of an infant with sudden death. Pediatrics 1979; 63(6): 837–843.
21. Kahn A, Franco P, Kato I, et al. Breathing during sleep in infancy. In: Loughlin GM, Carroll JL, Marcus CL, eds. Sleep and breathing in children: a developmental approach. New York: Marcel Dekker, Inc., 2000:405–422.
22. Don GW, Kirjavainen T, Broome C, et al. Site and mechanics of spontaneous, sleep-associated obstructive apnea in infants. J Appl Physiol 2000; 89(6):2453–2462.
23. Brouillette RT, Fernbach SK, Hunt CE. Obstructive sleep apnea in infants and children. J Pediatr 1982; 100(1):31–40.
24. Leiberman A, Tal A, Brama I, Sofer S. Obstructive sleep apnea in young infants. Int J Pediatr Otorhinolaryngol 1988; 16(1):39–44.
25. Guilleminault C, Ariagno R, Korobkin R, et al. Mixed and obstructive sleep apnea and near miss for sudden infant death syndrome: 2. Comparison of near miss and normal control infants by age. Pediatrics 1979; 64(6):882–891.
26. Guilleminault C, Souquet M, Ariagno RL, et al. Five cases of near-miss sudden infant death syndrome and development of obstructive sleep apnea syndrome. Pediatrics 1984; 73(1):71–78.
27. Mathur R, Douglas NJ. Relation between sudden infant death syndrome and adult sleep apnoea/hypopnoea syndrome. Lancet 1994; 344(8925):819–820.
28. Tishler PV, Redline S, Ferrette V, et al. The association of sudden unexpected infant death with obstructive sleep apnea. Am J Respir Crit Care Med 1996; 153 (6 pt 1):1857–1863.
29. Mixter RC, David DJ, Perloff WH, et al. Obstructive sleep apnea in Apert's and Pfeiffer's syndromes: more than a craniofacial abnormality. Plast Reconstr Surg 1990; 86(3):457–463.
30. Sculerati N, Gottlieb MD, Zimbler MS, et al. Airway management in children with major craniofacial anomalies. Laryngoscope 1998; 108(12):1806–1812.
31. Spier S, Rivlin J, Rowe RD, et al. Sleep in Pierre Robin syndrome. Chest 1986; 90 (5):711–715.
32. Abramson DL, Marrinan EM, Mulliken JB. Robin sequence: obstructive sleep apnea following pharyngeal flap. Cleft Palate Craniofac J 1997; 34(3):256–260.
33. Shprintzen RJ. Pierre Robin, micrognathia, and airway obstruction: the dependency of treatment on accurate diagnosis. Int Anesthesiol Clin 1988; 26(1):64–71.
34. Sher AE. Mechanisms of airway obstruction in Robin sequence: implications for treatment. Cleft Palate Craniofac J 1992; 29(3):224–231.
35. Johnston C, Taussig LM, Koopmann C, et al. Obstructive sleep apnea in Treacher-Collins syndrome. Cleft Palate J 1981; 18(1):39–44.

36. Donaldson JD, Redmond WM. Surgical management of obstructive sleep apnea in children with Down syndrome. J Otolaryngol 1988; 17(7):398–403.
37. Marcus CL, Keens TG, Bautista DB, et al. Obstructive sleep apnea in children with Down syndrome. Pediatrics 1991; 88(1):132–139.
38. Southall DP, Stebbens VA, Mirza R, et al. Upper airway obstruction with hypoxaemia and sleep disruption in Down syndrome. Dev Med Child Neurol 1987; 29(6):734–742.
39. Stebbens VA, Dennis J, Samuels MP, et al. Sleep related upper airway obstruction in a cohort with Down's syndrome. Arch Dis Child 1991; 66(11):1333–1338.
40. Jacobs IN, Gray RF, Todd NW. Upper airway obstruction in children with Down syndrome. Arch Otolaryngol Head Neck Surg 1996; 122(9):945–950.
41. Uong EC, McDonough JM, Tayag-Kier CE, et al. Magnetic resonance imaging of the upper airway in children with Down syndrome. Am J Respir Crit Care Med 2001; 163(3 pt 1):731–736.
42. Leighton SE, Papsin B, Vellodi A, et al. Disordered breathing during sleep in patients with mucopolysaccharidoses. Int J Pediatr Otorhinolaryngol 2001; 58(2): 127–138.
43. Kotoku R, Kinouchi K, Fukumitsu K, et al. A neonate with Beckwith-Wiedemann syndrome who developed upper airway obstruction after glossopexy. Masui 2002; 51(1):46–48.
44. Liao YF, Chuang ML, Chen PK, et al. Incidence and severity of obstructive sleep apnea following pharyngeal flap surgery in patients with cleft palate. Cleft Palate Craniofac J 2002; 39(3):312–316.
45. de Serres LM, Deleyiannis FW, Eblen LE, et al. Results with sphincter pharyngoplasty and pharyngeal flap. Int J Pediatr Otorhinolaryngol 1999; 48(1):17–25.
46. Jennum P, Borgesen SE. Intracranial pressure and obstructive sleep apnea. Chest 1989; 95(2):279–283.
47. Guilleminault C, Korobkin R, Winkle R. A review of 50 children with obstructive sleep apnea syndrome. Lung 1981; 159(5):275–287.
48. Gozal D, Arens R, Omlin KJ, et al. Peripheral chemoreceptor function in children with myelomeningocele and Arnold-Chiari malformation type 2. Chest 1995; 108(2): 425–431.
49. Gilmore RL, Falace P, Kanga J, et al. Sleep-disordered breathing in Mobius syndrome. J Child Neurol 1991; 6(1):73–77.
50. Ali NJ, Pitson DJ, Stradling JR. Snoring, sleep disturbance, and behaviour in 4–5 year olds. Arch Dis Child 1993; 68(3):360–366.
51. Redline S, Tishler PV, Schluchter M, et al. Risk factors for sleep-disordered breathing in children. Associations with obesity, race, and respiratory problems. Am J Respir Crit Care Med 1999; 159(5 pt 1):1527–1532.
52. Corbo GM, Fuciarelli F, Foresi A, et al. Snoring in children: association with respiratory symptoms and passive smoking. BMJ 1989; 299(6714):1491–1494.
53. Jeans WD, Fernando DC, Maw AR, et al. A longitudinal study of the growth of the nasopharynx and its contents in normal children. Br J Radiol 1981; 54(638): 117–121.
54. Vogler RC, Ii FJ, Pilgram TK. Age-specific size of the normal adenoid pad on magnetic resonance imaging. Clin Otolaryngol 2000; 25(5):392–395.

55. Goldbart AD, Goldman JL, Veling MC, et al. Leukotriene modifier therapy for mild sleep-disordered breathing in children. Am J Respir Crit Care Med 2005; 172(3): 364–370.
56. Isono S, Shimada A, Utsugi M, et al. Comparison of static mechanical properties of the passive pharynx between normal children and children with sleep-disordered breathing. Am J Respir Crit Care Med 1998; 157(4 pt 1):1204–1212.
57. Arens R, McDonough JM, Costarino AT, et al. Magnetic resonance imaging of the upper airway structure of children with obstructive sleep apnea syndrome. Am J Respir Crit Care Med 2001; 164(4):698–703.
58. Monahan KJ, Larkin EK, Rosen CL, et al. Utility of noninvasive pharyngometry in epidemiologic studies of childhood sleep-disordered breathing. Am J Respir Crit Care Med 2002; 165(11):1499–1503.
59. Kulnis R, Nelson S, Strohl K, et al. Cephalometric assessment of snoring and nonsnoring children. Chest 2000; 118(3):596–603.
60. Gozal D, Burnside MM. Increased upper airway collapsibility in children with obstructive sleep apnea during wakefulness. Am J Respir Crit Care Med 2004; 169 (2):163–167.
61. Croft CB, Brockbank MJ, Wright A, et al. Obstructive sleep apnoea in children undergoing routine tonsillectomy and adenoidectomy. Clin Otolaryngol 1990; 15 (4):307–314.
62. Fernbach SK, Brouillette RT, Riggs TW, et al. Radiologic evaluation of adenoids and tonsils in children with obstructive sleep apnea: plain films and fluoroscopy. Pediatr Radiol 1983; 13(5):258–265.
63. Liu J, Udupa JK, Odhner D, et al. System for upper airway segmentation and measurement with MR imaging and fuzzy connectedness. Acad Radiol 2003; 10:13–24.
64. Donnelly LF, Casper KA, Chen B. Correlation on cine MR imaging of size of adenoid and palatine tonsils with degree of upper airway motion in asymptomatic sedated children. AJR Am J Roentgenol 2002; 179(2):503–508.
65. Fregosi RF, Quan SF, Kaemingk KL, et al. Sleep-disordered breathing, pharyngeal size and soft tissue anatomy in children. J Appl Physiol 2003; 95(5):2030–2038.
66. Arens R, McDonough JM, Corbin AM, et al. Upper airway size analysis by magnetic resonance imaging of children with obstructive sleep apnea syndrome. Am J Respir Crit Care Med 2003; 167(1):65–70.
67. Arens R, Sin S, McDonough JM, et al. Changes in upper airway size during tidal breathing in children with obstructive sleep apnea syndrome. Am J Respir Crit Care Med 2005; 171(11):1298–1304.
68. Marcus CL, McColley SA, Carroll JL, et al. Upper airway collapsibility in children with obstructive sleep apnea syndrome. J Appl Physiol 1994; 77(2):918–924.
69. Fujioka M, Young LW, Girdany BR. Radiographic evaluation of adenoidal size in children: adenoidal-nasopharyngeal ratio. AJR Am J Roentgenol 1979; 133(3): 401–404.
70. Marcus CL. Sleep-disordered breathing in children. Am J Respir Crit Care Med 2001; 164(1):16–30.
71. Brodsky L, Adler E, Stanievich JF. Naso- and oropharyngeal dimensions in children with obstructive sleep apnea. Int J Pediatr Otorhinolaryngol 1989; 17(1):1–11.
72. Guilleminault C, Eldridge FL, Simmons FB, et al. Sleep apnea in eight children. Pediatrics 1976; 58(1):23–30.

73. Suen JS, Arnold JE, Brooks LJ. Adenotonsillectomy for treatment of obstructive sleep apnea in children. Arch Otolaryngol Head Neck Surg 1995; 121(5):525–530.
74. Rosen GM, Muckle RP, Mahowald MW, et al. Postoperative respiratory compromise in children with obstructive sleep apnea syndrome: can it be anticipated? Pediatrics 1994; 93(5):784–788.
75. Tal A, Bar A, Leiberman A, Tarasiuk A. Sleep characteristics following adeno-tonsillectomy in children with obstructive sleep apnea syndrome. Chest 2003; 124 (3):948–953.
76. Marcus CL, Ward SL, Mallory GB, et al. Use of nasal continuous positive airway pressure as treatment of childhood obstructive sleep apnea. J Pediatr 1995; 127 (1):88–94.
77. Brodsky L, Moore L, Stanievich JF. A comparison of tonsillar size and oropharyngeal dimensions in children with obstructive adenotonsillar hypertrophy. Int J Pediatr Otorhinolaryngol 1987; 13(2):149–156.
78. Ryan CF, Lowe AA, Li D, et al. Magnetic resonance imaging of the upper airway in obstructive sleep apnea before and after chronic nasal continuous positive airway pressure therapy. Am Rev Respir Dis 1991; 144(4):939–944.
79. Hamans EP, Van Marck EA, De Backer WA, et al. Morphometric analysis of the uvula in patients with sleep-related breathing disorders. Eur Arch Otorhinolaryngol 2000; 257(4):232–236.
80. Sekosan M, Zakkar M, Wenig BL, et al. Inflammation in the uvula mucosa of patients with obstructive sleep apnea. Laryngoscope 1996; 106(8):1018–1020.
81. Shintani T, Asakura K, Kataura A. Adenotonsillar hypertrophy and skeletal morphology of children with obstructive sleep apnea syndrome. Acta Otolaryngol Suppl 1996; 523:222–224.
82. Shintani T, Asakura K, Kataura A. Evaluation of the role of adenotonsillar hypertrophy and facial morphology in children with obstructive sleep apnea. ORL J Otorhinolaryngol Relat Spec 1997; 59(5):286–291.
83. Kawashima S, Niikuni N, Chia-hung L, et al. Cephalometric comparisons of craniofacial and upper airway structures in young children with obstructive sleep apnea syndrome. Ear Nose Throat J 2000; 79(7):499–502, 505–5066.
84. Agren K, Nordlander B, Linder-Aronsson S, et al. Children with nocturnal upper airway obstruction: postoperative orthodontic and respiratory improvement. Acta Otolaryngol 1998; 118(4):581–587.
85. Kawashima S, Peltomaki T, Sakata H, et al. Craniofacial morphology in preschool children with sleep-related breathing disorder and hypertrophy of tonsils. Acta Paediatr 2002; 91(1):71–77.
86. Zucconi M, Caprioglio A, Calori G, et al. Craniofacial modifications in children with habitual snoring and obstructive sleep apnoea: a case-control study. Eur Respir J 1999; 13(2):411–417.
87. Behlfelt K. Enlarged tonsils and the effect of tonsillectomy. Characteristics of the dentition and facial skeleton. Posture of the head, hyoid bone and tongue. Mode of breathing. Swed Dent J Suppl; 72:1–35.
88. Hultcrantz E, Larson M, Hellquist R, et al. The influence of tonsillar obstruction and tonsillectomy on facial growth and dental arch morphology. Int J Pediatr Otorhinolaryngol 1991; 22(2):125–134.
89. Schiffman PH, Rubin NK, Dominguez T, et al. Mandibular dimensions in children with obstructive sleep apnea. Sleep 2004; 27:959–965.

90. Marcus CL, Carroll JL, Koerner CB, et al. Determinants of growth in children with the obstructive sleep apnea syndrome. J Pediatr 1994; 125(4):556–562.

91. Dietz WH. Health consequences of obesity in youth: childhood predictors of adult disease. Pediatrics 1998; 101(3 pt 2):518–525.

92. Wang G, Dietz WH. Economic burden of obesity in youths aged 6 to 17 years: 1979–1999. Pediatrics 2002; 109(5):E81–E91.

93. Mallory GB Jr., Fiser DH, Jackson R. Sleep-associated breathing disorders in morbidly obese children and adolescents. J Pediatr 1989; 115(6):892–897.

94. Brooks LJ, Stephens BM, Bacevice AM. Adenoid size is related to severity but not the number of episodes of obstructive apnea in children. J Pediatr 1998; 132 (4):682–686.

95. Silvestri JM, Weese-Mayer DE, Bass MT, et al. Polysomnography in obese children with a history of sleep-associated breathing disorders. Pediatr Pulmonol 1993; 16(2):124–129.

96. Marcus CL, Curtis S, Koerner CB, et al. Evaluation of pulmonary function and polysomnography in obese children and adolescents. Pediatr Pulmonol 1996; 21 (3):176–183.

97. Rosen CL. Clinical features of obstructive sleep apnea hypoventilation syndrome in otherwise healthy children. Pediatr Pulmonol 1999; 27(6):403–409.

98. Kahn A, Mozin MJ, Rebuffat E, et al. Sleep pattern alterations and brief airway obstructions in overweight infants. Sleep 1989; 12(5):430–438.

99. Kalra M, Inge T, Garcia V, et al. Obstructive sleep apnea in extremely overweight adolescents undergoing Bariatric Surgery. Obes Res 2005; 13(7):1175–1179.

100. Clinical practice guideline: diagnosis and management of childhood obstructive sleep apnea syndrome. Pediatrics 2002; 109(4):704–712.

101. Guilleminault C, Li KK, Khramtsov A, et al. Sleep disordered breathing: surgical outcomes in prepubertal children. Laryngoscope 2004; 114(1):132–137.

102. Spector A, Scheid S, Hassink S, et al. Adenotonsillectomy in the morbidly obese child. Int J Pediatr Otorhinolaryngol 2003; 67(4):359–364.

103. Chay OM, Goh A, Abisheganaden J, et al. Obstructive sleep apnea syndrome in obese Singapore children. Pediatr Pulmonol 2000; 29(4):284–290.

104. Wing YK, Hui SH, Pak WM, et al. A controlled study of sleep related disordered breathing in obese children. Arch Dis Child 2003; 88(12):1043–1047.

105. Gordon JE, Hughes MS, Shepherd K, et al. Obstructive sleep apnoea syndrome in morbidly obese children with tibia vara. J Bone Joint Surg Br 2006; 88(1):100–103.

106. Mitchell RB, Kelly J. Adenotonsillectomy for obstructive sleep apnea in obese children. Otolaryngol Head Neck Surg 2004; 131(1):104–108.

107. Horner RL, Mohiaddin RH, Lowell DG, et al. Sites and sizes of fat deposits around the pharynx in obese patients with obstructive sleep apnoea and weight matched controls. Eur Respir J 1989; 2(7):613–622.

108. Orenstein DM, Boat TF, Stern RC, et al. Progesterone treatment of the obesity hypoventilation syndrome in a child. J Pediatr 1977; 90(3):477–479.

109. Sanchez-Armengol A, Fuentes-Pradera MA, Capote-Gil F, et al. Sleep-related breathing disorders in adolescents aged 12 to 16 years: clinical and polygraphic findings. Chest 2001; 119(5):1393–1400.

110. Morton S, Rosen C, Larkin E, et al. Predictors of sleep-disordered breathing in children with a history of tonsillectomy and/or adenoidectomy. Sleep 2001; 24 (7):823–829.

111. Tasker C, Crosby JH, Stradling JR. Evidence for persistence of upper airway narrowing during sleep, 12 years after adenotonsillectomy. Arch Dis Child 2002; 86(1):34–37.

112. Guilleminault C, Partinen M, Praud JP, Quera-Salva MA, et al. Morphometric facial changes and obstructive sleep apnea in adolescents. J Pediatr 1989; 114 (6):997–999.

113. Guilleminault C, Pelayo R, Leger D, et al. Recognition of sleep-disordered breathing in children. Pediatrics 1996; 98(5):871–882.

114. Ogden CL, Flegal KM, Carroll MD, et al. Prevalence and trends in overweight among US children and adolescents, 1999–2000. JAMA 2002; 288(14):1728–1732.

115. Steinberger J, Steffen L, Jacobs DR, et al. Relation of leptin to insulin resistance syndrome in children. Obes Res 2003; 11(9):1124–1130.

116. Steinberger J. Diagnosis of the metabolic syndrome in children. Curr Opin Lipidol 2003; 14(6):555–559.

117. Steinberger J, Daniels SR. Obesity, insulin resistance, diabetes, and cardiovascular risk in children: an American Heart Association scientific statement from the Atherosclerosis, Hypertension, and Obesity in the Young Committee (Council on Cardiovascular Disease in the Young) and the Diabetes Committee (Council on Nutrition, Physical Activity, and Metabolism). Circulation 2003; 107(10): 1448–1453.

20

Pathophysiology of Childhood OSAS: Neuromotor Factors

CAROLE L. MARCUS
University of Pennsylvania School of Medicine, Philadelphia, Pennsylvania, U.S.A.

I. Introduction

This chapter discusses the neuromotor factors that play a role in the pathophysiology of the childhood obstructive sleep apnea syndrome (OSAS). Please see chapter 19 for a discussion of the role of structural factors in the pathophysiology of OSAS, and chapter 6 for a discussion on upper airway physiology.

Many studies have shown that patients with OSAS, irrespective of age, tend to have a smaller upper airway than controls. In adults, the usual cause of upper airway narrowing is obesity. In children, the commonest cause is adenotonsillar hypertrophy, although obesity is becoming more common (1). A small proportion of children with OSAS have craniofacial anomalies. However, neuromotor factors also play a critical role in the development of upper airway collapse. This is evidenced by the fact that obstructive apnea only occurs during sleep, when upper airway muscle tone is diminished, even though the same structural factors are present during both wakefulness and sleep. Furthermore, structural factors cannot account totally for airway collapse. For example, in one study, the degree of adenotonsillar hypertrophy could only explain approximately 25% of the variance in the apnea hypopnea index (2). Although most children with

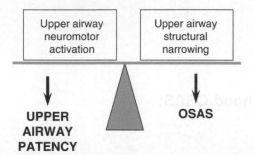

Figure 1 OSAS occurs when there is an imbalance between upper airway neuromotor tone (which is affected by factors such as the ventilatory drive, arousal threshold and upper airway reflexes), and the upper airway structural load.

OSAS are cured by tonsillectomy and adenoidectomy (T&A), approximately 15% do not resolve (3). In addition, there is preliminary evidence that OSAS may recur during adolescence in patients who were successfully treated by T&A during childhood (4,5). Thus, it can be hypothesized that certain children are at risk for the development of OSAS due to subtle abnormalities in upper airway neuromotor control. These individuals remain asymptomatic until they develop upper airway narrowing due to superimposition of a structural load, such as adenotonsillar hypertrophy. During wakefulness, they compensate for this load by increasing upper airway tone (6). Depending on the age of the individual and the degree of central nervous system and upper airway neuromotor control, this compensation may be lost during sleep, resulting in OSAS (Fig. 1). The neuromotor components leading to upper airway collapse during sleep are discussed below.

II. Factors Affecting Neuromotor Function During Sleep

A. Central Ventilatory Drive

Changes in Ventilatory Drive with Age

The evaluation of the development of ventilatory drive is controversial, as it is unclear how best to correct for differences in body size. It is especially difficult to compare infants to older subjects due to the difference in technique used for the different age groups (see Ref. 7 for a more detailed review). Nevertheless, the preponderance of evidence suggests that there is a continuum in ventilatory responses, which decline from childhood through adolescence, adulthood, and old age (8–14). The reason for the elevated ventilatory responses found in children is not known, but may be related to their high basal metabolic rate, which is one of the factors determining ventilatory drive. This increased central ventilatory drive may be one factor accounting for the increased upper airway reflexes during sleep in children compared with adults (see section on "Upper airway neuromotor tone and reflexes").

Ventilatory Drive During Sleep

Classically, the central ventilatory response to hypoxia and hypercapnia has been thought to be lower during sleep than wakefulness (15). However, newer studies suggest that this may not be true. Although there is less of an increase in ventilation in response to a hypoxic or hypercapnic stimulus during sleep compared to wakefulness, this may be due to the mechanical changes that occur during sleep, such as the increase in upper airway resistance, and changes in cerebral blood flow, rather than on a central basis (16).

Ventilatory Drive in OSAS

The role of the ventilatory drive in patients with OSAS remains unclear. Patients with OSAS have a high gain ventilatory control system, resulting in ventilatory instability and hence apnea (17,18). Clinically, most studies of the ventilatory drive in OSAS have evaluated rebreathing hypoxic/hypercapnic responses in adults, and were performed only during wakefulness. These studies have shown conflicting results. Some studies found a blunted drive (often improving after treatment), others found a normal drive, and others found abnormalities only in subsets of patients (19–28). These studies were confounded by comorbidities, including obesity, chronic obstructive pulmonary disease, and awake hypoventilation. In contrast, studies in children have shown normal overall ventilatory responses to hypoxia and hypercapnia during both wakefulness (29) and sleep (30). The differences in children compared with adults may be due to the decreased number of confounding factors in the children (in the pediatric studies, 10–40% of the OSAS children were obese, compared with 0–10% of controls), to the fact that OSAS in children is likely to have been milder and of shorter duration than in the adults, or to a true difference in pathophysiology between the age groups. Although the overall rebreathing ventilatory responses are normal in children with OSAS, subtle abnormalities may exist. Gozal et al. performed repetitive hypercapnic challenges during wakefulness early in the morning in children with OSAS who were hypercapnic during sleep (31). The children with OSAS mounted a respiratory response to the CO_2 challenge, but did not show the same adaptive changes in respiratory pattern over the course of multiple challenges as did the normal children. When studied later in the day or after treatment of OSAS, the OSAS group had a similar respiratory pattern to the controls, suggesting that these deficits were due to habituation to nocturnal hypercapnia or other sleep/circadian related factors. This is supported by data from children with OSAS showing an inverse correlation between the duration of hypercapnia during polysomnography and the awake hypercapnic ventilatory response (29).

In one small study, the occlusion pressure in 100 milliseconds ($P_{0.1}$) was measured in children and adults during wakefulness and sleep (32). The results were compared to the slope of the upper airway pressure-flow curve during sleep, which is a marker of upper airway collapsibility (see section on "Upper airway neuromotor tone and reflexes"). No correlation was found between the $P_{0.1}$ during wakefulness and the slope of the pressure-flow curve. However, there was a significant inverse correlation between $P_{0.1}$ asleep and the slope of the pressure-flow curve. This suggests that the central ventilatory drive affects upper airway collapsibility. The fact that the slope of the pressure-flow curve correlated with $P_{0.1}$ during sleep but not during wakefulness demonstrates that deficits in ventilatory drive may be sleep state specific.

Ventilatory drive has not been evaluated specifically in infants with OSAS. In general, infants have a strong biphasic response to hypoxemia, with an initial increase in ventilation, followed by a sustained depression of ventilation. This ventilatory roll-off is much more pronounced in infants than in adults (33). Theoretically, it can lead to ventilatory instability, and may be one of the reasons for the high prevalence of apnea (both central and obstructive) in the preterm infant.

Changes in Ventilatory Drive in Disease States

The importance of the central ventilatory drive during sleep is evidenced most clearly by the sleep-related hypoventilation seen in children with the congenital central hypoventilation syndrome. Many patients with disorders of ventilatory control have an obstructive component in addition to central apnea/hypoventilation, e.g., 30% of children with spina bifida and Arnold Chiari malformations have obstructive apnea (34), and patients with Prader-Willi syndrome are more likely to have obstructive then central apnea. It is possible that the obstructive component is due to associated comorbidities, e.g., glossopharyngeal nerve involvement in Arnold Chiari malformation and obesity in Prader-Willi syndrome.

B. Arousal Responses

Arousal is an important defense mechanism in response to upper airway obstruction. Arousal in response to respiratory stimuli appears to be mediated via mechanoreceptor stimulation and the degree of respiratory effort (35,36). However, this is not the only mechanism, as in patients with abnormal respiratory sensation, such as children with congenital central hypoventilation syndrome (37) or adults with quadriplegia (38), exogenous hypercapnia can cause arousal from sleep without an increase in respiratory effort. Moderate hypoxemia (Sao_2 of $\sim$75%) is a poor stimulus to arousal in humans of all ages, from infants to adults (30,39–41). In contrast, hypercapnia is a potent stimulus to arousal in all age groups, although the hypercapnic threshold may differ between ages. Small studies have shown arousal at a mean end-tidal Pco_2 of 52 mmHg in infants, 59 mmHg in prepubertal children, 46 mmHg in adolescents, and 49 mmHg in adults (30,37,41–44). Interestingly, exogenous hypoxic hypercapnia is a potent stimulus to arousal in children with OSAS (30), despite the fact that these children frequently have spontaneous obstructive apneas that are associated with hypoxic hypercapnia and yet do not result in cortical arousals.

The arousal response to obstructive apnea differs markedly between children and adults. In adults, obstructive apnea termination is associated with an EEG arousal in approximately 70% of non–rapid eye movement (NREM) events (45,46), whereas in children, arousals frequently do not occur. Several studies have shown that only half of obstructive events are associated with EEG arousals in children (47–49). In infants, arousals to obstructive apneas are even less common: in one study, only 18% of quiet (NREM) and 12% of active (REM) sleep obstructions terminated in arousal (47). EEG arousals are even less likely to occur after central apnea (47). The lack of cortical arousal in children with OSAS may explain why children can have extended, uninterrupted periods of obstructive hypoventilation (prolonged periods of partial upper airway obstruction associated with hypercapnia) (50). Because children with OSAS often do not arouse in response to obstructive apnea, sleep architecture is preserved in these patients (51), and daytime sleepiness is less common than in adults with OSAS (52). Infants with apnea, however, may have decreased REM time (53).

Although children may not manifest cortical arousals, there is evidence that they do have a subcortical or autonomic response to most obstructive apneas. The vast majority of obstructive apneas in children terminate with movement, even in the absence of EEG arousals (54,55). Analysis of spectral EEG characteristics has shown changes during obstructions (56). Autonomic responses, such as changes in the pulse transit time or in peripheral arterial tonometry, occur with most obstructions (48,49). Thus, it appears as if there is subcortical activation of the brain in children in response to upper airway obstruction. It is possible that these subcortical arousals account for some of the autonomic abnormalities seen in children with OSAS (e.g., hypertension) and may also contribute to the neurobehavioral sequelae of this syndrome.

Why do children often not have cortical arousals to obstructive apnea? Children have a higher arousal threshold than adults; the younger the child, the higher the arousal threshold (57). Concordant with this, the number of spontaneous arousals during sleep increases with age, from childhood to the elderly (58). Age-related changes in the arousal threshold, however, do not appear to be the sole reason for the lack of arousal in children with OSAS. Children with OSAS have been shown to have a specific arousal deficit in response to respiratory stimuli, such as hypercapnia (30) or inspiratory resistance loading (59), but normal arousal to nonrespiratory (e.g., acoustic) stimuli (60) when compared with age-matched controls. Children with the highest apnea indices have the highest hypercapnic arousal threshold (30). The hypercapnic arousal threshold decreases following treatment in both infants and older children, suggesting that the blunted arousal threshold is secondary to chronic nocturnal hypercapnia (30,61). Thus, it is possible that children with OSAS do not arouse in response to respiratory derangements, and thus prevent sleep fragmentation at the expense of incurring gas exchange abnormalities.

C. Ventilatory Response to Inspiratory Loading

Normal Subjects

Sleep onset is associated with a marked increase in upper airway resistance (62). This is one of the reasons for the relative hypoventilation that occurs during sleep compared to wakefulness. To understand the effects of this increase in resistance, studies have evaluated the response to exogenous inspiratory loads during wakefulness and sleep. During wakefulness in normal adults, there is an immediate perception of the load coupled with an immediate ventilatory compensatory response. This is thought to be cortically mediated. As a result, there is a prolonged inspiratory time (T_I), resulting in an increased ratio of T_I to the respiratory cycle (T_T), and maintenance of normal ventilation. During sleep, there is a prompt ventilatory response to total airway occlusion, which is frequently associated with arousal (63,64). However, there is no immediate response to an increased inspiratory load short of total occlusion. Instead, there is a decrease in minute ventilation resulting in hypoventilation. This is followed by a delayed compensatory response that is thought to develop secondary to gas exchange abnormalities, rather than to the load itself (63).

In normal children, the T_I/T_T ratio during sleep is increased in response to inspiratory loading, but even with this compensatory response, there is a marked decrease in minute ventilation. In one study, the minute ventilation dropped by as much as 40% in response to an inspiratory resistive load of 15 $cmH_2O/L/min$ (59). In contrast to adults, the minute ventilation failed to improve substantially over time (for at least 3 minutes).

Most studies of inspiratory loading in infants have focused on the premature infant, and were conducted during sleep. Although preterm infants show a brisk genioglossal EMG response to upper airway occlusion or increased resistance (65,66) and have an increase in the T_I/T_T ratio (65,67,68), they have an immediate and sustained decline in minute ventilation (67). Full-term infants have also been shown to have a decrease in minute ventilation in response to increased upper airway resistance (69).

Thus, all age groups fail to compensate immediately in response to inspiratory resistive loading during sleep, but normal adults tend to have a late (3–4 minutes) compensatory response, whereas normal infants and children do not.

Subjects with OSAS

Both adult and pediatric patients with OSAS have abnormal responses to inspiratory resistive loading. Studies comparing adult patients with OSAS to weight-matched controls showed that the OSAS group had a decreased perception of inspiratory resistive loads during wakefulness (70,71), and a decreased compensatory response to inspiratory resistive loading (72,73). Both the load perception and the ventilatory response to loading improved following CPAP therapy, suggesting that the impaired response to inspiratory resistive loading was a consequence rather than a cause of OSAS (71,73). In preterm infants with either central or obstructive apnea, imposed upper airway occlusion results in a prolongation of T_I similar to that seen in controls, but a reduced genioglossal EMG response (65). School-age children with OSAS arouse at a significantly higher inspiratory resistive load than controls, particularly during REM sleep (59), which is when most obstructive apnea events in children occur (51). This blunted arousal response may contribute to the presence of prolonged obstructive hypoventilation in children.

D. Upper Airway Neuromotor Tone and Reflexes

Upper airway neuromotor tone is discussed extensively in chapter 6. Pertinent aspects will be briefly reviewed here.

Upper Airway Neuromotor Tone During Sleep

The upper airway is a complex area, with more than 30 pairs of muscles involved in a myriad of activities, such as breathing, swallowing, coughing, sneezing, facial expressions etc. (7). Thus, abnormalities of upper airway neuromotor tone or function will have a profound effect on breathing, particularly during sleep.

Upper airway muscle tone decreases with sleep onset. As a result of the decrease in upper airway tone, upper airway resistance increases during sleep. In adults, the upper airway resistance during sleep may be double that of wakefulness (62). Because the upper airway resistance comprises nearly half of the total pulmonary resistance (74), small increases in upper airway resistance can have a significant impact on breathing. A question remains as to whether patients with OSAS have a relatively greater decrement in upper airway tone on sleep onset compared to normals and therefore develop obstructive apnea or whether they have a "normal" decrement in tone on sleep onset but an increased structural load, and therefore obstruct.

Although the overall ventilatory drive appears to be normal in children with OSAS, it is possible that central augmentation of upper airway neuromotor function is abnormal. The upper airway muscles are accessory muscles of respiration and, as such, are activated by stimuli such as hypoxemia, hypercapnia, and upper airway subatmospheric pressure (75,76). Previous studies have shown that when upper airway muscle function is decreased or absent, e.g., in postmortem preparations, the airway is prone to collapse (77). Conversely, stimulation of the upper airway muscles with hypercapnia or electrical stimulation in an isolated upper airway model results in decreased collapsibility (78,79). These studies confirm that the tendency of the upper airway to collapse is inversely related to the level of activity of the upper airway dilator muscles. Therefore, increased upper airway neuromotor tone may be one way that patients can compensate for a narrow upper airway. Indeed, this has been shown in adults. Mezzanotte et al. demonstrated that adult patients with OSAS compensated for their narrow upper airway during wakefulness by increasing their upper airway muscle tone (6). This compensatory mechanism was lost during sleep (80). Children with OSAS have been shown to have greater genioglossal EMG activity (expressed as percentage of maximal awake activity) during wakefulness than controls, and a greater decline in EMG activity during sleep onset (81). During stable NREM sleep, EMG activity remained below the waking baseline in the controls but increased above the baseline in a few of the subjects with OSAS, suggesting the presence of a compensatory mechanism in some individuals.

During REM sleep, upper airway motor tone decreases. EMG activity during REM sleep in OSAS has not been well studied due to technical difficulties, but this would be key as OSA occurs so frequently during REM sleep in children.

Measurements of Upper Airway Collapsibility

Techniques to measure upper airway collapsibility are reviewed in detail in chapter 6. In brief, assessment of the atonic airway by endoscopically measuring the upper airway cross-sectional area at different nasal pressure levels during general anesthesia with muscle paralysis provides information on upper airway structure (82–84). The upper airway can also be studied during natural sleep by measuring the change in maximal inspiratory airflow in response to changes in nasal pressure (85). Applying increasingly negative (subatmospheric) levels of nasal pressure results in activation of the upper airway muscles, i.e., an activated state, whereas dropping the nasal pressure from positive to subatmospheric levels for only a few breaths results in a hypotonic upper airway (86,87). Upper airway collapsibility is characterized using both the closing pressure (also termed the critical closing pressure, or P_{crit}) and the properties of the pressure-flow/area curve, such as the slope.

Normal Developmental Changes in Upper Airway Neuromotor Tone and Reflexes

Changes in upper airway collapsibility with age are illustrated in Figures 2 to 4. Using the atonic technique, Isono et al. have shown that normal young children have an airway that is more resistant to collapse than that of either infants or adults (82,83,88) (Fig. 2). This is presumably due to the fact that an infant has a number of craniofacial factors that result in a narrow airway (see chap. 6 for details), whereas an adult has increased soft tissue surrounding the upper airway. It is also possible that young children have a stiff airway due to differences in the intrinsic upper airway tissue properties. As expected, measurements of upper airway collapsibility in the activated state during normal sleep show less collapsibility than in the atonic state, due to the presence of increased muscle tone

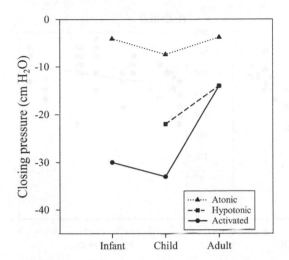

Figure 2 A schematic diagram of the closing pressure under atonic, hypotonic, and activated conditions is shown for infants, children, and adults. Note that the closing pressure for the atonic condition is derived using different techniques then in the hypotonic and activated conditions. Hypotonic data are not shown for infants, as the infant upper airway is not hypotonic under the experimental conditions used for the older age groups. *Source*: Data derived from Refs. 82, 83, 86, 88, and 110.

(Fig. 2). In the activated state, children have an upper airway that is extremely resistant to collapse compared to that of adults (32) (Fig. 3). In contrast to the atonic state, upper airway collapsibility during the activated state does not differ between infants and school-age children (86) (Fig. 2). Studies comparing the hypotonic to the activated state, as well as studies evaluating the upper airway response to hypercapnia, indicate the presence of active reflexes in school-age children during sleep (86). In contrast, these reflexes are diminished in adults (86,89). Infants have a very brisk upper airway reflex in response to subatmospheric pressure or upper airway occlusion, which manifests in the first one to two breaths after the stimulus is applied, compared with three to five breaths in older subjects (66,86). Overall, there is a strong correlation between age and the activated slope of the pressure-flow curve, showing that upper airway neuromotor tone during sleep decreases with age (Fig. 4). It can be speculated that infants and children have increased upper airway reflexes during sleep due to an increased ventilatory drive (90) and that this is a protective mechanism to compensate for a relatively narrower upper airway. With aging, this compensatory mechanism is lost. Interestingly, this change with age is gradual and continuous rather than showing an abrupt change at puberty, and the slope during adolescence is predicated by age rather than the degree of pubertal development (91). Thus, it does not appear as if the physiologic changes in sex hormones during puberty are the cause of the increased upper airway collapsibility.

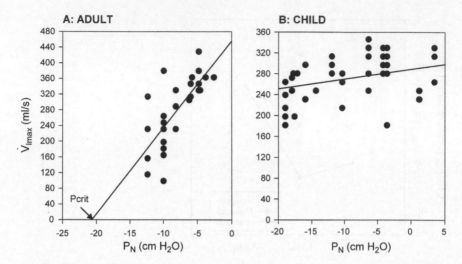

Figure 3 Pressure-flow relationships are shown for a normal, non-snoring 42-year-old adult and 6-year-old child. Maximal inspiratory flow (V_{Imax}) is plotted against nasal pressure (P_N). Note that the adult curve has a steep slope (22 mL/sec/cmH$_2$O) and a measurable P_{crit} (-21 cmH$_2$O). In contrast, the child curve has a flat slope (2 mL/sec/cmH$_2$O) and an unmeasurable P_{crit}. *Source*: From Ref. 32.

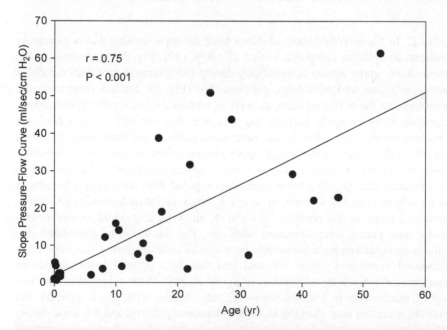

Figure 4 The slope of individual pressure-flow curves during sleep is plotted against age. There is a significant correlation between age and slope. *Source*: Data derived from Refs. 32, 93, and 110.

Upper Airway Neuromotor Tone and Reflexes in OSAS

As expected, children with OSAS have a more collapsible upper airway than age-matched controls, whether it be in the atonic, hypotonic, or activated state (82,92,93). This indicates the presence of both structural and neuromotor abnormalities, which predispose to OSAS. Unlike normal children, however, children with OSAS do not manifest reflex responses to either hypercapnia or subatmospheric pressure during sleep (93). Thus, their upper airway functions similar to that of the normal adult. As a result, there is no compensation for structural loads, such as adenotonsillar hypertrophy, and OSAS ensues. Several small studies have shown that the upper airway in children with OSAS continues to manifest increased collapsibility following adenotonsillectomy, especially in the hypotonic state, compared with that of normal, age-matched children (92,93). This indicates a recovery of neuromotor reflexes, but a persistent underlying abnormality in upper airway structure, in children with OSAS. However, larger studies are needed to confirm this.

Upper Airway Neuromotor Tone in Other Disease States

Children with disorders involving neuromotor control have an increased prevalence of OSAS. Thus, OSAS frequently occurs in patients with muscular dystrophy, such as Duchenne muscular dystrophy (94), due to upper airway muscle weakness. This frequently predates the onset of general respiratory failure. OSAS can also be seen in children with cerebral palsy (95). Although these patients may actually have increased muscle tone (i.e., spasticity), the muscles are incoordinated, resulting in the development of OSAS. Some of these patients improve after T&A, again demonstrating the interaction between structural and neuromotor factors.

E. Accessory Muscles of Ventilation

In addition to hypotonia of the upper airway muscles, other accessory muscles of ventilation, such as the intercostal muscles, also manifest a decrease in tone during sleep, particularly during REM sleep. This results in a decreased functional residual capacity, and therefore more rapid hypoxemia with apnea. This is especially apparent in young children in whom the decrease in muscle tone, combined with the increased compliance of the chest wall, results in paradoxical inward rib cage motion. This paradoxical breathing pattern is normal during REM sleep until at least three years of age (96).

F. Respiratory Sensation

The afferent (sensory) loop of the upper airway negative pressure reflex also plays a role in promoting airway stability. During wakefulness, topical nasopharyngeal anesthesia results in increased upper airway collapsibility in both children (97) and adults (98). Similarly, during sleep, the application of topical nasopharyngeal anesthesia in adults results in increased upper airway collapsibility, leading to obstructive apnea (99–102). The resultant worsening of apnea appears to be not only due, to changes in muscle tone (103) but also to blunting of the arousal response (99,102).

There also appears to be a defect in upper airway sensation during wakefulness in adult patients with OSAS. A number of studies have shown decreased pharyngeal sensation in response to stimuli, such as temperature, touch, and vibration (104–106). It is speculated that this is due to sensory nerve damage secondary to vibrational trauma from years of snoring (107). Similar studies have not been performed in children. It is possible that children have normal upper airway sensation due to the shorter duration of snoring in these patients.

Respiratory perception during sleep has been tested using respiratory-related evoked potentials (RREP). RREP are the averaged EEG responses to multiple, brief occlusions of the upper airway. Studies have shown blunted RREP during sleep in both adults and children with OSAS (108,109). It is possible that patients with OSAS have an underlying defect in respiratory perception, thereby inhibiting their ability to respond immediately to upper airway occlusion, resulting in clinically significant obstructive apneas. Alternatively, it is possible that the blunted RREP are secondary to chronic hypoxemia and hypercapnia during sleep, or to sleep fragmentation.

G. Summary of Neuromotor Factors

In summary, the overall ventilatory drive in response to hypoxia and hypercapnia is probably normal in otherwise healthy patients of all ages with OSAS. However, the central ventilatory drive plays a role in augmenting upper airway neuromotor reflexes and tone. Normal infants and children have brisker upper airway reflexes during sleep than adults, perhaps due to their greater central ventilatory drive. These reflexes appear to be blunted in children with OSAS; it is not known whether this blunting is a primary or secondary phenomenon. Both children and adults with OSAS have blunted respiratory perception of upper airway occlusion during sleep. Children and infants are less likely to arouse in response to upper airway obstruction than adults. Unlike adults, children and infants do not compensate for prolonged increases in inspiratory resistive load. These pathophysiologic features help explain some of the characteristic manifestations of OSAS in children, such as the preservation of sleep architecture and lack of excessive daytime sleepiness, the pattern of obstructive hypoventilation that may occur rather than discrete, cyclic obstructive apneas, and the preponderance of obstructive events during REM sleep.

III. Natural Course of Childhood OSAS

The natural course of childhood OSAS is not known. Specifically, it is not known whether childhood OSAS is a precursor of adult OSAS, or whether these are two diverse diseases affecting discrete populations. There are very few longitudinal studies of childhood OSAS. Guilleminault et al. reevaluated adolescents who had been successfully treated with adenotonsillectomy during childhood (4). They studied 49 subjects, of whom 23 returned for reevaluation. Of these 23 subjects, 5 snored and 3 (13%) had recurrence of OSAS. All patients with recurrences were male. In another long-term study, 20 of 61 children who had undergone adenoidectomy and/or tonsillectomy as treatment for OSAS were reevaluated as adolescents, using oximetry, snoring, and pulse transit time measurements during sleep (5). Subjects with previous OSAS were found to have more snoring and greater inspiratory effort (as measured by pulse transit time) during sleep than controls. Both of these studies can be criticized for methodologic problems, such as obtaining subjects retrospectively, lack of follow-up of all potential subjects, lack of evaluation for possible adenoidal regrowth, and incomplete diagnostic techniques. However, they do suggest that a subsection of children with OSAS may be at risk for recurrence of the disease in later life. This is supported by small physiologic studies showing residual abnormalities in upper airway collapsibility in prepubertal children with OSAS following adenotonsillectomy (92,97). Thus, it can be theorized that some children with OSAS have subtle abnormalities of central ventilatory control or upper airway neuromotor tone, or predisposing anatomic factors other than adenotonsillar hypertrophy (Fig. 1). These abnormalities may be clinically inapparent until the adenotonsillar hypertrophy results in an increased mechanical load on a marginal upper airway, thus precipitating clinical OSAS. Following surgical treatment, patients may again become asymptomatic. However, it is possible that these high-risk children will develop a recurrence of OSAS during adulthood if they acquire additional risk factors, such as weight gain or androgen secretion at puberty. Well-designed, large scale, long-term epidemiologic studies are needed to confirm this hypothesis.

References

1. Ogden CL, Carroll MD, Curtin LR, et al. Prevalence of overweight and obesity in the United States, 1999–2004. JAMA 2006; 295:1549–1555.
2. Arens R, McDonough JM, Costarino AT, et al. Magnetic resonance imaging of the upper airway structure of children with obstructive sleep apnea syndrome. Am J Respir Crit Care Med 2001; 164:698–703.
3. Suen JS, Arnold JE, Brooks LJ. Adenotonsillectomy for treatment of obstructive sleep apnea in children. Arch Otolaryngol Head Neck Surg 1995; 121:525–530.
4. Guilleminault C, Partinen M, Praud JP, et al. Morphometric facial changes and obstructive sleep apnea in adolescents. J Pediatr 1989; 114:997–999.
5. Tasker C, Crosby JH, Stradling JR. Evidence for persistence of upper airway narrowing during sleep, 12 years after adenotonsillectomy. Arch Dis Child 2002; 86:34–37.
6. Mezzanotte WS, Tangel DJ, White DP. Waking genioglossal electromyogram in sleep apnea patients versus normal controls (a neuromuscular compensatory mechanism). J Clin Invest 1992; 89:1571–1579.

7. Arens R, Marcus CL. Pathophysiology of upper airway obstruction: a developmental perspective. Sleep 2004; 27:997–1019.
8. Gaultier C, Perret L, Boule M, et al. Occlusion pressure and breathing pattern in healthy children. Respir Physiol 46:71–80.
9. Cosgrove JF, Neunburger N, Bryan MH, et al. A new method of evaluating the chemosensitivity of the respiratory center in children. Pediatrics 1975; 56:973–980.
10. Marcus CL, Glomb WB, Basinski DJ, et al. Developmental pattern of hypercapnic and hypoxic ventilatory responses from childhood to adulthood. J Appl Physiol 1994; 76:314–320.
11. Springer C, Wasserman K. Evidence that maturation of the peripheral chemoreceptors is not complete in childhood. Resp Physiol 1988; 74:55–64.
12. Kawakami Y, Yamamoto H, Yoshikawa T, et al. Age-related variation of respiratory chemosensitivity in monozygotic twins. Am Rev Respir Dis 1985; 132:89–92.
13. Kronenberg RG, Drage CW. Attenuation of the ventilatory and heart rate responses to hypoxia and hypercapnia with aging in normal man. J Clin Invest 1973; 52:1812–1819.
14. Nishimura M, Yamamoto M, Yoshioka A, et al. Longitudinal analyses of respiratory chemosensitivity in normal subjects. Am Rev Respir Dis 1991; 143:1278–1281.
15. Douglas NJ. Respiratory physiology: control of ventilation. In: Kryger M, Roth T, Dement WC, eds. Principles and Practice of Sleep Medicine. Philadelphia: W.B. Saunders, 2000:221–228.
16. Parisi RA, Edelman NH, Santiago TV. Central respiratory carbon dioxide chemosensitivity does not decrease during sleep. Am Rev Respir Dis 1992; 145:832–836.
17. Longobardo GS, Gothe B, Goldman MD, et al. Sleep apnea considered as a control system abnormality. Respir Physiol 1982; 50:311–333.
18. Hudgel DW, Gordon EA, Thanakitcharu S, et al. Instability of ventilatory control in patients with obstructive sleep apnea. Am J Respir Crit Care Med 1998; 158:1142–1149.
19. Bayadi SE, Millman RP, Tishler PV, et al. A family study of sleep apnea. Chest 1990; 98:554–559.
20. Benlloch E, Cordero P, Morales P, et al. Ventilatory pattern at rest and response to hypercapnic stimulation in patients with obstructive sleep apnea syndrome. Respiration 1995; 62:4–9.
21. Osanai S, Akiba Y, Fujiuchi S, et al. Depression of peripheral chemosensitivity by a dopaminergic mechanism in patients with obstructive sleep apnoea syndrome. Eur Respir J 1999; 13:418–423.
22. Kunitomo F, Kimura H, Tatsumi K, et al. Abnormal breathing during sleep and chemical control of breathing during wakefulness in patients with sleep apnea syndrome. Am Rev Respir Dis 1989; 139:164–169.
23. Lin C. Effect of nasal CPAP on ventilatory drive in normocapnic and hypercapnic patients with obstructive sleep apnoea syndrome. Eur Respir J 1994; 7:2005–2010.
24. Radwan L, Maszczyk Z, Koziorowski A, et al. Control of breathing in obstructive sleep apnoea and in patients with the overlap syndrome. Eur Respir J 1995; 8:542–545.
25. Garay SM, Rapoport D, Sorkin B, et al. Regulation of ventilation in the obstructive sleep apnea syndrome. Am Rev Respir Dis 1981; 124:451–457.
26. Zwillich CW, Sutton FD, Pierson DJ, et al. Decreased hypoxic ventilatory drive in the obesity-hypoventilation syndrome. Am J Med 1975; 59:343–348.

27. Rochester DF, Enson Y. Current concepts in the pathogenesis of the obesity-hypoventilation syndrome. Mechanical and circulatory factors. Am J Med 1974; 57:402–420.

28. Sullivan CE, Grunstein RR, Marrone O, et al. Sleep apnea - pathophysiology: upper airway and control of breathing. In: Guilleminault C, ed. Obstructive Sleep Apnea Syndrome. New York: Raven Press, 1990:49–71.

29. Marcus CL, Gozal D, Arens R, et al. Ventilatory responses during wakefulness in children with obstructive sleep apnea. Am J Respir Crit Care Med 1994; 149(3 pt 1): 715–721.

30. Marcus CL, Lutz J, Carroll JL, et al. Arousal and ventilatory responses during sleep in children with obstructive sleep apnea. J Appl Physiol 1998; 84:1926–1936.

31. Gozal D, Arens R, Omlin KJ, et al. Ventilatory response to consecutive short hypercapnic challenges in children with obstructive sleep apnea. J Appl Physiol 1995; 79:1608–1614.

32. Marcus CL, Lutz J, Hamer A, et al. Developmental changes in response to sub-atmospheric pressure loading of the upper airway. J Appl Physiol 1999; 87:626–633.

33. Rigatto H. Maturation of breathing control in the fetus and newborn infant. In: Beckerman RC, Brouillette RT, Hunt CE, eds. Respiratory Control Disorders in Infants and Children. Baltimore: Williams & Wilkins, 1992:61–75.

34. Waters KA, Forbes P, Morielli A, et al. Sleep-disordered breathing in children with myelomeningocele. J Pediatr 1998; 132:672–681.

35. Gleeson K, Zwillich CW, White DP. The influence of increasing ventilatory effort on arousal from sleep. Am Rev Respir Dis 1990; 142:295–300.

36. Kimoff RJ, Cheong TH, Olha AE, et al. Mechanisms of apnea termination in obstructive sleep apnea. Role of chemoreceptor and mechanoreceptor stimuli. Am J Respir Crit Care Med 1994; 149(3 pt 1):707–714.

37. Marcus CL, Bautista DB, Amihyia A, et al. Hypercapneic arousal responses in children with congenital central hypoventilation syndrome. Pediatrics 1991; 88:993–998.

38. Ayas NT, Brown R, Shea SA. Hypercapnia can induce arousal from sleep in the absence of altered respiratory mechanoreception. Am J Respir Crit Care Med 2000; 162(3 pt 1):1004–1008.

39. Davidson Ward SL, Bautista DB, Keens TG. Hypoxic arousal responses in normal infants. Pediatrics 1992; 89:860–864.

40. Berthon-Jones M, Sullivan CE. Ventilatory and arousal responses to hypoxia in sleeping humans. Am Rev Respir Dis 1982; 125:632–639.

41. Hedemark LL, Kronenberg RS. Ventilatory and heart rate responses to hypoxia and hypercapnia during sleep in adults. J Appl Physiol 1982; 53:307–312.

42. van der Hal A, Rodriguez AM, Sargent CW, et al. Hypoxic and hypercapneic arousal responses and prediction of subsequent apnea in apnea of infancy. Pediatrics 1985; 75:848–854.

43. Douglas NJ, White DP, Weil JV, et al. Hypercapnic ventilatory response in sleeping adults. Am Rev Respir Dis 1982; 126:758–762.

44. Livingston FR, Arens R, Bailey SL, et al. Hypercapnic arousal responses in Prader-Willi syndrome. Chest 1995; 108:1627–1631.

45. Rees K, Spence DP, Earis JE, et al. Arousal responses from apneic events during non-rapid-eye-movement sleep. Am J Respir Crit Care Med 1995; 152:1016–1021.

46. O'Malley EB, Norman RG, Farkas D, et al. The addition of frontal EEG leads improves detection of cortical arousal following obstructive respiratory events. Sleep 2003; 26:435–439.

47. McNamara F, Issa FG, Sullivan CE. Arousal pattern following central and obstructive breathing abnormalities in infants and children. J Appl Physiol 1996; 81:2651–2657.

48. Katz ES, Lutz J, Black C, et al. Pulse transit time as a measure of arousal and respiratory effort in children with sleep-disordered breathing. Pediatr Res 2003; 53:580–588.

49. Tauman R, O'Brien LM, Mast BT, et al. Peripheral arterial tonometry events and electroencephalographic arousals in children. Sleep 2004; 27:502–506.

50. American Thoracic Society. Standards and indications for cardiopulmonary sleep studies in children. Am J Respir Crit Care Med 1996; 153:866–878.

51. Goh DY, Galster P, Marcus CL. Sleep architecture and respiratory disturbances in children with obstructive sleep apnea. Am J Respir Crit Care Med 2000; 162(2 pt 1): 682–686.

52. Gozal D, Wang M, Pope DW Jr. Objective sleepiness measures in pediatric obstructive sleep apnea. Pediatrics 2001; 108:693–697.

53. McNamara F, Sullivan CE. Sleep-disordered breathing and its effects on sleep in infants. Sleep 1996; 19:4–12.

54. Praud JP, d'Allest AM, Nedelcoux H, et al. Sleep-related abdominal muscle behavior during partial or complete obstructed breathing in prepubertal children. Pediatr Res 1989; 26:347–350.

55. Mograss MA, Ducharme FM, Brouillette RT Movement/arousals. Description, classification, and relationship to sleep apnea in children. Am J Respir Crit Care Med 1994; 150(6 pt 1):1690–1696.

56. Bandla HPR, Gozal D. Dynamic changes in EEG spectra during obstructive apnea in children. Pediatr Pulmonol 1999; 29:359–365.

57. Busby KA, Mercier L, Pivik RT Ontogenetic variations in auditory arousal threshold during sleep. Psychophysiology 1994; 31:182–188.

58. Boselli M, Parrino L, Smerieri A, et al. Effect of age on EEG arousals in normal sleep. Sleep 1998; 21:351–357.

59. Marcus CL, Moreira GA, Bamford O, et al. Response to inspiratory resistive loading during sleep in normal children and children with obstructive apnea. J Appl Physiol 1999; 87:1448–1454.

60. Moreira GA, Tufik S, Nery LE, et al. Acoustic arousal responses in children with obstructive sleep apnea. Pediatr Pulmonol 2005; 40:300–305.

61. McNamara F, Sullivan CE. Effects of nasal CPAP therapy on respiratory and spontaneous arousals in infants with OSA. J Appl Physiol 1999; 87:889–896.

62. Lopes JM, Tabachnik E, Muller NL, et al. Total airway resistance and respiratory muscle activity during sleep. J Appl Physiol 1983; 54:773–777.

63. Henke KG, Badr MS, Skatrud JB, et al. Load compensation and respiratory muscle function during sleep. J Appl Physiol 1992; 72:1221–1234.

64. Issa FG, Sullivan CE. Arousal and breathing responses to airway occlusion in healthy sleeping adults. J Appl Physiol 1983; 55:1113–1119.

65. Gauda EB, Miller MJ, Carlo WA, et al. Genioglossus response to airway occlusion in apneic versus nonapneic infants. Pediatr Res 1987; 22:683–687.

66. Carlo WA, Miller MJ, Martin RJ. Differential response of respiratory muscles to airway occlusion in infants. J Appl Physiol 1985; 59:847–852.
67. Abbasi S, Duara S, Shaffer T, et al. Effect of external inspiratory loading on ventilation of premature infants. Pediatr Res 1984; 18:150–154.
68. Duara S, Silva NG, Claure N. Role of respiratory muscles in upper airway narrowing induced by inspiratory loading in preterm infants. J Appl Physiol 1994; 77:30–36.
69. Purcell M. Response in the newborn to raised upper airway resistance. Arch Dis Child 1976; 51:602–607.
70. Clerk AA, Dunan SR, Guilleminault C. Load detection in subjects with sleep-induced upper airway obstruction. Am J Respir Crit Care Med 1994; 149(3 pt 1): 727–730.
71. Tun Y, Hida W, Okabe S, et al. Inspiratory effort sensation to added resistive loading in patients with obstructive sleep apnea. Chest 2000; 118:1332–1338.
72. Rajagopal KR, Abbrecht PH, Tellis CJ. Control of breathing in obstructive sleep apnea. Chest 1984; 85:174–180.
73. Greenberg HE, Scharf SM. Depressed ventilatory load compensation in sleep apnea. Reversal by nasal CPAP. Am Rev Respir Dis 1993; 148(6 pt 1):1610–1615.
74. Ferris BG, Mead J, Opie LH. Partitioning of respiratory flow resistance in man. J Appl Physiol 1964; 19:653–658.
75. Weiner D, Mitra J, Salamone J, et al. Effects of chemical stimuli on nerves supplying upper airway muscles. J Appl Physiol 1982; 52:530–536.
76. Aronson RM, Onal E, Carley DW, et al. Upper airway and respiratory muscle responses to continuous negative airway pressure. J Appl Physiol 1989; 66:1373–1382.
77. Wilson SL, Thach BT, Brouillette RT, et al. Upper airway patency in the human infant: influence of airway pressure and posture. J Appl Physiol 1980; 48:500–504.
78. Schwartz AR, Thut DC, Russ B, et al. Effect of electrical stimulation of the hypoglossal nerve on airflow mechanics in the isolated upper airway. Am Rev Respir Dis 1993; 147:1144–1150.
79. Schwartz AR, Thut DC, Brower RG, et al. Modulation of maximal inspiratory airflow by neuromuscular activity: effect of CO2. J Appl Physiol 1993; 74:1597–1605.
80. Mezzanotte WS, Tangel DJ, White DP. Influence of sleep onset on upper-airway muscle activity in apnea patients versus normal controls. Am J Respir Crit Care Med 1996; 153(6 pt 1):1880–1887.
81. Katz ES, White DP. Genioglossus activity in children with obstructive sleep apnea during wakefulness and sleep onset. Am J Respir Crit Care Med 2003; 168:664–670.
82. Isono S, Shimada A, Utsugi M, et al. Comparison of static mechanical properties of the passive pharynx between normal children and children with sleep-disordered breathing. Am J Respir Crit Care Med 1998; 157(4 pt 1):1204–1212.
83. Isono S, Tanaka A, Ishikawa T, et al. Developmental changes in collapsibility of the passive pharynx during infancy. Am J Respir Crit Care Med 2000; 162(3 pt 1): 832–836.
84. Isono S, Morrison DL, Launois SH, et al. Static mechanics of the velopharynx of patients with obstructive sleep apnea. J Appl Physiol 1993; 75:148–154.
85. Smith PL, Wise RA, Gold AR, et al. Upper airway pressure-flow relationships in obstructive sleep apnea. J Appl Physiol 1988; 64:789–795.
86. Marcus CL, Fernandes do Prado LB, Lutz J, et al. Developmental changes in upper airway dynamics. J Appl Physiol 2004; 97:98–108.

87. Katz ES, Marcus CL, White DP. Influence of Airway Pressure on Genioglossus Activity During Sleep in Normal Children. Am J Respir Crit Care Med 2006; 173:902–909.

88. Isono S, Remmers JE, Tanaka A, et al. Anatomy of pharynx in patients with obstructive sleep apnea and in normal subjects. J Appl Physiol 1997; 82:1319–1326.

89. Pillar G, Malhotra A, Fogel RB, et al. Upper airway muscle responsiveness to rising PCO2 during NREM sleep. J Appl Physiol 2000; 89:1275–1282.

90. Glomb WB, Marcus CL, Keens TG, et al. Hypercapnic and hypoxic ventilatory and cardiac responses in school- aged siblings of sudden infant death syndrome victims. J Pediatr 1992; 121:391–397.

91. Bandla P, Pepe M, Samuel, J, et al. The effect of puberty on upper airway collapsibility. Am J Respir Crit Care Med 2006; 3:A374.

92. Marcus CL, McColley SA, Carroll JL, et al. Upper airway collapsibility in children with obstructive sleep apnea syndrome. J Appl Physiol 1994; 77:918–924.

93. Marcus CL, Katz ES, Lutz J, et al. Upper Airway Dynamic Responses in Children with the Obstructive Sleep Apnea Syndrome. Pediatr Res 2005; 57:99–107.

94. Khan Y, Heckmatt JZ. Obstructive apnoeas in Duchenne muscular dystrophy. Thorax 1994; 49:157–161.

95. Kotagal S, Gibbons VP, Stith JA Sleep abnormalities in patients with severe cerebral palsy. Dev Med Child Neurol 1994; 36:304–311.

96. Gaultier C, Praud JP, Canet E, et al. Paradoxical inward rib cage motion during rapid eye movement sleep in infants and young children. Journal of Developmental Physiology 1987; 9:391–397.

97. Gozal D, Burnside MM. Increased Upper Airway Collapsibility in Children with Obstructive Sleep Apnea During Wakefulness. Am J Respir Crit Care Med 2003; 169:163–167.

98. Fogel RB, Malhotra A, Shea SA, et al. Reduced genioglossal activity with upper airway anesthesia in awake patients with OSA. J Appl Physiol 2000; 88:1346–1354.

99. Berry RB, Kouchi KG, Bower JL, et al. Effect of upper airway anesthesia on obstructive sleep apnea. Am J Respir Crit Care Med 1995; 151:1857–1861.

100. Chadwick GA, Crowley P, Fitzgerald MX, et al. Obstructive sleep apnea following topical oropharyngeal anesthesia in loud snorers. Am Rev Respir Dis 1991; 143(4 pt 1): 810–813.

101. McNicholas WT, Coffey M, McDonnell T, et al. Upper airway obstruction during sleep in normal subjects after selective topical oropharyngeal anesthesia. Am Rev Respir Dis 1987; 135:1316–1319.

102. Basner RC, Ringler J, Garpestad E, et al. Upper airway anesthesia delays arousal from airway occlusion induced during human NREM sleep. J Appl Physiol 1992; 73:642–648.

103. Berry RB, McNellis MI, Kouchi K, et al. Upper airway anesthesia reduces phasic genioglossus activity during sleep apnea. Am J Respir Crit Care Med 1997; 156:127–132.

104. Larsson H, Carlsson-Nordlander B, Lindblad LE, et al. Temperature thresholds in the oropharynx of patients with obstructive sleep apnea syndrome. Am Rev Respir Dis 1992; 146(5 pt 1):1246–1249.

105. Guilleminault C, Li K, Chen NH, et al. Two-point palatal discrimination in patients with upper airway resistance syndrome, obstructive sleep apnea syndrome, and normal control subjects. Chest 2002; 122:866–870.

106. Kimoff RJ, Sforza E, Champagne V, et al. Upper airway sensation in snoring and obstructive sleep apnea. Am J Respir Crit Care Med 2001; 164:250–255.
107. Svanborg E Upper airway nerve lesions in obstructive sleep apnea. Am J Respir Crit Care Med 2001; 164:187–189.
108. Gora J, Trinder J, Pierce R, et al. Evidence of a sleep-specific blunted cortical response to inspiratory occlusions in mild obstructive sleep apnea syndrome. Am J Respir Crit Care Med 2002; 166:1225–1234.
109. Huang J, Marcus CL, Melendres MC, et al. Cortical processing of respiratory afferent stimuli during sleep in children with the obstructive sleep apnea syndrome. Sleep 2007 (in press).
110. Katz ES, Marcus CL. Obstructive sleep apnea: children *versus* adults. In: Pack AI, ed. Sleep apnea: Pathogenesis, Diagnosis and Treatment. New York: Taylor & Francis, 2007.

21

Cognitive and Behavioral Consequences of Childhood OSAS

LOUISE M. O'BRIEN and RONALD D. CHERVIN
University of Michigan, Ann Arbor, Michigan, U.S.A.

I. Introduction

Cognitive deficits and behavioral problems are among the most common morbidities associated with obstructive sleep apnea syndrome (OSAS) in children. Reports of impaired intellectual function in children with adenotonsillar hypertrophy date back to 1889 when Hill reported on "some causes of backwardness and stupidity in children" (1). Interest in this area was renewed in the 1970s when the first detailed report of a small group of children with OSAS was published (2). Data also now suggest that some of the cognitive and behavioral deficits observed in children with OSAS may be reversible with treatment. This chapter will highlight current understanding of both behavior and cognition in childhood OSAS and examine evidence for and against OSAS as an important contributor to neurobehavioral problems.

II. Behavioral Regulation in Children with OSAS

Starting three decades ago, Guilleminault et al. (2–4) reported that inattention, hyperactivity, and aggression were all important comorbidities of OSAS. Since then, and especially in the last 10 years, considerable new research has been performed on these relationships. In children with typical symptoms of OSAS behavioral problems are consistently documented by parental report or objective testing (5–26). Most studies have provided evidence for robust associations between OSAS and hyperactivity/impulsivity, attention deficit, and other externalizing behaviors such as aggression, although the implication—that OSAS may cause these outcomes—has yet to be proven in a definitive manner. Table 1 summarizes results from many of the studies on OSAS and behavior.

A. Hyperactivity/Impulsivity

In children with OSAS, hyperactivity is probably the most commonly reported behavioral problem. Multiple studies have described hyperactive/impulsive behaviors in children with parentally reported symptoms of OSAS (5,6,12, 14,15,20,23,24,26), polysomnographically confirmed OSAS (8,13,17,18,22), and primary snoring (19,21,23). The majority of studies have used well-validated tools, such as the Conners' Parent Rating Scales (5,12,14,17,20,21,24,26,29), the Child Behavior Checklist (13,21,22,26,30), or the Behavioral Assessment Scale for Children (8,18,31) to assess behavioral morbidity. Furthermore, hyperactive behaviors have been reported to improve in children whose snoring had spontaneously ceased at one- or two-year follow-up (23,32) with no difference in behavior between ex-snorers and controls. However, neither of these latter studies was able to demonstrate the time sequence of snoring and the associated behaviors.

Several studies have also obtained behavioral information from teachers. However, teacher as opposed to parent rating scales are less consistently supportive of a relationship between OSAS and behavioral problems. Ali et al. (5) found that both hyperactivity and inattention scores were elevated on the Conners' teacher ratings in children with OSAS symptoms whereas externalizing behaviors defined as aggression, oppositionality, or conduct problems were not. However, another study by the same group a few years later did not find any teacher-reported differences between children with and without OSAS symptoms (33), and neither did Arman et al. (24) using the Conners' instrument. Another study (18) found that externalizing behaviors were elevated on the Behavioral Assessment Scale for Children, although hyperactivity was not, and findings regarding attention were somewhat inconsistent. Teacher report scales, while helpful, are also subject to recall bias, particularly if the teacher does not know the child well. The limited number of studies that have included teacher reports make it difficult to assess their value in children with OSAS. Larger studies are warranted before conclusions can be drawn about discrepancies between teacher and parent reports in children with OSAS.

B. Inattention

Attention is the ability to remain on task and appropriately respond to stimuli. It can be considered a building block for other more complex forms of cognitive activity and therefore plays an important role in development. Inattentive

Table 1 Summary of Reviewed Studies Regarding Sleep and Parental Report of Behavior

Author (references)	Sample	Parental report of behavior in OSAS
Ali et al. (5)	$n = 132$ (66 high risk for OSAS) from community	Increased hyperactivity, externalizing problems, inattention
Chervin et al. (6)	$n = 70$ from psychiatric clinics (27 ADHD); $n = 73$ from general pediatric clinics	ADHD more likely to snore; snoring associated with hyperactivity and inattention
Blunden et al. (27)	$n = 16$ ENT (for evaluation of snoring); $n = 16$ controls	No significant differences in behavior
Owens et al. (8)	$n = 18$ from sleep clinic with confirmed OSAS	Substantial proportion of scores in clinical range Mild OSAS most hyperactive and inattentive
Chervin and Archbold (10)	$n = 113$ suspected OSAS	No difference in OSAS and non-OSAS; hyperactivity associated with periodic limb movements only when OSAS present
Chervin et al. (12)	$n = 866$ from general pediatric clinics	Snoring associated with hyperactivity and inattention
Lewin et al. (13)	$n = 20$ OSAS from sleep clinic; $n = 10$ controls	Externalizing problems in mild OSAS
Chervin et al. (14)	$n = 872$ from general pediatric clinics	Threefold increase in aggressive behavior
Gottlieb et al. (15)	$n = 3019$ from the community	Twofold increase in hyperactivity, inattention, and aggression
Kaemingk et al. (16)	$n = 77$ OSAS; $n = 72$ controls	No differences in behavior
O'Brien et al. (17)	$n = 44$ ADHD; $n = 27$ mild ADHD; $n = 39$ controls	Fivefold increase in snoring in mild ADHD
Beebe et al. (18)	$n = 15$ OSAS, $n = 17$ primary snoring; $n = 17$ controls	Increased hyperactivity and attention, especially mild OSAS

(Continued)

Table 1 Summary of Reviewed Studies Regarding Sleep and Parental Report of Behavior (*Continued*)

Author (references)	Sample	Parental report of behavior in OSAS
Melendres et al. (20)	$n = 108$ from sleep clinic; $n = 72$ controls	Hyperactivity
O'Brien et al. (21)	$n = 87$ primary snoring; $n = 31$ controls all from community	Primary snoring more hyperactive
O'Brien et al. (28)	$n = 35$ OSAS with matched controls all from community	No differences in behavior
Rosen et al. (22)	$n = 829$ from community	Primary snoring and mild OSAS more externalizing problems, hyperactivity, and aggression.
Urschitz et al. (23)	$n = 1144$ from community	Snoring associated with hyperactivity and inattention
Arman et al. (24)	$n = 96$ habitual snoring; $n = 190$ controls all from community	Snoring associated with hyperactivity, inattention, conduct prob.
Blunden et al. (25)	$n = 20$ snorers; $n = 31$ controls	Externalizing problems
Mulvaney et al. (26)	$n = 403$ from community	High RDI, more inattention, and aggression but not hyperactivity

Abbreviations: ADHD, attention-deficit/hyperactivity disorder; ENT, ear, nose, throat conditions; OSAS, obstructive sleep apnea syndrome.

behaviors have been reported in habitually snoring children (12,21,24) and in those with documented OSAS (18,25,26,28), but less consistently than hyperactive/ impulsive behaviors. This may be due, in part, to the inability to discriminate between inattentive and impulsive behaviors by some validated measures, such as the Child Behavior Checklist. Objective measures of attention can also be used, often in the form of auditory or visual continuous performance tests (34–36). Such tests are able to differentiate different aspects of attention, such as selective or sustained attention. Children with OSAS, even when mild, show objective attention deficits when compared to healthy children (27,37,38).

C. Aggression

Aggressive behavior is a frequent component of conduct disorder, a condition estimated to affect approximately 2–9% of U.S. children (39). Aggressive behavior in childhood OSAS has not been studied as much as hyperactivity and inattention, but strong associations have been described between parentally reported symptoms of OSAS and aggressiveness (5,14,15). Each of these studies included a large number of children; in total, over 4600 parents responded to the questionnaires. Chervin et al. (14) surveyed parents of 872 children aged between 2 and 14 years at two general pediatric clinics with validated instruments, the pediatric sleep questionnaire (PSQ) (40), and the Conners' Parent Rating Scales (41). Children at high risk for sleep-disordered breathing (SDB) were found to be two to three times more likely to be bullying, constantly fighting, quarrelsome, and cruel, in comparison to other children, even after adjustment for comorbid hyperactivity or the use of stimulants. In addition, the SDB score and the conduct problem index showed a significant dose-dependent relationship. In another study, in-home polysomnograms in 403 school-age children showed that respiratory disturbance indices within the top 15% (mean index = 12.4 ± 8.8) were associated with higher Child Behavior Checklist scores for aggression, with a small-to-medium effect size of 0.35 (26). Aggressive behaviors in schools are highly prevalent and likely to arise from a number of social, environmental, and biological factors, but the extent to which undiagnosed and untreated OSAS may contribute remains unknown.

III. Evidence for a Relationship Between OSAS and ADHD

Attention-deficit/hyperactivity disorder (ADHD) is the most frequently encountered pediatric neurobehavioral disorder. Prevalence rates are difficult to ascertain, partly because of the changing diagnostic criteria over time and partly because of the differences in settings and samples from which data have been obtained (42). However, the prevalence of ADHD in community school-age populations is generally thought to be about 8–10% (42). Sleep disturbance was a criterion for the diagnosis of ADHD in previous editions of the Diagnostic and Statistical Manual of Mental Disorders (43). Interest in sleep of children with ADHD has renewed with the realization that core features of ADHD—inattention, hyperactivity, and impulsivity—are also frequently encountered in childhood OSAS.

A. Data from Parental Report

Parents of children with ADHD observe a variety of sleep-related problems (44–49), and in comparison to parents of children without ADHD, they report a five-fold increase in sleep disturbances (50). Snoring is common among children with ADHD, with about one-third snoring more than half the time, compared with only 9–11% of control children (6). LeBourgeios et al. (51) did not find that snoring was more common in children with ADHD than in children without ADHD, but did find that snoring was common among children with the hyperactive/impulsive subtype. These findings are in concordance with others that report associations between hyperactive/impulsive behaviors (even in the absence of ADHD) and symptoms of OSAS.

B. Objective Data

Early studies that recorded sleep among children with and without ADHD initially showed no consistent differences. However, two more recent studies that specifically tested for SDB found OSAS to be much more common in ADHD than in healthy controls (52,53). At least one study (54) did not confirm this finding, perhaps in part because the threshold used to define sleep apnea was higher than that used in the two other studies (55). Interestingly, the frequency of OSAS was found to be five times higher in children with mild hyperactivity than in those with more severe levels (17), leading some to speculate that OSAS may result in mild, subclinical forms of ADHD rather than the full spectrum of symptoms required to make the diagnosis. Remarkably few studies have used thorough, structured interviews by child psychiatrists to determine the frequency of ADHD in children with OSAS. One study that did use structured interviews found formal diagnoses of ADHD in 22 (28%) of 78 children scheduled for adenotonsillectomy because of clinical suspicion for OSAS (37).

In a meta-analysis of the literature to date, Sadeh et al. (56) suggested that factors, such as age, gender, inclusion of an adaptation night, and comorbidity may play moderating roles in a complex relationship between sleep and ADHD. A recent systematic review (57) excluded all studies without rigorous diagnostic evaluations, pooled data from objective sleep assessments, and concluded that children with ADHD have significantly higher apnea-hypopnea indices than controls, albeit in a range suggestive of mild OSAS. One speculative explanation for the findings of mild rather than severe OSAS in children with ADHD may be that severe OSAS is associated with sleepiness that could mask the hyperactive behaviors (55).

IV. Cognitive Deficits in Children with OSAS

Cognitive findings among children with OSAS are somewhat less clear than the behavioral manifestations. In his comprehensive review, Beebe (58) suggested that factors, such as prematurity, socioeconomic status, and the age of the child may each play an important role in a variable relationship between OSAS and cognition. For example, associations have been reported between OSAS and cognitive achievement deficits in children born prematurely, but the differences were attenuated when socioeconomic status was taken into account. After adjustment for covariates, no associations between OSAS and cognitive achievement were found for children born at term (59). Socioeconomic status is an important, although frequently omitted, variable in studies of OSAS and can have an important confounding influence on the relationship of sleep apnea to school performance (60). Conclusions of all correlative studies are limited by what potential confounders may not have considered, and studies of cognition and OSAS are no exception.

A. Intelligence

Standardized IQ scores are likely to be lower in children with either subjective or objective evidence of OSAS in comparison to controls (27,28,61–63). Some studies did not confirm full-scale IQ differences between these groups (13,16,59), but did report deficits in more specific domains, such as verbal IQ scale, in association with increasing levels of OSAS (13). The status of verbal abilities in OSAS remains somewhat unclear though. This may be due, in part, to differing measures of language abilities (e.g., expressive language, vocabulary, phonological processing) in the relevant studies. Interestingly, intelligence may also be reduced in children with habitual snoring in the absence of OSAS (1,19,27).

One challenge in this research is that while children with OSAS often have lower cognitive scores than controls, they often perform close to the mean, whereas control children perform above average (58). Recruitment bias could arise if volunteer control families, with little to gain personally from participation, in comparison to case families, are atypical and have overly intelligent children. This could artificially inflate scores and produce a group difference unrelated to OSAS. However, an alternative explanation is that OSAS could impair the cognitive function in highly performing children only to a point that their scores appear average. Thus, studies that search for only cognitive deficits per se may underestimate the scope and prevalence of OSAS morbidity.

Findings on cognitive abilities of children with and without OSAS may also be affected by the age of the subjects. Younger children may be more vulnerable to cognitive deficits. Most studies reporting an association between cognitive dysfunction and symptoms of OSAS were conducted in young children (preschool- or early-school-age). Even infants who snore but do not have OSAS perform worse on the Mental Development Index of the Bayley Scales of Infant Development (64,65). Older children tend to show weaker associations (16,18,59), possibly suggesting a window of vulnerability in the developing brain. This concept has some support from work in rodents (see below).

B. Memory

Studies on memory in childhood OSAS have yielded inconsistent results. Memory deficits have been reported (16,19,61), with Rhodes et al. (61) suggesting a dose-response relationship whereby children with more severe OSAS show greater memory disturbances. However, other studies have failed to find memory impairment even in large samples with variable degrees of OSAS severity (21,25,28). Differences in aspects of memory that were measured (e.g., declarative memory, verbal memory, or working memory) may have contributed to these discrepancies.

C. Executive Functioning

Executive functioning underlies the ability to plan, develop, and sustain an organized and flexible approach to problem solving. Executive functioning allows a child to inhibit actions and restrain or delay responses. This cognitive domain is crucial for normal psychological and social development (66). Such problem-solving processes are invoked when tasks are non-automatic and novel (67). Close relationships exist between executive functioning, attention, and working memory (68,69).

Deficits in executive functioning are reported commonly in adults with OSAS (70) and in children (13,18,25,28,62,71). Executive functioning may suffer in OSAS in a dose-dependent manner (13), with more severe OSAS related to worse measures particularly in verbal abilities. Among mild apneics in one study, sustained attention and vigilance were impaired but verbal ability was not (71). Executive functioning is complex and covers many abilities that may go some way to explaining the inconsistencies in findings, particularly since the isolation of executive functioning from other cognitive abilities is difficult. Deficits in executive functioning can alter recruitment of other cognitive abilities and give rise to problematic behaviors such as those observed in children with OSAS. The prefrontal cortex, which develops throughout childhood (72), has been implicated in executive dysfunction observed after sleep disruption (73–75).

D. School Performance

Poor school performance (23,60,76–79) and learning problems (63,80–82) can appear in children with OSAS symptoms. A six- to ninefold increase in sleep-associated gas exchange abnormalities was found among poorly performing first graders (76). Frequent snoring has shown an association with poor performance in mathematics and spelling (78). Habitual snorers in this latter study had twice the risk of poor school performance, and the association was stronger with increasing snoring frequency. This did not appear to be mediated by hypoxemia since the associations were not diminished after children with mild oxyhemoglobin desaturations were excluded. However, low socioeconomic status or associated increases in body mass index may account for deficits in academic performance observed in some studies (60).

Preliminary data using objective measures of OSAS severity suggested that in the absence of hypoxemia, a respiratory disturbance index >5 was associated with parent-reported learning problems in young children; if hypoxemia was used to define the respiratory event, learning problems were associated with a respiratory disturbance index >1 (82). Only one question was used to identify learning problems and some potential confounders such as socioeconomic status were not taken into account, but the results suggest that polysomnographic variables correspond with cognitive morbidity in OSAS. While hypoxemia may mediate some of the cognitive deficits observed in OSAS, it is also possible that attention problems may underlie learning difficulties or poor academic achievement. Blunden et al. (27) suggested that since learning is dependent on the ability to rehearse, encode, store, and retrieve information, impaired attention may render these processes inefficient and thus adversely impact performance. This may help to account for cognitive deficits that are observed in children with primary snoring in the absence of hypoxemia.

V. Moving Beyond Associations: Does OSAS Directly Cause or Contribute to Neurobehavioral Morbidity?

Despite the large number of investigations into the relationship between OSAS and neurobehavioral deficits, studies to date have not proven definitively that OSAS causes such deficits in large numbers of children. Conclusions are limited by lack of consistent definitions across studies, differences in populations that have been studied (e.g., clinical vs. community-based samples), and a dearth of longitudinal studies. Although virtually all published studies suggest some relationship between OSAS, behavior, and cognition, the question remains whether these associations represent a causal relationship. This question can only be answered in a definitive manner by randomized controlled intervention trials, which to this date have not been performed. Current data provide ample evidence for, but also some evidence against, the hypothesis that childhood OSAS causes or contributes to neurobehavioral deficits.

A. Evidence for a Causal Relationship

Data from cross-sectional studies, such as those we have reviewed, even when strong associations are found, cannot by themselves prove that a risk factor causes an outcome. Additional evidence accrues from several longitudinal studies that establish a consistent temporal relationship between snoring and behavioral problems (77,83). Some of the strongest longitudinal evidence to date to support the hypothesis that OSAS causes hyperactive behavior comes from a recent four-year prospective study in Michigan, U.S.A. (83). Snoring and other symptoms of OSAS were strong risk factors for the future development or exacerbation of hyperactive behavior, with habitual snoring at baseline increasing the risk for hyperactivity at follow-up by more than fourfold. These findings were particularly strong for boys under the age of eight years and were independent of hyperactivity at baseline and stimulant use at follow-up. The findings also remained similar after accounting for OSAS symptoms at follow-up, suggesting that damage done four years earlier may have been visible as a hyperactive phenotype only later in life. Consistent results emerged from a case-control study of seventh and eighth grade children with poor school performance: these children were more likely than others in their grades to have snored frequently and loudly during their early childhood (77). While these data still do not prove that OSAS induces behavioral problems, they do at least suggest that OSAS precedes hyperactivity.

Improvement of Behavior and Cognition with Treatment for OSAS

Evidence in favor of causality can be gained from intervention studies: if OSAS causes behavioral and cognitive deficits, then treatment of OSAS should result in improvement, to the extent that neurobehavioral deficits are reversible. A number of nonrandomized studies now have suggested that therapeutic surgical intervention, in the form of adenotonsillectomy, results in significant improvement in both behavior and cognition (33,37,38,76,84–87). In a small study of children before and after adenotonsillectomy, Ali et al. (33) showed that following surgery, children with OSAS experienced a significant reduction in aggression, inattention, and hyperactivity on the Conners' Parent Rating Scale and an improvement in vigilance on the Continuous Performance Test. A group of snoring children without OSAS also improved, showing less hyperactive behavior and better vigilance, while a control group of children who underwent unrelated surgical procedures did not exhibit any discernable change in behavior. While parental reports are subjective, objective measures of attention on a continuous performance task have also shown substantial improvement in two months in the postoperative period (86). Figure 1 depicts the effect sizes for changes in several cognitive measures after surgical intervention.

Friedman et al. (85) further reported that the sequential and simultaneous mental processing scales and the overall mental processing composite (as a measure of general intelligence) improved to control levels in children aged between five and nine years when studied again six to ten months after adenotonsillectomy, further supporting the contention that such deficits are in fact reversible. More recently, Chervin et al. (37) found 78 children scheduled to undergo adenotonsillectomy much more likely to be hyperactive than controls whereas no group differences retained significance one year after surgery. Additional evidence for reversibility comes from school grades of poorly performing children with OSAS (76). Children whose parents opted for

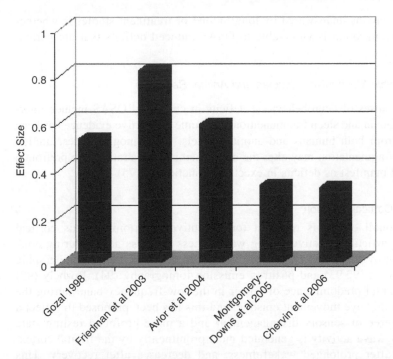

Figure 1   The impact of adenotonsillectomy on cognitive ability. The effect size was calculated for treatment studies from raw data given in the individual manuscripts. Gozal (76) reported improved school grades one year following adenotonsillectomy; Friedman et al. (85) reported increased mental processing composite score, as a proxy for total intelligence, from the Kaufman Assessment Battery for Children (88); Montgomery-Downs et al. (63) reported increased General Conceptual Ability, as a proxy for IQ, from the Differential Ability Scales (89); Avior et al. (86) and Chervin et al. (37) both found increases in cognitive attention using the Test of Variables of Attention (34) and the Integrated Visual and Auditory (90) continuous performance tests respectively.

surgical intervention showed significantly improved school grades one year later, while those whose parents pursued no treatment showed school grades that remained low. A limitation to these treatment studies is that the full potential of these children in the absence of any OSAS during their development remains unknown, and therefore the extent to which their deficits are fully reversible remains unclear. In preschool children from low-income families, not all the subtests of cognitive assessment improved following surgery for OSAS (63). Furthermore, some children with OSAS who do not meet the criteria for ADHD before adenotonsillectomy do meet these criteria one year later, again suggesting that damage to the brain earlier in life may only emerge as a visible phenotype later in life (37). A critical question that therefore remains unanswered by longitudinal or treatment studies is whether the developing brain is vulnerable to OSAS-induced deficits that are permanent (91).

Feasible Mechanisms: Human and Animal Research

Proposed causes of neurobehavioral deficits in childhood OSAS include intermittent hypoxia and sleep fragmentation, and some supportive evidence has been obtained from both humans and animal models. Oxyhemoglobin desaturation and sleep fragmentation may alter the neurochemical substrate of the prefrontal cortex and manifest as deficits in executive functioning (75).

Prefrontal Cortical Function

The prefrontal cortex is required for executive functioning. This cortical region is particularly active during wakefulness and less active during non–rapid eye movement sleep, as shown by quantitative electroencephalographic (EEG) studies (92,93) and positron emission tomography (94). Borbely (92) noted a frontal predominance of power in the low-frequency band during the first non–rapid eye movement episode, and this has been proposed to reflect a greater degree of sensory disengagement and a more profound resting state (95). Slow wave activity is generated most prominently by the frontal cortex, increases after prolonged wakefulness, and decreases after recovery. This provides additional evidence that the prefrontal cortex is sensitive to sleep deprivation. Furthermore, the hypoxia observed during sleep in OSAS is also associated with a persistent increase in slow EEG frequencies and with excessive sleepiness during the daytime, both of which improve with continuous positive airway pressure (96,97). Studies of children with OSAS show that breath-to-breath changes in slow wave EEG spectral power, in addition to power in other frequencies, may predict subsequent sleepiness and inattention (98). One speculation is that OSAS may impede homeostatic sleep drive dissipation that is dependent on uninterrupted slow wave activity. Such activity may be forced into other sleep and wake states, with a negative impact on daytime performance (98).

Dysfunction of the prefrontal cortex, particularly the dorsolateral region, is well recognized as a sequel to disrupted sleep (74,99,100). In a recent functional magnetic resonance imaging (fMRI) study, adults with OSAS performed worse on working memory tasks and had reduced activation within the prefrontal cortex compared with controls (101). However, changes in cerebral responses can be either reduced activation or increased activation depending on the task administered. For example, increased activation is observed during verbal learning tasks in fMRI studies after sleep deprivation (100,102), and fMRI studies in adults with OSAS support this finding (103). Increased activation is associated with better cognitive performance and is consistent with studies observing no impairment in short-term verbal memory in OSAS (70). Thus, it is possible that the lack of cognitive impairment in some adults with OSAS may be secondary to compensatory recruitment of other brain regions as reflected by increased activation in these areas (103).

No fMRI studies have been reported in children with OSAS. However, the prefrontal cortex is believed to play a critical role in the regulation of arousal, sleep, affect, and attention in children (73). Disturbances of prefrontal inhibitory functions have been implicated in deficits observed in children with ADHD (69,104), and fMRI studies in children with ADHD have supported specific impairments in prefrontal cortical functioning (105). Whether similar patterns of activation suggestive of compensatory recruitment also occur in children with OSAS remains unknown.

Other imaging techniques may also prove informative. Magnetic resonance imaging shows morphological changes in the frontal cortex, the parietal cortex, and the hippocampus, among other structures, in adults with OSAS (106,107). Proton magnetic resonance spectroscopy imaging in six children aged 9 to 16 years with severe OSAS and six similarly aged controls recently showed significant differences in the ratios of neuronal metabolites (*N*-acetyl aspartate/ choline) in the left hippocampus and the right frontal cortex (108). Together these data begin to provide neurochemical and neuroanatomical evidence of damage to the brain in areas that correspond to functional deficits observed in OSAS.

Sleep Fragmentation

Excessive daytime sleepiness induced by sleep fragmentation, such as that caused by multiple respiratory-related arousals from sleep, results in daytime performance deficits similar to those seen after sleep deprivation (109–111). Such findings are supported by animal models in which sleep deprivation and restriction impair hippocampal-dependent learning processes (112), and sleep fragmentation hampers spatial learning in rats (113).

Until recently, sleep architecture in childhood OSAS was often thought to be normal because discreet EEG arousals that are more obvious in adult OSAS were commonly absent. However, more sensitive techniques such as EEG signal analysis (114–116) and autonomic measures (117,118) show that normal sleep physiology is not preserved in children and that sleep fragmentation is associated with neurobehavioral outcomes (119,120). For example, in a study that used a novel computerized signal-processing algorithm, respiratory cycle-related EEG changes invisible to visual inspection diminished after adenotonsillectomy to an extent predictive of improvement in Multiple Sleep Latency Tests for daytime sleepiness (98). Interestingly, changes in auditory attention scores after surgery were correlated with changes in delta respiratory cycle-related EEG changes more robustly than with changes in apnea indices, again suggesting that measurement of nonvisually recognizable alterations in the EEG may have clinical implications. Indeed, data from fMRI studies have suggested that fragmented sleep may contribute to cognitive deficits more than hypoxia does (101).

Other Sleep Disorders Associated with Similar Behavioral Phenotypes.
Restless legs syndrome and periodic limb movements during sleep in children
are strongly associated with hyperactivity (10,11,121). A high prevalence of
ADHD has been found in children with periodic limb movements (122), and,
conversely, children with ADHD are more likely to have periodic limb movements during sleep (123,124). Children with ADHD also have an increased risk
for restless legs syndrome or a family history of this condition (122,124). One
possibility is that restless legs syndrome and periodic limb movements may
disrupt sleep and lead to symptoms similar to ADHD. Both restless legs syndrome and periodic limb movements respond to dopaminergic therapy. Interestingly, Walters et al. (121) found that dopaminergic therapy was associated
with improved behavior, with three of seven children with ADHD no longer
qualifying for a diagnosis of ADHD. As the mechanisms that link periodic limb
movements and behavioral problems have not been fully delineated, explan-
ations for the behavioral improvement could include restoration of consolidated
sleep or a common dopaminergic deficit shared by periodic limb movements and
ADHD.

Daytime behavioral problems also have been reported in children with
narcolepsy (125,126) and circadian rhythm disorders, such as delayed sleep
phase insomnia (127). In adolescents, developmental influences can produce a
delayed sleep phase–like profile with an inability to get out of bed, falling asleep
at school, and poor academic achievement. Many of these adolescents are
labeled as having behavioral problems, but if they are allowed to sleep until late
in the morning, their symptoms abate (128).

Inadequate sleep, secondary to poor sleep hygiene, can impair cognition
and performance. In their review, Wolfson and Carskadon (129) showed that
shortened sleep time and irregular sleep schedules are associated with poor
school performance in adolescents. In younger school-age children, Fallone et al.
(130) also found that sleep restriction had a direct effect on school performance
and attention even among children with no prior history of academic or
behavioral problems. Sleep disruption as measured by actigraphy is associated
with deficits in complex neurobehavioral tasks, such as selective attention in
otherwise healthy children (119). Sleep disruption outside the context of OSAS
is an often overlooked factor that can contribute to daytime deficits. A recent
review (131) concluded that sleep deprivation, sleep disruption, and intermittent
hypoxia independently may be sufficient to cause daytime neurobehavioral
effects in vulnerable children, and that the combination of two or more of these
factors may result in particular impairment of daytime functioning.

Moreover, treatment of sleep disorders other than OSAS may similarly
improve daytime behavior. The mechanism by which these disorders may contribute to behavioral manifestations is unknown, but a shared feature, such as
sleepiness, could play a role. Excessive daytime sleepiness is common in many
sleep disturbances at older ages but typically is not believed to be a common,

overt symptom of pediatric OSAS. However, recent work suggests that it may be more common and important than previously believed (20,116). Snoring and other symptoms of OSAS correlate with subjective daytime sleepiness in children (12). Polysomnographic measures of OSAS severity predict objective measures of sleepiness in children and improvement of those measures after adeno-tonsillectomy (116). Hyperactive children unselected for sleep complaints are sleepier than other children (52,132), and conversely experimental sleep restriction produces ADHD-like behaviors (133). Children who are sleepy—whether as a result of ADHD, OSAS, any other sleep disorder, or even poor sleep hygiene—may have strong drives to stay awake, to the extent that they develop hyperactive, stimulus-seeking behavior. Insufficient or inadequate sleep may, through the induction of sleepiness, impair executive functioning, regulation of impulsivity, and control of emotions (73).

Intermittent Hypoxia

Intermittent hypoxemia is associated with impaired cognitive function in adults (134,135) and has been implicated in the cognitive deficits observed in OSAS. Hypoxia is associated with neurobehavioral problems in children: for a comprehensive review see Bass et al. (136). Even mild desaturations can be associated with adverse effects (84). Nonetheless, hypoxia is unlikely to be the sole cause of neurobehavioral deficits observed in OSAS because children with primary snoring and other sleep disorders that involve no hypoxemia can show similar problems (21,23,25).

In young rodents, intermittent hypoxia during sleep, in the absence of significant sleep fragmentation, induces neuronal cell loss and impairs spatial memory (137). Developing rats may be uniquely vulnerable (138,139). Interestingly, the window of vulnerability in developing rats corresponds to a period of development in humans during early childhood, when the prevalence of OSAS is at its peak.

Intermittent hypoxia and sleep fragmentation in animals can trigger inflammatory responses and oxidative stress that seem to contribute to neurocognitive dysfunction, while antioxidants may be neuroprotective (140). Systemic markers of inflammation and oxidative stress are also present in humans with OSAS and may play a role in the pathogenesis of performances deficits (141–143). Moreover, interactions between environmental factors may modify susceptibility to the effects of intermittent hypoxia (140,144–146). Not all children with OSAS have clear neurobehavioral morbidity, which suggests that genetic variation may also play a role in individual susceptibility.

B. Evidence Against a Causal Relationship

Not all evidence implicates OSAS as a cause of neurobehavioral deficits. Several arguments against a causal relationship are discussed below.

Neurobehavioral Phenotype Is Not Consistent

While behavioral morbidities are typically found, not all studies have revealed the same problematic behaviors. For example, using the Conners' Parent Rating Scale, the hyperactivity index is elevated in many studies but not all, and similar findings are reported for externalizing behaviors as measured by the Child Behavior Checklist. Cognitive deficits in particular have implicated different domains in different studies of children with OSAS. Beeb has summarized this finding in a recent review (58). For example, verbal deficits have been reported in some studies (21,27,59), as well as visuospatial deficits (21,27,85), memory deficits (62,85), or attention and executive dysfunction (13,18,27,59,71).

Lack of Expected Relationships Between Objective Measures of OSAS and Behavior

Owens et al. (8) reported that some behavioral problems, including hyper-activity, were more common in children with mild OSAS compared to severe OSAS when assessed with the Conners' Rating Scale but not with the Behavioral Assessment Scale for Children. Such results may have occurred because the sample size was small, yet Lewin et al. (13) used the Child Behavior Checklist in a referred sample and found similar results. As mentioned above, a large community-based study found mild behavioral problems to be five times more closely associated with OSAS than were severe behavioral problems (17). In short, while a strong relationship between OSAS and hyperactive behavior is commonly reported, a dose-dependent relationship is not clearly evident.

Measures obtained from polysomnograms, such as the apnea/hypopnea index or oxyhemoglobin desaturation, generally do not correlate with neuro-behavioral outcomes. In a comparison of 77 children aged 6 to 12 years who had polysomnographic evidence of OSAS with 72 children without OSAS, an extensive battery of cognitive tests showed no differences between groups for most domains, and behavioral ratings showed no differences (16). In a study of 205 five-year-old children, OSAS symptoms predicted cognitive deficits even after children with polysomnographic evidence of OSAS were excluded (62). Among 113 children referred for suspected OSAS, many were found to have elevated hyperactivity scores but hyperactivity showed no association with the apnea/hypopnea index, extent of oxyhemoglobin desaturation, or minimal esophageal pressure (10). Instead, periodic limb movements during sleep more readily showed a relationship to hyperactivity. This suggests that other factors may play an important role in behavioral problems experienced by children with OSAS. Another possibility is that behavioral deficits seen at any given time point reflect permanent damage done years before by a disorder that has since resolved in many cases (83). If so, correlations between measures of OSAS and behavior or cognition might well be weak at any single time point. In another study, deficits in attention and executive function also appeared unrelated to poly-somnographic measures of OSAS, although some aspects of attention and executive function could be predicted by the proportion of slow wave sleep and parent-reported sleepiness (18). Parental report of snoring, rather than any objective variable, may show greater association with daytime deficits (18,20).

In short, if OSAS does cause behavioral morbidities, then the expected dose-response relationship with polysomnographic OSAS measures has been elusive, and some studies have suggested, in fact, that children with mild OSAS perform worse than those with severe OSAS (8,13,17). More sensitive measures of OSAS may be required to show associations with outcomes. Several newer approaches that may have potential include characterization of the cyclic alternating pattern (147), respiratory and nonrespiratory arousals (148), and respiratory cycle-related EEG changes (115).

OSAS Measures Do Not Predict Neurobehavioral Improvement After Treatment

Treatment of OSAS generally leads to improvement in behavior and cognition, yet baseline polysomnographic measures may not predict improvement. Chervin et al. (37) found that one year following adenotonsillectomy, behavior improved in a group of children with OSAS, but common laboratory measures of OSAS severity at enrollment did not predict neurobehavioral outcomes except for reduced sleepiness. Again, the lack of significant associations could reflect methodological limitations that newer approaches (115,147,148) may address in the future. The clinical predictive value of respiratory cycle-related EEG changes, thought to represent respiratory micro-arousals with each breath, appears promising (115,116,149).

Challenges of Developmental Context in Children

The relationship between sleep and behavior at any age is far from simple, and children bring an added dimension of complexity that arises from rapid developmental changes. Most pediatric OSAS studies have been conducted in prepubertal children when the tonsils are largest in size relative to the airway and the prevalence of OSAS peaks. This is also a time of intense brain development when any insult such as intermittent hypoxia or sleep fragmentation could have long-lasting impact. Conversely, adaptive or compensatory mechanisms may occur more easily at certain stages of brain development than at others. Taken together, these maturational changes and differences in age groups must remain suspect as factors that might explain inconsistencies, within and between different studies, in reported relationships between pediatric OSAS, behavior, and cognition.

VI. Summary and Future Directions

Relationships between OSAS, behavioral problems, and cognitive deficits are strong and clinically relevant. In particular, consistent cross-sectional and longitudinal evidence supports a relationship between OSAS and hyperactivity/impulsivity, attention deficit, and other externalizing behaviors. Considerable evidence, though perhaps less consistent, exists for cognitive deficits. An important consequence of cognitive ability and behavior—academic achievement—appears likely to be sensitive to OSAS. In addition, treatment of OSAS seems to result in improvements in both behavior and cognition. Nonetheless, the large majority of studies have been cross-sectional, and standard laboratory measures of OSAS have not shown close relationships with behavioral or cognitive outcomes. Although biologically plausible, from multiple perspectives, that OSAS could cause daytime neurobehavioral deficits, no randomized controlled clinical trials or other accumulated evidence have proven this hypothesis.

A.   How Clinicians Can Make Best Use of Current Data

OSAS is highly prevalent in children and probably remains undiagnosed in most cases (150). Clinicians should be aware that neurobehavioral problems are common morbidities in pediatric OSAS. Patients who have some of the most common neurobehavioral problems of childhood—including symptoms of ADHD, other externalizing behavior, or learning deficits—should be screened for symptoms of OSAS. If OSAS does contribute to neurobehavioral problems, the proportion of all hyperactive children who might stand to benefit from assessment and treatment of habitual snoring or any underlying OSAS remains unknown, but estimates have ranged from 15% to 25% (6,12). Despite proof at this time that treatment for OSAS improves neurobehavioral problems, accumulating evidence suggests that parents and physicians need to consider this possibility along with chronic medication or other approaches otherwise used to control these conditions.

B.   What Remains as Research Priorities in This Area

Randomized controlled treatment trials are needed to confirm suspected causal relationships between OSAS and neurobehavioral problems. Studies from infancy through childhood to adulthood will be needed to understand relationships that may vary prominently with age or express their consequences only years later. The roles of other risk factors such as socioeconomic status, race, and obesity need to be further investigated. Additional research also must focus on the development of new objective measures of OSAS that provide maximal clinical predictive value at the lowest cost and most widespread availability. Translational research should remain a priority to better define the neural substrates and biological mechanisms that explain cognitive and behavioral deficits in OSAS. Large epidemiological studies of OSAS have been performed on adults but are needed in children to define the prevalence of OSAS, the levels that raise concern for neurobehavioral and other morbidity, and the findings necessary to define a treatable condition. The relationship between OSAS and neurobehavioral morbidity could have substantial public health impact and offers a critical opportunity to improve the health of many children for years to come.

References

1. Hill W. On some causes of backwardness and stupidity in children: and the relief of the symptoms in some instances by nasopharyngeal scarifications. BMJ 1889; 2:711–712.
2. Guilleminault C, Eldridge FL, Simmons FB, et al. Sleep apnea in eight children. Pediatrics 1976; 58:23–31.
3. Guilleminault C, Korobkin R, Winkle R. A review of 50 children with obstructive sleep apnea syndrome. Lung 1981; 159:275–287.
4. Guilleminault C, Winkle R, Korobkin R, et al. Children and nocturnal snoring—evaluation of the effects of sleep related respiratory resistive load and daytime functioning. Eur J Pediatr 1982; 139:165–171.
5. Ali NJ, Pitson D, Stradling JR. Snoring, sleep disturbance and behaviour in 4-5 year olds. Arch Dis Child 1993; 68:360–366.
6. Chervin R, Dillon J, Bassetti C, et al. Symptoms of sleep disorders, inattention, and hyperactivity in children. Sleep 1997; 20:1185–1192.
7. Owens J, Opipari L, Nobile C, et al. Sleep and daytime behavior in children with obstructive sleep apnea and behavioral sleep disorders. Pediatrics 1998; 102: 1178–1184.
8. Owens J, Spirito A, Marcotte A, et al. Neuropsychological and behavioral correlates of obstructive sleep apnea syndrome in children: a preliminary study. Sleep Breath 2000; 4(2):67–78.
9. Blunden S, Lushington K, Kennedy D. Cognitive and behavioural performance in children with sleep-related obstructive breathing disorders. Sleep Med Rev 2001; 5(6):447–461.
10. Chervin RD, Archbold KH. Hyperactivity and polysomnographic findings in children evaluated for sleep-disordered breathing. Sleep 2001; 24(3):313–320.
11. Chervin RD, Archbold KH, Dillon JE, et al. Associations between symptoms of inattention, hyperactivity, restless legs, and periodic leg movements. Sleep 2002; 25(2):213–218.
12. Chervin RD, Archbold KH, Dillon JE, et al. Inattention, hyperactivity, and symptoms of sleep-disordered breathing. Pediatrics 2002; 109(3):449–456.
13. Lewin DS, Rosen RC, England SJ, et al. Preliminary evidence of behavioral and cognitive sequelae of obstructive sleep apnea in children. Sleep Med 2002; 3(1): 5–13.
14. Chervin RD, Dillon JE, Archbold KH, et al. Conduct problems and symptoms of sleep disorders in children. J Am Acad Child Adolesc Psychiatry 2003; 42(2): 201–208.
15. Gottlieb DJ, Vezina RM, Chase C, et al. Symptoms of sleep-disordered breathing in 5-year-old children are associated with sleepiness and problem behaviors. Pediatrics 2003; 112(4):870–877.
16. Kaemingk KL, Pasvogel AE, Goodwin JL, et al. Learning in children and sleep disordered breathing: findings of the Tucson Children's Assessment of Sleep Apnea (tuCASA) prospective cohort study. J Int Neuropsychol Soc 2003; 9(7): 1016–1026.
17. O'Brien LM, Holbrook CR, Mervis CB, et al. Sleep and neurobehavioral characteristics in 5–7 year old children with parentally reported symptoms of ADHD. Pediatrics 2003; 111:554–563.

18. Beebe DW, Wells CT, Jeffries J, et al. Neuropsychological effects of pediatric obstructive sleep apnea. J Int Neuropsychol Soc 2004; 10(7):962–975.

19. Kennedy JD, Blunden S, Hirte C, et al. Reduced neurocognition in children who snore. Pediatr Pulmonol 2004; 37(4):330–337.

20. Melendres MC, Lutz JM, Rubin ED, et al. Daytime sleepiness and hyperactivity in children with suspected sleep-disordered breathing. Pediatrics 2004; 114(3):768–775.

21. O'Brien LM, Mervis CB, Holbrook CR, et al. Neurobehavioral implications of habitual snoring in children. Pediatrics 2004; 114:44–49.

22. Rosen CL, Storfer-Isser A, Taylor HG, et al. Increased behavioral morbidity in school-aged children with sleep-disordered breathing. Pediatrics 2004; 114 (6):1640–1648.

23. Urschitz MS, Eitner S, Guenther A, et al. Habitual snoring, intermittent hypoxia, and impaired behavior in primary school children. Pediatrics 2004; 114(4): 1041–1048.

24. Arman AR, Ersu R, Save D, et al. Symptoms of inattention and hyperactivity in children with habitual snoring: evidence from a community-based study in Istanbul. Child Care Health Dev 2005; 31(6):707–717.

25. Blunden S, Lushington K, Lorenzen B, et al. Neuropsychological and psychosocial function in children with a history of snoring or behavioral sleep problems. J Pediatr 2005; 146(6):780–786.

26. Mulvaney SA, Goodwin JL, Morgan WJ, et al. Behavior problems associated with sleep disordered breathing in school-aged children—the Tucson children's assessment of sleep apnea study. J Pediatr Psychol 2006; 31(3):322–330.

27. Blunden S, Lushington K, Kennedy D, et al. Behavior and neurocognitive performance in children aged 5–10 years who snore compared to controls. J Clin Exp Neuropsychol 2000; 22(5):554–568.

28. O'Brien LM, Mervis CB, Holbrook CR, et al. Neurobehavioral correlates of OSA in children. J Sleep Res 2004; 13:165–172.

29. Conners CK. Conners' Rating Scales-Revised: Technical Manual, North Tonawanda, NY: Multi-Health Systems Publishing, 1997.

30. Achenbach TM. Manual for the Revised Child Behavior Checklist. Burlington, VT: University of Vermont, Department of Psychiatry, 1991.

31. Reynolds CR, Kamphaus RW. BASC—Behavioral Assessment System for Children Manual. Circle Pines, MN: American Guidance Service Publishing, 1992.

32. Ali NJ, Pitson D, Stradling JR. Natural history of snoring and related behaviour problems between the ages of 4 and 7 years. Arch Dis Child 1994; 71(1):74–76.

33. Ali NJ, Pitson D, Stradling JR. Sleep disordered breathing: effects of adenotonsillectomy on behaviour and psychological functioning. Eur J Pediatr 1996; 155 (1):56–62.

34. Greenberg LM. Tests of Variables of Attention Interpretation Manual. Minneapolis: Lawrence M. Greenberg, 1991.

35. Keith RW. Auditory Continuous Performance Test (ACPT). San Antonio, TX: The Psychological Corporation, 1994.

36. Conners CK. Conners' Continuous Performance Test II. Technical guide and software manual. Toronto, ON, Canada: Multi-Health Systems Inc., 2000.

37. Chervin RD, Ruzicka DL, Giordani BJ, et al. Sleep-disordered breathing, behavior, and cognition in children before and after adenotonsillectomy. Pediatrics 2006; 117 (4):e769–e778.

38. Galland BC, Dawes PJ, Tripp EG, et al. Changes in behavior and attentional capacity after adenotonsillectomy. Pediatr Res 2006; 59(5):711–716.
39. Costello EJ. Child psychiatric epidemiology: implications for clinical research and practice. In: Lahey BB, Kazdin AE, eds. Advances in Clinical Child Psychology. Vol 13. New York: Plenum Press, 1990:53–90.
40. Chervin RD, Hedger K, Dillon JE, et al. Pediatric sleep questionnaire (PSQ): validity and reliability of scales for sleep-disordered breathing, snoring, sleepiness, and behavioral problems. Sleep Med 2000; 1(1):21–32.
41. Conners CK, Barkley RA. Rating scales and checklists for child psychopharmacology. Psychopharmacol Bull 1985; 21:809–868.
42. American academy of pediatrics, committee on quality improvement and subcommittee on attention-deficit/hyperactivity disorder diagnosis and evaluation of the child with attention-deficit/hyperactivity disorder. Pediatrics 2000; 105:1158–1170.
43. American Psychiatric Association. Diagnostic and Statistical Manual of Mental Disorders. 3rd ed. Washington, D.C.: American Psychiatric Association, 1980.
44. Marcotte AC, Thacher PV, Butters M, et al. Parental report of sleep problems in children with attentional and learning disorders. J Dev Behav Pediatr 1998; 19(3): 178–186.
45. Ring A, Stein D, Barak Y, et al. Sleep disturbances in children with attention-deficit/hyperactivity disorder: a comparative study with healthy siblings. J Learn Disabil 1998; 31(6):572–578.
46. Corkum P, Moldofsky H, Hogg-Johnson S, et al. Sleep problems in children with attention-deficit/hyperactivity disorder: impact of subtype, comorbidity, and stimulant medication. J Am Acad Child Adolesc Psychiatry 1999; 38(10):1285–1293.
47. Mick E, Biederman J, Jetton J, et al. Sleep disturbances associated with attention deficit hyperactivity disorder: the impact of psychiatric comorbidity and pharmacotherapy. J Child Adolesc Psychopharmacol 2000l; 10(3):223–231.
48. Owens JA, Maxim R, Nobile C, et al. Parental and self-report of sleep in children with attention-deficit/hyperactivity disorder. Arch Pediatr Adolesc Med 2000; 154 (6):549–555.
49. Corkum P, Tannock R, Moldofsky H, et al. Actigraphy and parental ratings of sleep in children with attention-deficit/hyperactivity disorder (ADHD). Sleep 2001; 24 (3):303–312.
50. Corkum P, Tannock R, Moldofsky H. Sleep disturbances in children with attention-deficit/hyperactivity disorder. J Am Acad Child Adolesc Psychiatry 1998; 37 (6):637–646.
51. LeBourgeios MK, Avis K, Mixon M, et al. Snoring, sleep quality, and sleepiness across attention-deficit/hyperactivity disorder subtypes. Sleep 2004; 27(3):520–525.
52. Golan N, Shahar E, Ravid S, et al. Sleep disorders and daytime sleepiness in children with attention-deficit/hyperactive disorder. Sleep 2004; 27(2):261–266.
53. Huang YS, Chen NH, Li HY, et al. Sleep disorders in Taiwanese children with attention deficit/hyperactivity disorder. J Sleep Res 2004; 13(3):269–277.
54. Sangal RB, Owens JA, Sangal J. Patients with attention-deficit/hyperactivity disorder without observed apneic episodes in sleep or daytime sleepiness have normal sleep on polysomnography. Sleep 2005; 28(9):1143–1148.
55. Chervin RD. How many children with ADHD have sleep apnea or periodic limb movements on polysomnography? Sleep 2005; 28(9):1041–1042.

56. Sadeh A, Pergamin L, Bar-Haim Y. Sleep in children with attention-deficit hyperactivity disorder: a meta-analysis of polysomnographic studies. Sleep Med Rev 2006; 10(6):381–398.

57. Cortese S, Konofal E, Yateman N, et al. Sleep and alertness in children with attention-deficit/hyperactivity disorder: a systematic review of the literature. Sleep 2006; 29(4):504–511.

58. Beebe DW. Neurobehavioral morbidity associated with disordered breathing during sleep in children: a comprehensive review. Sleep 2006; 29(9):1115–1134.

59. Emancipator JL, Storfer-Isser A, Taylor HG, et al. Variation of cognition and achievement with sleep-disordered breathing in full-term and preterm children. Arch Pediatr Adolesc Med 2006; 160(2):203–210.

60. Chervin RD, Clarke DF, Huffman JL, et al. School performance, race, and other correlates of sleep-disordered breathing in children. Sleep Med 2003; 4(1):21–27.

61. Rhodes SK, Shimoda KC, Waid LR, et al. Neurocognitive deficits in morbidly obese children with obstructive sleep apnea. J Pediatr 1995; 127(5):741–744.

62. Gottlieb DJ, Chase C, Vezina RM, et al. Sleep-disordered breathing symptoms are associated with poorer cognitive function in 5-year-old children. J Pediatr 2004; 145(4):458–464.

63. Montgomery-Downs HE, Crabtree VM, Gozal D. Cognition, sleep and respiration in at-risk children treated for obstructive sleep apnoea. Eur Respir J 2005; 25 (2):336–342.

64. Bayley N. Bayley Scales of Infant Development. San Antonio, TX: Psychological Corporation, 1993.

65. Montgomery-Downs HE, Gozal D. Snore-associated sleep fragmentation in infancy: mental development effects and contribution of secondhand cigarette smoke exposure. Pediatrics 2006; 117(3):e496–e502.

66. Lezak M. Neuropsychological assessment. New York: Oxford University Press, 1995.

67. Hayes SC, Gifford EY, Ruckstuhl LE Jr. Relational frame theory and executive function: a behavioral approach. In: Lyon GR, Krasnegor NA, eds. Attention, Memory, and Executive Function. Baltimore, MD: Paul H Brookes, 1996:279–305.

68. Eslinger PJ. Conceptualizing, describing, and measuring components of executive function: a summary. In: Lyon GR, Krasnegor NA, eds. Attention, Memory, and Executive Function. Baltimore, Maryland: Paul H Brookes, 1996:367–395.

69. Barkley RA. Behavioral inhibition, sustained attention, and executive functions: constructing a unifying theory of ADHD. Psychol Bull 1997; 121(1):65–94.

70. Beebe DW, Groesz L, Wells C, et al. The neuropsychological effects of obstructive sleep apnea: a meta-analysis of norm-referenced and case-controlled data. Sleep 2003; 26(3):298–307.

71. Archbold KH, Giordani B, Ruzicka DL, et al. Cognitive executive dysfunction in children with mild sleep-disordered breathing. Biol Res Nurs 2004; 5(3):168–176.

72. Welsh MC, Pennington BF. Assessing frontal lobe functioning in children: views from developmental psychology. Dev Neuropsychol 1988; 4:199–230.

73. Dahl RE. The impact of inadequate sleep on children's daytime cognitive function. Semin Pediatr Neurol 1996; 3(1):44–50.

74. Harrison Y, Horne JA. Sleep loss impairs short and novel language tasks having a prefrontal focus. J Sleep Res 1998; 7(2):95–100.

75. Beebe DW, Gozal D. Obstructive sleep apnea and the prefrontal cortex: towards a comprehensive model linking nocturnal upper airway obstruction to daytime cognitive and behavioral deficits. J Sleep Res 2002; 11(1):1–16.
76. Gozal D. Sleep-disordered breathing and school performance in children. Pediatrics 1998; 102:616–620.
77. Gozal D, Pope Jr. DW. Snoring during early childhood and academic performance at ages 13–14 years. Pediatrics 2001; 107:1394–1399.
78. Urschitz MS, Guenther A, Eggebrecht E, et al. Snoring, intermittent hypoxia and academic performance in primary school children. Am J Respir Crit Care Med 2003; 168(4):464–468.
79. Urschitz MS, Wolff J, Sokollik C, et al. Nocturnal arterial oxygen saturation and academic performance in a community sample of children. Pediatrics 2005; 115(2): e204–e209.
80. Weissbluth M, Davis AT, Poncher J, et al. Signs of airway obstruction during sleep and behavioral, developmental, and academic problems. J Dev Behav Pediatr 1983; 4(2):119–121.
81. Goodwin JL, Babar SI, Kaemingk KL, et al. Symptoms related to sleep-disordered breathing in white and Hispanic children: the Tucson Children's Assessment of Sleep Apnea Study. Chest 2003; 124(1):196–203.
82. Goodwin JL, Kaemingk KL, Fregosi RF, et al. Clinical outcomes associated with sleep-disordered breathing in Caucasian and Hispanic children—the Tucson Children's Assessment of Sleep Apnea Study (TuCASA). Sleep 2003; 26(5): 587–591.
83. Chervin RD, Ruzicka DL, Archbold KH, et al. Snoring predicts hyperactivity four years later. Sleep 2005; 28(7):885–890.
84. Stradling JR, Thomas G, Warley ARH, et al. Effect of adenotonsillectomy on nocturnal hypoxaemia, sleep disturbance, and symptoms in snoring children. Lancet 1990; 335:249–253.
85. Friedman BC, Hendeles-Amitai A, Kozminsky E, et al. Adenotonsillectomy improves neurocognitive function in children with obstructive sleep apnea syndrome. Sleep 2003; 26(8):999–1005.
86. Avior G, Fishman G, Leor A, et al. The effect of tonsillectomy and adenoidectomy on inattention and impulsivity as measured by the Test of Variables of Attention (TOVA) in children with obstructive sleep apnea syndrome. Otolaryngol Head Neck Surg 2004; 131(4):367–371.
87. Roemmich JN, Barkley JE, D'Andrea L, et al. Increases in overweight after adenotonsillectomy in overweight children with obstructive sleep-disordered breathing are associated with decreases in motor activity and hyperactivity. Pediatrics 2006; 117(2):e200–e208.
88. Kaufman SA, Kaufman NL. Kaufman Assessment Battery for Children—Israeli Version. Interpretive Manual. Jerusalem: Ministry of Education, Culture and Sports, 1996.
89. Elliott CD. Differential Ability Scales: Introductory and Technical Handbook. San Antonio, TX: The Psychological Corporation, Harcourt Brace Jovanovich, Inc., 1983.
90. Sandford JA, Turner A. Manual for the Integrated Visual and Auditory Continuous Performance Test. Richmond, VA: Braintrain, 1995.

91. Halbower AC, Mahone EM. Neuropsychological morbidity linked to childhood sleep-disordered breathing. Sleep Med Rev 2006; 10(2):97–107.

92. Borbely AA. From slow waves to sleep homeostasis: new perspectives. Arch Ital Biol 2001; 139(1–2):53–61.

93. Finelli LA, Borbely AA, Achermann P. Functional topography of the human nonREM sleep electroencephalogram. Eur J Neurosci 2001; 13(12):2282–2290.

94. Nofzinger EA, Price JC, Meltzer CC, et al. Towards a neurobiology of dysfunctional arousal in depression: the relationship between beta EEG power and regional cerebral glucose metabolism during NREM sleep. Psychiatry Res 2000; 98(2): 71–91.

95. Horne JA. Human sleep, sleep loss and behaviour. Implications for the prefrontal cortex and psychiatric disorder. Br J Psychiatry 1993; 162:413–419.

96. Chervin RD, Aldrich MS. Characteristics of apneas and hypopneas during sleep and relation to excessive daytime sleepiness. Sleep 1998; 21(8):799–806.

97. Morisson F, Decary A, Petit D, et al. Daytime sleepiness and EEG spectral analysis in apneic patients before and after treatment with continuous positive airway pressure. Chest 2001; 119(1):45–52.

98. Chervin RD, Burns JW, Subotic NS, et al. Correlates of respiratory cycle-related EEG changes in children with sleep-disordered breathing. Sleep 2004; 27(1): 116–121.

99. Harrison Y, Horne JA. The impact of sleep deprivation on decision making: a review. J Exp Psychol Appl 2000; 6(3):236–249.

100. Drummond SP, Brown GG, Gillin JC, et al. Altered brain response to verbal learning following sleep deprivation. Nature 2000; 403(6770):655–657.

101. Thomas RJ, Rosen BR, Stern CE, et al. Functional imaging of working memory in obstructive sleep-disordered breathing. J Appl Physiol 2005; 98(6):2226–2234.

102. Drummond SP, Meloy MJ, Yanagi MA, et al. Compensatory recruitment after sleep deprivation and the relationship with performance. Psychiatry Res 2005; 140 (3):211–223.

103. Ayalon L, Ancoli-Israel S, Klemfuss Z, et al. Increased brain activiation during verbal learning in obstructive sleep apnea. Neuroimage 2006; 31(4):1817–1825.

104. Chelune GJ, Ferguson W, Koon R, et al. Frontal lobe disinhibition in attention deficit disorder. Child Psychiatry Hum Dev 1986; 16(4):221–234.

105. Rubia K, Overmeyer S, Taylor E, et al. Hypofrontality in attention deficit hyperactivity disorder during higher-order motor control: a study with functional MRI. Am J Psychiatry 1999; 156:891–896.

106. Macey PM, Henderson LA, Macey KE, et al. Brain morphology associated with obstructive sleep apnea. Am J Respir Crit Care Med 2002; 166(10):1382–1387.

107. Morrell MJ, McRobbie DW, Quest RA, et al. Changes in brain morphology associated with obstructive sleep apnea. Sleep Med 2003; 4(5):451–454.

108. Halbower AC, Degaonkar M, Barker PB, et al. Childhood obstructive sleep apnea associates with neuropsychological deficits and neuronal brain injury. PLoS Med 2006; 3(8):e301–e311.

109. Stepanski EJ, Lamphere P, Badia P. Sleep fragmentation and daytime sleepiness. Sleep 1984; 7:18–26.

110. Stepanski EJ, Lamphere J, Roehrs T. Experimental sleep fragmentation in normal subjects. Int J Neurosci 1987; 33:207–214.

111. Martin SE, Engleman HM, Deary IJ, et al. The effect of sleep fragmentation on daytime function. Am J Respir Crit Care Med 1996; 153(4 pt 1):1328–1332.

112. Hairston IS, Little MT, Scanlon MD, et al. Sleep restriction suppresses neurogenesis induced by hippocampus-dependent learning. J Neurophysiol 2005; 94(6): 4224–4233.

113. Tartar JL, Ward CP, McKenna JT, et al. Hippocampal synaptic plasticity and spatial learning are impaired in a rat model of sleep fragmentation. Eur J Neurosci 2006; 23(10):2739–2748.

114. Bandla HP, Gozal D. Dynamic changes in EEG spectra during obstructive apnea in children. Pediatr Pulmonol 2000; 29(5):359–365.

115. Chervin RD, Burns JW, Subotic NS, et al. Method for detection of respiratory cycle-related EEG changes in sleep-disordered breathing. Sleep 2004; 27(1): 110–115.

116. Chervin RD, Weatherly RA, Ruzicka DL, et al. Subjective sleepiness and polysomnographic correlates in children scheduled for adenotonsillectomy vs other surgical care. Sleep 2006; 29(4):495–503.

117. Tauman R, O'Brien LM, Mast BT, et al. Peripheral arterial tonometry events and electroencephalographic arousals in children. Sleep 2004; 27(3):502–506.

118. O'Brien LM, Gozal D. Potential usefulness of non-invasive autonomic monitoring in recognition of arousals in normal healthy children. J Clin Sleep Med 2007; 15; 3 (1):41–47.

119. Sadeh A, Gruber R, Raviv A. Sleep, neurobehavioral functioning, and behavior problems in school-age children. Child Dev 2002; 73:405–417.

120. O'Brien LM, Tauman R, Gozal D. Sleep pressure correlates of cognitive and behavioral morbidity in snoring children. Sleep 2004; 27:279–282.

121. Walters AS, Mandelbaum DE, Lewin DS, et al. Dopaminergic therapy in children with restless legs/periodic limb movements in sleep and ADHD. Dopaminergic Therapy Study Group. Pediatr Neurol 2000; 22(3):182–186.

122. Picchietti DL, Walters AS. Moderate to severe periodic limb movement disorder in childhood and adolescence. Sleep 1999; 22(3):297–300.

123. Picchietti DL, England SJ, Walters AS, et al. Periodic limb movement disorder and restless legs syndrome in children with attention-deficit hyperactivity disorder. J Child Neurol 1998; 13(12):588–594.

124. Picchietti DL, Underwood DJ, Farris WA, et al. Further studies on periodic limb movement disorder and restless legs syndrome in children with attention-deficit hyperactivity disorder. Mov Disord 1999; 14(6):1000–1007.

125. Dahl RE, Holttum J, Trubnick L. A clinical picture of child and adolescent narcolepsy. J Am Acad Child Adolesc Psychiatry 1994; 33(6):834–841.

126. Guilleminault C, Pelayo R. Narcolepsy in prepubertal children. Ann Neurol 1998; 43(1):135–142.

127. Dahl RE, Pelham WE, Wierson M. The role of sleep disturbances in attention deficit disorder symptoms: a case study. J Pediatr Psychol 1991; 16(2):229–239.

128. Millman RP. Working Group on Sleepiness in Adolescents/Young Adults; AAP Committee on Adolescence. Excessive sleepiness in adolescents and young adults: causes, consequences, and treatment strategies. Pediatrics 2005; 115(6):1774–1786.

129. Wolfson AR, Carskadon MA. Understanding adolescents' sleep patterns and school performance: a critical appraisal. Sleep Med Rev 2003; 7(6):491–506.
130. Fallone G, Acebo C, Seifer R, et al. Experimental restriction of sleep opportunity in children: effects on teacher ratings. Sleep 2005; 28(12):1561–1567.
131. Blunden SL, Beebe DW. The contribution of intermittent hypoxia, sleep debt and sleep disruption to daytime performance deficits in children: consideration of respiratory and non-respiratory sleep disorders. Sleep Med Rev 2006; 10(2):109–118.
132. Lecendreux M, Konofal E, Bouvard M, et al. Sleep and alertness in children with ADHD. J Child Psychol Psychiatry 2000; 41(6):803–812.
133. Fallone G, Acebo C, Arnedt JT, et al. Effects of acute sleep restriction on behavior, sustained attention, and response inhibition in children. Percept Mot Skills 2001; 93 (1):213–229.
134. Findley LJ, Barth JT, Powers DC, et al. Cognitive impairment in patients with obstructive sleep apnea and associated hypoxemia. Chest 1986; 90(5):686–690.
135. Naegele B, Thouvard V, Pepin JL, et al. Deficits of cognitive executive functions in patients with sleep apnea syndrome. Sleep 1995; 18:43–52.
136. Bass JL, Corwin M, Gozal D, et al. The effect of chronic or intermittent hypoxia on cognition in childhood: a review of the evidence. Pediatrics 2004; 114(3):805–816.
137. Gozal D, Daniel JM, Dohanich GP. Behavioral and anatomical correlates of chronic episodic hypoxia during sleep in the rat. J Neurosci 2001; 21:2442–2450.
138. Gozal E, Row BW, Schurr A, et al. Developmental differences in cortical and hippocampal vulnerability to intermittent hypoxia in the rat. Neurosci Lett 2001; 305:197–201.
139. Row BW, Kheirandish L, Neville JJ, et al. Impaired spatial learning and hyperactivity in developing rats exposed to intermittent hypoxia. Pediatr Res 2002; 52:449–453.
140. Row BW, Liu R, Xu W, et al. Intermittent hypoxia is associated with oxidative stress and spatial learning deficits in the rat. Am J Respir Crit Care Med 2003; 167 (11):1548–1553.
141. Shamsuzzaman AS, Winnicki M, Lanfranchi P, et al. Elevated C-reactive protein in patients with obstructive sleep apnea. Circulation 2002; 105(21):2462–2464.
142. Lavie L. Obstructive sleep apnoea syndrome—an oxidative stress disorder. Sleep Med Rev 2003; 7(1):35–51.
143. Tauman R, Ivanenko A, O'Brien LM, et al. Plasma C-reactive protein in children with sleep-disordered breathing. Pediatrics 2004; 113:e564–e569.
144. Yehuda S, Rabinovitz S, Mostofsky DI. Mediation of cognitive function by high fat diet following stress and inflammation. Nutr Neurosci 2005; 8(5–6):309–315.
145. Goldbart AD, Row BW, Kheirandish-Gozal L, et al. High fat/refined carbohydrate diet enhances the susceptibility to spatial learning deficits in rats exposed to intermittent hypoxia. Brain Res 2006; 1090(1):190–196.
146. Gozal D, Kheirandish L. Oxidant stress and inflammation in the snoring child: confluent pathways to upper airway pathogenesis and end-organ morbidity. Sleep Med Rev 2006; 10(2):83–96.
147. Bruni O, Ferri R, Miano S, et al. Sleep cyclic alternating pattern in normal school-age children. Clin Neurophysiol 2002; 113(11):1806–1814.

148. Tauman R, O'Brien LM, Holbrook CR, et al. Sleep pressure score: a new index of sleep disruption in snoring children. Sleep 2004; 27:274–278.
149. Chervin RD, Burns JW, Ruzicka DL. Electroencephalographic changes during respiratory cycles predict sleepiness in sleep apnea. Am J Respir Crit Care Med 2005; 171(6):652–658.
150. Chervin RD, Archbold KH, Panahi P, et al. Sleep problems seldom addressed at two general pediatric clinics. Pediatrics 2001; 107(6):1375–1380.

22

Inflammatory Association with Childhood Obstructive Sleep Apnea Syndrome

RAOUF AMIN
University of Cincinnati, Cincinnati, Ohio, U.S.A.

I. Introduction

In 1877, W.H. Broadbent, a British physician, provided one of the earliest descriptions of obstructive sleep apnea syndrome (OSAS) (1) in the journal *Lancet*. He characterized the condition as failure of inspiration to overcome the resistance in the pharynx leading to snoring and periods of perfect silence during several respiratory periods. It was not until the mid to late 1900s that the high prevalence of this condition in children and adults was recognized by the medical community. The mounting knowledge of OSAS and of its pathogenesis evolved over time as we began learning about the association of the disorder with serious adverse health outcomes. Significant progress has been made over the last two decades in our understanding of the mechanisms mediating adverse health outcomes due to OSAS. Such progress was supported by the technological advances in the study of sleep, in the continuous monitoring of ventilatory parameters, and finally in the revolution in molecular techniques. Specifically, these advances supported the investigation of the inflammatory and metabolic disease mechanisms in children and adults with OSAS.

The link between inflammation and OSAS has been addressed in multiple studies, which have implicated local and systemic inflammation in the pathophysiology of the seemingly all mechanical problem. This concept has evolved over time from that of a regional inflammation in upper airway tissues to that of a systemic inflammation that may contribute to end organ damage. This chapter will review the new concepts of regional and systemic inflammation as they relate to OSAS. While focusing primarily on pediatric literature, the chapter will refer to adult studies when the pediatric evidence is missing.

II. Local Inflammation

Airway mucosa is known to play an important role in modulating lower airway patency (2). However, its role in modulating upper airway collapsibility in patients with OSAS has not been fully investigated. Various invasive and noninvasive techniques have been utilized to describe the inflammatory state of upper airway mucosa, submucosa, and musculature. To establish the association between airway inflammation and OSAS in children, investigators have relied on noninvasive techniques, such as the measurements of inflammatory mediators in induced sputum and in exhaled breath condensates. Analysis of induced sputum in children with OSAS showed that the percentage of sputum neutrophils was markedly increased compared with controls and that the degree of neutrophilic inflammation correlated significantly and positively with the severity of the disorder (3). Similar observations were made in adult patients with OSAS. Compared with control subjects, adult patients with OSAS had a higher percentage of neutrophils in their sputum (4) and nasal lavage fluid (5). They also had greater concentrations of bradykinin and vasoactive intestinal peptide (6). Goldbart et al. examined the level of leukotrienes C4, B4, D4, E4, and prostaglandin E2 in children's exhaled breath condensate (7). Leukotrienes are short-lived lipid mediators that have potent pro-inflammatory biological activities. Following their formation at the nuclear membrane of inflammatory cells (macrophages, neutrophils, eosinophils, and mast cells) in response to diverse immune and inflammatory stimuli, leukotrienes are secreted into the extracellular space through specific transporters. Leukotrienes then bind to specific G-protein-coupled receptors on various target cells and elicit their well-recognized anaphylactic, edema-causing, and pro-inflammatory actions. In Goldbart's study, children with OSAS had higher levels of leukotrienes than controls. There was a dose-dependent increase in the level of leukotriene B4 with increased severity of the disorder. The implications of elevated neutrophil count and pro-inflammatory mediators, such as leukotrienes, in upper airway secretions are yet to be defined.

In an effort to determine whether inflammatory processes extend to upper airway tissues, histological analysis of samples obtained from patients undergoing uvulopalatopharyngoplasty for OSAS was performed. The analysis showed that the number of leukocytes in the lamina propria of the uvula mucosa was significantly higher in patients with OSAS than in controls (8,9). The majority of the cells were plasma cells and lymphocytes. The plasma cells were predominantly cells bearing immunoglobulin G while the lymphocytes were B and T cells. Furthermore, other studies that examined the histopathological changes in the soft palate showed that myelinated nerves and striated muscles were damaged in uvulas removed surgically from patients with OSAS (10). Morphometric analysis of the uvula in patients with sleep apnea showed a higher percentage of connective tissue and intercellular space, a lower proportion of muscle tissue, and a significantly thicker epithelium than controls (9,11). Boyd et al. described an inflammatory cell infiltration in the muscular layer of the pharynx in patients with OSAS (10). A significant increase in activated T-cell infiltration was observed in OSAS patients in comparison with the control tissue sample. Immunolocalization of protein gene product 9.5 (PGP 9.5), a pan-neuronal marker that stains all types of afferent and efferent nerve fibers, and immunostaining with neural cell adhesion molecule (N-CAM) CD56, a cell surface marker expressed on denervated muscle fibers, were significantly higher in patients with OSAS than in controls. Thus, the simultaneous increase in a marker of nerve regeneration, PGP 9.5, and in a marker of nerve degeneration, N-CAM, suggests an active process of denervation and reinnervation in upper airway muscles of patients with OSAS (Figs. 1 and 2). In summary, these studies demonstrated that upper airway inflammation involves both the muscular and the mucosal tissue compartments and that the inflammatory cells consist predominantly of activated T lymphocytes. Active processes of nerve degeneration and regeneration and muscular damage in this patient population suggest that inflammation might negatively impact the function of upper airway tissues. However, data that quantify the degree of airway tissue injury across the spectrum of severity of the disorder could shed light on the nature of the association between OSAS and local inflammation.

A. Significance of Upper Airway Inflammation

The role of upper airway inflammation in the pathophysiology of airway occlusion during sleep is not very well defined. In many publications, the local inflammatory response described in the upper airway was attributed to the mechanical trauma induced by large intraluminal pharyngeal pressure swings, tissue vibration, and eccentric muscle contraction. However, several studies have also suggested that upper airway inflammation could exacerbate upper airway obstruction. McNicholas et al. showed that in patients with acute exacerbations of allergic rhinitis, a condition associated with upper airway inflammation, obstructive apneas lasted longer and were more frequent than those recorded during remission (12). Increased vasodilatation in anesthetized animals, a characteristic feature of inflammation, has been shown to decrease pharyngeal cross-sectional area and promote upper airway collapsibility. Furthermore, stimulation of upper

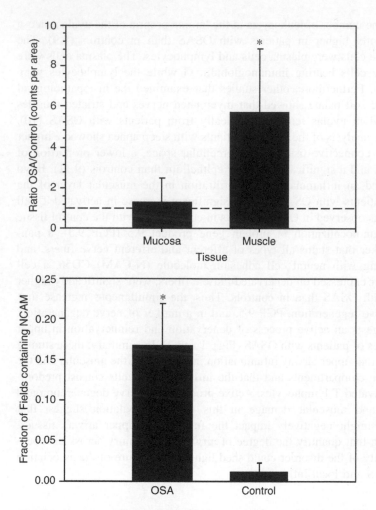

Figure 1 The upper panel shows the ratio of counts per area for PGP 9.5 in upper airway muscle and mucosa in OSA versus control subjects. Values over one (*above dashed line*) indicate increased nerve in patients with OSA. The lower panel shows the fraction of fields containing N-CAM-positive fibers in OSA versus control. A dramatic increase in both nerves PGP9.5 and denervated muscle fibers N-CAM was demonstrated for OSA versus control in muscle. *$p < 0.05$ OSA versus control. *Abbreviations*: PGP 9.5, protein gene product 9.5; OSA, obstructive sleep apnea syndrome; N-CAM, neural cell adhesion molecule. *Source*: From Ref. 10.

airway secretions in rabbits made a collapsed airway more difficult to reopen (13,14). This effect could be ascribed to the high viscoelasticity of the induced secretions and the increased surface tension of the upper airway lining fluid. The causal relationship between local inflammation and airway collapsibility has been

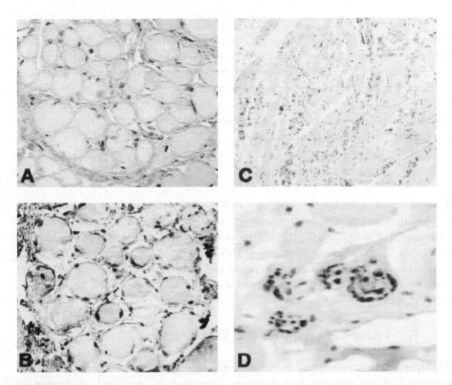

Figure 2 (A) Control upper airway muscle stained for N-CAM (negative). (B) OSAS upper airway muscle heavily positive for N-CAM. Note the subsarcolemmal staining of myocytes. (C) Patient with OSAS with abundant intramuscular PGP 9.5-positive nerve. (D) High-power cross-section of nerve fibers in OSAS. All positive structures are brown corresponding to the common secondary peroxidase antibody system. *Abbreviations*: N-CAM, neural cell adhesion molecule; OSAS, obstructive sleep apnea syndrome; PGP 9.5, protein gene product 9.5. *Source*: From Ref. 10.

recently investigated. Findings from several studies suggest that surface tension plays a role in modulating upper airway patency and may also be a marker for disturbances in airway neuromuscular control (15–18). In dogs, instillation of substances with surface tension-lowering properties into the upper airway was associated with a reduction in airflow resistance (19) and in the degree of genioglossus muscle recruitment required to reopen the closed upper airway (20). The instillation of surface tension-lowering substances also decreased both upper airway opening and closing pressures. These observations were extended to humans by demonstrating that the instillation of exogenous surfactant significantly decreased upper airway opening pressure (18). These findings support the hypothesis that surface tension of upper airway lining fluid generates a force that hinders airway opening. Such force could be minimized through the instillation of surface active agents into the upper airway lumen.

The exact mechanisms underlying the upregulation of inflammatory processes within the upper airway require further investigation. Whether these processes are the results or the triggers of OSAS are critical questions to our understanding of the pathophysiology of this disorder. Before markers of inflammation in sputum or breath condensate are considered correlates of OSAS, the relation of upper airway inflammation to lower airway structural and functional abnormalities and to mediators of inflammation measured in the peripheral circulation should be further defined.

III. Systemic Inflammation

The observed association between OSAS, cardiovascular disease, metabolic dysfunction, and neurocognitive deficits, which all share common inflammatory pathways, led to the investigation of mechanisms mediating these adverse health outcomes. With the assumption that OSAS mediates its adverse health outcomes through exposure to intermittent hypoxia and through its effect on sleep, efforts were made to understand how the sequelae of OSAS create a milieu that promotes inflammation.

IV. Intermittent Hypoxia and Inflammation

Multiple studies attempted to answer the question of whether intermittent hypoxia-induced inflammation develops secondary to increased production of reactive oxygen species (ROS) from inflammatory cells. To that end, investigators have used the same paradigm of ischemia/reperfusion injury, where the reoxygenation phase is characterized by intense inflammatory response causing organ injury and failure. Although the generation of ROS cannot be directly measured in biological systems, several biomarkers have been identified that provide a measure of oxidative damage to biomolecules. These include oxidative damage to DNA (8-OH-2-deoxyguanosine), amino acid oxidation products (homocysteine, dityrosine), arachidonic acid derivatives (F2 isoprostanes), and chemical modification of proteins subsequent to lipid oxidation [malondialdehyde (MDA)]. Furthermore, the activity of the antioxidant defense system can be estimated, including enzymes such as superoxide dismutase (SOD), glutathione peroxidase (GPX), glutathione reductase (GR), nonenzymatic plasma antioxidants (albumin, bilirubin, and urate), and melatonin, the chief secretory product of the pineal gland, which is known to be one of the most effective endogenous free radical scavengers.

A. Amino Acid Oxidation

Homocysteine is a thiol-containing amino acid that is an intermediate substance produced during intracellular demethylation of methionine. Elevated levels of homocysteine are found in patients with cardiovascular diseases. A clear correlation was shown between mildly elevated total blood homocysteine concentrations and premature coronary artery diseases, stroke, peripheral artery diseases, and venous thrombosis (21,22). The initial observation of elevated homocysteine in patients with OSAS was demonstrated in adults with ischemic heart disease and OSAS (23). However, subsequent studies did not show consistent differences in homocysteine levels between subjects with OSAS and controls (24). The response to continuous positive airway pressure (CPAP) was also inconsistent. While some studies showed a decrease in homocysteine level with treatment (25), others showed no significant change (24).

B. Lipid Peroxidation

The extent of lipid oxidation can be determined by measuring the losses of unsaturated fatty acids, the amounts of primary peroxidation products, and the amounts of secondary products, such as hydrocarbon gases (26). Analysis of fatty acids by gradient and high performance liquid chromatography was found to be a useful tool for assessing lipid peroxidation. The peroxidation of unsaturated fatty acids is accompanied by the formation of conjugated diene structures, which absorb ultraviolet (UV) light in the 230- to 235-nm wavelength range. Measurement of this UV absorbance is useful in studies of pure lipids, detecting an early stage in the peroxidation process. One of the most commonly applied assays is the thiobarbituric acid (TBA) test. The method is based on the reaction of TBA with MDA, one of the aldehyde products of lipid peroxidation. However, its application to body fluids and tissue extracts has been problematic. Several substances not related to lipid peroxidation can react with TBA to form chromogen with absorbance of around 530 to 535 nm, and this possibility of interference has prompted severe doubts about the validity of the test (27). Nevertheless, one of the most reliable and highly specific TBA assays is the one in which the whole TBA reaction mixture is separated by high-performance liquid chromatography and the peak of the MDA–TBA adduct is quantified. In a study by Lavie et al., TBA-reactive substances were significantly correlated with the frequency of respiratory events (28). However, this was not reproduced in other studies (29).

Analysis of isoprostanes has emerged as a credible approach to the study of lipid peroxidation in vivo. Isoprostanes are formed from arachidonic acid by a free radical mechanism and are chemically stable. They are generated initially at the site of free radical attack in cell membranes from which they are cleaved, presumably by phospholipases, then circulated, and excreted in urine. Besides blood and urine, they have also been reported in body fluids, such as pericardial fluid (30), bile (31), lung condensates (32), and cerebrospinal fluid (33). Several isoprostanes are known to have biological effects in vitro via membrane receptors for prostaglandins. Isoprostane F2a-III is a potent smooth muscle cell constrictor and a mitogen. It modulates platelet as well as other cell functions in vitro (34–37). Animals exposed to intermittent hypoxia show elevated levels of isoprostanes and lipid peroxidation, which are dependent on inducible nitric oxide activity. In humans, altered generation of isoprostanes has been reported in a variety of syndromes putatively associated with oxidant stress. These include coronary ischemia-reperfusion syndromes (38,39), Alzheimer's disease (33,40), adult respiratory distress syndrome, and chronic obstructive pulmonary disease (38,39,41–43). As a marker of oxidative stress, 8-isoprostane was found to be significantly higher in blood, urine, and breath condensate of adult patients with OSAS compared with controls. The level of isoprostane correlated positively with the frequency of respiratory events and with indices of hypoxemia. Treatment of OSAS with CPAP was associated with reduction in isoprostane. Such response to treatment suggested that in patients with OSAS, CPAP functioned as an antioxidant by reducing markers of lipid peroxidation. However, in a subset analysis of normotensive, nonsmoking, newly diagnosed, and untreated OSAS patients who had no comorbidities, there was no significant difference measured in markers of lipid peroxidation between OSAS patients and a control group matched for body mass index, age, and lipid profile.

C. Chemical Modification of Proteins

The reactions of ROS with polyunsaturated fatty acids yield lipid hydroperoxides. A variety of aldehydes can be formed in the breakdown of such hydroperoxides. MDA, one of the major aldehyde species, is commonly accepted as a measure of the degree of lipid peroxidation. In a study of the changes in MDA in healthy subjects exposed to hypoxia, Freudenthaler et al. demonstrated that there was a significant increase in the level of MDA after exposure to 13% oxygen for a period of six hours, which was not altered by treatment with thioctic acid, N-acetylcysteine 600 mg, or placebo (0.9% sodium chloride) (44). Small cross-sectional studies showed higher levels of MDA in adults with OSAS than in controls and a time-dependent increase of MDA levels during sleep. MDA levels showed a highly significant correlation with degree and duration of nocturnal oxygen desaturation (44–46). To demonstrate causality between hypoxia and elevated MDA, several studies in animal models exposed to intermittent hypoxia showed increased MDA in brain, myocardium, and liver tissues (47–49). These data suggested that periods of reoxygenation following hypoxia are likely to be responsible for the elevation of MDA levels observed in patients with OSAS.

D. Antioxidant Defense

The study of antioxidants in OSAS is based on the hypothesis that repeated hypoxemia in patients with OSAS creates an imbalance between reactive oxygen intermediate molecules and the antioxidant reserve that is essential for their detoxification. Young adult male Sprague–Dawley rats exposed to hypoxia, at levels commonly occurring in human patients with OSAS, had induction of antioxidant responses in the cerebellum and pons. This was indicated by increased activities of the antioxidant enzymes, SOD and GR, and elevated levels of the lipid oxidation products, TBA-reactive substances, in response to severe intermittent hypoxia (50). In a small group of 14 patients with OSAS, Kostas et al. showed a negative correlation between the antioxidant capacity in their blood samples and frequency of obstructive events. However, conflicting results were demonstrated by Wali et al. who did not show any difference in the susceptibility of low-density lipoprotein to oxidative stress between hypoxic and nonhypoxic OSAS Furthermore, treatment with CPAP did not significantly change the level of the antioxidant enzymes (51).

E. Melatonin

There is abundant evidence that melatonin has a protective effect against cellular oxidative stress. Melatonin is capable of enhancing glucose metabolism through the pentose phosphate shunt pathway, increasing production of nicotinamide adenine dinucleotide phosphate hydrogen (NADPH), and thereby influencing the cellular redox potential (52). In addition, melatonin stimulates production of glutathione—a metabolite that helps to protect cells from oxidative stress (53). However, studies of melatonin in OSAS are scarce and, to date, do not provide sufficient evidence that melatonin levels or rhythms are altered by OSAS.

In summary, there are significant inconsistencies in the investigations of oxidative stress in patients with OSAS. Such conflicting results might be the results of differences in study populations and methods of approach. It is also likely that in the absence of significant comorbidities sleep apnea does not, in and of itself, initiate the generation of oxidative stress or lipid peroxidation.

F. Transcription Factors and OSAS

Transcription is controlled by regulatory proteins known as transcription factors, which bind to specific DNA sequences in the gene promoter and activate or inhibit transcription. One such important transcription factors is nuclear factor kappa B (NF-κB), which governs the expression of early response genes involved in cell-to-cell interaction, intercellular communication, cell recruitment or transmigration, and amplification or spreading of primary pathogenic signals.

The central role of NF-κB in human defense and disease has made it an interesting transcription factor, whose biology is very complex due to several mechanisms involved in its activation, nuclear transport, and finally DNA binding. Activation of the NF-κB/Rel family by nuclear translocation of cytoplasmic complexes plays a central role in inflammatory diseases through its ability to induce transcription of pro-inflammatory, inflammatory, and immune genes (54,55). These include genes encoding at least 27 different cytokines, chemokines, and receptors involved in immune recognition, such as members of the major histocompatability complex (MHC), proteins involved in antigen presentation, and receptors required for neutrophil adhesion and migration (56). Cytokines that are stimulated by NF-κB, such as IL-1b and tumor necrosis factor-alpha (TNF-α), can also directly activate the NF-κB pathway, thus establishing a positive autoregulatory cycle that can amplify the inflammatory response and increase the duration of chronic inflammation (54,55). NF-κB also stimulates the expression of enzymes, whose products contribute to the pathogenesis of the inflammatory processes, including the inducible form of nitric oxide synthase that generates nitric oxide and the inducible cyclooxygenase that in turn generates prostanoids (56).

Activation of NF-κB in response to hypoxia was first examined in mice exposed to chronic intermittent hypoxia for up to 14 days. A study by Greenberg et al. demonstrated increased NF-κB binding activity in aorta, heart, and lung tissues in an exposure time-dependent manner. The induction of the inducible form of nitric oxide synthase expression by chronic intermittent hypoxia was temporally correlated with activation of NF-κB. In a small cross-sectional study, which included five subjects with OSAS and five healthy controls, monocytes from OSAS patients showed a 3.7-fold increase in NF-κB band intensity compared with controls. This difference was reduced by 56.4% after one month of CPAP therapy (57).

G. NF-κB-Dependent Genes and OSAS

Circulating NF-κB-dependent genes, interleukin 6 (IL-6) and TNF-α were found to be higher in adult patients with OSAS compared with controls (58–60). IL-6 is a pleiotropic cytokine with a variety of biological activities, including the ability to induce B- and T-cell differentiation and activation of macrophages and natural killer cells.

IL-6 is secreted by endothelial cells, macrophages, lymphocytes, and adipocytes. It exerts its biological actions through the IL-6 receptor complex. The IL-6 receptor complex consists of two membrane-bound glycoproteins, an 80 kDa ligand-binding component (termed IL-6R) and a 130 kDa signal-transducing component (termed gp130). It also activates a soluble IL-6R (sIL-6R). The activated IL-6/sIL-6R complex serves as a potent agonist that binds the signal-transducing component of the membrane-bound receptor, gp130, with high affinity. Through this mechanism, IL-6 is believed to exert effects in cells that lack the IL-6R per se. IL-6 stimulates hepatocytes to produce acute-phase proteins, such as C-reactive protein (CRP), which is an important activator of neutrophil production of the soluble IL-6R. As such, CRP acts not only as an acute-phase reactant, but may also have a profound effect on distal IL-6-mediated events that occur during the inflammatory process. The unequivocal evidence that IL-6 plays a central role in mediating cardiovascular disease elicited interest in examining the association between this cytokine, its receptors and OSAS.

Specifically, several epidemiological studies have demonstrated the predictive role of IL-6 in the future development of arthrosclerosis in adults (61–63). In a 12-year follow-up study of 392 adults, high levels of IL-6 CRP predicted carotid atherosclerosis. This association was independent of multiple biological and behavioral risk factors for atherosclerosis (61).

In adults with OSAS, levels of IL-6 in breath condensates correlated with the severity of the disorder (64). In a cohort of adults with a variable degree of severity of OSAS, IL-6 was significantly higher in subjects with moderate to severe OSAS compared with subjects without OSAS. However, after adjustments for demographic characteristics, these differences were no longer significant. Soluble IL-6R demonstrated a significant association with the severity of OSAS after adjustments for demographic characteristics (58).

Another circulating NF-κB-dependent gene with potential role in the development of cardiovascular disease, TNF-α, was also found to be elevated in subjects with OSAS. TNF belongs to a family of signaling molecules that exist as Type II membrane proteins characterized by an extracytoplasmic C-terminus. Currently, two isoforms of TNF have been identified and share similar inflammatory activities. TNF-α, the smaller and more abundant of the two peptides, is thought to be the peptide that mediates cardiovascular homeostasis. Several animal studies have demonstrated that TNF-α binding to its cognate receptor and the subsequent activation of the downstream signaling cascade play a role in the postnatal adaptive myocardial growth response to multiple biomechanical stresses. TNF-α expression and peptide production are upregulated in the adult heart in response to pressure overload and to stretch in isolated cardiac myocytes. Physiologically relevant concentrations of TNF-α provoke a hypertrophic response by increasing the synthesis of both structural and contractile proteins in adult feline cardiac myocytes (65). Additional in vivo evidence in transgenic mice overexpressing TNF-α specifically in the heart supports the role of TNF-α in the induction of cardiac hypertrophy (66,67). In support of the requirement of TNF-α for hypertrophic adaptive cardiac growth, Smith et al. showed that mice deficient in TNF-α have a significantly reduced right ventricular hypertrophic response to chronic hypoxia compared with wild type litter mate controls (68).

TNF-α has been identified throughout the full spectrum of atherosclerotic development. In fact, in humans TNF-α has been identified in the endothelial and smooth muscle cells from the early intimal thickening stage of atherosclerosis to subjects with established occlusive atherosclerosis. Large scale epidemiological studies conducted in adult populations showed an independent association between levels of TNF-α and cardiovascular events and mortality (69–71).

In adults with OSAS, circulating TNF-α levels were higher than that in control subjects and significantly decreased with CPAP therapy. In a multivariate analysis, TNF-α was independently associated with the desaturation index, Epworth sleepiness score, and cholesterol level (72,73).

H. Acute-Phase Reactants and OSAS

CRP is a normal plasma protein that belongs to the evolutionary ancient and highly conserved pentraxin family. It is a highly soluble serum protein that shows calcium-dependent affinity for phosphate monoesters; in particular, phosphocholine. Other intrinsic ligands include native and modified plasma lipoproteins, damaged cell membranes, small ribonucleoprotein particles, apoptotic cells, and fibronectin. Among extrinsic ligands are components of bacteria, fungi, and parasites as well as plant products. When bound to these ligands, CRP is recognized by C1q, leading to activation of the classical complement pathway. In addition, bound CRP also regulates alternative-pathway amplification and C5 convertases. The half-life of CRP is approximately 19 hours and appears to be similar under physiological and pathological conditions. The CRP gene in hepatocytes is predominantly under transcriptional control by the cytokine IL-6 and to a lesser degree IL-1β and TNF-α.

The introduction of high-sensitivity assays for serum CRP (hs-CRP) has permitted routine measurements of baseline CRP levels and initiated numerous studies investigating CRP as a risk factor for cardiovascular disease. To date, over two dozen large-scale prospective studies have shown baseline levels of hs-CRP to independently predict future myocardial infarction, stroke, cardiovascular death, and incident peripheral arterial disease (74,75). Moreover, eight major prospective studies have had adequate power to evaluate hs-CRP after adjustment for all Framingham covariates and all have confirmed the independence of hs-CRP as a risk factor for cardiovascular disease (76–82).

The independent association between CRP and sleep-disordered breathing (SDB) in adults has been described initially by Shamsuzzaman et al. (83) and further confirmed by multiple studies (84–90). Similarly, in children two studies demonstrated a positive association between acute-phase reactant and SDB (91,92). Nevertheless, a few well-designed studies did not find a significant association between CRP and SDB (93–95) The conflicting results were in part attributed to the difference in the degree of adiposity among the study populations. Since obesity is considered a pro-inflammatory condition, it is plausible that a critical threshold of background inflammation must exist before an independent association between CRP and SDB can be observed.

In contrast to studies in adults, in which CRP concentration has been associated with smoking, blood pressure, blood lipid concentrations, and hyperglycemia, CRP concentration in children does not correlate consistently with these risk factors (96). In children as in adults, excess weight is a consistent and an important determinant of circulating CRP concentration. Thus, the predictive significance of elevated CRP in adults might differ substantially from its significance in children.

V. Summary

The evidence for increased systemic inflammatory markers in children with SDB is emerging. Since the end-points of SDB morbidity are age dependent, the long-term inference that could be derived from elevated markers of inflammation should be investigated in the pediatric population.

References

1. Broadbent WH. Cheyne-Stokes respiration in cerebral hemorrhage. Lancet 1877; 3: 307–309.
2. Dusser DJ, Djokic TD, Borson DB, et al. Cigarette smoke induces bronchoconstrictor hyperresponsiveness to substance P and inactivates airway neutral endopeptidase in the guinea pig. Possible role of free radicals. J Clin Invest 1989; 84(3): 900–906.
3. Li AM, Hung E, Tsang T, et al. Induced sputum inflammatory measures correlate with disease severity in children with obstructive sleep apnoea. Thorax 2007; 62(1): 75–79.
4. Salerno FG, Carpagnano E, Guido P, et al. Airway inflammation in patients affected by obstructive sleep apnea syndrome. Respir Med 2004; 98(1):25–28.
5. Rubinstein I. Nasal inflammation in patients with obstructive sleep apnea. Laryngoscope 1995; 105(2):175–177.
6. Li H, Meng X, Yang H. The relationship between content of substance P, VIP in pharyngeal tissue and narrow pharyngeal cavity of patients with OSAS. Lin Chuang Er Bi Yan Hou Ke Za Zhi 2001; 15(12):539–541.
7. Goldbart A, Krishna DJ, Li RC, et al. Inflammatory mediators in exhaled breath condensate of children with obstructive sleep apnea syndrome. Chest 2006; 130(1): 143–148.
8. Sekosan M, Zakkar M, Wenig BL, et al. Inflammation in the uvula mucosa of patients with obstructive sleep apnea. Laryngoscope 1996; 106(8):1018–1020.
9. Hamans EP, Van Marck EA, De Backer WA, et al. Morphometric analysis of the uvula in patients with sleep-related breathing disorders. Eur Arch Otorhinolaryngol 2000; 257(4):232–236.
10. Boyd JH, Petrof BJ, Hamid Q, et al. Upper airway muscle inflammation and denervation changes in obstructive sleep apnea. Am J Respir Crit Care Med 2004; 170(5):541–546.
11. Zhou B, Ji C, Zhou D. Clinical study on oropharyngeal fatty infiltration on the pathogenesis of obstructive sleep apnea syndrome. Lin Chuang Er Bi Yan Hou Ke Za Zhi 2003; 17(9):535–538.
12. McNicholas W T, Tarlo S, Cole P, et al. Obstructive apneas during sleep in patients with seasonal allergic rhinitis. Am Rev Respir Dis 1982; 126(4):625–628.
13. Olson LG, Strohl KP. Airway secretions influence upper airway patency in the rabbit. Am Rev Respir Dis 1988; 137(6):1379–1381.
14. Olson LG, Strohl KP. Non-muscular factors in upper airway patency in the rabbit. Respir Physiol 1988; 71(2):147–155.
15. Kirkness JP, Amis TC, Wheatley JR, et al. Determining the surface tension of microliter amounts of liquid. J Colloid Interface Sci 2000; 232(2):408–409.

16. Kirkness JP, Christenson HK, Garlick SR, et al. Decreased surface tension of upper airway mucosal lining liquid increases upper airway patency in anaesthetised rabbits. J Physiol 2003; 547(pt 2):603–611.

17. Kirkness JP, Eastwood PR, Szollosi I, et al. Effect of surface tension of mucosal lining liquid on upper airway mechanics in anesthetized humans. J Appl Physiol 2003; 95(1):357–363.

18. Kirkness JP, Madronio M, Stavrinou R, et al. Relationship between surface tension of upper airway lining liquid and upper airway collapsibility during sleep in obstructive sleep apnea hypopnea syndrome. J Appl Physiol 2003; 95(5):1761–1766.

19. Widdicombe JG, Davies A. The effects of a mixture of surface-active agents (Sonarex) on upper airways resistance and snoring in anaesthetized dogs. Eur Respir J 1988; 1(9):785–791.

20. Miki H, Hida W, Kikuchi Y, et al. Effects of pharyngeal lubrication on the opening of obstructed upper airway. J Appl Physiol 1992; 72(6):2311–2316.

21. Troughton JA, Woodside JV, Young IS, et al. Homocysteine and coronary heart disease risk in the PRIME study. Atherosclerosis 2007; 191(1):90–97.

22. Haim M, Tanne D, Goldbourt U, et al. Serum homocysteine and long-term risk of myocardial infarction and sudden death in patients with coronary heart disease. Cardiology 2007; 107(1):52–56.

23. Lavie L, Perelman A, Lavie P. Plasma homocysteine levels in obstructive sleep apnea: association with cardiovascular morbidity. Chest 2001; 120(3):900–908.

24. Svatikova A, Wolk R, Magera MJ, et al. Plasma homocysteine in obstructive sleep apnoea. Eur Heart J 2004; 25(15):1325–1329.

25. Jordan W, Berger C, Cohrs S, et al. CPAP-therapy effectively lowers serum homocysteine in obstructive sleep apnea syndrome. J Neural Transm 2004; 111(6): 683–689.

26. Kadiiska MB, Gladen BC, Baird DD, et al. Biomarkers of oxidative stress study III. Effects of the nonsteroidal anti-inflammatory agents indomethacin and meclofenamic acid on measurements of oxidative products of lipids in CCl4 poisoning. Free Radic Biol Med 2005; 38(6):711–718.

27. Korchazhkina O, Exley C, Andrew Spencer S. Measurement by reversed-phase high-performance liquid chromatography of malondialdehyde in normal human urine following derivatisation with 2,4-dinitrophenylhydrazine. J Chromatogr B Analyt Technol Biomed Life Sci 2003; 794(2):353–362.

28. Lavie L, Vishnevsky A, Lavie P. Evidence for lipid peroxidation in obstructive sleep apnea. Sleep 2004; 27(1):123–128.

29. Svatikova A, Wolk R, Lerman LO, et al. Oxidative stress in obstructive sleep apnoea. Eur Heart J 2005; 26(22):2435–2439.

30. Mallat Z, Philip I, Lebret M, et al. Elevated levels of 8-iso-prostaglandin F2alpha in pericardial fluid of patients with heart failure: a potential role for in vivo oxidant stress in ventricular dilatation and progression to heart failure. Circulation 1998; 97 (16):1536–1539.

31. Leo MA, Aleynik SI, Siegel JH, et al. F2-isoprostane and 4-hydroxynonenal excretion in human bile of patients with biliary tract and pancreatic disorders. Am J Gastroenterol 1997; 92(11):2069–2072.

32. Montuschi P, Barnes PJ. Analysis of exhaled breath condensate for monitoring airway inflammation. Trends Pharmacol Sci 2002; 23(5):232–237.

33. Montine TJ, Markesbery WR, Morrow JD, et al. Cerebrospinal fluid F2-isoprostane levels are increased in Alzheimer's disease. Ann Neurol 1998; 44(3):410–413.

34. Morrow JD, Minton TA, Roberts LJ II. The F2-isoprostane, 8-epi-prostaglandin F2 alpha, a potent agonist of the vascular thromboxane/endoperoxide receptor, is a platelet thromboxane/endoperoxide receptor antagonist. Prostaglandins 1992; 44(2): 155–163.

35. Yin K, Halushka PV, Yan YT, et al. Antiaggregatory activity of 8-epi-prostaglandin F2 alpha and other F-series prostanoids and their binding to thromboxane A2/ prostaglandin H2 receptors in human platelets. J Pharmacol Exp Ther 1994; 270(3): 1192–1196.

36. Pratico D, Smyth EM, Violi F, et al. Local amplification of platelet function by 8-Epi prostaglandin F2alpha is not mediated by thromboxane receptor isoforms. J Biol Chem 1996; 271(25):14916–14924.

37. Elmhurst JL, Betti PA, Rangachari PK. Intestinal effects of isoprostanes: evidence for the involvement of prostanoid EP and TP receptors. J Pharmacol Exp Ther 1997; 282(3):1198–1205.

38. Delanty N, Reilly MP, Pratico D, et al. 8-epi PGF2 alpha generation during coronary reperfusion. A potential quantitative marker of oxidant stress in vivo. Circulation 1997; 95(11):2492–2499.

39. Reilly MP, Delanty N, Roy L, et al. Increased formation of the isoprostanes IPF2alpha-I and 8-epi-prostaglandin F2alpha in acute coronary angioplasty: evidence for oxidant stress during coronary reperfusion in humans. Circulation 1997; 96(10):3314–3320.

40. Pratico D, Lee V M-Y, Trojanowski JQ, et al. Increased F2-isoprostanes in Alzheimer's disease: evidence for enhanced lipid peroxidation in vivo. FASEB J 1998; 12(15):1777–1783.

41. Pratico D, Basili S, Vieri M, et al. Chronic obstructive pulmonary disease is associated with an increase in urinary levels of isoprostane F2alpha-III, an index of oxidant stress. Am J Respir Crit Care Med 1998; 158(6):1709–1714.

42. Roberts LJ II, Moore KP, Zackert WE, et al. Identification of the major urinary metabolite of the F2-isoprostane 8-iso-prostaglandin F2alpha in humans. J Biol Chem 1996; 271(34):20617–20620.

43. Chiabrando C, Valagussa A, Rivalta C, et al. Identification and measurement of endogenous beta-oxidation metabolites of 8-epi-Prostaglandin F2alpha. J Biol Chem 1999; 274(3):1313–1319.

44. Freudenthaler SM, Schreeb KH, Wiese A, et al. Influence of controlled hypoxia and radical scavenging agents on erythropoietin and malondialdehyde concentrations in humans. Acta Physiol Scand 2002; 174(3):231–235.

45. Dikmenoglu N, Ciftci B, Ileri E, et al. Erythrocyte deformability, plasma viscosity and oxidative status in patients with severe obstructive sleep apnea syndrome. Sleep Med 2006; 7(3):255–261.

46. Jordan W, Cohrs S, Degner D, et al. Evaluation of oxidative stress measurements in obstructive sleep apnea syndrome. J Neural Transm 2006; 113(2):239–254.

47. Row BW, Kheirandish L, Neville JJ, et al. Impaired spatial learning and hyperactivity in developing rats exposed to intermittent hypoxia. Pediatr Res 2002; 52(3): 449–453.

48. Chen L, Einbinder E, Zhang Q, et al. Oxidative stress and left ventricular function with chronic intermittent hypoxia in rats. Am J Respir Crit Care Med 2005; 172(7): 915–920.

49. Li J, Savransky V, Nanayakkara A, et al. Hyperlipidemia and lipid peroxidation are dependent on the severity of chronic intermittent hypoxia. J Appl Physiol 2007; 102 (2):557–563.

50. Ramanathan L, Gozal D, Siegel JM. Antioxidant responses to chronic hypoxia in the rat cerebellum and pons. J Neurochem 2005; 93(1):47–52.

51. Wali SO, Bahammam AS, Massaeli H, et al. Susceptibility of LDL to oxidative stress in obstructive sleep apnea. Sleep 1998; 21(3):290–296.

52. Winiarska K, Drozak J, Wegrzynowicz M, et al. Diabetes-induced changes in glucose synthesis, intracellular glutathione status and hydroxyl free radical generation in rabbit kidney-cortex tubules. Mol Cell Biochem 2004; 261(1–2):91–98.

53. Rodriguez-Reynoso S, Leal C, Portilla-de Buen E, et al. Melatonin ameliorates renal ischemia/reperfusion injury. J Surg Res; 116(2):242–247.

54. Tak PP, Firestein GS. NF-kappaB: a key role in inflammatory diseases. J Clin Invest 2001; 107(1):7–11.

55. Yamamoto Y, Gaynor RB. Therapeutic potential of inhibition of the NF-kappaB pathway in the treatment of inflammation and cancer. J Clin Invest 2001; 107(2): 135–142.

56. Pahl HL. Activators and target genes of Rel/NF-kappaB transcription factors. Oncogene 1999; 18(49):6853–6866.

57. Greenberg H, Ye X, Wilson D, et al. Chronic intermittent hypoxia activates nuclear factor-kappaB in cardiovascular tissues in vivo. Biochem Biophys Res Commun 2006; 343(2):591–596.

58. Mehra R, Storfer-Isser A, Kirchner HL, et al. Soluble interleukin 6 receptor: a novel marker of moderate to severe sleep-related breathing disorder. Arch Intern Med 2006; 166(16):1725–1731.

59. Ciftci TU, Kokturk O, Bukan N, Bilgihan A. The relationship between serum cytokine levels with obesity and obstructive sleep apnea syndrome. Cytokine 2004; 28(2):87–91.

60. Vgontzas AN, Bixler EO, Chrousos GP. Metabolic disturbances in obesity versus sleep apnoea: the importance of visceral obesity and insulin resistance. J Intern Med 2003; 254(1):32–44.

61. Lee WY, Allison MA, Kim DJ, et al. Association of interleukin-6 and C-reactive protein with subclinical carotid atherosclerosis (the Rancho Bernardo Study). Am J Cardiol 2007; 99(1):99–102.

62. Orbe J, Montero I, Rodriguez JA, et al. Independent association of matrix metalloproteinase-10, cardiovascular risk factors and subclinical atherosclerosis. J Thromb Haemost 2007; 5(1):91–97.

63. Amar J, Fauvel J, Drouet L, et al. Interleukin 6 is associated with subclinical atherosclerosis: a link with soluble intercellular adhesion molecule 1. J Hypertens 2006; 24(6):1083–1088.

64. Carpagnano GE, Kharitonov SA, Resta O, et al. Increased 8-isoprostane and interleukin-6 in breath condensate of obstructive sleep apnea patients. Chest 2002; 122(4):1162–1167.

65. Yokoyama T, Nakano M, Bednarczyk JL, et al. Tumor necrosis factor-alpha provokes a hypertrophic growth response in adult cardiac myocytes. Circulation 1997; 95(5): 1247–1252.

66. Kubota T, McTiernan CF, Frye CS, et al. Cardiac-specific overexpression of tumor necrosis factor-alpha causes lethal myocarditis in transgenic mice. J Card Fail 1997; 3(2):117–124.

67. Kubota T, Miyagishima M, Alvarez RJ, et al. Expression of proinflammatory cytokines in the failing human heart: comparison of recent-onset and end-stage congestive heart failure. J Heart Lung Transplant 2000; 19(9):819–824.

68. Smith RM, McCarthy J, Sack MN. TNF alpha is required for hypoxia-mediated right ventricular hypertrophy. Mol Cell Biochem 2001; 219(1–2):139–143.

69. Tuomisto K, Jousilahti P, Sundvall J, et al. C-reactive protein, interleukin-6 and tumor necrosis factor alpha as predictors of incident coronary and cardiovascular events and total mortality. A population-based, prospective study. Thromb Haemost 2006; 95(3):511–518.

70. Cesari M, Penninx BW, Newman AB, et al. Inflammatory markers and onset of cardiovascular events: results from the Health ABC study. Circulation 2003; 108 (19):2317–2322.

71. Cesari M, Penninx BW, Newman AB, et al. Inflammatory markers and cardiovascular disease [The Health, Aging and Body Composition (Health ABC) Study]. Am J Cardiol 2003; 92(5):522–528.

72. Ryan S, Taylor CT, McNicholas WT. Selective activation of inflammatory pathways by intermittent hypoxia in obstructive sleep apnea syndrome. Circulation 2005; 112(17): 2660–2667.

73. Ryan S, Taylor CT, McNicholas WT. Predictors of elevated nuclear factor-kappaB-dependent genes in obstructive sleep apnea syndrome. Am J Respir Crit Care Med 2006; 174(7):824–830.

74. Ridker PM, Stampfer MJ, Rifai N. Novel risk factors for systemic atherosclerosis: a comparison of C-reactive protein, fibrinogen, homocysteine, lipoprotein(a), and standard cholesterol screening as predictors of peripheral arterial disease. JAMA 2001; 285(19):2481–2485.

75. Ridker PM. Clinical application of C-reactive protein for cardiovascular disease detection and prevention. Circulation 2003; 107(3):363–369.

76. Ridker PM, Cushman M, Stampfer MJ, et al. Inflammation, aspirin, and the risk of cardiovascular disease in apparently healthy men. N Engl J Med 1997; 336(14): 973–979.

77. Ridker PM, Rifai N, Rose L, et al. Comparison of C-reactive protein and low-density lipoprotein cholesterol levels in the prediction of first cardiovascular events. N Engl J Med 2002; 347(20):1557–1565.

78. Pai JK, Pischon T, Ma J, et al. Inflammatory markers and the risk of coronary heart disease in men and women. N Engl J Med 2004; 351(25):2599–2610.

79. Ballantyne CM, Hoogeveen RC, Bang H, et al. Lipoprotein-associated phospholipase A2, high-sensitivity C-reactive protein, and risk for incident coronary heart disease in middle-aged men and women in the Atherosclerosis Risk in Communities (ARIC) study. Circulation 2004; 109(7):837–842.

80. Koenig W, Khuseyinova N, Lowel H, et al. Lipoprotein-associated phospholipase A2 adds to risk prediction of incident coronary events by C-reactive protein in apparently healthy middle-aged men from the general population: results from the 14-year follow-up of a large cohort from southern Germany. Circulation 2004; 110 (14):1903–1908.

81. Danesh J, Wheeler JG, Hirschfield GM, et al. C-reactive protein and other circulating markers of inflammation in the prediction of coronary heart disease. N Engl J Med 2004; 350(14):1387–1397.

82. Cushman M, Arnold AM, Psaty BM, et al. C-reactive protein and the 10-year incidence of coronary heart disease in older men and women: the cardiovascular health study. Circulation 2005; 112(1):25–31.

83. Shamsuzzaman AS, Winnicki M, Lanfranchi P, et al. Elevated C-reactive protein in patients with obstructive sleep apnea. Circulation 2002; 105(21):2462–2464.

84. Yokoe T, Minoguchi K, Matsuo H, et al. Elevated levels of C-reactive protein and interleukin-6 in patients with obstructive sleep apnea syndrome are decreased by nasal continuous positive airway pressure. Circulation 2003; 107(8):1129–1134.

85. Teramoto S, Yamamoto H, Ouchi Y. Increased C-reactive protein and increased plasma interleukin-6 may synergistically affect the progression of coronary atherosclerosis in obstructive sleep apnea syndrome. Circulation 2003; 107(5):E40–E50.

86. Kokturk O, Ciftci TU, Mollarecep E, et al. Elevated C-reactive protein levels and increased cardiovascular risk in patients with obstructive sleep apnea syndrome. Int Heart J 2005; 46(5):801–809.

87. Minoguchi K, Yokoe T, Tazaki T, et al. Increased carotid intima-media thickness and serum inflammatory markers in obstructive sleep apnea. Am J Respir Crit Care Med 2005; 172(5):625–630.

88. Hayashi M, Fujimoto K, Urushibata K, et al. Hypoxia-sensitive molecules may modulate the development of atherosclerosis in sleep apnoea syndrome. Respirology 2006; 11(1):24–31.

89. Kageyama N, Nomura M, Nakaya Y, et al. Relationship between adhesion molecules with hs-CRP and changes therein after ARB (Valsartan) administration in patients with obstructive sleep apnea syndrome. J Med Invest 2006; 53(1–2):134–139.

90. Punjabi NM, Beamer BA. C-reactive protein is associated with sleep disordered breathing independent of adiposity. Sleep 2007; 30(1):29–34.

91. Tauman R, Ivanenko A, O'Brien LM, et al. Plasma C-reactive protein levels among children with sleep-disordered breathing. Pediatrics 2004; 113(6):e564–e569.

92. Larkin EK, Rosen CL, Kirchner HL, et al. Variation of C-reactive protein levels in adolescents: association with sleep-disordered breathing and sleep duration. Circulation 2005; 111(15):1978–1984.

93. Guilleminault C, Li KK, Khramtsov A, et al. Sleep disordered breathing surgical outcomes in prepubertal children. Laryngoscope 2004; 114(1):132–137.

94. Akashiba T, Akahoshi T, Kawahara S, et al. Effects of long-term nasal continuous positive airway pressure on C-reactive protein in patients with obstructive sleep apnea syndrome. Intern Med 2005; 44(8):899–900.

95. Kaditis AG, Alexopoulos EI, Kalampouka E, et al. Morning levels of C-reactive protein in children with obstructive sleep-disordered breathing. Am J Respir Crit Care Med 2005; 171(3):282–286.

96. Ford ES. C-reactive protein concentration and cardiovascular disease risk factors in children: findings from the National Health and Nutrition Examination Survey 1999–2000. Circulation 2003; 108(9):1053–1058.

23

Metabolic Aspects of Sleep Apnea in Children

RIVA TAUMAN
Tel Aviv University, Tel Aviv, Israel

DAVID GOZAL
University of Louisville School of Medicine, Louisville, Kentucky, U.S.A.

I. Introduction

During the past decade the childhood obstructive sleep apnea syndrome (OSAS) has become widely recognized as a common disorder with potentially serious clinical implications. Considerable insights have been gained into the morbidities associated with OSAS, and into their underlying mechanisms.

Concomitant with the evolving knowledge and awareness on childhood OSAS, our society is facing a dramatic increase in the prevalence of obesity worldwide. The classic presentation of children with OSAS as underweight children with adenotonsillar hypertrophy is being substantially replaced by an increasing proportion of young patients who are either overweight or obese (1). This trend allows for the prediction of a marked increase in the incidence of OSAS, occurrence of which would then lead to a corresponding increase in the prevalence of obesity-associated morbidities, particularly those involving the metabolic and cardiovascular systems.

The metabolic syndrome is an emerging public health problem that essentially comprises a constellation of cardiovascular risk factors for which obesity plays a critical role. The close analogy between the known risk factors of metabolic syndrome and those of OSAS have led to the hypothesis that OSAS may constitute an important risk factor contributing to the initiation and magnitude of metabolic syndrome, and that this process most likely involves potentiation of inflammatory cascades. The complex interactions between OSAS, obesity, and the metabolic syndrome most probably represent the additive and even synergistic consequences of the interaction between the biologic responses of adipose tissue and those of hypoxia and sleep disruption. Indeed, adipose tissue and sleep are viewed as "metabolic regulators," and both of these may recruit or modulate a large host of inflammatory pathways, which in turn regulate and effect many aspects of metabolic control. For example, systemic low-grade inflammation has been increasingly implicated in a large number of the morbidities associated with either increased ponderal indices, reduced sleep, or conditions leading to disrupted sleep such as OSAS.

II. OSAS

OSAS in children is characterized by recurrent events of partial or complete upper airway obstruction during sleep, resulting in disruption of normal gas exchange [intermittent hypoxia (IH) and hypercapnia] and sleep fragmentation (2). The clinical spectrum of obstructive sleep disordered breathing includes overt, fully-established OSAS at the one end of the severity spectrum, and then in decremental order, obstructive alveolar hypoventilation, upper airway resistance syndrome (UARS; traditionally associated with overall normal oxygenation patterns in the presence of increased respiratory-related arousals, i.e., sleep fragmentation), and finally a condition that has been termed either primary or habitual snoring, the latter consisting of snoring in the absence of apnea, gas exchange abnormalities, and/or disruption of sleep architecture, and that is believed to represent a relatively more benign manifestation of increased upper airway resistance during sleep.

The cumulative evidence collected over the last several decades indicates that the consequences of untreated OSAS in young children can be serious. These include excessive daytime sleepiness; learning and behavioral problems that include aggression, hyperactivity, restlessness, and decreased school performance; impaired somatic growth; pulmonary hypertension and cor pulmonale; systemic hypertension and left ventricular dysfunction; decreased quality of life; depressive mood; and global increases in health related costs. The prevalence of OSAS in children is currently estimated at up to 3% among two to eight-year-old children (3–5). However, habitual snoring during sleep, the hallmark indicator of increased upper airway resistance is much more frequent in children, and may affect up to 27% of all school-age children (6–8).

The vast majority of OSAS occurrences in children are due, at least to some extent, to the presence of enlarged tonsils and adenoids. However, our current understanding of childhood OSAS supports the existence of alterations in structural and anatomical characteristics, protective reflexes, and neuromotor abnormalities of the upper airway, all of which are implicated to a greater or lesser extent in any given child. In support of such a working model, several reports have suggested that pediatric OSAS is more common in those children with a family history of OSAS, children with allergy, children born prematurely, in African-American children, and in children with chronic upper and lower respiratory tract diseases (5,9–14).

III. Obesity as a Risk Factor for OSAS

Obesity is by far the most prominent risk factor for sleep apnea in adults, and has now clearly emerged as a leading risk factor for sleep apnea in children as well. The prevalence and severity of increased body fat in children and adolescents is dramatically increasing worldwide, and is currently affecting 15–17% of all children and adolescents (15–20). Childhood obesity is associated with a higher risk for development of OSAS, and the severity of OSAS appears to be proportional to some extent to the degree of obesity (5,21–25).

Adenotonsillar hyperplasia/hypertrophy is not always the main contributing factor to the development of OSAS in obese children (22,24–27). The exact mechanisms by which obesity may increase the risk of OSAS or vice versa are unclear. Fatty infiltration of upper airway structures, decreased lung volumes and oxygen reserve, and increased work of breathing during sleep have all been implicated (28–32). Although obesity may affect the anatomy of the respiratory system including that of the upper airway, central mechanisms regulating ventilatory control and pharyngeal airway tone may also explain the link between obesity and sleep-disordered breathing. In addition, the metabolic activity of the visceral fat in obese individuals may further contribute to the pathogenesis of OSAS. Specifically, the potential role of leptin as an endocrine-mediated link between obesity and OSAS has begun to emerge and will be discussed below.

IV. The Metabolic Consequences of OSAS

One of the morbidities associated with OSAS in adults is type 2 diabetes mellitus and metabolic dysfunction. In the past, type 2 diabetes was a condition that occurred almost exclusively in adults; however, over the past decade an alarming increase in the prevalence of type 2 diabetes mellitus in children has been noted, and now it has surpassed type 1 diabetes to become the most frequent endocrine disorder affecting glucose homeostasis in children (33,34) (Fig. 1).

The emergence of overt diabetes is usually preceded by long periods of insulin resistance during which blood glucose is maintained at near normal levels by compensatory hyperinsulinemia. Insulin resistance per se is an important component of the metabolic syndrome (35). When β cells are no longer able to compensate for underlying insulin resistance through incremental insulin

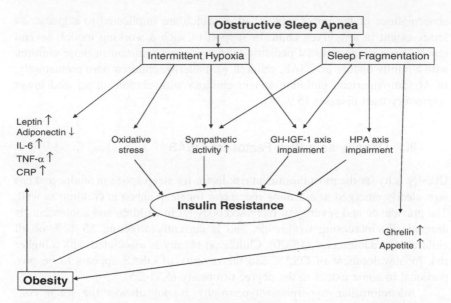

Figure 1 Schematic diagram on the multiple interactions between OSA and obesity in the pathophysiology of insulin resistance. *Abbreviations*: IL-6, interleukin-6; TNF-α, tumor necrosis factor-α; CRP, C-reactive protein; GH-IGF, growth hormone-insulin growth factor-1; HPA axis, hypothalamic-pituitary-adrenal axis.

production, impaired glucose tolerance (IGT) will emerge (36), and is characterized by an excessive blood glucose concentration in the postprandial phase, with fasting glucose levels in the normal range. Under these circumstances, prolonged imbalance between caloric intake and expenditure will eventually lead to the presence of overt diabetes, the latter being characterized by high-fasting and postprandial glycemic levels.

All the three conditions, i.e., insulin resistance, IGT, and overt diabetes, increase the risk of cardiovascular disease. Insulin resistance seems to play a key role in the mechanisms responsible for the metabolic syndrome (37), which represents the clustering of insulin resistance, dyslipidemia, hypertension, and obesity. Although no clear cut definition of the metabolic syndrome has been agreed upon for the pediatric age group (38), the overall prevalence of the metabolic syndrome among 12 to 19-year-old children in the United States has been estimated at 4.2% if adult criteria are applied (39). Using alternatively modified criteria, Weiss et al. found that the risk of the metabolic syndrome was nearly 50% in severely obese youngsters, and that such a risk increased linearly in relation to body mass index (BMI) (40). Elevation of fasting insulin levels and increased BMI during childhood further emerged as the most likely predictors of the metabolic syndrome in adulthood (41,42). Moreover, insulin resistance in childhood was associated with an increased risk for later cardiovascular morbidity and mortality (43–45).

An epidemiologic link between OSAS and metabolic syndrome in adult patients has been reported (46–49). Indeed, habitual snoring was independently associated with abnormalities in glucose tolerance and serum insulin levels or even with overt diabetes mellitus in studies involving large population cohorts (50). Moreover, in a study by Ip et al., patients with OSAS had significantly higher levels of fasting glucose and insulin resistance compared to those without OSAS, independent of the degree of adiposity (51). The severity of OSAS was, in fact, closely correlated with increased insulin resistance (51). In addition, Punjabi et al. demonstrated a significant trend across AHI severity groups for adiposity, glucose intolerance, and calculated indices of insulin resistance. Impairment of glucose tolerance was related to the degree of hypoxemia and the severity of the respiratory disturbance, even after controlling for obesity (52). Indeed, adults with OSAS and those with the metabolic syndrome share many of the same features, namely systemic hypertension, central obesity, and insulin resistance. Therefore, some investigators have proposed to include OSAS within the cluster of the metabolic syndrome (syndrome Z) (53). However, while several reports have found OSAS to be an independent predictor of insulin resistance, i.e., after controlling for BMI (51,52), this association has not been consistently confirmed (54,55). Furthermore, the effect of treatment with continuous positive airway pressure (CPAP) on the metabolic disturbances associated with SDB has yielded conflicting results (56–59).

In children, we are aware of only a few studies that have thus far examined the relationships between OSAS, obesity, and the metabolic syndrome. In a large cohort of snoring children, we have recently shown that both insulin resistance [measured by Insulin/Glucose ratio and HOMA (homeostatic model assessment)] and lipid dysregulation (evidence of increased plasma triglycerides and decreased plasma high density lipoprotein concentrations) are primarily determined by the degree of adiposity, and that OSAS plays a minimal, if any, role in the occurrence of insulin resistance (60). These findings have been subsequently confirmed in a study of Greek children (61). In two other studies conducted in obese children with OSAS, insulin resistance was found to correlate with the severity of the respiratory disease (62,63). However, in a study of nonobese children we found evidence for altered lipid homeostasis in pediatric OSAS, thereby confirming some of the findings in rodent models of sleep apnea (64). Thus, the relative contribution of OSAS to glucose metabolism seems to be negligible in the absence of obesity, while OSAS does appear to alter lipid homeostasis independent of obesity.

The exact pathophysiologic mechanisms linking SDB to insulin resistance and dyslipidemia are not well understood. However, there is growing evidence from clinical and experimental studies suggesting that the metabolic abnormalities observed in OSAS are most likely the result of sleep disruption/fragmentation and IH through alteration of the autonomic and hypothalamic-pituitary-adrenal (HPA) axes and through potentiation of pathways involving inflammatory cytokines and adipokines.

V. Sleep Disruption and Glucose Homeostasis

Clinical and epidemiologic studies have suggested that the sleep disruption that characterizes OSAS plays an important role in the development of the metabolic abnormalities associated with the disorder. Sleep disruption could contribute to the development of insulin resistance and type 2 diabetes mellitus either directly, through deleterious effects on components of glucose regulation, or indirectly, by its effects on appetite regulatory mechanisms leading to increased food ingestion, and consequent weight gain and obesity, the latter then providing a major risk factor for insulin resistance and diabetes.

There have been several epidemiologic studies in recent years reporting on an inverse relationship between sleep duration and body weight in both pediatric (65–68) and adult populations (69–72). In addition, an association between short sleep duration and the development of diabetes has also been described, even after controlling for BMI (73–75). Note that the physiologic studies below were all performed in adults.

In a series of elegant laboratory studies, Spiegel et al. have shown that recurrent partial sleep restriction in healthy young adults induced marked alterations in glucose metabolism, such as decreased glucose tolerance and insulin sensitivity (76,77). The neuroendocrine regulation of appetite was also affected as the levels of the anorexigenic hormone leptin were decreased, whereas the levels of orexigenic factor ghrelin were increased. Importantly, these neuroendocrine abnormalities were correlated with increased hunger and appetite, which ultimately may lead to overeating and increased weight gain (77). Taheri et al. reported similar findings in a large epidemiologic study of more than 1000 adults (69).

Several mechanisms may underlie the association between sleep disruption and glucose homeostasis. Sleep restriction is associated with increased sympathetic activity, and since β-cell function is influenced by autonomic nervous system tone, it is possible that the altered insulin reactivity observed in sleep restriction conditions is related to the increase in tonic sympathetic activity associated with sleep restriction. Another possible explanation involves disturbances in the secretory profiles of the counter-regulatory hormones, growth hormone and cortisol. Indeed, short-term sleep restriction in normal subjects has been shown to worsen glucose tolerance, increase levels of evening cortisol and heighten sympathetic activity (78,79).

Similar to short sleepers, patients with OSAS display higher ghrelin levels, and these increased circulating ghrelin levels have been shown to decrease to nearly those of BMI-matched controls after only 2 days of CPAP treatment (69,80). However, in contrast to short sleepers, patients with OSAS have elevated leptin levels, which are corrected following treatment with CPAP (51,80–83).

One of the immediate, acute, and long-standing consequences of OSAS is sleep fragmentation. To date, there are only very few studies that have specifically examined the possible role of sleep fragmentation or altered sleep architecture on metabolic disturbances. It has been shown that sleep disruption is associated with increased metabolic rate throughout the night compared with nondisrupted sleep (84). In another experimental study, using acoustic stimuli in healthy subjects, sleep fragmentation and suppression of slow wave sleep resulted in elevation of plasma catecholamine levels that correlated with the degree of sleep fragmentation (85). Moreover, sleep fragmentation was also associated with increased morning cortisol levels and hyperlipidemia, with a positive correlation between arousal frequency and morning levels of serum and salivary cortisol (86). Thus, activation of the HPA axis and the presence of abnormally high sympathetic output due to sleep fragmentation (87) have been proposed as the most likely mechanism underlying the metabolic abnormalities observed in OSAS. Further studies are critically needed to validate the hypothesis that sleep fragmentation without reduction in total sleep time may adversely affect metabolic and endocrine function, and plays a pathogenetic role in the metabolic abnormalities observed in patients with OSAS.

VI. IH and Metabolic Abnormalities

To investigate the mechanisms underlying the association between sleep apnea and impaired glucose metabolism, several investigators have used IH as a surrogate model. Humans exposed to hypoxia either in the setting of higher altitude or in the context of an experimental paradigm in the laboratory demonstrate alterations in glucose homeostasis (88–91). Elevations in fasting insulin levels following exposure to hypoxia have also been demonstrated in several animal models (92,93). Using a mouse model of IH, Polotsky et al. have shown that long-term exposure to IH is associated with time-dependent increases in fasting serum insulin levels, along with worsening of glucose tolerance (94). The response to hypoxia, however, was only evident in obese leptin-deficient mice, suggesting that disruption of leptin pathways may be important for hypoxia-mediated alterations in glucose metabolism. The repetitive cycles of hypoxia-reoxygenation with IH increase oxidative stress and induce a number of reactive mechanisms that are regulated, in part, by hypoxia-inducible factor-1α (HIF-1α) (95). HIF-1α induces the expression of several genes that encode numerous glycolytic enzymes (96–99) and glucose transporters. Thus, the IH component of sleep apnea may influence glucose homeostasis through modulation of glucose transport and utilization, and these effects may be due, at least in part, to HIF-1α-mediated transcriptional regulation.

Multiple studies have thus far consistently shown that both adults and children with OSAS exhibit elevated levels of sympathetic activation. Hypoxemia is an important stimulus for altering autonomic activity, with larger desaturations causing greater increases in sympathetic activity (100). However, other factors like hypercapnia can also increase autonomic output (87,101,102). Sympathetic hyperactivity can influence glucose homeostasis by increasing glycogen breakdown and gluconeogenesis. Autonomic activation in sleep apnea may also increase corticotropin releasing hormone and cortisol production (103). However, studies on CPAP effects on cortisol levels have thus far revealed conflicting results (103–105).

While several studies have focused on the effects of IH on glucose homeostasis and insulin metabolism, little information is currently available on the impact of IH on lipid metabolism. This is of particular importance because abnormalities in lipid profile may act to increase cardiovascular risk in susceptible populations. In a series of clinical studies, IH and obesity were shown to interact and alter lipid metabolism in sleep apnea patients (81,106–108). Recent work in a mouse model of IH demonstrated that IH exposures during sleep alter lipid biosynthesis and cholesterol uptake in the liver and lead to lipid abnormalities in lean mice, and further showed that obesity can mask the effects of IH on lipid metabolism (109). Moreover, the degree of the metabolic dysregulation was dependent on the severity of the hypoxic stimulus (110) and was mediated by HIF-1α related pathways (111).

VII. IGF-1—A Possible Link Between OSAS and Impaired Glucose Metabolism

Another important factor linking sleep apnea to impaired glucose metabolism is insulin growth factor-1 (IGF-1). Indeed, lower circulating levels of IGF-1 and its main binding protein in the serum, IGF-binding protein 3, predict the subsequent risk for development of impaired glucose tolerance and type 2 diabetes mellitus (112). As in obesity, impairments in the GH/IGF-1 axis activity are observed in patients with OSAS (104,113–115). This appears to be independent of the degree of adiposity, since these abnormalities are restored following treatment by nocturnal CPAP treatment, in the absence of any change in body weight (104,113,114). Of note, studies in children have also shown impaired activity of the GH/IGF-1 axis, with significant improvement following adenotonsillectomy (116). It is currently postulated that both the sleep disruption and IH associated with OSAS are potential mechanisms mediating GH/IGF-1 axis dysfunction.

VIII. Inflammation

Systemic subclinical inflammation could be yet another link underlying the associations between OSAS, obesity, and the metabolic syndrome. Inflammatory cytokines play an important role in mediating peripheral insulin resistance by inhibiting glucose uptake by fat and muscle, increasing the level of counter-regulatory hormones, and inducing the release of free fatty acid via stimulation of lipolysis (117–120). Obese children of all ages have evidence of a low-grade inflammatory state, and the degree of inflammation, as measured by circulating cytokines like interleukin-6 (IL-6) and tumor necrosis factor-α (TNF-α) and acute phase reactants like C-reactive protein (CRP), is often correlated with the presence of insulin resistance and dyslipidemia (121–123). OSAS-related IH and sleep fragmentation may alter glucose metabolism by promoting the release of inflammatory cytokines, such as IL-6, from either liver or adipocyte sources. Indeed, clinical studies have shown that plasma levels of IL-6 and TNF-α are higher in adult patients with OSAS compared with normal subjects, and correlate with both the degree of excessive daytime sleepiness and with fasting plasma insulin levels (124,125). In children, plasma IL-6 levels were found to be elevated in children with OSAS, with a linear correlation with the severity of the disease, independent of obesity (126). Plasma TNF-α levels were also found to be elevated in children with OSAS, and were highly correlated with the degree of sleep fragmentation (127). TNF-α is a key intermediate in the development of insulin resistance and metabolic syndrome (128). For example, although obese mice with homozygous null mutations of either TNF-α or TNF receptors remain obese, they appear to be protected from developing obesity-related insulin resistance (129,130). Additionally, both in vitro (131) and in vivo (132) studies have shown that TNF-α can impair insulin signaling and lead to derangements in insulin mediated glucose uptake and storage, such that inhibition of TNF-α improves insulin sensitivity.

IL-6 is another cytokine that has been implicated in the pathogenesis of insulin resistance and type 2 diabetes mellitus. IL-6 is a pro-inflammatory cytokine that largely controls the synthesis of CRP, and is also an important risk factor for atherosclerosis and cardiovascular morbidity (133,134). In addition to its inflammatory cell sources, IL-6 is also released from adipose tissue, and therefore IL-6 plasma levels reflect to some extent the degree of adiposity (135,136). As mentioned above, increased plasma levels of IL-6 and CRP are found in adults and children with OSAS (124–126,137–141), in obese subjects (135,136), as well as in those with type 2 diabetes mellitus and the metabolic syndrome (141–146). However, the exact role of IL-6 in disorders of glucose metabolism is still unclear.

Taken together, the recurring hypoxemia and arousals that occur during the night in patients with OSAS induces a heightened level of systemic inflammation, which is manifested through elevated circulating inflammatory cytokines and other related substances. The addition of sleep deprivation and obesity burdens, in the context of OSAS, operates therefore to amplify the global cytokine response, and this contributes to the metabolic derangements described heretofore.

IX. Adipokines

Our understanding of adipocyte biology has dramatically changed in the last decade. Adipose tissue is considered today to be an extremely active and responsive endocrine tissue whose activity is modulated and controlled through a host of afferent messages from several different tissue sources, including the autonomic nervous system and the HPA axis. Furthermore, adipose tissue responses consist of the release of several cytokines that convey precise efferent messages to target organs. These findings have launched a resurgence of interest in the complex interactions among OSAS, obesity, and the metabolic syndrome.

In a series of studies involving both humans and animal models, the potential role of leptin as an endocrine link between obesity, metabolic dysfunction, and SDB has begun to emerge. Leptin, an adipocyte-derived hormone regulating energy expenditure and food intake (147), is readily found in the circulation, and its levels appear to be determined by the degree of obesity. Indeed, obesity is associated with peripheral and central leptin resistance, which in turn leads to relatively ineffective elevation of circulating leptin levels (148). Plasma leptin levels appear to be determined as well by the severity of OSAS, particularly by the degree and duration of hypoxemia (51,124,125,149–151). Conversely, plasma leptin levels are decreased following weight loss (152) or treatment of OSAS with CPAP (56,58), the latter effect occurring independently from changes in BMI (81,82).

In snoring children, both obesity and OSAS severity were found to contribute to the elevation of plasma leptin levels. In a recent study, we found that plasma leptin levels were elevated in children with OSAS independent of obesity, and were significantly lower in those children with OSAS but with minimal hypoxemia compared with children with OSAS and with more pronounced hypoxemia. Furthermore, and as anticipated from the aforementioned considerations, plasma leptin levels were also found to correlate with the degree of insulin resistance among snoring children (153).

Animal studies have clearly demonstrated that hypoxia induces increases in both leptin gene expression (via nuclear binding and transcriptional activation of HIF-1α) and plasma leptin levels (94,154,155). Moreover, in leptin-deficient mice, pharmacologically increased leptin bioavailability protected against development of glucose intolerance and insulin resistance during intermittent hypoxia (94). Thus, the elevation of leptin levels in children with OSAS may represent an important compensatory mechanism aiming to minimize metabolic dysfunction and preserve glucose homeostasis. In addition, leptin is a powerful respiratory stimulant (156,157). Plasma leptin levels are higher in adult sleep apnea patients than in controls matched for BMI (158). Furthermore, hypercapnic patients with OSAS have higher leptin levels than eucapnic, BMI-matched controls with sleep apnea (159). Therefore, leptin release could provide an adaptive mechanism aiming to enhance ventilation in patients with respiratory depression subsequent to obesity (156,157) and in those with respiratory impairment due to OSAS. It is, of course, possible that the elevation of plasma leptin levels in OSAS may reflect a respiratory compensatory mechanism to the alveolar hypoventilation induced by increased upper airway resistance. Conversely, high circulating leptin levels suggest increased leptin resistance at the level of the central nervous system.

In addition to its now rather well established functions in energy balance, leptin clearly possesses pro-inflammatory properties (160,161). Recent evidence further suggests that leptin is also involved in several aspects of cardiovascular morbidity, including ventricular hypertrophy, systemic hypertension, and angiogenesis, with increased leptin levels being associated with decreased arterial distensibility as well as with increased CRP levels, all of these remaining valid after controlling for adiposity (162–166). Indeed, plasma leptin levels were found to correlate with plasma CRP levels in snoring children (153). Increased sympathetic activity and hypertension are present in both adults and children with OSAS (87,167–171). It has been suggested that OSAS-induced sympathetic activity may lead to alteration in leptin expression, and that these relationships between autonomic nervous system recruitment and leptin pathways may explain the almost immediate reduction in leptin levels and concomitant improvements in sympathetic tone following 24 hours of treatment with CPAP (51,171). On the other hand, leptin can induce increased sympathetic activity, as well as elevated heart rate and blood pressure (77,171–173). Thus, elevated leptin levels in subjects with OSAS are likely to contribute either directly or indirectly to the cardiovascular morbidity associated with the disorder.

Adiponectin is the most abundant adipose tissue-specific protein and is exclusively expressed and secreted from adipocytes. Adiponectin has anti-inflammatory, anti-atherogenic, and insulin-sensitizing properties (175). Reduced plasma adiponectin levels increase the risk for cardiovascular morbidity and insulin resistance, and paradoxically also increases the risk for obesity (176–183). Previous studies concerning plasma adiponectin levels in adults with OSAS have thus far revealed conflicting results (183–187). In snoring children, circulating adiponectin levels are primarily linked to obesity, and are inversely correlated with the severity of insulin resistance and plasma CRP levels (153).

In contrast to leptin and adiponectin, the role of resistin in human is still unclear. Although initially described as a fat tissue–derived hormone that increased insulin resistance (thereby its designation), more recent studies have thus far failed to demonstrate any association between resistin levels and insulin resistance (188,189). Of note, Harsch et al. recently reported a significant, albeit weak, correlation between plasma resistin levels and insulin resistance in obese adult patients with OSAS (190). However, while insulin resistance improved with CPAP treatment, there were no concomitant changes in plasma resistin levels (190). In children, no association has emerged between plasma resistin concentrations and either the severity of OSAS or the degree of obesity (153).

In summary, in the context of obesity-related contributions to the development of SDB in children, the role of adipokines in general, and more particularly that played by leptin, merits further study. More particularly, the role of leptin in the pathophysiology of metabolic and cardiac morbidity and in upper airway dysfunction and altered ventilatory responses to increased upper resistance remains to be fully elucidated.

X. Summary

The spectrum of OSAS in children is rapidly evolving. There is clearly an increased body of evidence pointing to a multiplicity of OSAS-induced end-organ morbidities, and certainly one of these consequences is reflected through substantial metabolic alterations. Furthermore, many of the OSAS-associated morbidities appear to be mediated, at least in part, by the systemic recruitment of inflammatory and oxidant pathways. The increased prevalence of obesity among children with OSAS is further likely to enhance the magnitude of OSAS and its associated consequences, and reciprocally, the presence of OSAS may amplify obesity and its related morbidities.

Acknowledgments

Parts of this work were supported by the National Institutes of Health (grant HL-65270), The Children's Foundation Endowment for Sleep Research, and the Commonwealth of Kentucky Challenge for Excellence Trust Fund.

References

1. Gozal D, Simakajornboon N, Holbrook CR, et al. Secular trends in obesity and parentally-reported daytime sleepiness among children referred to a pediatric sleep center for snoring and suspected sleep-disordered breathing (SDB). Sleep 2006; 29: A74 (abstr).
2. American Thoracic Society. Standards and indications for cardiopulmonary sleep studies in children. Am J Crit Care Med 1995; 153:866–878.
3. Ali NJ, Pitson DJ, Stradling JR. Snoring, sleep disturbance, and behaviour in 4-5 year olds. Arch Dis Child 1993; 68:360–363.
4. Gislason T, Benediktsdottir B. Snoring, apneic episodes, and nocturnal hypoxemia among children 6 months to 6 years old. An epidemiologic study of lower limit of prevalence. Chest 1995; 107:963–966.
5. Redline S, Tishler PV, Schluchter M, et al. Risk factors for sleep-disordered breathing in children. Associations with obesity, race, and respiratory problems. Am J Respir Crit Care Med 1999; 159:1527–1532.
6. Corbo GM, Fuciarelli F, Foresi A, et al. Snoring in children: association with respiratory symptoms and passive smoking. BMJ 1989; 299:1491–1494.
7. Owen GO, Canter RJ, Robinson A. Snoring, apnoea and ENT symptoms in the paediatric community. Clin Otolaryngol Allied Sci 1996; 21:130–134.

8. Ferreira AM, Clemente V, Gozal D, et al. Snoring in Portuguese primary school children. Pediatrics 2000; 106:e64.

9. Redline S, Tishler PV, Hans MG, et al. Racial differences in sleep-disordered breathing in African-Americans and Caucasians. Am J Respir Crit Care Med 1997; 155:186–192.

10. Urschitz MS, Guenther A, Eitner S, et al. Risk factors and natural history of habitual snoring. Chest 2004; 126:790–800.

11. Mitchell EA, Thompson JM. Snoring in the first year of life. Acta Pediatr 2003; 92:425–429.

12. Montgomery-Downs HE, Gozal D. Sleep habits and risk factors for sleep-disordered breathing in infants and young toddlers in Louisville, Kentucky. Sleep Med 2006; 7:211–219.

13. Montgomery-Downs HE, Gozal D. Primary snoring in infancy: mental development effects and contribution of secondhand smoke exposure. Pediatrics 2006; 117: e496–e502.

14. Rosen CL, Larkin EK, Kirchner HL, et al. Prevalence and risk factors for sleep-disordered breathing in 8- to 11-year-old children: association with race and prematurity. J Pediatr 2003; 142:383–389.

15. Dietz WH, Robinson TN. Clinical practice. Overweight children and adolescents. N Eng J Med 2005; 352:2100–2109.

16. Magarey AM, Daniels LA, Boulton TJ. Prevalence of overweight and obesity in Australian children and adolescents: reassessment of 1985 and 1995 data against new standard international definitions. Med J Aust 2001; 174:561–564.

17. Lobstein T, Baur L, Uauy R. IASO International Obesity Task Force. Obesity in children and young people: a crisis in public health. Obes Rev 2004; 5(suppl 1): 1–4.

18. Ogden CL, Kuczmarski RJ, Flegal KM, et al. Centers for Disease Control and Prevention 2000 growth charts for the United States: improvements to the 1977 National Center for Health Statistics version. Pediatrics 2002; 109:45–60.

19. Ogden CL, Flegal KM, Carroll MD, et al. Prevalence and trends in overweight among US children and adolescents, 1999–2000. JAMA 2002; 288:1728–1732.

20. Guilleminault C, Korobkin R, Winkle R. Review of 50 children with obstructive sleep apnea syndrome. Lung 1981; 159:275–287.

21. Marcus CL, Curtis S, Koerner CB, et al. Evaluation of pulmonary function and polysomnography in obese children and adolescents. Pediatr Pulmonol 1996; 21: 176–183.

22. Young T, Peppard PE, Gottlieb DJ. Epidemiology of obstructive sleep apnea – a population health perspective. Am J Respir Crit Care Med 2002; 165:1217–1239.

23. Mallory GB Jr., Fiser DH, Jackson R. Sleep-associated breathing disorders in morbidly obese children and adolescents. J Pediatr 1989; 115:892–897.

24. Silvestri JM, Weese-Mayer DE, Bass MT, et al. Polysomnography in obese children with a history of sleep-associated breathing disorders. Pediatr Pulmonol 1993; 16:124–129.

25. Sogut A, Altin R, Uzun L, et al. Prevalence of obstructive sleep apnea syndrome and associated symptoms in 3-11-year-old Turkish children. Pediatr Pulmonol 2005; 39:251–256.

26. Kahn A, Mozin MJ, Rebuffat E, et al. Sleep pattern alterations and brief airway obstructions in overweight infants. Sleep 1989; 12:430–438.

27. Shine NP, Coates HL, Lannigan FJ. Obstructive sleep apnea, morbid obesity, and adenotonsillar surgery: a review of the literature. Int J Ped Otolaryngol 2005; 69:1475–1482.
28. Horner RL, Mohiaddin RH, Lowell DG, et al. Sites and size of fat deposits around the pharynx in obese patients with obstructive sleep apnoea and weight matched controls. Eur Respire J 1989; 2:613–622.
29. Suratt PM, Wilhoit SC, Atkinson RL. Elevated pulse flow resistance in awake obese subjects with obstructive sleep apnea. Am Rev Respir Dis 1983; 127:162–165.
30. White DP, Lombard RM, Cadieux RJ, et al. Pharyngeal resistance in normal humans: influence of gender, age, and obesity. J Appl Physiol 1985; 58:365–371.
31. Mallory GB Jr., Beckerman RC. Relationships between obesity and respiratory control abnormalities. In: Beckerman RC, Brouillette RT, Hunt CE, eds. Respiratory Control Disorders in Infants and Children. Baltimore: Williams & Wilkins, 1992: 342–351.
32. Naimark A, Cherniack RM. Compliance of the respiratory system and its components in health and obesity. J Appl Physiol 1960; 15:377–382.
33. Vivian EM. Type 2 diabetes in children and adolescents–the next epidemic? Curr Med Res Opin 2006; 22:297–306.
34. Pinhas-Hamiel O, Dolan LM, Daniels SR, et al. Increased incidence of non-insulin-dependent diabetes mellitus among adolescents. J Pediatr 1996; 128:608–615.
35. Haffner SM, Stern MP, Hazuda HP, et al. Cardiovascular risk factors in confirmed prediabetic individuals. Does the clock for coronary heart disease start ticking before the onset of clinical diabetes? JAMA 1990; 263:2893–2898.
36. Kahn SE. The relative contributions of insulin resistance and beta-cell dysfunction to the pathophysiology of type 2 diabetes. Diabetologia 2003; 46:3–19.
37. Sowers JR, Frohlich ED. Insulin and insulin resistance: impact on blood pressure and cardiovascular disease. Med Clin North Am 2004; 88:63–82.
38. Tresaco B, Bueno G, Pineda I, et al. Homeostatic model assessment (HOMA) index cut-off values to identify the metabolic syndrome in children. J Physiol Biochem 2005; 61:381–388.
39. Cook S, Weitzman M, Auinger P, et al. Prevalence of a metabolic syndrome phenotype in adolescents: findings from the third National Health and Nutrition Examination Survey, 1988–1994. Arch Pediatr Adolesc Med 2003; 157:821–827.
40. Weiss R, Dziura J, Burgert TS, et al. Obesity and the metabolic syndrome in children and adolescents. N Eng J Med 2004; 350:2362–2374.
41. Srinivasan SR, Myers L, Berenson GS. Predictability of childhood adiposity and insulin for developing insulin resistance syndrome (syndrome X) in young adulthood: the Bogalusa Heart Study. Diabetes 2002; 51:204–209.
42. Steinberger J, Moorehead C, Katch V, et al. Relationship between insulin resistance and abnormal lipid profile in obese adolescents. J Pediatr 1995; 126:690–695.
43. Bao W, Srinivasan SR, Berenson GS. Persistent elevation of plasma insulin levels is associated with increased cardiovascular risk in children and young adults. The Bogalusa Heart Study. Circulation 1996; 93:54–59.
44. Berenson GS, Srinivasan SR, Bao W, et al. Association between multiple cardiovascular risk factors and atherosclerosis in children and young adults. The Bogalusa Heart Study. N Eng J Med 1998; 338:1650–1656.
45. Cruz ML, Huang TT, Johnson MS, et al. Insulin sensitivity and blood pressure in black and white children. Hypertension 2002; 40:18–22.

46. Strohl KP, Novak RD, Singer W, et al. Insulin levels, blood pressure and sleep apnea. Sleep 1994; 17:614–618.
47. Strohl KP. Diabetes and sleep apnea. Sleep 1996; 19:S225–S228.
48. Grunstein RR, Stenlof K, Hedner J, et al. Impact of obstructive sleep apnea and sleepiness on metabolic and cardiovascular risk factors in the Swedish Obese Subjects (SOS) Study. Int J Obes Relat Metab Disord 1995; 19:410–418.
49. Grunstein RR. Metabolic aspects of sleep apnea. Sleep 1996; 19: S218–S220.
50. Enright PL, Newman AB, Wahl PW, et al. Prevalence and correlates of snoring and observed apneas in 5,201 older adults. Sleep 1996; 19:531–538.
51. Ip MS, Lam B, Ng MM, et al. Obstructive sleep apnea is independently associated with insulin resistance. Am J Respir Crit Care Med 2002; 165:670–676.
52. Punjabi NM, Sorkin JD, Katzel LI, et al. Sleep-disordered breathing and insulin resistance in middle-aged and overweight men. Am J Respir Crit Care Med 2002; 165:677–682.
53. Wilcox I, McNamara SG, Collins FL, et al. "Syndrome Z": the interaction of sleep apnea, vascular risk factors and heart disease. Thorax 1998; 53(suppl 3): s25–s28.
54. Stoohs RA, Facchini F, Guilleminault C. Insulin resistance and sleep-disordered breathing in healthy humans. Am J Respir Crit Care Med 1996; 154:170–174.
55. Davies RJ, Turner R, Crosby J, et al. Plasma insulin and lipid levels in untreated obstructive sleep apnoea and snoring; their comparison with matched controls and response to treatment. J Sleep Res 1994; 3:180–185.
56. Harsch IA, Schahin SP, Radespiel-Troger M, et al. Continuous positive airway pressure treatment rapidly improves insulin sensitivity in patients with obstructive sleep apnea syndrome. Am J Respir Crit Care Med 2004; 169:156–162.
57. Brooks B, Cistulli PA, Borkman M, et al. Obstructive sleep apnea in obese noninsulin-dependent diabetic patients: effect of continuous positive airway pressure treatment on insulin responsiveness. J Clin Endocrinol Metab 1994; 79:1681–1685.
58. Saarelainen S, Lahtela J, Kallonen E. Effect of nasal CPAP treatment on insulin sensitivity and plasma leptin. J Sleep Res 1997; 6:146–147.
59. Smurra M, Philip P, Taillard J, et al. CPAP treatment does not affect glucose-insulin metabolism in sleep apneic patients. Sleep Med 2001; 2:207–213.
60. Tauman R, O'Brien LM, Ivanenko A, et al. Obesity rather than severity of sleep-disordered breathing as the major determinant of insulin resistance and altered lipidemia in snoring children. Pediatrics 2005; 116(1):e66–e73.
61. Kaditis AG, Alexopoulos EI, Damani E, et al. Obstructive sleep-disordered breathing and fasting insulin levels in nonobese children. Pediatr Pulmonol 2005; 40:515–523.
62. de la Eva RC, Baur LA, Donaghue KC, et al. Metabolic correlates with obstructive sleep apnea in obese subjects. J Pediatr 2002; 140:641–643.
63. Waters KA, Sitha S, O'brien LM, et al. Follow-up on metabolic markers in children treated for obstructive sleep apnea. Am J Respir Crit Care Med 2006; 174(4): 455–60.
64. Sans Capdevila O, Kheirandish-Gozal L, Tauman R, et al. Sleep disordered breathing and metabolic dysfunction in children: a pre- vs. postadenotonsillectomy study. Sleep 2006; 29:A74.
65. Reilly JJ, Armstrong J, Dorosty AR, et al. Avon Longitudinal Study of Parents and Children Study Team. Early life risk factors for obesity in childhood: cohort study. Br Med J 2005; 330(7504):1357.

66. Sekine M, Yamagami T, Handa K, et al. A dose-response relationship between short sleeping hours and childhood obesity: results of the Toyama Birth Cohort Study. Child Care Health Dev 2002; 28:163–170.

67. Locard E, Mamelle N, Billette A, et al. Risk factors of obesity in a five year old population. Parental versus environmental factors. Int J Obes Relat Metab Disord 1992; 16:721–729.

68. Gupta NK, Mueller WH, Chan W, et al. Is obesity associated with poor sleep quality in adolescents? Am J Hum Biol 2002; 14:762–768.

69. Taheri S, Lin L, Austin D, et al. Short sleep duration is associated with reduced leptin, elevated ghrelin, and increased body mass index. PLoS Med 2004; 1:e62.

70. Hasler G, Buysse DJ, Klaghofer R, et al. The association between short sleep duration and obesity in young adults: a 13-year prospective study. Sleep 2004; 27:661–666.

71. Vioque J, Torres A, Quiles J. Time spent watching television, sleep duration and obesity in adults living in Valencia, Spain. Int J Obes Relat Metab Disord 2000; 24:1683–1688.

72. Vorona RD, Winn MP, Babineau TW, et al. Overweight and obese patients in a primary care population report less sleep than patients with a normal body mass index. Arch Intern Med 2005; 165:25–30.

73. Ayas NT, White DP, Al-Delaimy WK, et al. A prospective study of self-reported sleep duration and incident diabetes in women. Diabetes Care 2003; 26:380–384.

74. Nilsson PM, Roost M, Engstrom G, et al. Incidence of diabetes in middle-aged men is related to sleep disturbances. Diabetes Care 2004; 27:2464–2469.

75. Meisinger C, Heier M, Loewel H; MONICA/KORA Augsburg Cohort Study. Sleep disturbance as a predictor of type 2 diabetes mellitus in men and women from the general population. Diabetologia 2005; 48:235–238.

76. Spiegel K, Leproult R, L'hermite-Baleriaux M, et al. Leptin levels are dependent on sleep duration: relationships with sympathovagal balance, carbohydrate regulation, cortisol, and thyrotropin. J Clin Endocrinol Metab 2004; 89:5762–5771.

77. Spiegel K, Tasali E, Penev P, et al. Brief communication: Sleep curtailment in healthy young men is associated with decreased leptin levels, elevated ghrelin levels, and increased hunger and appetite. Ann Intern Med 2004; 141:846–850.

78. Spiegel K, Leproult R, Van Cauter E. Impact of sleep debt on metabolic and endocrine function. Lancet 1999; 354:1435–1439.

79. Spiegel K, Knutson K, Leproult R, et al. Sleep loss: a novel risk factor for insulin resistance and Type 2 diabetes. J Appl Physiol 2005; 99:2008–2019.

80. Harsch IA, Konturek PC, Koebnick C, et al. Leptin and ghrelin levels in patients with obstructive sleep apnoea: effect of CPAP treatment. Eur Respir J 2003; 22:251–257.

81. Chin K, Shimizu K, Nakamura T, et al. Changes in intra-abdominal visceral fat and serum leptin levels in patients with obstructive sleep apnea syndrome following nasal continuous positive airway pressure therapy. Circulation 1999; 100:706–712.

82. Sanner BM, Kollhosser P, Buechner N, et al. Influence of treatment on leptin levels in patients with obstructive sleep apnoea. Eur Respir J 2004; 23:601–604.

83. Shimizu K, Chin K, Nakamura T, et al. Plasma leptin levels and cardiac sympathetic function in patients with obstructive sleep apnoea-hypopnoea syndrome. Thorax 2002; 57:429–434.

84. Bonnet MH, Berry RB, Arand DL. Metabolism during normal, fragmented, and recovery sleep. J Appl Physiol 1991; 71:1112–1118.

85. Tiemeier H, Pelzer E, Jonck L, et al. Plasma catecholamines and selective slow wave sleep deprivation. Neuropsychobiology 2002; 45:81–86.

86. Ekstedt M, Akerstedt T, Soderstrom M. Microarousals during sleep are associated with increased levels of lipids, cortisol, and blood pressure. Psychosom Med 2004; 66:925–931.

87. Somers VK, Dyken ME, Clary MP, et al. Sympathetic neural mechanisms in obstructive sleep apnea. J Clin Invest 1995; 96:1897–1904.

88. Larsen JJ, Hansen JM, Olsen NV, et al. The effect of altitude hypoxia on glucose homeostasis in men. J Physiol 1997; 504:241–249.

89. Braun B, Rock PB, Zamudio S, et al. Women at altitude: short-term exposure to hypoxia and/or alpha(1)-adrenergic blockade reduces insulin sensitivity. J Appl Physiol 2001; 91:623–631.

90. Davidson MB, Aoki VS. Fasting glucose homeostasis in rats after chronic exposure to hypoxia. Am J Physiol 1970; 219:378–383.

91. Oltmanns KM, Gehring H, Rudolf S, et al. Hypoxia causes glucose intolerance in humans. Am J Respir Crit Care Med 2004; 169:1231–1237.

92. Cheng N, Cai W, Jiang M, et al. Effect of hypoxia on blood glucose, hormones, and insulin receptor functions in newborn calves. Pediatr Res 1997; 41:852–856.

93. Raff H, Bruder ED, Jankowski BM, et al. Effect of neonatal hypoxia on leptin, insulin, growth hormone and body composition in the rat. Horm Metab Res 2001; 33:151–155.

94. Polotsky VY, Li J, Punjabi NM, et al. Intermittent hypoxia increases insulin resistance in genetically obese mice. J Physiol 2003; 552:253–264.

95. Semenza GL. Hypoxia-inducible factor 1: master regulator of O2 homeostasis. Curr Opin Genet Dev 1998; 8:588–594.

96. Iyer NV, Kotch LE, Agani F, et al. Cellular and developmental control of O2 homeostasis by hypoxia-inducible factor 1 alpha. Genes Dev 1998; 12:149–162.

97. Minchenko A, Leshchinsky I, Opentanova I, et al. Hypoxia-inducible factor-1-mediated expression of the 6-phosphofructo-2-kinase/fructose-2,6-bisphosphatase-3 (PFKFB3) gene. Its possible role in the Warburg effect. J Biol Chem 2002; 277:6183–6187.

98. Minchenko O, Opentanova I, Minchenko D, et al. Hypoxia induces transcription of 6-phosphofructo-2-kinase/fructose-2,6-biphosphatase-4 gene via hypoxia-inducible factor-1alpha activation. FEBS Lett 2004; 576:14–20.

99. Minchenko O, Opentanova I, Caro J. Hypoxic regulation of the 6-phosphofructo-2-kinase/fructose-2,6-bisphosphatase gene family (PFKFB-1-4) expression in vivo. FEBS Lett 2003; 554:264–270.

100. Smith ML, Niedermaier ON, Hardy SM, et al. Role of hypoxemia in sleep apnea-induced sympathoexcitation. J Auton Nerv Syst 1996; 56:184–190.

101. Somers VK, Mark AL, Zavala DC, et al. Contrasting effects of hypoxia and hypercapnia on ventilation and sympathetic activity in humans. J Appl Physiol 1989; 67:2101–2106.

102. Somers VK, Mark AL, Zavala DC, et al. Influence of ventilation and hypocapnia on sympathetic nerve responses to hypoxia in normal humans. J Appl Physiol 1989; 67:2095–2100.

103. Bratel T, Wennlund A, Carlstrom K. Pituitary reactivity, androgens and catecholamines in obstructive sleep apnoea. Effects of continuous positive airway pressure treatment (CPAP). Respir Med 1999; 93:1–7.
104. Grunstein RR, Handelsman DJ, Lawrence SJ, et al. Neuroendocrine dysfunction in sleep apnea: reversal by continuous positive airways pressure therapy. J Clin Endocrinol Metab 1989; 68:352–358.
105. Grunstein RR, Stewart DA, Lloyd H, et al. Acute withdrawal of nasal CPAP in obstructive sleep apnea does not cause a rise in stress hormones. Sleep 1996; 19:774–782.
106. Newman AB, Nieto FJ, Guidry U, et al. Relation of sleep-disordered breathing to cardiovascular disease risk factors: the Sleep Heart Health Study. Am J Epidemiol 2001; 154:50–59.
107. Chin K, Nakamura T, Shimizu K, et al. Effects of nasal continuous positive airway pressure on soluble cell adhesion molecules in patients with obstructive sleep apnea syndrome. Am J Med 2000; 109:562–567.
108. Robinson GV, Pepperell JC, Segal HC, et al. Circulating cardiovascular risk factors in obstructive sleep apnoea: data from randomised controlled trials. Thorax 2004; 59:777–782.
109. Li J, Thorne LN, Punjabi NM, et al. Intermittent hypoxia induces hyperlipidemia in lean mice. Circ Res 2005; 97:698–706.
110. Li J, Savransky V, Nanayakkara A, et al. Hyperlipidemia and lipid peroxidation are dependent on the severity of chronic intermittent hypoxia. J Appl Physiol 2007; 102(2):557–563.
111. Li J, Bosch-Marce M, Nanayakkara A, et al. Altered metabolic responses to intermittent hypoxia in mice with partial deficiency of hypoxia-inducible factor-1alpha. Physiol Genomics 2006; 25:450–457.
112. Sandhu MS, Heald AH, Gibson JM, et al. Circulating concentrations of insulin-like growth factor-I and development of glucose intolerance: a prospective observational study. Lancet 2002; 359:1740–1745.
113. Saini J, Krieger J, Brandenberger G, et al. Continuous positive airway pressure treatment. Effects on growth hormone, insulin and glucose profiles in obstructive sleep apnea patients. Horm Metab Res 1993; 25:375–381.
114. Cooper BG, White JE, Ashworth LA, et al. Hormonal and metabolic profiles in subjects with obstructive sleep apnea syndrome and the acute effects of nasal continuous positive airway pressure (CPAP) treatment. Sleep 1995; 18:172–179.
115. McArdle N, Hillman D, Beilin L, et al. Metabolic Risk Factors for Vascular Disease in Obstructive Sleep Apnea: A Matched Controlled Study. Am J Respir Crit Care Med 2007; 175:190–195.
116. Bar A, Tarasiuk A, Segev Y, et al. The effect of adenotonsillectomy on serum insulin-like growth factor-I and growth in children with obstructive sleep apnea syndrome. J Pediatr 1999; 135:76–80.
117. Hotamisligil GS, Shargill NS, Spiegelman BM. Adipose expression of tumor necrosis factor-alpha: direct role in obesity-linked insulin resistance. Science 1993; 259:87–91.
118. Hotamisligil GS, Spiegelman BM. Tumor necrosis factor alpha: a key component of the obesity-diabetes link. Diabetes 1994; 43:1271–1278.
119. Stumvoll M, Haring H. Insulin resistance and insulin sensitizers. Horm Res 2001; 55:3–13.

120. Hotamisligil GS, Murray DL, Choy LN, et al. Tumor necrosis factor alpha inhibits signaling from the insulin receptor. Proc Natl Acad Sci 1994; 91:4854–4858.
121. Schwarzenberg SJ, Sinaiko AR. Obesity and inflammation in children. Ped Respir Rev 2006; 7:239–246.
122. Moon YS, Kim DH, Song DK. Serum tumor necrosis factor-alpha levels and components of the metabolic syndrome in obese adolescents. Metabolism 2004; 53:863–867.
123. Lambert M, Delvin EE, Paradis G, et al. C-reactive protein and features of the metabolic syndrome in a population-based sample of children and adolescents. Clin Chem 2004; 50:1762–1768.
124. Vgontzas AN, Papanicolaou DA, Bixler EO, et al. Sleep apnea and daytime sleepiness and fatigue: relation to visceral obesity, insulin resistance, and hyper-cytokinemia. J Clin Endocrinol Metab 2000; 85:1151–1158.
125. Vgontzas AN, Bixler EO, Chrousos GP. Metabolic disturbances in obesity versus sleep apnoea: the importance of visceral obesity and insulin resistance. J Intern Med 2003; 254:32–44.
126. Tauman R, O'Brien LM, Gozal D. Hypoxemia and obesity modulate plasma C-reactive protein and interleukin-6 levels in sleep-disordered breathing. Sleep Breath 2007; 11(2):77–84.
127. Serpero LD, Kheirandish L, Sans Capevila O, Tauman R, Gozal D. Sleep Fragmentation and Circulating TNFα Levels in Children with Sleep Disordered Breathing. Presented at: 2005 ALA/ATS International Conference, May 19–24, 2005, San Diego, CA. Abstracted in: Proc. Am. Thor Soc. 2005; 3:A555.
128. Hotamisligil GS. Mechanisms of TNF-alpha-induced insulin resistance. Exp Clin Endocrinol Diabetes 1999; 107:119–125.
129. Uysal KT, Wiesbrock SM, Marino MW, et al. Protection from obesity-induced insulin resistance in mice lacking TNF-alpha function. Nature 1997; 389:610–614.
130. Ventre J, Doebber T, Wu M, et al. Targeted disruption of the tumor necrosis factor-alpha gene: metabolic consequences in obese and nonobese mice. Diabetes 1997; 46:1526–1531.
131. Halse R, Pearson SL, McCormack JG, et al. Effects of tumor necrosis factor-alpha on insulin action in cultured human muscle cells. Diabetes 2001; 50:1102–1109.
132. Youd JM, Rattigan S, Clark MG. Acute impairment of insulin-mediated capillary recruitment and glucose uptake in rat skeletal muscle in vivo by TNF-alpha. Diabetes 2000; 49:1904–1909.
133. Castell J, Gomez-Lechion M, David M. Acute phase response of human hepatocyte: regulation of acute phase protein synthesis by interleukin-6. Hepatology 1990; 12: 1179–1186.
134. Haddy N, Sass C, Droesch S, et al. IL-6, TNF-alpha and atherosclerosis risk indicators in a healthy family population: the STANISLAS cohort. Atherosclerosis 2003, 170:277–283.
135. Roytblat L, Rachinsky M, Fisher A, et al. Raised interleukin-6 levels in obese patients. Obes Res 2000, 8:673–675.
136. Kern PA, Ranganathan S, Li C, et al. Adipose tissue tumor necrosis factor and interleukin-6 expression in human obesity and insulin resistance. Am J Physiol Endocrinol Metab 2001; 280:E745–E751.
137. Tauman R, Ivanenko A, O'Brien LM, et al. Plasma C-reactive protein levels among children with sleep-disordered breathing. Pediatrics 2004; 113:e564–e569.

138. Kheirandish-Gozal L, Sans Capdevila O, Tauman R, et al. Plasma C-reactive protein in non-obese children with obstructive sleep apnea before and after adenotonsillectomy. J. Clin. Sleep Med 2006; 2:301–304.

139. Larkin EK, Rosen CL, Kirchner HL, Storfer-Isser A, et al. Variation of C-reactive protein levels in adolescents: association with sleep-disordered breathing and sleep duration. Circulation 2005; 111:1978–1984.

140. Yokoe T, Minoguchi K, Matsuo H, et al. Elevated levels of C-reactive protein and interleukin-6 in patients with obstructive sleep apnea syndrome are decreased by nasal continuous positive airway pressure. Circulation 2003, 107:1129–1134.

141. Shamsuzzaman ASM, Winnicki M, Lanfranchi P, et al. Elevated C-reactive protein in patients with obstructive sleep apnea. Circulation 2002; 105:2462–2464.

142. Festa A, D'Agostino R Jr., Howard G, et al. Chronic subclinical inflammation as part of the insulin resistance syndrome: the Insulin Resistance Atherosclerosis Study (IRAS). Circulation 2000; 102:42–47.

143. Pradhan AD, Manson JE, Rifai N, et al. C-reactive protein, interleukin 6, and risk of developing type 2 diabetes mellitus. JAMA 2001; 286:327–334.

144. Spranger J, Kroke A, Mohlig M, et al. Inflammatory cytokines and the risk to develop type 2 diabetes: results of the prospective population-based European Prospective Investigation into Cancer and Nutrition (EPIC)-Potsdam Study. Diabetes 2003; 52:812–817.

145. Pickup JC, Chusney GD, Thomas SM, et al. Plasma interleukin-6, tumour necrosis factor alpha and blood cytokine production in type 2 diabetes. Life Sci 2000; 67:291–300.

146. Laaksonen DE, Niskanen L, Nyyssonen K, et al. C-reactive protein and the development of the metabolic syndrome and diabetes in middle-aged men. Diabetologia 2004; 47:1403–1410.

147. Friedman JM. Leptin, leptin receptors and the control of body weight. Nutr Rev 1998; 56:s38–s46.

148. Considine RV, Sinha MK, Heiman ML, et al. Serum immunoreactive - leptin concentrations in normal-weight and obese humans. NEJM 1996; 334:292–295.

149. Ulukavak CT, Kokturk O, Bukan N, et al. Leptin and ghrelin levels in patients with obstructive sleep apnea syndrome. Respiration 2005; 72:395–401.

150. Ozturk L, Unal M, Tamer L, et al. The association of the severity of obstructive sleep apnea with plasma leptin levels. Arch Otolaryngol Head Neck Surg 2003; 129:538–540.

151. Tatsumi K, Kasahara Y, Kurosu K, et al. Sleep oxygen desaturation and circulating leptin in obstructive sleep apnea hypopnea syndrome. Chest 2005, 127:716–721.

152. Havel PJ, Kasim-Karakas S, Mueller W, et al. Relationship of plasma leptin to plasma insulin and adiposity in normal weight and overweight women: effects of dietary fat content and sustained weight loss. J Clin Endocrinol Metab 1996; 81: 4406–4413.

153. Tauman R, Serpero LD, Sans Capdevilla O, et al. Adipokines in children with sleep disordered breathing. Sleep 2007; 30(4):443–449.

154. Ambrosini G, Nath AK, Sierra-Honigmann MR, et al. Transcriptional activation of the human leptin gene in response to hypoxia. Involvement of hypoxia-inducible factor 1. J Biol Chem 2002; 277:34601–34609.

155. Grosfeld A, Andre J, Hauguel-De Mouzon S, et al. Hypoxia-inducible factor 1 transactivates the human leptin gene promoter. J Biol Chem 2002; 277: 42953–42957.
156. O'Donnell CP, Tankersley CG, Polotsky VP, et al. Leptin obesity and respiratory function. Respir Physiol 2000, 119:163–170.
157. O'Donnell CP, Schaub CD, Haines AS, et al. Leptin prevents respiratory depression in obesity. Am J Respir Crit Care Med 1999; 159:1477–1484.
158. Phillips BG, Kato M, Narkiewicz K, et al. Increases in leptin levels, sympathetic drive, and weight gain in obstructive sleep apnea. Am J Physiol Heart Circ Physiol 2000; 279:H234–H237.
159. Phipps PR, Starritt E, Caterson I, et al. Association of serum leptin with hypoventilation in human obesity. Thorax 2002; 57:75–76.
160. Peelman F, Waelput W, Iserentant H, et al. Leptin: linking adipocyte metabolism with cardiovascular and autoimmune diseases. Prog Lipid Res 2004; 43:283–301.
161. Otero M, Lago R, Lago F, et al. Leptin, from fat to inflammation: old questions and new insights. FEBS Lett 2005; 579:295–301.
162. Paolisso G, Tagliamonte MR, Galderisi M, et al. Plasma leptin level is associated with myocardial wall thickness in hypertensive insulin-resistant men. Hypertension 1999; 34:1047–1052.
163. Agata J, Masuda A, Takada M, et al. High plasma immunoreactive leptin level in essential hypertension. Am J Hypertens 1997; 10:1171–1174.
164. Sierra-Honigmann MR, Nath AK, Murakami C, et al. Biological action of leptin as an angiogenic factor. Science 1998; 281:1683–1686.
165. Singhal A, Farooqi IS, Cole TJ, et al. Influence of leptin on arterial distensibility: a novel link between obesity and cardiovascular disease? Circulation 2002; 106: 1919–1924.
166. Shamsuzzaman ASM, Winnicki M, Wolk R, et al. Independent association between plasma leptin and C-reactive protein in healthy humans. Circulation 2004, 109: 2181–2185.
167. Marcus CL, Greene MG, Carroll JL. Blood pressure in children with obstructive sleep apnea. Am J Respir Crit Care Med 1998, 157:1098–1103.
168. Amin RS, Carroll JL, Jeffries JL, et al. Twenty-four hour ambulatory blood pressure in children with sleep-disordered breathing. Am J Respir Crit Care Med 2004, 169:950–956.
169. Loredo JS, Ziegler MG, Ancoli-Israel S, et al. Relationship of arousals from sleep to sympathetic nervous system activity and BP in obstructive sleep apnea. Chest 1999; 116:655–659.
170. Aljadeff G, Gozal S, Schechtman VL, et al. Heart rate variability in children with obstructive sleep apnea. Sleep 1997; 20:151–157.
171. Phillips BG, Somers VK. Neural and humeral mechanisms mediating cardiovascular responses to obstructive sleep apnea. Respir Physiol 2000; 119:181–187.
172. Haynes WG. Interaction between leptin and sympathetic nervous system in hypertension. Curr Hypertens Rep 2000; 2:311–318.
173. Shek EW, Brands MW, Hall JE. Chronic leptin infusion increases arterial pressure. Hypertension 1998; 31:409–414.
174. Kubota N, Terauchi Y, Yamauchi T, et al. Disruption of adiponectin causes insulin resistance and neointimal formation. J Biol Chem 2002; 277:25863–25866.

175. Ouchi N, Kihara S, Arita Y, et al. Novel modulator for endothelial adhesion molecules: adipocyte-derived plasma protein adiponectin. Circulation 1999; 100: 2473–2476.

176. Kumada M, Kihara S, Sumitsuji S, et al. Association of hypoadiponectinemia with coronary artery disease in men. Arterioscler Thromb Vasc Biol 2003; 23:85–89.

177. Pilz S, Horejsi R, Moller R, et al. Early atherosclerosis in obese juveniles is associated with low serum levels of adiponectin. J Clin Endocrinol Metab 2005; 90:4792–4796.

178. Maahs DM, Ogden LG, Kinney GL, et al. Low plasma adiponectin levels predict progression of coronary artery calcification. Circulation 2005; 111:747–753.

179. Nakamura Y, Shimada K, Fukuda D, et al. Implications of plasma concentrations of adiponectin in patients with coronary artery disease. Heart 2004; 90:528–533.

180. Weyer C, Funahashi T, Tanaka S, et al. Hypoadiponectinemia in obesity and type 2 diabetes: close association with insulin resistance and hyperinsulinemia. J Clin Endocrinol Metab 2001; 86:1930–1935.

181. Reinehr T, Roth C, Menke T, et al. Adiponectin before and after weight loss in obese children. J Clin Endocrinol Metab 2004; 89:3790–3794.

182. Asayama K, Hayashibe H, Dobashi K, et al. Decrease in serum adiponectin level due to obesity and visceral fat accumulation in children. Obes Res 2003; 11:1072–1079.

183. Arita Y, Kihara S, Ouchi N, et al. Paradoxical decrease of an adipose-specific protein, adiponectin, in obesity. Biochem Biophys Res Commun 1999; 257:79–83.

184. Harsch IA, Wallaschofski H, Koebnick C, et al. Adiponectin in patients with obstructive sleep apnea syndrome: course and physiological relevance. Respiration 2004; 71:580–586.

185. Zhang XL, Yin KS, Wang H, et al. Serum adiponectin levels in adult male patients with obstructive sleep apnea hypopnea syndrome. Respiration 2006; 73:73–77.

186. Wolk R, Svatikova A, Nelson CA, et al. Plasma levels of adiponectin, a novel adipocyte-derived hormone, in sleep apnea. Obes Res 2005; 13:186–190.

187. Makino S, Handa H, Suzukawa K, et al. Obstructive sleep apnea syndrome, plasma adiponectin levels and insulin resistance. Clin Endocrinol 2006, 64:12–19.

188. Janke J, Engeli S, Gorzelniak K, et al. Resistin gene expression in human adipocytes is not related to insulin resistance. Obes Res 2002; 10:1–5.

189. Lee JH, Chan JL, Yiannakouris N, et al. Circulating resistin levels are not associated with obesity or insulin resistance in humans and are not regulated by fasting or leptin administration: cross-sectional and interventional studies in normal, insulin-resistant, and diabetic subjects. J Clin Endocrinol Metab 2003; 88:4848–4856.

190. Harsch IA, Koebnick C, Wallaschofski H, et al. Resistin levels in patients with obstructive sleep apnea syndrome – the link to subclinical inflammation? Med Sci Monit 2004; 10:CR510–CR515.

24

Cardiovascular Complications of Childhood OSAS

ATHANASIOS G. KADITIS
University of Thessaly School of Medicine and Larissa University Hospital,
Larissa, Greece

I. Overview

Reports of pulmonary hypertension and cor pulmonale in children with severe obstructive sleep apnea had appeared in the literature several years before the Sleep Heart Health Study revealed an increased prevalence of heart failure, stroke, and coronary artery disease in adults with obstructive sleep-disordered breathing (SDB) (1–3). Obstructive sleep apnea syndrome (OSAS) is due to intermittent upper airway obstruction during sleep, and it is characterized by increased work of breathing, more negative than usual intrathoracic pressure during inspiration, arousals and sleep disruption, and blood gas exchange abnormalities (4).

The above noted immediate consequences of intermittent upper airway obstruction during sleep are associated with a second series of sustained abnormalities that can be classified as (*i*) endothelial dysfunction and decreased arterial distensibility (5,6), (*ii*) chronic inflammation and metabolic disturbances (7–12), (*iii*) blood pressure abnormalities (13–15), and (*iv*) changes in cardiac structure and function (5,16–19). When the previous alterations persist over long periods of time, cardiovascular complications can potentially emerge, specifically

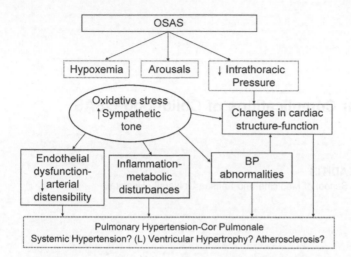

Figure 1 OSAS is associated with gas exchange abnormalities, arousals from sleep, and exaggerated negative intrathoracic pressure swings (immediate consequences). These abnormalities lead to a second series of sustained alterations (e.g., endothelial dysfunction, inflammation, metabolic disturbances), probably via oxidative stress and increased sympathetic tone. If OSAS remains untreated, cardiovascular complications (mainly pulmonary hypertension and cor pulmonale) can occur. *Abbreviation*: OSAS, obstructive sleep apnea syndrome.

(*i*) systemic arterial hypertension, (*ii*) pulmonary hypertension and cor pulmonale, (*iii*) left ventricular hypertrophy and diastolic dysfunction, and (*iv*) development of atherosclerosis. Figure 1 represents a simplified approach to the chain of events leading from obstructive sleep apnea to the development of cardiovascular complications.

In this chapter, evidence regarding cardiovascular complications of pediatric OSAS will be reviewed and compared with relevant findings from studies with adult participants. Pathogenetic mechanisms leading from intermittent upper airway obstruction during sleep to cardiovascular morbidity will also be presented. Detailed discussions of the detrimental inflammatory and metabolic pathways activated by OSAS in children can be found in chapters 22 and 23, respectively.

II. From Intermittent Upper Airway Obstruction to Cardiovascular Complications: Proposed Chain of Events

Data from both children and adults have been accumulating in the literature regarding the immediate consequences of obstructive sleep apnea (blood gas exchange abnormalities, exaggerated negative intrathoracic pressure swings, arousals from sleep and sleep fragmentation) and its subsequent sustained abnormalities (insulin and leptin resistance, blood pressure elevation, changes in cardiac structure and function). Moreover, strong epidemiologic evidence suggests that OSAS constitutes a major risk factor for systemic arterial hypertension, coronary artery disease, heart failure, and stroke in adults (13,20–22).

Nevertheless, our understanding of the exact chain of pathophysiologic events leading from intermittent upper airway obstruction during sleep to cardiovascular morbidity is incomplete. Three main hypotheses have been proposed to explain why obstructive sleep apnea has adverse effects on the cardiovascular system: (*i*) sympathetic nervous system activation; (*ii*) effects of upper airway obstruction on preload and afterload of the cardiac ventricles (cardiac strain); and (*iii*) the oxidative stress hypothesis. Impairment of the hypothalamic-pituitary-adrenal (HPA) axis is a fourth potential pathogenetic pathway, but currently there are no data supporting its role in pediatric OSAS.

A. Sympathetic Nervous System Activation

Evidence for Increased Sympathetic Activity in OSAS

In healthy humans, sympathetic output, heart rate, and levels of blood pressure decline from wakefulness to non–rapid eye movement (NREM) sleep and increase again during rapid eye movement (REM) sleep (23). Arousal stimuli are accompanied by bursts of sympathetic nerve activity and transient increases in blood pressure (23,24). Sympathetic activity can also be increased by hypoxia and hypercapnia via stimulation of peripheral and central chemoreceptors, especially in the absence of the inhibitory effect of normal ventilation (25). It is therefore reasonable to speculate that intermittent gas exchange abnormalities and arousals from sleep related to obstructive sleep apnea will augment the sympathetic tone (26–29). Activity of the sympathetic nervous system can be evaluated either directly by recording muscle sympathetic nerve output (peroneal microneurography) (23) or indirectly by measuring urine concentrations of catecholamines (norepinephrine, epinephrine) and their metabolic products (normetanephrine, metanephrine, vanilmandelic acid) (30).

With the use of peroneal microneurography, it was shown that adults with OSAS have high levels of sympathetic activity compared with control subjects during both sleep and wakefulness (26,28). Increased levels of sympathetic activity can be attenuated by treatment with nasal continuous positive airway pressure (CPAP) (26). Furthermore, in adults with OSAS, several studies have shown that urine or plasma catecholamines correlate with polysomnographic indices (27,31–34). Most studies have found a relationship between the severity of OSAS and plasma and urine norepinephrine concentration but not with epinephrine levels (35). Healthy subjects exposed acutely to hypoxia in vitro, or after rapid transport from sea level to high altitude, experience an immediate and short-lasting increase in plasma epinephrine levels and a delayed elevation in plasma norepinephrine concentration (36,37). This differential effect of hypoxia on the release of catecholamines could explain why mostly increased urine norepinephrine (but not epinephrine) has been reported in sleep apneics (35). Treatment of OSAS in adults is accompanied by a reduction in plasma or urine catecholamine levels, a finding supporting the concept that intermittent upper airway obstruction during sleep leads to increased sympathetic activity (38–41).

Very few investigations have evaluated autonomic function in children with OSAS (42–44). O'Brien and Gozal used peripheral arterial tonometry to measure sympathetic responses during wakefulness in 28 children with OSAS and 29 healthy controls (42). They demonstrated exaggerated sympathetic responses following vital capacity sighs and hand immersion in ice-cold water in the former group compared with the latter. Baharav et al. (43) performed power spectrum analysis of instantaneous fluctuations in heart rate in 10 children with OSAS and 10 healthy controls; their analysis revealed enhanced sympathetic activity in the former group compared with the latter. Aljadeff et al. (44) studied heart rate variability in seven children with OSAS and in seven subjects with primary snoring. Beat-to-beat variation at slow heart rates was significantly increased and variation at fast and intermediate heart rates was significantly decreased in participants with OSAS compared with subjects with primary snoring.

Impact of Increased Sympathetic Activity on the Cardiovascular System

Increased sympathetic nerve activity has been implicated in the pathogenesis of hypertension in subjects with OSAS (26). Overnight microneurography and blood pressure monitoring in adults with OSAS have shown a pattern of surges in muscle sympathetic nerve activity accompanying episodes of apnea, which are followed by transient rises in blood pressure when normal breathing resumes (recovery from apnea) (28). The transient rise in blood pressure is most likely due to vasoconstriction resulting from the intermittent surges of sympathetic activity (45). Additionally, obstructive sleep apnea is independently associated with insulin resistance, a predisposing factor for atherosclerosis (46). Activation of the sympathoadrenal system by nocturnal hypoxemia is one of the mechanisms mediating development of insulin resistance because it promotes glycogenolysis and gluconeogenesis (36).

B. Upper Airway Obstruction and Effects on Cardiac Preload and Afterload

Abnormalities in myocardial structure and function have been identified in children with OSAS, but the exact pathophysiologic mechanism is unclear (16–19). Chronic mechanical strain of the cardiac ventricles secondary to intermittent upper airway obstruction during sleep may play an important pathogenetic role (16–19,47). Monitoring of blood pressure and left ventricle stroke volume in adults with severe OSAS has demonstrated that at the end of an obstructive event (recovery from apnea) arterial pressure increases whereas stroke volume decreases (48). Similar changes have been reported for pulmonary artery pressure and right ventricle stroke volume (49). The increase in systemic blood pressure has been attributed to peripheral vasoconstriction resulting from sympathetic nervous system activation secondary to hypoxemia and microarousals (32).

Ventricular stroke volume is affected by changes in preload, afterload, or myocardial contractility. Reduction in stroke volume of the right and left ventricles could be the result of episodic rises in afterload due to oscillations in pulmonary and systemic arterial pressure accompanying obstructive events (28,50). Furthermore, exaggerated negative intrathoracic pressure swings during upper airway obstruction increase systemic venous return and end-diastolic volume of the right ventricle (preload), with displacement of the interventricular septum toward the left ventricle free wall (16,51–53). Displacement of the interventricular septum impairs left cardiac ventricle filling, and in combination with the increased afterload reduces stroke volume (45,48). It should be noted that left cardiac ventricle afterload is enhanced not only by peripheral vasoconstriction but also by the large negative swings in intrathoracic pressure (50,54). Chronic nocturnal increases in ventricular afterload may result in increased left cardiac ventricle mass, an important risk factor for future cardiovascular diseases such as congestive heart failure (55).

Cardiac strain in children with OSAS may be reflected by blood levels of brain natriuretic peptide (BNP). BNP is a neurohormone released by the cardiac ventricles in response to volume and pressure overload (ventricular strain), as occurs in adult subjects with congestive heart failure or acute myocardial infarction (56–58). It is produced mainly by myocytes of the cardiac ventricles as a prohormone, but received its name because it was initially detected in porcine brain (59,60). Acute overload of the cardiac ventricles promotes BNP gene expression and secretion of the peptide in the bloodstream (56). Increased levels of BNP have been found in children with heart failure due to various causes and with congenital cardiac anomalies causing left-to-right shunts or pulmonary hypertension (61). BNP tends to reduce cardiac ventricular overload by causing vasodilation and natriuresis (62).

In a recent pediatric investigation, evening and morning plasma BNP levels were measured in children with snoring and an apnea-hypopnea index (AHI) ≥ 5 episodes/hr, in snorers with an AHI <5 episodes/hr, and in control subjects without snoring (63). Overnight change in BNP (log-transformed ratio of morning-to-evening levels) was larger in the subjects with AHI ≥ 5 episodes/hr compared with the other two groups, and was associated with polysomnographic abnormalities. The correlation between the overnight increase in BNP and the severity of intermittent upper airway obstruction during sleep probably reflects the presence of nocturnal cardiac strain.

Studies exploring the presence of a correlation between BNP levels and severity of OSAS in adults have provided contradictory results (64–66). Kita et al. recorded increasing BNP levels in the second half of sleep time (2–6 AM) that correlated with the average apnea duration (65). Svatikova et al. did not identify a change in BNP concentration between 2 AM and 6 AM, but during this sleep period participants were undergoing a therapeutic CPAP trial (66). In a third study (64), adult subjects with OSAS and controls free of sleep disturbances were recruited. BNP levels were measured only in the morning and no difference was identified between study groups. Treatment with CPAP for 12 to 17 months did not affect morning BNP plasma concentrations.

The clinical usefulness of measuring plasma BNP levels in children with OSAS needs to be assessed further. More studies are necessary to investigate the possible correlation of cardiac ventricular anatomy and function with overnight changes in BNP plasma concentration, as well as the potential effect of adenotonsillectomy on BNP levels.

C. Oxidative Stress Hypothesis

The oxidative stress hypothesis provides a comprehensive interpretation of inflammatory abnormalities in OSAS (67). Nocturnal intermittent hypoxemia increases production of reactive oxygen species (68,69), activates redox-sensitive transcription factors (e.g., nuclear factor κB) (70–72), and results in release of inflammatory mediators (73) and increased expression of endothelial and leukocyte adhesion molecules (69). Leukocyte adherence to endothelial cells can probably cause endothelial dysfunction and vascular injury (5,69,74). In agreement with the above described hypothesis, a number of reports in adults with OSAS have described increased serum levels of adhesion molecules, a finding that may be a surrogate measure of endothelial activation (75–78).

Evidence for the role of oxidative stress and endothelial dysfunction in children with OSAS is very limited (79,80). In a group of children with mild to moderate or no SDB, there was no relationship between the urinary metabolite of F_2-isoprostanes and the severity of intermittent upper airway obstruction during sleep (79). F_2-isoprostanes are produced from peroxidation of cell membrane phospholipids or circulating low-density lipoproteins (81,82). O'Brien et al. assessed endothelial activation indirectly by measuring morning plasma levels of intercellular adhesion molecule-1 (ICAM-1) and P-selectin (both adhesion molecules) in children with OSAS (AHI > 5 episodes/hr), mild OSAS (AHI, 1–5episodes/hr) and in healthy controls (AHI < 1 episode/hr) (80). Subjects with an AHI >5 episodes/hr had higher levels of ICAM-1 and P-selectin than controls, but the difference in ICAM-1 did not persist after adjustment by body mass index.

Another study assessed the hypothesis that the overnight change of serum ICAM-1 levels in children with snoring was correlated with the severity of OSAS. Evening and morning serum levels of ICAM-1 were measured in children with AHI ≥5 episodes/hr, children with AHI <5 and >1 episodes/hr, and controls with snoring and AHI ≤1 episode/hr; the overnight change in ICAM-1 (ratio of morning-to-evening levels) was similar among the three study groups (83). In accordance with findings in healthy adults (84), serum concentrations of the adhesion molecule decreased overnight, but this expected physiologic overnight decrease was less pronounced for children with AHI ≥5 episodes/hr because they tended to have higher morning ICAM-1 levels compared with participants with a milder disorder. Thus, it is conceivable that if children with snoring had similar severity of SDB to that reported in adults, overnight change in ICAM-1 levels might have been affected significantly by intermittent nocturnal airway obstruction.

III. Cardiovascular Complications of OSAS

A. Effects on Systemic Blood Pressure

Evidence from Studies with Adult Subjects

Strong epidemiologic evidence supports an association between SDB and hypertension (13,21). Cross-sectional analyses of 6132 participants in the Sleep Heart Health Study (40 years of age or older) revealed that the odds ratio for hypertension in the group with an AHI ≥ 30 episodes/hr relative to the group with an index <1.5 episodes/hr was 1.37 (95% CI, 1.03–1.83) (13). In 709 participants of the Wisconsin Sleep Cohort Study, a dose-response relationship was identified between severity of SDB at first visit (baseline) and the presence of hypertension four years later (follow-up), which was independent of known confounding factors (21). After adjustment for baseline hypertension status, the odds ratios for the presence of hypertension at follow-up were: 1.42 (95% CI, 1.13–1.78) with an AHI of 0.1 to 4.9 events/hr at baseline and 2.89 (1.46–5.64) with an AHI ≥ 15.0 events per hour compared with no events per hour (reference). Thus, SDB in adults is a risk factor for the presence of hypertension or development of hypertension later in life.

Review of Published Pediatric Studies

Blood pressure in childhood changes with growth, and normative blood pressure values are based on age, gender, and height (85). To compare blood pressure among children of different ages, gender, and height, most pediatric studies have indexed measurements to the 95th percentile values (14,86,87). In the majority of pediatric studies, the correlation between the level of systemic arterial pressure and polysomnography indices was evaluated.

Marcus et al. compared 41 children with OSAS and 26 children with primary snoring who underwent polysomnography (14). Blood pressure was measured every 15 minutes in the sleep laboratory using an automated system. Diastolic blood pressure indexed for age, gender, and height was higher in children with OSAS than in those with primary snoring during both sleep and during wakefulness. No differences were identified between the two study groups regarding systolic blood pressure.

Kohyama et al. recruited 23 children with suspected OSAS and adeno-tonsillar hypertrophy who were divided into two groups based on the AHI using a cutoff value of 10 episodes/hr (87). Systolic and diastolic blood pressures indexed for age during REM sleep and during wakefulness were higher in the group with more severe OSAS. However, in multivariable analysis, AHI was predictive only of systolic blood pressure during REM sleep.

In a third study of 30 children with primary snoring and 30 healthy controls matched for age, gender, and body size, significantly higher mean (nonindexed) systolic and diastolic daytime blood pressures were identified in the former group compared with the latter (6). The presence of primary snoring, age, and body mass index were significant determinants of systolic blood pressure; primary snoring and age were significant determinants of diastolic blood pressure.

In one of the two published series with community-based samples of children, 239 subjects underwent overnight home polysomnography, and blood pressure was measured in the evening (15). Logistic regression analysis revealed that subjects with systolic and diastolic blood pressure over the 90th percentile (adjusted for age, height, and gender) were more likely to have a higher AHI and poorer sleep efficiency.

The second population-based study recruited 760 children attending nursery, elementary, and high schools (88). Children were screened for symptoms of OSAS using a questionnaire, and morning blood pressure measurements were obtained. Fifty of 760 (6.6%) participants snored more than three nights per week (habitual snorers). While age, gender, and body mass index were significant predictors of systolic blood pressure in a general linear model, snoring was not. Similarly, gender and body mass index, but not snoring, were significant predictors of diastolic blood pressure. Narrowing of the upper airway during sleep occurs to a variable degree within a population (89,90). It is likely that most children with snoring in a population sample have mild OSAS in contrast to symptomatic subjects referred for polysomnography who probably have more severe disease. Thus, large population samples are probably required to detect a significant association between the presence of snoring and elevated blood pressure.

Two studies used 24-hour ambulatory blood pressure monitoring in children with snoring who underwent polysomnography (86,91). Amin et al. studied 39 children with OSAS and 21 subjects with primary snoring by overnight polysomnography and 24-hour ambulatory blood pressure recording (86). The investigators did not identify a significant difference in average systolic blood pressure during wakefulness or sleep, or in average diastolic blood pressure during sleep, between subjects with OSAS and primary snoring. An unexpected finding was that the average diastolic blood pressure during wakefulness was inversely related to the AHI. Children with more severe OSAS had increased blood pressure variability and decreased nocturnal blood pressure dipping, both of which are risk factors for cardiovascular disease in adults (92,93).

In contrast to the study by Amin et al. (86), Leung et al. found that the desaturation index was a significant predictor of diastolic blood pressure during sleep in 96 children with snoring who underwent 24-hour ambulatory blood pressure monitoring and overnight polysomnography (91). There was no difference regarding nocturnal blood pressure dipping in subjects with high and low AHI (AHI > 5 episodes/hr vs. ≤ 5 episodes/hr). Children in the high AHI group were more likely to have systolic or diastolic hypertension (during sleep or wakefulness) compared with participants in the group with less severe OSAS (odds ratio, 3.20; 95% CI, 1.04–9.83). Among obese children, AHI >5 episodes/hr was a significant predictor of hypertension (odds ratio, 6.67; 95% CI, 1.04 to 44.29), supporting the concept that OSAS in children has detrimental effects on the health of the cardiovascular system, especially when it coexists with obesity (94).

Meta-analyses of Published Pediatric Studies

A meta-analysis of published pediatric studies (95) provided an estimate of the risk for elevated blood pressure in children with moderate to severe OSAS compared with mild or no OSAS. Studies of subjects with OSAS who were 18 years of age or younger were analyzed (14,15,86–88), except for the study by Leung et al. (91), which was published concurrently with the meta-analysis. The meta-analysis revealed a lack of significant association between systolic or diastolic blood pressure and OSAS (Fig. 2). During wakefulness, moderate to severe OSAS was associated with an 87% and 121% higher risk for elevated systolic and diastolic blood pressures, respectively, compared with mild or no OSAS, but the association was not significant [random effects odds ratio, 1.87 (95% CI, 0.73–4.80) and 2.21 (95% CI, 0.80–6.10), respectively]. During sleep, the random effects odds ratio for elevated systolic blood pressure was 1.20 (95% CI, 0.29–5.02) and the fixed effects odds ratio for elevated diastolic blood pressure was 2.23 (95% CI, 0.61–8.16).

Significant heterogeneity was detected among the analyzed studies. Variable definitions of severity of OSAS and of elevated blood pressure in each report potentially contributed to the large heterogeneity between published investigations. Also, the methods of diagnosis of OSAS and the frequency of blood pressure recording were not the same in all reports. For example, blood pressure was measured at home in the evening prior to polysomnography (15), at school in the morning (88), every 15 minutes during polysomnography (14,87), or every 15 minutes over 24 hours (86). All included studies except for one (15) were designed to assess the potential correlation of blood pressure values with the severity of OSAS and not the risk (odds ratio) for elevated blood pressure according to AHI.

It should be noted that because of the small number of participants in each pediatric study, only Enright et al. (15) were able to establish significant differences in the prevalence of hypertension between study groups with a high and low AHI. In a meta-analysis (96) of three pediatric studies (14,18,97), the calculated odds ratio for hypertension among children with high AHI relative to those with a low AHI was 2.93 (95% CI, 1.18–7.29).

In summary, most pediatric studies have recruited small numbers of subjects with and without OSAS. It is difficult to combine results of individual published reports due to different methodologies, but the trend seems to be that

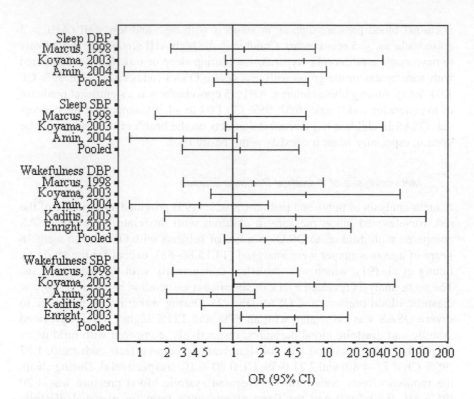

Figure 2 Risk for elevated DBP or SBP during sleep or wakefulness in children with moderate to severe OSAS compared with those with mild or no OSAS. Each study is shown by an OR estimate with the corresponding 95% CI. The random effects pooled ORs are presented. The horizontal axis is plotted on a log scale and the vertical line corresponds to an OR of 1.00. *Abbreviations*: SBP, systolic blood pressure; DBP, diastolic blood pressure; OSAS, obstructive sleep apnea syndrome; CI, confidence interval; OR, odds ratio. *Source*: From Ref. 95.

the greater the severity of OSAS, the higher the systemic blood pressure (especially the diastolic component). It is unknown to what extent intermittent upper airway obstruction during sleep contributes to the development of hypertension. Large, population-based studies using overnight polysomnography and 24-hour ambulatory blood pressure monitoring are necessary to clarify whether long-term persistence of OSAS is connected to elevation of systemic blood pressure above the normotensive range, especially in obese children.

OSAS and Elevated Blood Pressure: Potential Pathophysiologic Mechanisms

It is not well understood how the repetitive nocturnal oscillations in blood pressure related to obstructive apnea result in sustained daytime blood pressure elevation (98). One potential explanation is that patients with OSAS have high levels of sympathetic traffic even during daytime normoxic wakefulness (26). Activation of the renin-angiotensin-aldosterone system by nocturnal episodic hypoxemia may also contribute to sustained systemic hypertension in subjects with OSAS (64,99,100).

Genetic predisposition may determine which patients with OSAS will respond to nocturnal intermittent upper airway obstruction with systemic blood pressure elevation. Recent publications have focused on the role of the insertion/ deletion (I/D) polymorphism of the angiotensin-converting enzyme (ACE) gene. A dose-response relationship was reported between the number of D alleles and blood pressure in Caucasian adults with OSAS (101). A second study (102) confirmed that the interaction between the ACE gene DD polymorphism and OSAS is an important mechanism in the development of hypertension, particularly in Caucasian men. In contrast, Zhang et al. (103) showed that the I allele and the II ACE genotypes were associated with OSAS in Chinese adults with hypertension. The above data indicate that genetic predisposition for elevated blood pressure in response to OSAS probably varies with ethnic origin.

B. Changes in Cardiac Structure and Function

As was discussed earlier in this chapter, hypoxemia, sympathetic nervous system activation, and exaggerated negative intrathoracic pressure during inspiration against an obstructed upper airway are important OSAS-related consequences that have an impact on preload and afterload of the cardiac ventricles (Fig. 1). Supposedly, chronic ventricular strain results in changes in cardiac structure and function. Animal experiments have also shown that long-term intermittent hypoxia increases the myocardial mass of the left ventricle (104,105). In this section, studies reporting cardiac abnormalities associated with OSAS are summarized.

Evidence from Studies of Adults

OSAS has a negative impact on the myocardial structure and function (5,106–110). Diastolic dysfunction (abnormal relaxation pattern) has been reported in patients with OSAS: more severe OSAS is related to more severe left ventricular diastolic dysfunction (106,110). Hypertrophic interventricular septum, lower left ventricle ejection fraction, and stroke volume have been detected in patients with OSAS and without known cardiac morbidity, relative to controls (5,107,109). The right ventricle in patients with OSAS has larger dimensions than in controls (109). Of note, both left and right ventricle morphologic and functional abnormalities can be reversed partially or completely after treatment with CPAP (107,109,111).

Review of Published Pediatric Studies

Older studies and case reports pointed out that children with severe OSAS can present with cor pulmonale and pulmonary hypertension (1–3,16,47). Sofer et al. described four children with cor pulmonale, pulmonary edema, and respiratory

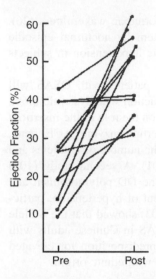

Figure 3 Right ventricular ejection fraction measured by radionuclide ventriculography in 11 children with OSAS before and after adenotonsillectomy. *Abbreviation*: OSAS, obstructive sleep apnea syndrome. *Source*: From Ref. 17.

distress due to chronic upper airway obstruction caused by adenoidal or tonsillar hypertrophy (16). Right ventricular dilatation and reduced ejection fraction were documented by echocardiography and radionuclide angiography, and resolved after adenotonsillectomy. Tal et al. evaluated ventricular function by radionuclide ventriculography in 27 children with OSAS and oropharyngeal obstruction (17). Right ventricular ejection fraction was reduced in 37% of children and improved following adenotonsillectomy (Fig. 3).

Recently, it was recognized that not only the right but also the left cardiac ventricle may be affected in children with OSAS (18,19). Amin et al. reported that in children with snoring, the higher the AHI, the higher the risk for increased right cardiac ventricle end-diastolic dimension and increased left ventricle mass index (18). The same investigators found a negative correlation between the severity of OSAS and left cardiac ventricle diastolic function (19). In an older study of adolescents with snoring who underwent polysomnography and echo-cardiography, deceleration of early diastolic flow and isovolumetric relaxation time (both measures of diastolic function) were predicted by the AHI (112).

C. Effects on Vascular Wall and Predisposition to Atherosclerosis

It is likely that long-term persistence of oxidative stress and sympathetic nervous system activation resulting from intermittent upper airway obstruction during sleep promotes blood pressure elevation, insulin resistance, chronic inflammation, endothelial dysfunction, and decreased arterial distensibility, and ultimately leads to development of atherosclerosis (Fig. 1). In this section, published studies supporting the previous hypothesis will be reviewed.

Evidence from Studies with Adult Subjects

In the Sleep Heart Health Study, Shahar et al. presented a cross-sectional association between OSAS diagnosed by unattended home polysomnography and self-reported cardiovascular disease (20). When participants were stratified by AHI, it was apparent that OSAS was associated with self-reported heart failure and stroke, while the association with coronary heart disease did not reach statistical significance. In an observational study by Marin et al. (22), 264 healthy men, 377 simple snorers, 403 subjects with untreated mild to moderate OSAS, 235 with untreated severe disease, and 372 with OSAS treated with CPAP were followed up at least once per year for a mean period of 10.1 years. Participants with untreated severe disease had a higher incidence of fatal and nonfatal cardiovascular events relative to untreated patients with mild to moderate OSAS, simple snorers, patients treated with CPAP, and healthy controls. The remarkable finding of the study was that treatment with CPAP reduced the incidence of cardiovascular events.

Apart from evidence collected from epidemiologic studies, in a number of investigations, OSAS has been related to early signs of vascular disease. Atherosclerosis is not only a process of lipid accumulation in the vascular wall, but is also characterized by low-grade vascular inflammation (113). Elevated serum or plasma C-reactive protein (CRP) has been associated with increased cardiovascular risk in healthy individuals (114), and it probably reflects chronic vascular inflammation related to atherosclerosis (113). For this reason, a number of studies have assessed the potential pathogenetic role of inflammation in the association between OSAS and cardiovascular disease, with conflicting results (7,115–119). Some investigations have identified a positive correlation of CRP levels with severity of OSAS (7,116,117), while other reports have not confirmed these findings (115,118,119). It has been argued that, since obesity is correlated with both severity of OSAS and elevated serum CRP, it is probably a confounding factor in the association between OSAS and CRP (120,121).

Endothelial dysfunction precedes or accelerates atherosclerosis (122). Normal endothelium releases nitric oxide (NO) in response to reactive hyperemia after transient forearm ischemia produced by inflation of a pneumatic cuff (endothelium-dependent flow-mediated vasodilation) (123). Subjects with OSAS have abnormal branchial artery flow-mediated vasodilation (5,74,124,125), a known predictor of cardiovascular disease (123). Compared to healthy subjects, patients with OSAS have higher numbers of circulating apoptotic endothelial cells, which correlate with the degree of abnormality in vascular function (126). Circulating apoptotic endothelial cells are an early sign of endothelial injury and their numbers in adults with obstructive sleep apnea decrease following treatment with CPAP (126). Moreover, patients with OSAS have reduced brachial artery dilation after intra-arterial infusion of acetylcholine, but normal responses to sodium nitroprusside, which is a donor of NO (endothelium-independent vasodilation) (74). Since acetylcholine stimulates endothelial release of NO, the previous finding is consistent with decreased NO availability in OSAS due to oxidative stress (67,127). The reduced endothelial-dependent vasodilation in untreated patients with OSAS improves with the administration of the free radical scavenger vitamin C (128). For this reason, it has been proposed that antioxidant strategies should be explored for the treatment of OSAS-related cardiovascular disease (128).

Other investigations have identified subtle vascular changes in adults with OSAS (129). Carotid-femoral pulse wave velocity, which is inversely related to arterial distensibility, is increased in subjects with OSAS but without clinically apparent cardiovascular disease (129). Increased intima-media thickness of large vessels and changes in the elastic properties of the aorta (increased stiffness) have also been described (129–132).

Review of Published Pediatric Studies

Data supporting an association between OSAS in children and the development of atherosclerosis are extremely limited. A few studies assessed the potential presence of chronic systemic inflammation in children with OSAS as reflected by serum or plasma levels of CRP (8,133–135). In most studies, body mass index was a significant predictor of CRP levels. Kaditis et al. (133) measured CRP mainly in nonobese children with an AHI up to 20 events per hour and did not find an association between the two variables. Tam et al. (135) recruited a total of 113 children (44 with OSAS and 69 controls), most of whom were lean. The authors found no association between CRP levels with polysomnography indices. Tauman et al. (8) recruited children and adolescents with a similar severity of OSAS as compared to the children in the study by Kaditis et al. (133). However, many subjects and especially those with an AHI >5 episodes/hr were obese. A correlation of CRP with AHI was documented and remained significant after adjustment for the degree of adiposity. In a fourth study, Larkin et al. (134) included mostly nonobese adolescents (29% of subjects were obese) but some of the participants had an AHI as high as 50 events/hr. Correlation of CRP values with AHI was identified for subjects with AHI >5 episodes/hr, but not for those with less severe disease. Therefore, it seems that obese children with more severe OSAS are more likely to have chronic systemic inflammation relative to lean subjects with mild OSAS (94).

CRP provides an overall picture of proinflammatory cytokine activation (136). It may have a direct role in the pathogenesis of atherosclerosis due to effects, such as complement activation (137), induction of adhesion molecules expression (138), and promotion of monocyte recruitment into the vascular wall (139). Synthesis of CRP in the liver is regulated mainly by interleukin-6, which is released from monocytes, adipocytes, and other cells in response to hypoxia, sleep disruption, and sleep deprivation related to obstructive sleep apnea (140).

It is unknown whether long-term elevation of CRP levels associated with OSAS in childhood contributes to the development of atherosclerosis in adulthood. One study identified decreased brachioradial arterial distensibility in children with primary snoring relative to controls, by measuring pulse wave velocity (6). Arterial distensibility is an important determinant of the afterload presented to the left ventricle.

IV. Conclusions and Unanswered Questions for Future Research

Older reports indicate that severe OSAS due to adenotonsillar hypertrophy is associated with cor pulmonale and pulmonary hypertension.

A number of methodologically heterogeneous studies, including mainly hospital-referred children, reveal that OSAS may contribute to elevation of systemic arterial blood pressure (mostly of the diastolic component).

Insufficient data exist regarding sympathetic activation in children with OSAS and its potential importance for the development of hypertension and abnormalities in cardiac structure and function.

Although there is evidence on the inflammatory and metabolic consequences of childhood OSAS, the role of oxidative stress in the pathogenesis of future cardiovascular morbidity has not been adequately studied.

There are no long-term, population-based investigations assessing the contribution of OSAS to the development of atherosclerosis, especially in children with coexisting cardiovascular risk factors such as obesity.

The following are important unanswered research questions:

What is the risk for hypertension in children with OSAS in population-based samples? Does adenotonsillectomy reduce the risk for hypertension?

Are structural and functional cardiac changes detected by echocardiography in children with OSAS of clinical importance? Do they resolve after successful treatment of the disturbance in respiration during sleep?

Does sympathetic activation and surges of negative intrathoracic pressure affect cardiac preload, afterload, and stroke volume?

Is the oxidative stress hypothesis applicable in children with OSAS? In what way does oxidative stress affect inflammatory and metabolic pathways?

Are there early signs of vascular disease, such as decreased arterial distensibility and abnormal flow-mediated vasodilation, in children with OSAS? Do they resolve with treatment? Is there decreased NO availability in children with OSAS?

What is the risk for future cardiovascular morbidity in children with untreated OSAS and other coexisting risk factors for atherosclerosis (e.g., obesity)?

References

1. Massumi RA, Sarin RK, Pooya M, et al. Tonsillar hypertrophy, airway obstruction, alveolar hypoventilation, and cor pulmonale in twin brothers. Dis Chest 1969; 55(2): 110–114.
2. Levine OR, Simpser M. Alveolar hypoventilation and cor pulmonale associated with chronic airway obstruction in infants with Down syndrome. Clin Pediatr (Phila) 1982; 21(1):25–29.
3. Steier M, Shapiro SC. Cor pulmonale from airway obstruction in children. JAMA 1973; 225(1):67.
4. Marcus CL. Pathophysiology of childhood obstructive sleep apnea: current concepts. Respir Physiol 2000; 119(2–3):143–154.
5. Kraiczi H, Caidahl K, Samuelsson A, et al. Impairment of vascular endothelial function and left ventricular filling: association with the severity of apnea-induced hypoxemia during sleep. Chest 2001; 119(4):1085–1091.
6. Kwok KL, Ng DK, Cheung YF. BP and arterial distensibility in children with primary snoring. Chest 2003; 123(5):1561–1566.
7. Yokoe T, Minoguchi K, Matsuo H, et al. Elevated levels of C-reactive protein and interleukin-6 in patients with obstructive sleep apnea syndrome are decreased by nasal continuous positive airway pressure. Circulation 2003; 107(8):1129–1134.
8. Tauman R, Ivanenko A, O'Brien LM, et al. Plasma C-reactive protein levels among children with sleep-disordered breathing. Pediatrics 2004; 113(6):e564–e569.
9. Kaditis AG, Alexopoulos EI, Kalampouka E, et al. Morning levels of fibrinogen in children with sleep-disordered breathing. Eur Respir J 2004; 24(5):790–797.
10. Punjabi NM, Shahar E, Redline S, et al. Sleep-disordered breathing, glucose intolerance, and insulin resistance: the Sleep Heart Health Study. Am J Epidemiol 2004; 160(6):521–530.
11. de la Eva RC, Baur LA, Donaghue KC, et al. Metabolic correlates with obstructive sleep apnea in obese subjects. J Pediatr 2002; 140(6):654–659.
12. Ip MS, Lam KS, Ho C, et al. Serum leptin and vascular risk factors in obstructive sleep apnea. Chest 2000; 118(3):580–586.
13. Nieto FJ, Young TB, Lind BK, et al. Association of sleep-disordered breathing, sleep apnea, and hypertension in a large community-based study. Sleep Heart Health Study. JAMA 2000; 283(14):1829–1836.
14. Marcus CL, Greene MG, Carroll JL. Blood pressure in children with obstructive sleep apnea. Am J Respir Crit Care Med 1998; 157(4):1098–1103.
15. Enright PL, Goodwin JL, Sherrill DL, et al. Blood pressure elevation associated with sleep-related breathing disorder in a community sample of white and Hispanic children: the Tucson Children's Assessment of Sleep Apnea study. Arch Pediatr Adolesc Med 2003; 157(9):901–904.
16. Sofer S, Weinhouse E, Tal A, et al. Cor pulmonale due to adenoidal or tonsillar hypertrophy or both in children. Noninvasive diagnosis and follow-up. Chest 1988; 93(1):119–122.
17. Tal A, Leiberman A, Margulis G, et al. Ventricular dysfunction in children with obstructive sleep apnea: radionuclide assessment. Pediatr Pulmonol 1988; 4(3): 139–143.

18. Amin RS, Kimball TR, Bean JA, et al. Left ventricular hypertrophy and abnormal ventricular geometry in children and adolescents with obstructive sleep apnea. Am J Respir Crit Care Med 2002; 165(10):1395–1399.
19. Amin RS, Kimball TR, Kalra M, et al. Left ventricular function in children with sleep-disordered breathing. Am J Cardiol 2005; 95(6):801–804.
20. Shahar E, Whitney CW, Redline S, et al. Sleep-disordered breathing and cardiovascular disease: cross-sectional results of the Sleep Heart Health Study. Am J Respir Crit Care Med 2001; 163(1):19–25.
21. Peppard PE, Young T, Palta M, et al. Prospective study of the association between sleep-disordered breathing and hypertension. N Engl J Med 2000; 342(19): 1378–1384.
22. Marin JM, Carrizo SJ, Vicente E, et al. Long-term cardiovascular outcomes in men with obstructive sleep apnoea-hypopnoea with or without treatment with continuous positive airway pressure: an observational study. Lancet 2005; 365(9464):1046–1053.
23. Somers VK, Dyken ME, Mark AL, et al. Sympathetic-nerve activity during sleep in normal subjects. N Engl J Med 1993; 328(5):303–307.
24. Hornyak M, Cejnar M, Elam M, et al. Sympathetic muscle nerve activity during sleep in man. Brain 1991; 114(pt 3):1281–1295.
25. Somers VK, Mark AL, Zavala DC, et al. Contrasting effects of hypoxia and hypercapnia on ventilation and sympathetic activity in humans. J Appl Physiol 1989; 67(5):2101–2106.
26. Somers VK, Dyken ME, Clary MP, et al. Sympathetic neural mechanisms in obstructive sleep apnea. J Clin Invest 1995; 96(4):1897–1904.
27. Loredo JS, Ziegler MG, Ancoli-Israel S, et al. Relationship of arousals from sleep to sympathetic nervous system activity and BP in obstructive sleep apnea. Chest 1999; 116(3):655–659.
28. Leuenberger U, Jacob E, Sweer L, et al. Surges of muscle sympathetic nerve activity during obstructive apnea are linked to hypoxemia. J Appl Physiol 1995; 79 (2):581–588.
29. Carlson JT, Hedner J, Elam M, et al. Augmented resting sympathetic activity in awake patients with obstructive sleep apnea. Chest 1993; 103(6):1763–1768.
30. Esler M, Jennings G, Korner P, et al. Assessment of human sympathetic nervous system activity from measurements of norepinephrine turnover. Hypertension 1988; 11(1):3–20.
31. Dimsdale JE, Coy T, Ziegler MG, et al. The effect of sleep apnea on plasma and urinary catecholamines. Sleep 1995; 18(5):377–381.
32. Peled N, Greenberg A, Pillar G, et al. Contributions of hypoxia and respiratory disturbance index to sympathetic activation and blood pressure in obstructive sleep apnea syndrome. Am J Hypertens 1998; 11(11 pt 1):1284–1289.
33. Elmasry A, Lindberg E, Hedner J, et al. Obstructive sleep apnoea and urine catecholamines in hypertensive males: a population-based study. Eur Respir J 2002; 19(3):511–517.
34. Jennum P, Schultz-Larsen K, Christensen N. Snoring, sympathetic activity and cardiovascular risk factors in a 70 year old population. Eur J Epidemiol 1993; 9(5): 477–482.
35. Coy TV, Dimsdale JE, Ancoli-Israel S, et al. Sleep apnea and sympathetic nervous system activity: a review. J Sleep Res 1996; 5(1):42–50.

36. Oltmanns KM, Gehring H, Rudolf S, et al. Hypoxia causes glucose intolerance in humans. Am J Respir Crit Care Med 2004; 169(11):1231–1237.
37. Kanstrup IL, Poulsen TD, Hansen JM, et al. Blood pressure and plasma catecholamines in acute and prolonged hypoxia: effects of local hypothermia. J Appl Physiol 1999; 87(6):2053–2058.
38. Minemura H, Akashiba T, Yamamoto H, et al. Acute effects of nasal continuous positive airway pressure on 24-hour blood pressure and catecholamines in patients with obstructive sleep apnea. Intern Med 1998; 37(12):1009–1013.
39. Fletcher EC, Miller J, Schaaf JW, et al. Urinary catecholamines before and after tracheostomy in patients with obstructive sleep apnea and hypertension. Sleep 1987; 10(1):35–44.
40. Baruzzi A, Riva R, Cirignotta F, et al. Atrial natriuretic peptide and catecholamines in obstructive sleep apnea syndrome. Sleep 1991; 14(1):83–86.
41. Marrone O, Riccobono L, Salvaggio A, et al. Catecholamines and blood pressure in obstructive sleep apnea syndrome. Chest 1993; 103(3):722–727.
42. O'Brien LM, Gozal D. Autonomic dysfunction in children with sleep-disordered breathing. Sleep 2005; 28(6):747–752.
43. Baharav A, Kotagal S, Rubin BK, et al. Autonomic cardiovascular control in children with obstructive sleep apnea. Clin Auton Res 1999; 9(6):345–351.
44. Aljadeff G, Gozal D, Schechtman VL, et al. Heart rate variability in children with obstructive sleep apnea. Sleep 1997; 20(2):151–157.
45. Garpestad E, Parker JA, Katayama H, et al. Decrease in ventricular stroke volume at apnea termination is independent of oxygen desaturation. J Appl Physiol 1994; 77(4): 1602–1608.
46. Ip MS, Lam B, Ng MM, et al. Obstructive sleep apnea is independently associated with insulin resistance. Am J Respir Crit Care Med 2002; 165(5):670–676.
47. Hunt CE, Brouillette RT. Abnormalities of breathing control and airway maintenance in infants and children as a cause of cor pulmonale. Pediatr Cardiol 1982; 3(3): 249–256.
48. Garpestad E, Katayama H, Parker JA, et al. Stroke volume and cardiac output decrease at termination of obstructive apneas. J Appl Physiol 1992; 73(5):1743–1748.
49. Bonsignore MR, Marrone O, Romano S, et al. Time course of right ventricular stroke volume and output in obstructive sleep apneas. Am J Respir Crit Care Med 1994; 149(1):155–159.
50. Ringler J, Basner RC, Shannon R, et al. Hypoxemia alone does not explain blood pressure elevations after obstructive apneas. J Appl Physiol 1990; 69(6):2143–2148.
51. Bradley TD, Hall MJ, Ando S, et al. Hemodynamic effects of simulated obstructive apneas in humans with and without heart failure. Chest 2001; 119(6):1827–1835.
52. Brinker JA, Weiss JL, Lappe DL, et al. Leftward septal displacement during right ventricular loading in man. Circulation 1980; 61(3):626–633.
53. Shiomi T, Guilleminault C, Stoohs R, et al. Obstructed breathing in children during sleep monitored by echocardiography. Acta Paediatr 1993; 82(10):863–871.
54. Morgan BJ, Denahan T, Ebert TJ. Neurocirculatory consequences of negative intrathoracic pressure vs. asphyxia during voluntary apnea. J Appl Physiol 1993; 74 (6):2969–2975.
55. Levy D, Garrison RJ, Savage DD, et al. Prognostic implications of echocardiographically determined left ventricular mass in the Framingham Heart Study. N Engl J Med 1990; 322(22):1561–1566.

56. Nakagawa O, Ogawa Y, Itoh H, et al. Rapid transcriptional activation and early mRNA turnover of brain natriuretic peptide in cardiocyte hypertrophy. Evidence for brain natriuretic peptide as an "emergency" cardiac hormone against ventricular overload. J Clin Invest 1995; 96(3):1280–1287.

57. Maeda K, Tsutamoto T, Wada A, et al. Plasma brain natriuretic peptide as a biochemical marker of high left ventricular end-diastolic pressure in patients with symptomatic left ventricular dysfunction. Am Heart J 1998; 135(5):825–832.

58. Morita E, Yasue H, Yoshimura M, et al. Increased plasma levels of brain natriuretic peptide in patients with acute myocardial infarction. Circulation 1993; 88(1):82–91.

59. Saito Y, Nakao K, Itoh H, et al. Brain natriuretic peptide is a novel cardiac hormone. Biochem Biophys Res Commun 1989; 158(2):360–368.

60. Sudoh T, Kangawa K, Minamino N, et al. A new natriuretic peptide in porcine brain. Nature 1988; 332(6159):78–81.

61. Nir A, Nasser N. Clinical value of NT-ProBNP and BNP in pediatric cardiology. J Card Fail 2005; 11(suppl 5):S76–S80.

62. Yoshimura M, Yasue H, Morita E, et al. Hemodynamic, renal, and hormonal responses to brain natriuretic peptide infusion in patients with congestive heart failure. Circulation 1991; 84(4):1581–1588.

63. Kaditis AG, Alexopoulos EI, Hatzi F, et al. Overnight change in brain natriuretic peptide levels in children with sleep-disordered breathing. Chest 2006; 130(5): 1377–1384.

64. Moller DS, Lind P, Strunge B, et al. Abnormal vasoactive hormones and 24-hour blood pressure in obstructive sleep apnea. Am J Hypertens 2003; 16(4):274–280.

65. Kita H, Ohi M, Chin K, et al. The nocturnal secretion of cardiac natriuretic peptides during obstructive sleep apnoea and its response to therapy with nasal continuous positive airway pressure. J Sleep Res 1998; 7(3):199–207.

66. Svatikova A, Shamsuzzaman AS, Wolk R, et al. Plasma brain natriuretic peptide in obstructive sleep apnea. Am J Cardiol 2004; 94(4):529–532.

67. Lavie L. Obstructive sleep apnoea syndrome—an oxidative stress disorder. Sleep Med Rev 2003; 7(1):35–51.

68. Schulz R, Mahmoudi S, Hattar K, et al. Enhanced release of superoxide from polymorphonuclear neutrophils in obstructive sleep apnea. Impact of continuous positive airway pressure therapy. Am J Respir Crit Care Med 2000; 162(2): 566–570.

69. Dyugovskaya L, Lavie P, Lavie L. Increased adhesion molecules expression and production of reactive oxygen species in leukocytes of sleep apnea patients. Am J Respir Crit Care Med 2002; 165(7):934–939.

70. Yamauchi M, Tamaki S, Tomoda K, et al. Evidence for activation of nuclear factor kappaB in obstructive sleep apnea. Sleep Breath 2006; 10(4):189–193.

71. Ryan S, Taylor CT, McNicholas WT. Selective activation of inflammatory pathways by intermittent hypoxia in obstructive sleep apnea syndrome. Circulation 2005; 112(17):2660–2667.

72. Htoo AK, Greenberg H, Tongia S, et al. Activation of nuclear factor kappaB in obstructive sleep apnea: a pathway leading to systemic inflammation. Sleep Breath 2006; 10(1):43–50.

73. Vgontzas AN, Papanicolaou DA, Bixler EO, et al. Sleep apnea and daytime sleepiness and fatigue: relation to visceral obesity, insulin resistance, and hypercytokinemia. J Clin Endocrinol Metab 2000; 85(3):1151–1158.

74. Kato M, Roberts-Thomson P, Phillips BG, et al. Impairment of endothelium-dependent vasodilation of resistance vessels in patients with obstructive sleep apnea. Circulation 2000; 102(21):2607–2610.

75. Ohga E, Nagase T, Tomita T, et al. Increased levels of circulating ICAM-1, VCAM-1, and L-selectin in obstructive sleep apnea syndrome. J Appl Physiol 1999; 87(1):10–14.

76. Chin K, Nakamura T, Shimizu K, et al. Effects of nasal continuous positive airway pressure on soluble cell adhesion molecules in patients with obstructive sleep apnea syndrome. Am J Med 2000; 109(7):562–567.

77. El-Solh AA, Mador MJ, Sikka P, et al. Adhesion molecules in patients with coronary artery disease and moderate-to-severe obstructive sleep apnea. Chest 2002; 121(5):1541–1547.

78. Ohga E, Tomita T, Wada H, et al. Effects of obstructive sleep apnea on circulating ICAM-1, IL-8, and MCP-1. J Appl Physiol 2003; 94(1):179–184.

79. Montgomery-Downs HE, Krishna J, Roberts LJ II, et al. Urinary F(2)-isoprostane metabolite levels in children with sleep-disordered breathing. Sleep Breath 2006; 10(4):211–215.

80. O'Brien LM, Serpero LD, Tauman R, et al. Plasma adhesion molecules in children with sleep-disordered breathing. Chest 2006; 129(4):947–953.

81. Morrow JD, Hill KE, Burk RF, et al. A series of prostaglandin F2-like compounds are produced in vivo in humans by a non-cyclooxygenase, free radical-catalyzed mechanism. Proc Natl Acad Sci U S A 1990; 87(23):9383–9387.

82. Lynch SM, Morrow JD, Roberts LJ II, et al. Formation of non-cyclooxygenase-derived prostanoids(F2-isoprostanes) in plasma and low density lipoprotein exposed to oxidative stress in vitro. J Clin Invest 1994; 93(3):998–1004.

83. Kaditis AG, Alexopoulos EI, Kalampouka E, et al. Nocturnal change of circulating intercellular adhesion molecule-1 levels in children with snoring. Sleep Breath 2007; 11(4):267–274.

84. Maple C, Kirk G, McLaren M, et al. A circadian variation exists for soluble levels of intercellular adhesion molecule-1 and E-selectin in healthy volunteers. Clin Sci (Lond) 1998; 94(5):537–540.

85. National High Blood Pressure Education Program Working Group on High Blood Pressure in Children and Adolescents. The fourth report on the diagnosis, evaluation, and treatment of high blood pressure in children and adolescents. Pediatrics 2004; 114(2 suppl):555–576.

86. Amin RS, Carroll JL, Jeffries JL, et al. Twenty-four-hour ambulatory blood pressure in children with sleep-disordered breathing. Am J Respir Crit Care Med 2004; 169 (8):950–956.

87. Kohyama J, Ohinata JS, Hasegawa T. Blood pressure in sleep disordered breathing. Arch Dis Child 2003; 88(2):139–142.

88. Kaditis AG, Alexopoulos EI, Kostadima E, et al. Comparison of blood pressure measurements in children with and without habitual snoring. Pediatr Pulmonol 2005; 39(5):408–414.

89. Grote L, Ploch T, Heitmann J, et al. Sleep-related breathing disorder is an independent risk factor for systemic hypertension. Am J Respir Crit Care Med 1999; 160(6):1875–1882.

90. Lavie P, Herer P, Hoffstein V. Obstructive sleep apnoea syndrome as a risk factor for hypertension: population study. BMJ 2000; 320(7233):479–482.

91. Leung LC, Ng DK, Lau MW, et al. Twenty-four-hour ambulatory BP in snoring children with obstructive sleep apnea syndrome. Chest 2006; 130(4):1009–1017.
92. Tozawa M, Iseki K, Yoshi S, et al. Blood pressure variability as an adverse prognostic risk factor in end-stage renal disease. Nephrol Dial Transplant 1999; 14(8): 1976–1981.
93. Verdecchia P, Schillaci G, Borgioni C, et al. Altered circadian blood pressure profile and prognosis. Blood Press Monit 1997; 2(6):347–352.
94. Kelly A, Marcus CL. Childhood obesity, inflammation, and apnea: what is the future for our children? Am J Respir Crit Care Med 2005; 171(3):202–203.
95. Zintzaras E, Kaditis AG. Sleep-disordered breathing and blood pressure in children: a meta-analysis. Arch Pediatr Adolesc Med 2007; 161(2):172–178.
96. Ng DK, Chan C, Chow AS, et al. Childhood sleep-disordered breathing and its implications for cardiac and vascular diseases. J Paediatr Child Health 2005; 41(12): 640–646.
97. Guilleminault C, Khramsov A, Stoohs RA, et al. Abnormal blood pressure in prepubertal children with sleep-disordered breathing. Pediatr Res 2004; 55(1):76–84.
98. Phillips BG, Somers VK. Neural and humoral mechanisms mediating cardiovascular responses to obstructive sleep apnea. Respir Physiol 2000; 119(2–3):181–187.
99. Fletcher EC, Bao G, Li R. Renin activity and blood pressure in response to chronic episodic hypoxia. Hypertension 1999; 34(2):309–314.
100. Barcelo A, Elorza MA, Barbe F, et al. Angiotensin converting enzyme in patients with sleep apnoea syndrome: plasma activity and gene polymorphisms. Eur Respir J 2001; 17(4):728–732.
101. Lin L, Finn L, Zhang J, et al. Angiotensin-converting enzyme, sleep-disordered breathing, and hypertension. Am J Respir Crit Care Med 2004; 170(12):1349–1353.
102. Bostrom KB, Hedner J, Melander O, et al. Interaction between the angiotensin-converting enzyme gene insertion/deletion polymorphism and obstructive sleep apnoea as a mechanism for hypertension. J Hypertens 2007; 25(4):779–783.
103. Zhang J, Zhao B, Gesongluobu, et al. Angiotensin-converting enzyme gene insertion/deletion (I/D) polymorphism in hypertensive patients with different degrees of obstructive sleep apnea. Hypertens Res 2000; 23(5):407–411.
104. Fletcher EC, Lesske J, Behm R, et al. Carotid chemoreceptors, systemic blood pressure, and chronic episodic hypoxia mimicking sleep apnea. J Appl Physiol 1992; 72(5):1978–1984.
105. Kraiczi H, Magga J, Sun XY, et al. Hypoxic pressor response, cardiac size, and natriuretic peptides are modified by long-term intermittent hypoxia. J Appl Physiol 1999; 87(6):2025–2031.
106. Fung JW, Li TS, Choy DK, et al. Severe obstructive sleep apnea is associated with left ventricular diastolic dysfunction. Chest 2002; 121(2):422–429.
107. Alchanatis M, Tourkohoriti G, Kosmas EN, et al. Evidence for left ventricular dysfunction in patients with obstructive sleep apnoea syndrome. Eur Respir J 2002; 20(5):1239–1245.
108. Laaban JP, Pascal-Sebaoun S, Bloch E, et al. Left ventricular systolic dysfunction in patients with obstructive sleep apnea syndrome. Chest 2002; 122(4):1133–1138.
109. Shivalkar B, Van de Heyning C, Kerremans M, et al. Obstructive sleep apnea syndrome: more insights on structural and functional cardiac alterations, and the effects of treatment with continuous positive airway pressure. J Am Coll Cardiol 2006; 47(7):1433–1439.

110. Arias MA, Garcia-Rio F, Alonso-Fernandez A, et al. Obstructive sleep apnea syndrome affects left ventricular diastolic function: effects of nasal continuous positive airway pressure in men. Circulation 2005; 112(3):375–383.

111. Dursunoglu N, Dursunoglu D, Ozkurt S, et al. Effects of CPAP on left ventricular structure and myocardial performance index in male patients with obstructive sleep apnoea. Sleep Med 2007; 8(1):51–59.

112. Sanchez-Armengol A, Rodriguez-Puras MJ, Fuentes-Pradera MA, et al. Echo-cardiographic parameters in adolescents with sleep-related breathing disorders. Pediatr Pulmonol 2003; 36(1):27–33.

113. Libby P, Ridker PM, Maseri A. Inflammation and atherosclerosis. Circulation 2002; 105(9):1135–1143.

114. Danesh J, Whincup P, Walker M, et al. Low grade inflammation and coronary heart disease: prospective study and updated meta-analyses. BMJ 2000; 321(7255): 199–204.

115. Guilleminault C, Kirisoglu C, Ohayon MM. C-reactive protein and sleep-disordered breathing. Sleep 2004; 27(8):1507–1511.

116. Shamsuzzaman AS, Winnicki M, Lanfranchi P, et al. Elevated C-reactive protein in patients with obstructive sleep apnea. Circulation 2002; 105(21):2462–2464.

117. Kokturk O, Ciftci TU, Mollarecep E, et al. Elevated C-reactive protein levels and increased cardiovascular risk in patients with obstructive sleep apnea syndrome. Int Heart J 2005; 46(5):801–809.

118. Barcelo A, Barbe F, Llompart E, et al. Effects of obesity on C-reactive protein level and metabolic disturbances in male patients with obstructive sleep apnea. Am J Med 2004; 117(2):118–121.

119. Akashiba T, Akahoshi T, Kawahara S, et al. Effects of long-term nasal continuous positive airway pressure on C-reactive protein in patients with obstructive sleep apnea syndrome. Intern Med 2005; 44(8):899–900.

120. Visser M, Bouter LM, McQuillan GM, et al. Elevated C-reactive protein levels in overweight and obese adults. JAMA 1999; 282(22):2131–2135.

121. Cheng TO. Could elevated C-reactive protein in patients with obstructive sleep apnea be due to obesity per se? Circulation 2003; 107(1):e9.

122. Shimokawa H. Primary endothelial dysfunction: atherosclerosis. J Mol Cell Cardiol 1999; 31(1):23–37.

123. Corretti MC, Anderson TJ, Benjamin EJ, et al. Guidelines for the ultrasound assessment of endothelial-dependent flow-mediated vasodilation of the brachial artery: a report of the International Brachial Artery Reactivity Task Force. J Am Coll Cardiol 2002; 39(2):257–265.

124. Nieto FJ, Herrington DM, Redline S, et al. Sleep apnea and markers of vascular endothelial function in a large community sample of older adults. Am J Respir Crit Care Med 2004; 169(3):354–360.

125. Ip MS, Tse HF, Lam B, et al. Endothelial function in obstructive sleep apnea and response to treatment. Am J Respir Crit Care Med 2004; 169(3):348–353.

126. El Solh AA, Akinnusi ME, Baddoura FH, et al. Endothelial Cell Apoptosis in Obstructive Sleep Apnea: A Link to Endothelial Dysfunction. Am J Respir Crit Care Med 2007; 175(11):1186–1191.

127. Ip MS, Lam B, Chan LY, et al. Circulating nitric oxide is suppressed in obstructive sleep apnea and is reversed by nasal continuous positive airway pressure. Am J Respir Crit Care Med 2000; 162(6):2166–2171.

128. Grebe M, Eisele HJ, Weissmann N, et al. Antioxidant vitamin C improves endothelial function in obstructive sleep apnea. Am J Respir Crit Care Med 2006; 173(8): 897–901.
129. Drager LF, Bortolotto LA, Lorenzi MC, et al. Early signs of atherosclerosis in obstructive sleep apnea. Am J Respir Crit Care Med 2005; 172(5):613–618.
130. Tanriverdi H, Evrengul H, Kaftan A, et al. Effect of obstructive sleep apnea on aortic elastic parameters: relationship to left ventricular mass and function. Circ J 2006; 70(6):737–743.
131. Suzuki T, Nakano H, Maekawa J, et al. Obstructive sleep apnea and carotid-artery intima-media thickness. Sleep 2004; 27(1):129–133.
132. Schulz R, Seeger W, Fegbeutel C, et al. Changes in extracranial arteries in obstructive sleep apnoea. Eur Respir J 2005; 25(1):69–74.
133. Kaditis AG, Alexopoulos EI, Kalampouka E, et al. Morning levels of C-reactive protein in children with obstructive sleep-disordered breathing. Am J Respir Crit Care Med 2005; 171(3):282–286.
134. Larkin EK, Rosen CL, Kirchner HL, et al. Variation of C-reactive protein levels in adolescents: association with sleep-disordered breathing and sleep duration. Circulation 2005; 111(15):1978–1984.
135. Tam CS, Wong M, McBain R, et al. Inflammatory measures in children with obstructive sleep apnoea. J Paediatr Child Health 2006; 42(5):277–282.
136. Ridker PM. High-sensitivity C-reactive protein: potential adjunct for global risk assessment in the primary prevention of cardiovascular disease. Circulation 2001; 103(13):1813–1818.
137. Bhakdi S, Torzewski M, Klouche M, et al. Complement and atherogenesis: binding of CRP to degraded, monoxidized LDL enhances complement activation. Arterioscler Thromb Vasc Biol 1999; 19(10):2348–2354.
138. Pasceri V, Cheng JS, Willerson JT, et al. Modulation of C-reactive protein-mediated monocyte chemoattractant protein-1 induction in human endothelial cells by anti-atherosclerosis drugs. Circulation 2001; 103(21):2531–2534.
139. Torzewski M, Rist C, Mortensen RF, et al. C-reactive protein in the arterial intima: role of C-reactive protein receptor-dependent monocyte recruitment in atherogenesis. Arterioscler Thromb Vasc Biol 2000; 20(9):2094–2099.
140. Castell JV, Gomez-Lechon MJ, David M, et al. Acute-phase response of human hepatocytes: regulation of acute-phase protein synthesis by interleukin-6. Hepatology 1990; 12(5):1179–1186.

25

Acoustic Reflectance

LEE J. BROOKS
University of Pennsylvania, Philadelphia, Pennsylvania, U.S.A.

I. Introduction

The size and mechanical properties of the upper airway may be important in understanding the pathophysiology of obstructive sleep apnea (OSA), central apnea (1), and sudden infant death syndrome (2). Such measurements may prove useful clinically in diagnosing patients and/or predicting or measuring response to therapy. Measurements of the upper airway are difficult, however, because it is a geometrically complex structure subject to considerable variability with changes in neuromuscular activation, sleep stages, position, and transmural pressure. Acoustic reflectance represents a unique and noninvasive technique to "image" the airways, and has been used to assess the properties of the lower airways, as well as the nose, pharynx, and trachea.

II. Basic Principles of the Technique

Studies of respiratory impedance by forced oscillation at the mouth at frequencies of 1–10 Hz found the respiratory system to have three lumped elements in a series: a resistance, a compliance, and an inertance (3). At these frequencies the acoustic

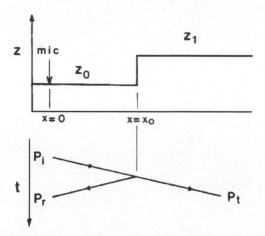

Figure 1 (*Top*) Characteristic impedance (z) of a hypothetical acoustic transmission line as a function of distance from the microphone (mic), with impedance discontinuity at $x = x_0$. (*Bottom*) Schematic diagram illustrating an incident pressure wave P_i, its reflection P_r from the discontinuity, and the transmitted wave P_t (5).

wavelength is greater than 24 m, which can be as much as 1000 times longer than the respiratory structures of interest. These measurements essentially reduce the lung to a point, with all the properties of central airways, peripheral airways, pulmonary parenchyma, and chest wall lumped into effective system compliances, resistances, and inertances (4). However, at frequencies above about 250 Hz, the response to a pressure wave excitation of the airways is no longer "lumped," but is more influenced by serially distributed properties along the length of the system (5). This fact allows us to infer the properties of that system at any point along its length. When an acoustic impulse encounters a discontinuity of impedance (such as a change in the cross-sectional area of the tube), a portion of the signal is reflected in the opposite direction while the rest of the signal is transmitted along its initial path (Fig. 1). In a complex structure, such as the airways that include changes in area, branching, etc., there are multiple reflections, all arriving back at the origin at different times (Fig. 2). Assuming lossless one-dimensional (planar) wave propagation, regular branching, and rigid walled tubes, the change in impedance is inversely proportional to the change in cross-sectional area of the structure. It is therefore possible to calculate the cross-sectional area of the system at any given distance down the tube (5). This technique was demonstrated by Jackson et al. using a spark to generate a pressure pulse, a wave tube through which the pressure wave is transmitted to the structure under study, and a microphone to measure the incident and reflected waves. The system was tested in physical models, in excised dog lungs (5), airway casts, (6) and anesthetized, mechanically ventilated dogs (7,8) under various conditions to simulate central airway constriction, air trapping, and changes induced by histamine and carbachol.

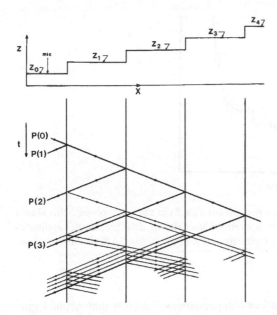

Figure 2 (*Top*) Characteristic impedance (z) of hypothetical acoustic transmission line with multiple impedance discontinuities plotted as a function of distance from the microphone (mic). (*Bottom*) Schematic diagram of reflections resulting from incident wave, P(0) (5).

The technique was modified by Fredberg et al. to use a horn driver rather than a spark to generate the incident pulse, and to use a gas mixture of 80% helium and 20% oxygen. This gas mixture has a higher wave speed, which allows for a higher frequency to maximize airway wall rigidity [tissues behave relatively rigidly at frequencies greater than 120 Hz (9)] as well as a longer wavelength to minimize cross-modes, that is, wave movement in other than the desired direction, and promote planar wave propagation. Using mouthpieces custom-made of dental materials to eliminate the large area of the mouth as a source of cross-modes, they demonstrated good agreement of acoustic measurements of tracheal cross-sectional area with roentgenographic measurements in six adult volunteers (10). The technique was further refined to allow for multiple pulses launched at rates up to 5/sec to allow measurements during various breathing maneuvers. A plot of airway area as a function of distance down the airway was generated (Fig. 3). There was good agreement with glass tube models, excised tracheas, and human volunteers breathing comfortably around functional residual capacity (FRC) (11). The technique showed good agreement with CT scans in seven adults with a history of upper airway abnormalities (12).

Brooks et al. used glass airway models, excised canine tracheas, and human volunteers to establish certain limits of the technique. In particular, a

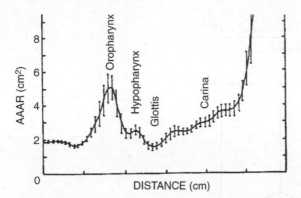

Figure 3 A plot of AAAR as a function of distance from the microphone. This shows mean ±SD of 90 measurements made at a rate of 5/sec during tidal breathing. Landmarks are indicated as identified roentgenographically (11). *Abbreviation*: AAAR, airway cross-sectional area by acoustic reflection.

small proximal structure, "glottis" or "upper airway," of less than about 1 cm^2 resulted in an overestimation of the size of distal structures, probably through viscous losses (11). This limitation was confirmed using a commercially available device in studies of plexiglass airway models and cadaver airways, where the signal was impaired when the cross-sectional area of the airway was less than 0.64 cm^2 (13). Very large proximal (upper airway) structures, greater than about 10 cm^2, resulted in an underestimation of distal structures, probably because of cross-modes (11). This finding supported their use of a dental mouthpiece to minimize the size of the oral cavity. A standard pulmonary function-type mouthpiece could also be used, but the measured size of the pharynx varied widely between the rubber and dental wax mouthpieces (14). Others found better agreement between measurements made with dental and rubber mouthpieces (15). These measurements were not affected by CO_2 concentrations as high as 10% (16).

The technique was further modified to obviate the need for a two-meter long wave tube by using two microphones (17). With "judicious signal processing," this technique was shown to yield similar results with human volunteers breathing air and a heliox gas mixture (18). Huang et al. used a different algorithm to measure the nasal septum and caliber of the pharynx using acoustic pulses launched through both nostrils (19).

In summary, since distal measurements can be affected by proximal measurements, if one is interested in the trachea or smaller airways, it is helpful to ensure that proximal measurements such as the pharynx and glottis are not too large and promoting cross-modes, or too small to promote viscous losses. However, the technique is more forgiving if one is focusing on proximal structures, such as the nasal passages or pharynx.

III. Applications

The acoustic reflections technique was rapidly applied to address physiological and clinical questions about the airways.

A. Trachea

Hoffstein used the technique to explore the relationship between tracheal size and lung volumes and expiratory flows in 24 healthy adults. He found a significant correlation between tracheal size and lung volume in women, but not in men, supporting the concept of dysanapsis, that is, differential rates of growth of the airways and lung parenchyma (20). Martin et al. studied 54 adults and found that men had larger tracheas than women, but there was no relationship between tracheal size and lung size in adults (21). This finding was confirmed by Brooks et al. who analyzed a mid-tracheal segment in a larger sample of 103 adults. Men had a larger trachea than women (2.48 cm^2 vs. 1.91 cm^2, $p < 0.001$) (22). They showed a significant correlation between tracheal size and vital capacity in men, but not in women, and suggested that this reflects differential growth patterns in the airways of males and females (23).

Acoustic reflections have been employed to study the elastic characteristics of the airways. Hoffstein et al. measured esophageal pressure and airway area by acoustic reflection (AAAR) to demonstrate the mechanical properties of the extrathoracic and intrathoracic airway. They found that the area of the trachea and bronchial segments increase with increasing lung volume and transpulmonary pressure. The trachea and bronchi demonstrated variable degrees of hysteresis, which may be greater or less than that of the lung parenchyma, and the specific compliance of the intrathoracic trachea was significantly smaller than that of the bronchial segment (24). Fouke et al. also defined regional differences in upper airway elasticity, and found significant differences between the extrathoracic and intrathoracic airways (25).

Measurements of tracheal size and dynamics have proven useful in clinical studies as well. Acoustic reflections identified the extent and position of segments of tracheal stenosis, and were superior to measurements of maximal expiratory flow (26). The stenotic segments were found to be less compliant than nearby nonstenotic segments. Children with cystic fibrosis were found to have more distensible tracheas than age and sex-matched controls, perhaps a result of airway inflammation (27). Raphael applied the technique in 10 adult patients under general anesthesia and neuromuscular blockade. He showed a rapid rise in the area-distance plot past the carina of patients who were tracheally intubated with a rapid fall beyond the endotracheal tube of patients who were intubated in the esophagus (28). Gucev et al. were able to correctly distinguish endobronchial, tracheal, and esophageal intubations in 20 of 21 children. In one child, a tracheal intubation was falsely identified as esophageal, presumably because the endotracheal tube abutted against the airway wall (29).

B. Nasal Cavity

The acoustic reflections technique has been proposed as a rapid and noninvasive way to quantify nasal obstruction, particularly in the anterior nasal cavity, which is the site of the nasal valve (30). The technique was validated in nasal casts, a human cadaver, and in living humans with water displacement, rhinomanometry, CT scans (31,32), and magnetic resonance imaging (33,34). Using low-pass filtering, Hilberg was able to get comparable results using air or a heliox mixture in nasal models (35). Features on the area-distance function generated by acoustic rhinometry corresponded to anatomical landmarks identified by rigid nasal endoscopy, but not in an exact point-to-point manner (36). Atypical large openings to the paranasal sinuses, such as after paranasal sinus surgery, may result in inaccurate acoustic nasal measurements (37).

Pedersen et al. studied the nasal cavities of 27 newborns and found a weak ($p = 0.036$) correlation between birth weight and the smallest area of the nasal cavities, but there was no relationship to race, sex, head circumference, or age (38). In adults, there were no differences in the decongested nasal dimensions of healthy men and women, but Asian and white subjects had a significantly smaller nasal cavity than black subjects (39).

Gungor measured nasal patency of normal volunteers every 15 minutes for 4 hours, along with a visual analog scale for the subjective feeling of nasal congestion. There were tremendous irregular variations in nasal patency over time, accompanied or counteracted by the other nasal cavity. Subjects were unaware of their nasal cycles and there was no relationship between nasal patency and the subjective congestion scores (40). Hilberg used acoustic rhinometry to measure the nasal patency of 12 nonallergic subjects and 12 with allergy to pollen out of the pollen season in a climatic chamber every 15 minutes for 7 hours on two consecutive days. They found the allergic subjects had more spontaneous variation in nasal patency than the nonallergic subjects ($p = 0.004$). Exercise increased nasal patency more in the nonallergic subjects ($p = 0.05$), while pharmacological decongestion tended to increase nasal patency more in the allergic subjects ($p = 0.08$) (41).

C. Pharynx and Upper Airway

Acoustic reflectance has been an important tool to study the pathophysiology of OSA. The size and mechanical properties of the pharynx are important factors in the pathophysiology of OSA; a smaller, more compliant pharynx increases the risk for OSA, especially in the supine position.

Postural Changes

Fouke and Strohl used acoustic measurements of the pharynx in 10 healthy volunteers to show that pharyngeal cross-sectional area decreases simply on changing from the upright to the supine posture, independent of changes in FRC

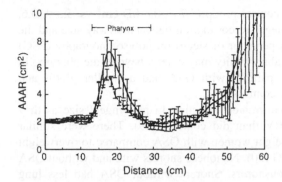

Figure 4 AAAR measured near FRC (*solid line*) and RV (*dashed line*). Vertical bars indicate ±SD. (45). *Abbreviations*: AAAR, airway cross-sectional area by acoustic reflection; FRC, functional residual capacity; RV, residual volume.

(42). Although nonapneic snorers and patients with OSA demonstrated the same phenomenon (43), patients with OSA had less of a change in pharyngeal area on assuming the supine position than did nonapneic snorers or nonsnoring controls (44), suggesting that patients with OSA defend their upper airway more on lying down than do snorers or normal subjects.

Gender Differences

Men have a greater prevalence of OSA. Brooks and Strohl performed acoustic measurements of the pharynx in 77 normal men and 98 normal women while slowly exhaling from total lung capacity (TLC) to residual volume (RV) (Fig. 4). They found that gender was the most important factor contributing to pharyngeal size; men had a significantly larger pharynx than women (3.63 ± 0.10 SEM cm^2 vs. 3.20 ± 0.09, $p < 0.01$). This would seem to place men at less risk for OSA than women. However, the men had a larger change in pharyngeal area with changing lung volume than the women, even after normalizing for pharyngeal size (45). This suggests that the increased risk of OSA in males may, at least in part, be attributed to a "floppier" pharynx. In a smaller study of 24 healthy volunteers, Brown et al. normalized pharyngeal size for body surface area and found no differences between men and women (46). This discrepancy is likely due to the small sample size, which prevented them from employing more powerful statistical methods.

Snorers and Patients with OSA

Patients with OSA generally have a smaller pharynx than controls. Rivlin et al. studied nine male patients with OSA and 10 age-matched obese subjects without OSA. Acoustic measurements of the upper airway were significantly smaller in the patients with OSA than the control group (3.7 ± 0.8 SD cm^2 vs. 5.3 ± 0.6, $p < 0.0001$) with a significant negative correlation between airway size and the apnea index (number of apneas per hour of sleep) on polysomnography (PSG) ($r = 0.87$, $p < 0.01$) (47). This abnormality may extend beyond the pharynx. In addition to a smaller pharynx, patients with OSA had a smaller glottis and cervical trachea than nonapneic controls (48).

Men with OSA also had a greater reduction in pharyngeal size as they slowly exhaled from TLC to RV than did controls (49). There were similar findings in a group of 14 overweight women with OSA compared to overweight female controls with normal PSG (50). Nonobese snorers with and without OSA had a smaller pharynx than nonsnorers. Snorers without OSA had less lung volume-dependent change in pharyngeal area, suggesting they may be protected from complete upper airway occlusion by a less compliant pharynx (51). Pharyngeal compliance was assessed more directly by measuring mouth pressure, while AAAR was measured with the distal wave tube occluded, enabling the construction of a pressure-area curve. Specific pharyngeal compliance was greater in 13 patients with OSA (0.094 ± 0.012) than in 7 snoring controls (0.036 ± 0.004, $p < 0.01$) (52). Ten patients with severe OSA but low-normal pharyngeal collapsibility as measured acoustically had paradoxical glottic narrowing during inspiration, suggesting the glottis may contribute to the pathophysiology of OSA, at least in some cases (53). Children with OSA had a smaller pharynx and a larger change in pharyngeal area following topical anesthesia with cetacaine than did snoring children without OSA. A change in pharyngeal area of 30% or greater was proposed to differentiate children with OSA from those with primary snoring. However, only two-third of the children studied normalized their pharyngeal collapsibility after adenotonsillectomy despite resolution of their sleep-disordered breathing (54).

Treatment seems to affect the properties of the pharynx. Twelve overweight patients with OSA showed a significant improvement in lung volume dependence of pharyngeal area along with improvement in sleep-disordered breathing after a 26 ± 18 kg weight loss (55). The three patients with paradoxical inspiratory narrowing of the glottis showed reversal of this phenomenon after weight loss. Patients with central sleep apnea had larger pharynges and a greater lung volume dependence of pharyngeal area than did weight-matched snoring controls without apnea (1). This suggests that pharyngeal size and compliance may play a role in central apnea, or may simply reflect differences in neuromuscular activation that affects both pharyngeal properties and respiratory drive independently.

IV. Summary

Acoustic reflectance provides a unique, noninvasive way to study the size and mechanical properties of the airways. Although it cannot provide specific anatomical details such as those that can be obtained by CT or magnetic resonance imaging, it does not involve radiation and sedation, which can be a concern in children with upper airway obstruction. Measurements can be made in the seated or recumbent positions. This technique has been useful in understanding airway mechanics in OSA, tracheal stenosis, and cystic fibrosis, and may have clinical applicability in these and other airway disorders as well. However, there must be careful attention to technique since the magnitude of measurements may be affected by the type of mouthpiece used, gas composition, lung volume, and head and body position.

References

1. Bradley TD, Brown IG, Zamel N, et al. Differences in pharyngeal properties between snorers with predominantly central sleep apnea and those without sleep apnea. Am Rev Respir Dis 1987; 135:387–391.
2. Guilleminault C, Heldt G, Powell N, et al. Small upper airway in near-miss sudden infant death syndrome infants and their families. Lancet 1986; 1:402–407.
3. DuBois AB, Brody AW, Lewis DH, et al. Oscillation mechanics of lungs and chest in man. J Appl Physiol 1956; 8:587–594.
4. Hoffstein V, Fredberg JJ. The acoustic reflection technique for non-invasive assessment of upper airway area. Eur Respir J 1991; 4(5):602–611.
5. Jackson AC, Butler JP, Millet EJ, et al. Airway geometry by analysis of acoustic pulse response measurements. J Appl Physiol 1977; 43(3):523–536.
6. Jackson AC, Olson DE. Comparison of direct and acoustical area measurements in physical models of human central airways. J Appl Physiol 1980; 48(5):896–902.
7. Jackson AC. Serial distribution of airway geometry from acoustic impedance data. Fed Proc 1980; 39:2741–2746.
8. Jackson AC, Krevans JR. Tracheal cross-sectional areas from acoustic reflections in dogs. J Appl Physiol 1984; 57(2):351–353.
9. Ishizaka K, French JH, Flanagan JM. Direct determination of vocal tract wall impedance. IEEE Trans Acoust Speech Signal Process 1975; 23:370–373.
10. Fredberg JJ, Wohl MEB, Glass GM, et al. Airway area by acoustic reflections measured at the mouth. J Appl Physiol 1980; 48(5):749–758.
11. Brooks LJ, Castile RG, Glass GM, et al. Reproducibility and accuracy of airway area by acoustic reflection. J Appl Physiol 1984; 57(3):777–787.
12. D'Urzo AD, Lawson G, Vassal KP, et al. Airway area by acoustic response measurements and computerized tomography. Am Rev Respir Dis 1987; 135:392–395.
13. Czaja JM, McCaffrey TV. Acoustic measurements of subglottic stenosis. Ann Otol Rhinol Laryngol 1996; 105:504–509.
14. Brooks LJ, Byard PJ, Fouke JM, et al. Reproducibility of measurements of upper airway area by acoustic reflection. J Appl Physiol 1989; 66(6):2901–2905.
15. Rubinstein I, McClean PA, Boucher R, et al. Effect of mouthpiece, noseclips, and head position on airway area by acoustic reflection. J Appl Physiol 1987; 63(4):1469–1474.
16. D'Urzo AD, Rebuck AS, Lawson VG, et al. Effect of CO_2 concentration on acoustic inferences of airway area. J Appl Physiol 1986; 60(2):398–401.

17. Louis B, Glass GM, Kresen B, et al. Airway area by acoustic reflection: the two microphone method. J Biomech Eng 1993; 115:278–285.
18. Louis B, Glass GM, Fredberg JJ. Pulmonary airway area by the two-microphone acoustic reflection method. J Appl Physiol 1994; 76(5):2234–2240.
19. Huang J, Itai N, Hoshiba T, et al. A new nasal acoustic reflection technique to estimate pharyngeal cross-sectional area during sleep. J Appl Physiol 2000; 88: 1457–1466.
20. Hoffstein V. Relationship between lung volume, maximal expiratory flow, forced expiratory volume in one second, and tracheal area in normal men and women. Am Rev Respir Dis 1986; 134:956–961.
21. Martin TR, Castile RG, Fredberg JJ, et al. Airway size is related to sex but not lung size in normal adults. J Appl Physiol 1987; 63(5):2042–2047.
22. Brooks LJ, Byard PJ, Helms RC, et al. Relationship between lung volume and tracheal area as assessed by acoustic reflection. J Appl Physiol 1988; 64(3):1050–1054.
23. Brooks LJ, Byard PJ, Fouke JM, et al. Central airway growth as measured by acoustic reflections. Am Rev Respir Dis 1986; 133:A189.
24. Hoffstein V, Castile RG, O'Donnell CR, et al. In vivo estimation of tracheal distensibility and hysteresis in normal adults. J Appl Physiol 1987; 63(6):2482–2489.
25. Fouke JM, Wolin AD, Strohl KP, et al. Elastic characteristics of the airway wall. J Appl Physiol 1989; 66(2):962–967.
26. Hoffstein V, Zamel N. Tracheal stenosis measured by the acoustic reflection technique. Am Rev Respir Dis 1984; 130:472–475.
27. Brooks LJ. Tracheal size and distensibility in patients with cystic fibrosis. Am Rev Respir Dis 1990; 141:513–516.
28. Raphael DT. Acoustic reflectometry profiles of endotracheal and esophageal intubation. Anesthesiology 2000; 92:1293–1299.
29. Gucev G, Raphael DT, Elspas S, et al. Pediatric airway and esophageal profiles with acoustic reflectometry. Anesth Analg 2006; 103:1126–1130.
30. Fisher EW, Lund VJ, Scadding GK. Acoustic rhinometry in rhinological practice. J Royal Soc Med 1994; 87:411–413.
31. Hilberg O, Jackson AC, Swift DL, et al. Acoustic rhinometry: evaluation of nasal cavity geometry by acoustic reflection. J Appl Physiol 1989; 66(1):295–303.
32. Terheyden H, Maune S, Mertens J, et al. Acoustic rhinometry: validation by three-dimensionally reconstructed computer tomographic scans. J Appl Physiol 2000; 89: 1013–1021.
33. Hilberg O, Jensen FT, Pedersen OF. Nasal airway geometry: comparison between acoustic reflections and magnetic resonance scanning. J Appl Physiol 1993; 75(6): 2811–2819.
34. Corey JP, Gungor A, Nelson R, et al. A comparison of the nasal cross-sectional areas and volumes obtained with acoustic rhinometry and magnetic resonance imaging. Otolaryngol Head Neck Surg 1997; 117:349–354.
35. Hilberg O, Lyholm B, Michelsen A, et al. Acoustic reflections during rhinometry: spatial resolution and sound loss. J Appl Physiol 1998; 84(3):1030–1039.
36. Corey JP, Nalbone VP, Ng BA. Anatomic correlates of acoustic rhinometry as measured by rigid nasal endoscopy. Otolaryngol Head Neck Surg 1999; 121:572–576.
37. Mlynski R, Grutzenmacher S, Mlynski G. Acoustic rhinometry and paranasal sinuses: a systematic study in models, anatomic specimens, and in vivo. Laryngoscope 2005; 115:837–843.

38. Pedersen OF, Berkowitz R, Yamagiwa M, et al. Nasal cavity dimensions in the newborn measured by acoustic reflections. Laryngoscope 1994; 104:1023–1028.

39. Corey JP, Gungor A, Nelson R, et al. Normative standards for nasal cross-sectional areas by race as measured by acoustic rhinometry. Otolaryngol Head Neck Surg 1998; 119:389–393.

40. Gungor A, Moinuddin R, Nelson RH, et al. Detection of the nasal cycle with acoustic rhinometry: techniques and applications. Otolaryngol Head Neck Surg 1999; 120:238–247.

41. Hilberg O, Grymer LF, Pedersen OF. Spontaneous variations in congestion of the nasal mucosa. Ann Allergy Asthma Immunol 1995; 74(6):516–521.

42. Fouke JM, Strohl KP. Effect of position and llund volume on upper airway geometry. J Appl Physiol 1987; 63(1):375–380.

43. Brown IB, McClean PA, Boucher R, et al. Changes in pharyngeal cross-sectional area with posture and application of continuous positive airway pressure in patients with obstructive sleep apnea. Am Rev Respir Dis 1987; 136:628–632.

44. Martin SE, Marshall I, Douglas NJ. The effects of posture on airway caliber with the sleep-apnea/hypopnea syndrome. Am J Respir Crit Care Med 1995; 152:721–724.

45. Brooks LJ, Strohl KP. Size and mechanical properties of the pharynx in healthy men and women. Am Rev Respir Dis 1992; 146:1394–1397.

46. Brown IG, Zamel N, Hoffstein V. Pharyngeal cross-sectional area in normal men and women. J Appl Physiol 1986; 61(3):890–895.

47. Rivlin J, Hoffstein V, Kalbfleisch J, et al. Upper airway morphology in patients with idiopathic obstructive sleep apnea. Am Rev Respir Dis 1984; 129:355–360.

48. Rubinstein I, Bradley TD, Zamel N, et al. Glottic and cervical tracheal narrowing in patients with obstructive sleep apnea. J Appl Physiol 1989; 67(6):2427–2437.

49. Hoffstein V, Zamel N, Phillipson EA. Lung volume dependence of pharyngeal cross-sectional area in patients with obstructive sleep apnea. Am Rev Respir Dis 1984; 130:175–178.

50. Rubinstein I, Hoffstein V, Bradley TD. Lung volume-related changes in the pharyngeal area of obese females with and without obstructive sleep apnea. Eur Respir J 1989; 2:344–351.

51. Bradley TD, Brown IG, Grossman RF, et al. Pharyngeal size in snorers, nonsnorers, and patients with obstructive sleep apnea. N Engl J Med 1986; 315:1327–1331.

52. Brown IG, Bradley TD, Phillipson EA, et al. Pharyngeal compliance in snoring subjects with and without obstructive sleep apnea. Am Rev Respir Dis 1985; 132: 211–215.

53. Rubinstein I, Slutsky AS, Zamel N, et al. Paradoxical glottic narrowing in patients with severe obstructive sleep apnea. J Clin Invest 1988; 81:1051–1055.

54. Gozal D, Burnside MM. Increased upper airway collapsibility in children with obstructive sleep apnea during wakefulness. Am J Respir Crit Care Med 2004; 169: 163–167.

55. Rubinstein I, Colapinto N, Rotstein LE, et al. Improvement in upper airway function after weight loss in patients with obstructive sleep apnea. Am Rev Respir Dis 1988; 138:1192–1195.

26

Pediatric Obstructive Sleep Apnea Syndrome: 30 Years of Progress

ROBERT T. BROUILLETTE
McGill University, Montreal, Quebec, Canada

I. Introduction

The present chapter will review the early history of sleep apnea in children, detail several of the seminal papers (Table 1) in this field, and propose challenges for the future.

In 1975–1976, Christian Guilleminault et al. published the first case series that clearly described sleep apnea, its clinical manifestations, consequences, diagnosis, and treatment in children aged 5 to 14 years (1,2). Loud, frequent snoring was present in all the children. Associated problems included daytime hypersomnolence, decreased school performance, mood and behavioral disturbances, hypertension, marked respiratory sinus arrhythmia, and weight abnormalities, including both underweight and obesity. Polysomnography was used as a diagnostic technique and demonstrated drops in oxygen saturation consequent to obstructive sleep apneas, dramatic fluctuations in esophageal pressure, and arousals terminating the obstructive events. They reported that apnea and hypopnea were most frequent in stages 1 and 2 of non–rapid eye movement (NREM) sleep. Upper airway examination revealed adenotonsillar hypertrophy in six of

Table 1 Seminal Papers in the Investigation of Pediatric OSAS

1951–1953	Aserinsky and Kleitman discover REM sleep
1965–1967	Cox, Menash, Noonan, Luke, Levy and their groups report cor pulmonale secondary to enlarged tonsils and adenoids
1965	Gastaut et al. and Jung and Kuhlo describe OSAS in adults
1976	Guilleminault et al. study a case series of 8 children with sleep apnea
1978	Remmers et al. show that in adult OSAS the upper airway obstructs when collapsing negative pressure is not balanced by dilating muscular force
1979,1980	Brouillette and Thach develop a model for airway collapse in OSAS
1983	Haponik et al. show that adults with OSAS have smaller pharynxes when awake
1984	Brouillette et al. prepare a questionnaire to distinguish children with OSAS from normals
1989	Mallory et al. report sleep-associated breathing disorders in morbidly obese children and adolescents
1991	Gleadhill et al. show that adults with OSAS have smaller, more collapsible pharynx when asleep
1992	Marcus et al. find normal values for polysomnography
1992,1994	McColley et al. and Rosen et al. delineate risk factors for respiratory compromise after adenotonsillectomy
1994	Marcus et al. apply Starling resistor model to airway collapse in sleeping children
1995	Carroll et al. study inability of clinical history to distinguish primary snoring from OSAS
1996	American Thoracic Society reports standards and indications for cardiopulmonary sleep studies
1997	Isono and Remmers show that adults with OSAS have smaller, more collapsible pharynx under anesthesia
1997	Chervin et al. report that habitual snoring was more frequent in children with ADHD than in children from psychiatry or general pediatric clinics.
1998	Isono et al. study airway collapse in anesthetized children
1998,2001	Gozal et al. show effects of OSAS on school performance
2000	Brouillette et al. demonstrate the usefulness of nocturnal pulse oximetry in confirming a suspicion of OSAS
2001,2003	Arens et al. use MRI to delineate the upper airway structure of children
2002	American Academy of Pediatrics issues Clinical Practice Guideline and Technical Document
2002	Chervin et al. find in general pediatric clinics an association of snoring and sleepiness with inattention and hyperactivity
2002,2005	Amin et al. show left heart changes in pediatric OSAS
2003	Schwimmer et al. report that OSAS adversely affects quality of life in severely obese children and adolescents
2003	O'Brien et al. report a high prevalence of snoring among a group of children showing mild symptoms of attention deficit hyperactivity disorder
2007	Chervin et al. prepare a pediatric sleep questionnaire that predicts outcomes of T&A better than polysomnography

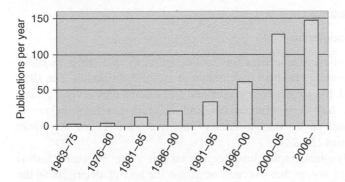

Figure 1 Publications on obstructive sleep apnea in children.

eight children, most of whom recovered after removal of the lymphoid tissue. Two children had tracheostomy with resolution of sleep-related obstructive events and clinical improvements in hypertension, enuresis, and daytime fatigue. Subsequently increasing numbers of papers have been published on sleep apnea in children (Fig. 1).

In the years preceding this first case series, a number of discoveries laid the groundwork for the description of sleep apnea in children. In 1952–1953, Aserinsky, a PhD student, was assigned to observe body movements and eye motility in infants. He noticed periods of jerky eye movements that have subsequently been called REM sleep (3). Further work by Dement and Kleitman in humans and by Jouvet in cats established a characteristic alternation between quiet sleep and the hypotonia of REM sleep (4,5). See Dement's article for an excellent review of the history of our understanding of sleep (6). About the same time, Burwell et al. published the association between morbid obesity and hypoventilation, terming it the Pickwickian syndrome (7). Several papers reported this association in children and adolescents (8,9).

Starting in the mid-1960s two key developments occurred. First, two groups described obstructive sleep apnea syndrome (OSAS) in adults (10,11). Most early patients were "Pickwickian," i.e., they were morbidly obese and hypersomnolent. These and subsequent papers reported that polygraphic recordings during sleep demonstrated repetitive obstructive apnea terminated by and alternating with arousal from sleep. Coccagna et al. were interested in "hypersomnia with periodic breathing" and described a 12-year-old with OSAS who responded to tracheostomy (12). David White has recently reviewed the history of OSAS in adults (13).

Second, several papers described an association between adenotonsillar hypertrophy and airway obstruction on the one hand and cor pulmonale, pulmonary hypertension, congestive heart failure, cardiomegaly, and pulmonary edema on the other (14–18).

II. Diagnosis

A. Polysomnography

The establishment of normative data for cardiorespiratory and sleep variables during sleep in children has been an important and useful contribution. The 1992 work of Marcus et al. has largely been confirmed and extended by several groups (19–24). This data has been summarized and incorporated into diagnostic guidelines and standards by the American Thoracic Society and American Academy of Pediatrics (25–28).

Although polysomnography has been used for over 30 years and is accepted as the most comprehensive and accurate method of determining the presence and severity of OSAS in children, important questions remain unanswered. First, normative data described above are just that, namely, reference values. It is clear that severely ill children who have polysomnographic metrics far from the norm, such as many of the children described in early case series, will benefit from treatment. However, the threshold for deciding on treatment for pediatric OSAS has not been established. Randomized controlled trials will be required to determine which metrics and what severities relate to clinically significant long-term benefits.

Second, different laboratories continue to use different methods to diagnose partial airway obstruction. The most accurate method to quantitate airflow through the upper airway is a pneumotachograph with integration to obtain tidal volume. Likewise the most accurate method of determining respiratory effort is esophageal pressure recording. Because these techniques are difficult to perform on children, most laboratories have used less accurate methodologies. Respiratory inductive plethysmography and nasal pressure bear the closest relations to tidal volume and airflow, respectively (29,30). By contrast, thermistor and nasal CO_2 measurements are qualitative measures of airflow; using these techniques, small amounts of expiratory airflow that would qualify as hypopnea using more quantitative techniques may appear normal. Trang and Serebrisky demonstrated the superiority of nasal pressure over thermistor for detection of hypopnea in children (31,32).

Third, it has been proposed that many children have an upper airway resistance syndrome (UARS) that has a similar pathophysiology and consequences to OSAS but does not meet diagnostic criteria for OSAS (33). Confirmation of this hypothesis has been slow in coming for two reasons. To make this diagnosis, a first level test, standard polysomnography must be negative for OSAS and it must have been performed with optimal noninvasive techniques. As described above, such a test should rely on a semiquantitative measure of flow such as nasal pressure and/or respiratory inductive plethysmography. Additionally, few laboratories have experience with esophageal pressure recordings in children (34).

B. History and Physical Examination

In the initial 1976 reports by Guilleminault et al., a detailed history and careful physical examination, particularly of the upper airway, was considered mandatory for making the diagnosis and deciding upon treatment. Virtually all subsequent papers have taken this position, but debate continues whether history and physical examination alone is adequate to diagnose some cases of OSAS. In a 1984 case-control study, Brouillette et al. compared the symptomatology of children with polysomnographically proven sleep apnea to normal controls (35). It was clear from this work that children with sleep apnea have signs and symptoms, such as snoring, difficulty in breathing during sleep, and parentally observed apneas, that are very different from other children presenting to pediatric clinics and offices. Numerous subsequent studies have shown that it is impossible to accurately predict which children referred to a pediatric sleep laboratory for possible OSAS will have polysomnographically proven disease (36,37). However, most adenotonsillectomies are performed for obstructive breathing and most otolaryngologists remove tonsils and adenoids without the benefit of polysomnography or other testing prior to surgery (38). Some reports have stressed that adenotonsillectomy may be beneficial even if polysomnography does not demonstrate OSA and a recent report suggests that a symptom questionnaire may better predict response to adenotonsillectomy than polysomnography (39,40).

C. Alternative or Abbreviated Testing

Polysomnography is an expensive medical test with current costs generally in the range of $1000 to $2000. Furthermore, there are relatively few pediatric sleep laboratories. By contrast, adenotonsillectomy is the most common surgical procedure in childhood and is most often performed for obstructive symptomatology. To test 400,000 children at $1500 per test would require $600 million annually in the United States. This would also require 800 pediatric sleep laboratories, each performing 500 studies per year. Not surprisingly, there has been interest in less expensive testing methods that could be more available. The American Academy of Pediatrics reviewed audio taping and videotaping, nap studies, home polysomnography, and pulse oximetry (26,28). Of these techniques, pulse oximetry has a number of advantages. When positive it can confirm a suspicion of OSAS (41). It is simple and inexpensive enough to be made widely available. Children who have had an abnormal nocturnal oximetry result are more likely to have perioperative respiratory compromise and need a lower narcotic dose for pain control postoperatively (42–44). Of importance, an inconclusive overnight oximetry test, like other abbreviated testing, does not rule out OSAS (41).

III. Pathogenesis

In Guilleminault's 1976 papers, six of eight children had adenotonsillar hypertrophy suggesting the importance of anatomic blockage of the upper airway (1,2). Pulmonary function during wakefulness was normal in all children suggesting that there was a physiologic difference between sleep and wakefulness (1). These two factors, anatomic and physiologic, have been further identified and understood in subsequent years. In the 1970s, after numerous descriptions of the OSAS in adults, respiratory physiologists and neurophysiologists became interested in understanding the upper airway collapse that occurred during sleep. Using electromyography, Sauerland and Harper studied activity of the genioglossus muscle that pulls the tongue forward and away from the oropharynx (45). Recordings of inspiratory pharyngeal pressure and genioglossal electromyography allowed Remmers et al. to propose the balance of forces model: "We speculate that genioglossal force acts to open the oropharynx and that negative pharyngeal pressure promotes pharyngeal closure" (46). Studies in animals demonstrated that a neuromuscular mechanism maintains pharyngeal airway patency and that muscles surrounding the upper airway act as accessory muscles of respiration (47,48). Another model of OSA is based on the pharyngeal airway acting as a collapsible segment or Starling resistor. Marcus et al. showed that during sleep, children have more stable or less collapsible pharyngeal airways than adults and that children with obstructive apnea have more collapsible airways than those with primary snoring (49). Isono et al. showed that when neuromuscular activity was eliminated by anesthesia and muscular paralysis, children with OSAS were more prone to collapse than controls leading them to conclude that "anatomic factors play a significant role in the pathogenesis of pediatric OSAS" (50). It is now understood that this physiologic propensity is sleep-related relaxation of upper airway maintaining musculature.

Similarly, studies of Aserinsky, Dement, and Kleitman in the 1950s demonstrated that sleep had two major stages, quiet and REM. Studies by Jouvet et al. showed that there was muscular hypotonia during REM sleep and studies by Sauerland, Harper, Remmers, and others showed that this hypotonia extended to muscles surrounding the pharyngeal airway. Some early reports suggested that sleep apnea was more frequent in light, quiet sleep, but subsequent studies have demonstrated a marked propensity for obstructive events during REM sleep in children, as would be predicted from the above (51–53).

In children, the most common anatomic contributor to OSAS is adenotonsillar hypertrophy. This was apparent from the earliest case series. Pediatric OSAS is most common in the age range of two to six years. In 1981, Jeans et al. presented radiographic data suggesting that the adenoidal and tonsillar lymphoid tissue grew more rapidly in young children than the skeletal box in which it was contained (54). This lymphoid overgrowth was therefore considered to narrow the upper airway and explain the prevalence of OSAS in preschool children. However, Arens et al., using magnetic resonance imaging (MRI) in children aged

1 to 11 years, found that soft tissues, including tonsils and adenoids, surrounding the upper airway grow proportionally to the skeletal structures (55–57). The tonsils and adenoids of most children with OSAS are larger than those of controls and therefore a fundamental question remains unanswered. What is the cause of adenotonsillar hypertrophy, which is so obviously maladaptive in cases of severe OSAS? Once we better understand the pathogenesis of the abnormal enlargement we may be better able to treat the problem medically and eliminate the need for surgery in many cases.

Early fluoroscopic studies showed the there were different patterns of pharyngeal airway collapse in different children with OSAS depending, at least in part, on the relative hypertrophy of adenoids versus tonsils (58,59). Recent MRI studies have suggested that the most common site of airway obstruction/air flow restriction is the area of overlap where both the tonsils and adenoids encroach upon the pharyngeal airway (57). MRI studies with respiratory gating and computational fluid mechanics suggest that the "restrictive segment" and the "collapsible segment" may overlap or may be identical (57,60). Clinicians still require a practical, widely available method of assessing the anatomic cause and the site of airway collapse in children who have OSAS but no obvious upper airway narrowing (61,62).

Other children with OSAS have an anatomic abnormality that either increases inspiratory upstream (nasal) resistance or narrows the collapsible (pharyngeal) airway. Crouzon and Pierre Robin syndromes are examples of these anatomic predispositions. OSAS is particularly frequent in Down syndrome (63–65). Uong et al. demonstrated that children with Down syndrome but without OSAS do not have adenotonsillar hypertrophy, but rather have reduced upper airway size caused by soft tissue crowding within a smaller mid- and lower face skeleton (66). Most commonly, they will benefit from adenotonsillectomy, but other airway operations are sometimes beneficial (67).

IV. Sequelae: Failure to Thrive

Five of eight patients of Guilleminault's 1976 study were underweight (1,2). In our series, 6 of 22 (27%) children with OSAS who had failure to thrive improved dramatically after surgical correction of airway obstruction (68). Many other papers have reported an increase in body weight, and sometimes height, after relief of sleep-related airway obstruction in children. Growth failure has been ascribed to three potential mechanisms, although the importance of each remains undetermined: inadequate caloric intake, increased metabolic rate, and abnormalities of growth hormone and insulin-related growth factor. Marcus et al. studied 14 children before and after adenotonsillectomy (69). They identified increases in body weight, no change in caloric intake, but a decrease of about 10% in sleeping energy expenditure after adenotonsillectomy. By contrast, Bland et al. found no significant difference in total energy expenditure measured by the doubly-labeled water method, although there was no consistent improvement in OSAS after adenotonsillectomy (70,71). Findings have been more consistent for growth hormone. Bar et al. reported increased weight and IGF-I after adenotonsillectomy for OSAS (72). Additional studies have shown increased weight for height, body mass index, body fat mass, fat-free mass, IGF-I and the IGFBP-3, weight and height standard deviation scores, and energy intake per kilogram (73,74). Unfortunately, postoperative weight gains are also seen in obese children with OSAS (75). A paradox remains: growth hormone is secreted during quiet sleep whereas the breathing disturbance in children with OSAS occurs primarily during REM sleep (52,53).

V. Sequelae: The Heart and Cardiovascular System

As mentioned above, reports in the 1960s associated adenotonsillar hypertrophy with pulmonary hypertension and cor pulmonale (14–18). In the 1950s, Burwell et al. had described an association of obesity and hypoventilation and called it the Pickwickian syndrome, after the character of Joe in Charles Dickens novel *The Posthumous Papers Of The Pickwick Club* (7). In fact, Joe would seem to have had the characteristics of a young adult with Prader-Willi syndrome— hyperphagia, obesity, hypersomnolence, intellectual limitations, and certain physical characteristics (76). There were several reports in the 1960s of the syndrome in children (8,9,77–79). The earliest reports of OSAS in children often had a high prevalence of right heart abnormalities that were ascribed to sleep-related hypoxemia. However, left heart problems were also seen and were sometimes ascribed to an increased afterload on the left heart related to working at low intrathoracic pressure during inspiration (80). Marcus et al. found more diastolic hypertension in children with OSAS than in children with primary snoring (81). Subsequent studies using larger subject numbers and 24-hour blood pressure recordings have confirmed a relationship between apnea severity and hypertension. Amin et al. reported lack of nocturnal dipping in blood pressure and increased blood pressure variability in children depending on severity of OSAS (82). Three studies have examined the interaction of obesity and OSA on hypertension (82–84).

Heart rate variability has been found to be elevated in children and adults with OSAS (85–88). Stradling et al. found heart rate to decrease after adenotonsillectomy and Constantin et al. found both pulse rate and pulse rate variability to decrease after adenotonsillectomy in children with moderate to severe OSAS (89,90). In adults, sympathetic nerve outflow increased during apnea and at arousal preceding rises in blood pressure and heart rate (91). High sympathetic nerve activity and plasma catecholamine levels are present during the day as well as at night in adults with OSAS (92). Amin et al. has suggested that effects on the heart and cardiovascular system could be either direct or indirect via cytokines (93,94).

To date, evidence of cardiovascular disease is primarily used as a marker for significant or serious OSAS. The most sensitive and practical methods of detecting cardiovascular disease secondary to OSAS need clarification. Further work is required to determine if nocturnal heart rate or heart rate variability can be used diagnostically (95). It is likely that both obesity and OSAS will contribute to the long-term morbidity of OSAS and this requires particularly careful study. Finally, an important but difficult challenge is to observe the long-term cardiovascular consequences of pediatric OSAS as individuals move through the lifecycle.

VI. Sequelae: Neurobehavioral Consequences of Sleep Apnea

In Guilleminault's 1976 paper, five of eight children had school problems and daytime sleepiness and six had behavior and/or emotional difficulties, particularly hyperactivity and bedtime refusal (1,2). They reported that school functioning improved but remained abnormal in two of five children after relief of airway obstruction. In the subsequent 30 years numerous papers have examined the topics of neurodevelopment, behavior, and learning in children with OSAS and/or snoring. The extensive literature in this area relates to the importance of the topic as well as the complexity of relating a wide variety of neurobehavioral outcomes to patients heterogeneous for age, gender, severity of OSAS, and accounting for potential confounders, such as socioeconomic status and craniofacial or neurologic disease that may relate to both the disease in question and to the outcomes of interest.

There have been a number of excellent reviews of this area; this section will not exhaustively review the entire area but simply mention some of the most important advances. The American Academy of Pediatrics Technical Report in 2002 found 12 publications that evaluated the association of behavioral problems with sleep-disordered breathing (SDB) (28). They estimated a threefold increase in behavior and neurocognitive abnormalities in children with SDB but indicated that most papers had not separated OSAS from primary snoring. In 2004, Ebert and Drake found 17 papers that assessed the relation of SDB to cognition and behavior in children (96) They focused on strengths and weaknesses from a methodologic standpoint. They reported numerous study design issues in the majority of these papers and suggested that "improvements in study design and methodology could initiate the development of a more complete understanding of this complex topic." In 2006, Halbrower and Mahone assessed 12 controlled studies of behavioral and cognitive function in children with SDB (97). They emphasized the need to focus on milder forms of SDB, such as snoring and upper airway resistance syndrome. They also pointed out the heterogeneity of results and the need to account for other factors that might affect performance on neuropsychological test scores including developmental stage, obesity, psychological/psychiatric disorders, poor sleep hygiene, and drugs.

In the 15 years following Guilleminault's 1976 papers, there was a paucity of rigorously designed clinical investigations assessing the relationship of developmental, behavioral and cognitive outcomes for sleep apnea or its treatment by adenotonsillectomy. Most studies in this era were case series that reported improvements in these domains after surgical treatment. The numerous additional case series and cross-sectional studies that have shown a relationship of neurobehavioral abnormalities to OSAS or resolution of such problems after adenotonsillectomy are appropriate for hypothesis generation but provide relatively weak evidence for a causal role of OSAS.

There is now substantial evidence that OSAS and snoring are associated with neurobehavioral problems. In a 1983 cross-sectional study, Weissbluth et al. associated snoring and other signs of airway obstruction with behavior, development, and academic problems (98). In 1993–1994, Ali et al., using a cohort design in over 500 children, showed that habitual snorers were more likely to be hyperactive, and have restless sleep and daytime sleepiness; however, over a two-year follow-up period, habitual snoring and the associated behavioral problems resolved spontaneously in about 50% cases (99,100). Chervin et al. found that habitual snoring was more frequent (33%) among children who carried a diagnosis of attention-deficit/hyperactivity disorder (ADHD) than among children at general pediatric clinics (9%) (101). Using a retrospective cohort design, Gozal reported that children with lower academic performance in middle school were more likely to have snored during early childhood (102).

Studies that assess neurobehavioral outcomes before and after surgery provide evidence of a causal relationship between OSAS and these important aspects of child development. Ali et al., in a 1996 case-control study, found that children with OSAS and those with primary snoring, but not those with other surgical problems, had improved hyperactivity and vigilance postoperatively (103). In 1998, Gozal et al. used a cohort of academically low-performing children, screened them for OSAS using oximetry and CO_2 recordings, and offered adenotonsillectomy to those thought to have OSAS (104). Children who had surgery, but not those whose parents declined operation, improved academically. By contrast, Harvey et al. reported that adenotonsillectomy did not modify temperament or development in neurologically normal children with OSAS (105). In one of the best studies to date, Chervin used a prospective cohort design to compare neurobehavioral outcomes of children scheduled for adenotonsillectomy to those undergoing other surgery. They found

> "children scheduled for adenotonsillectomy often have mild-to-moderate sleep-disordered breathing (SDB) and significant neurobehavioral morbidity, including hyperactivity, inattention, attention-deficit/hyperactivity disorder, and excessive daytime sleepiness, all of which tend to improve by 1 year after surgery."
> (105,106)

In contrast, Constantin et al. sent questionnaires to parents of children who had been evaluated for OSAS several years earlier. Parents of operated children were no more likely to report improvements in behavior than those of unoperated children (107).

It seems clear at this point that severe OSAS can cause such neurobehavioral problems as hyperactivity, sleep disturbance, school and learning problems, and daytime sleepiness. Randomized controlled trials of adenotonsillectomy and of medical therapy for mild OSAS, and for sleep-related airway obstruction that does not rise to the level currently defined as OSAS, will be required to prove a causal relationship between sleep-related breathing obstruction and neurobehavioral outcomes. Follow-up studies will be particularly important to show long-lasting, clinically significant benefits.

VII. Obesity

In Guilleminault's papers and in most other early reports of pediatric OSAS, failure to thrive was a frequent finding (1,2,68,108). However, two of eight children from the original case series were obese. Earlier, in the 1960s and 1970s several papers had reported the association of obesity, snoring, hypoventilation, and hypersomnolence (8). Mallory, Silvestri, and Marcus all reported a high prevalence, from 37–66%, of OSAS in morbidly obese children and adolescents (109–111). Redline et al. firmly established obesity as a risk factor for pediatric OSAS in a community survey (112). They estimated a fourfold increased risk of OSAS for obesity (BMI > 28) or a 12% increased risk for each kg/m^2 of BMI increase. As the prevalence of child and adolescent obesity and morbid obesity increase, obesity as a risk factor for OSAS is assuming increasing importance (113,114).

When failure to thrive was a common presenting problem in children with OSAS, weight gain after adenotonsillectomy or other correction of the sleep-related airway obstruction was considered positive (68,108). Subsequently, it has been reported that even obese children who have adenotonsillectomy often gain weight (75).

Children with obesity may be at increased perioperative risk for adenotonsillectomy and other operations. In 1994, Rosen et al. listed morbid obesity among the risk factors for postoperative upper airway obstruction after adenotonsillectomy for OSAS (115). Spector et al. reported that 6 of 14 morbidly obese patients required postoperative oxygen, intubation or noninvasive ventilation; surprisingly, they concluded that "routine PICU admission is not warranted for most morbidly obese patients" (116).

Both obesity and OSAS adversely affect a child's quality of life. Studies have evaluated both disease specific and global quality of life, sometimes providing comparisons to other pediatric disorders such as asthma, juvenile rheumatoid arthritis and cancer. Several groups have developed and validated disease-specific quality-of-life questionnaires (117–119). In 2002, Rosen et al., evaluating a community-based cohort, found OSAS related to overall physical health and complaints of bodily pain. They used obesity as a covariate (120). In 2003, Schwimmer et al. reported that severely obese children and adolescents had significantly lower health-related quality of life than controls (121). The only comorbid disorder that further impaired quality of life was OSAS. In 2004, Mitchell et al. reported that obese children with OSAS who underwent adenotonsillectomy showed a marked improvement in quality of life (122).

VIII. Surgical Treatment

Prior to the formal description of OSAS in children, it was recognized that adenotonsillectomy was effective in reversing congestive heart failure and pulmonary hypertension and that weight loss could have a salutary effect on children with the Pickwickian syndrome (14–18,123). Coccagna et al. reported improvement in a 12-year-old child with OSAS after tracheostomy (12). Of Guilleminault's original series, improvement or normalization of problems was reported after adenotonsillectomy in five of six patients; two patients required tracheostomy (1,2).

Adenotonsillectomy has remained the first-line treatment for pediatric OSAS (26,28). However, controversies persist. First, the minimal severity of OSAS or sleep-related airway obstruction justifying adenotonsillectomy has yet to be determined. Randomized controlled trials for mild disease will likely be needed to establish these guidelines. Second, the efficacy of adenotonsillectomy for OSAS requires further clarification. Some have reported that a significant percentage of patients undergoing operation have residual disease (124,125). It will be important to distinguish children who only have adenotonsillar hypertrophy from those who have significant comorbid disorders, such as obesity, craniofacial, genetic, and neurologic disorders. Third, there are debates about the need to keep all children with OSAS in hospital overnight after adenotonsillectomy and about the need to keep high-risk subjects in the pediatric intensive care unit after operation (115,126–131).

IX. Medical Treatments

In 1981, 10 years after it had been described for treating respiratory distress syndrome of the newborn, Collin Sullivan reported that continuous positive airway pressure (CPAP) delivered through a nasal mask could be used to treat adult OSAS (132,133).

Five years later Guilleminault reported use of CPAP in hospital and at home in 10 children, most with craniofacial and neurologic disorders (134). Case series have generally found CPAP to be an effective second-line treatment (135,136). Recent papers have stressed the need for a multidisciplinary approach to maximize effectiveness (137–139).

As OSAS in children is most often due to adenotonsillar hypertrophy and as surgery has inherent risks and discomforts, medical treatments to reduce the size of tonsils and adenoids are attractive. Al-Ghamdi et al. found that a short course of prednisone was ineffective in treating pediatric OSAS caused by adenotonsillar hypertrophy (140). Demain and Goetz demonstrated that nasal steroids could improve obstructive symptomatology and reduce the size of adenoids (141). In a randomized controlled trial evaluating a six-week course of nasal steroid treatment, Brouillette et al. showed a reduction in apnea hypopnea index and other polysomnographic measures of OSAS (142). Alexopolulos et al. found similar results (143). Criscouloli et al. found a reduced need for surgery in children with symptomatic adenotonsillar hypertrophy treated with a six-month course of nasal steroids (144). Goldbart et al. found glucocorticoid receptors in adenotonsillar tissue (145). They also found that over 16 weeks an oral leukotriene receptor antagonist induced significant reductions in adenoid size and respiratory-related sleep disturbances (146). Kheirandish et al. reported that combined anti-inflammatory therapy using oral montelukast and intranasal budesonide improved and/or normalized respiratory and sleep disturbances in children with residual

Table 2 OSAS Related Issues Confronting Pediatricians and Other Child Health Specialists

Allergy/immunology	Upper airway inflammation, allergic rhinitis
Anesthesiology	Pre- and intraoperative airway management
Cardiology	Cor pulmonale, ventricular dysfunction, hypertension
Critical care	Postoperative management including pulmonary edema following adenotonsillectomy and postoperative airway obstruction and desaturation
Developmental and general pediatrics	Developmental delay, failure to thrive, school and learning problems
Endocrine	Obesity, glucose intolerance, growth problems, puberty
Gastroenterology	Increase in gastroesophageal reflux
Genetics	Increased risk in African-Americans, gender differences
Hematology	Differential diagnosis of polycythemia
Infectious disease	Recurrent adenotonsillitis, pathogenesis of adenotonsillar hypertrophy
Nephrology	Hypertension
Neurology	Neurocognitive dysfunction
Neuroradiology	Changes in functional MRI associated with OSAS
Neurosurgery	Brainstem compression syndromes (achondroplasia, Chiari malformation)
Pulmonary	Abnormal respiration and gas exchange during sleep
Public health	Link to adult OSAS
Sleep medicine	Perhaps most common and clinically significant sleep disorder in children
Urology	Enuresis
Outcomes and health services research	Fertile area of research since at present there is little data on the natural history of OSAS in children, best approach to diagnosis and therapy, or treatment thresholds.

OSAS after adenotonsillectomy (147). These studies suggest the need to reevaluate adenotonsillectomy as first-line treatment for mild OSAS in children and to compare surgical with anti-inflammatory treatment for such cases.

Over the past 30 years, child health professionals have recognized that OSAS is an important problem that has consequences on the growth, development, and daily function of children at all ages. Clinical research has increased significantly with new findings that are now being reported weekly. However, significant deficits in our knowledge remain. A list of issues pediatricians may encounter as a consequence of OSAS is presented in Table 2. For clinicians these can be taken as problems to be solved at the bedside. For researchers, the challenges are to better understand the pathogenesis of the disorder, to elucidate the mechanisms of important sequelae, and to validate appropriate diagnostic and therapeutic modalities. Let us hope that we can meet these challenges in significantly less than the next 30 years.

References

1. Guilleminault C, Eldridge FL, Simmons FB, et al. Sleep apnea in eight children. Pediatrics 1976; 58(1):23–30.
2. Guilleminault C, Tilkian AG, Dement WC. Sleep and respiration in the syndrome "apnea during sleep" in the child. Electroencephalogr Clin Neurophysiol 1976; 41 (4):367–378.
3. Aserinsky E, Kleitman N. Regularly occurring periods of eye motility, and concomitant phenomena, during Sleep. Science 1953; 118(3062):273–274.
4. Dement W, Kleitman N. Cyclic variations in EEG during sleep and their relation to eye movements, body motility, and dreaming. Electroencephalogr Clin Neurophysiol Suppl 1957; 9(4):673–690.
5. Jouvet M, Michel F, Courjon J. EEG studies during physiological sleep in the cat, intact, decorticate and chronic mesencephalic. Electroencephal Clin Neurophysiol 1960; 12(2):536.
6. Dement WC. The study of human sleep: a historical perspective. Thorax 1998; 53: S2–S7.
7. Burwell CS, Robin ED, Whaley RD, et al. Extreme obesity associated with alveolar hypoventilation—Pickwickian Syndrome. Amer J Med 1959; 21(5):811–818.
8. Cayler GG, Mays J, Riley HD Jr. Cardiorespiratory syndrome of obesity (Pickwickian syndrome) in children. Pediatrics 1961; 27:237–245.
9. Finkelstein JW, Avery ME. The Pickwickian Syndrome. Studies on ventilation and carbohydrate metabolism: case report of a child who recovered. Am J Dis Child 1963; 106:251–257.
10. Gastaut H, Tassinari CA, Duron B. Polygraphic study of the episodic diurnal and nocturnal (hypnic and respiratory) manifestations of the Pickwick syndrome. Brain Res 1966; 1(2):167–186.
11. Jung R, Kuhlo W. Neurophysiological studies of abnormal night sleep and the Pickwickian Syndrome. Prog Brain Res 1965; 18:140–159.

12. Coccagna G, Mantovani M, Brignani F, et al. Tracheostomy in hypersomnia with periodic breathing. Bull Physiopathol Respir (Nancy). 1972; 8(5):1217–1227.

13. White DP. The pathogenesis of obstructive sleep apnea: advances in the past 100 years. Am J Respir Cell Mol Biol 2006; 34(1):1–6.

14. Cox MA, Schieble GL, Taylor WJ, et al. Reversible pulmonary hypertension in a child with respiratory obstruction and cor pulmonale. J Pediatr 1965; 67(2):192–197.

15. Menashe VD, Farrehi C, Miller M. Hypoventilation and cor pulmonale due to chronic upper airway obstruction. J Pediatr 1965; 67(2):198–203.

16. Noonan JA. Reversible cor pulmonale due to hypertrophied tonsils and adenoids— studies in 2 cases. Circulation 1965; 32(4 suppl 2):164.

17. Luke MJ, Mehrizi A, Folger GM, et al. Chronic nasopharyngeal obstruction as a cause of cardiomegaly cor pulmonale and pulmonary edema. Pediatrics 1966; 37 (5 pt 1):762–768.

18. Levy AM, Tabakin BS, Hanson JS, et al. Hypertrophied adenoids causing pulmonary hypertension and severe congestive heart failure. N Engl J Med 1967; 277(10): 506–511.

19. Marcus CL, Omlin KJ, Basinki DJ, et al. Normal polysomnographic values for children and adolescents. Am Rev Respir Dis 1992; 146(5 pt 1):1235–1239.

20. Moss D, Urschitz MS, von BA, et al. Reference values for nocturnal home poly-somnography in primary schoolchildren. Pediatr Res 2005; 58(5):958–965.

21. Quan SF, Goodwin JL, Babar SI, et al. Sleep architecture in normal Caucasian and Hispanic children aged 6-11 years recorded during unattended home poly-somnography: experience from the Tucson Children's Assessment of Sleep Apnea Study (TuCASA). Sleep Med 2003; 4(1):13–19.

22. Traeger N, Schultz B, Pollock AN, et al. Polysomnographic values in children 2-9 years old: additional data and review of the literature. Pediatr Pulmonol 2005; 40 (1): 22–30.

23. Uliel S, Tauman R, Greenfeld M, et al. Normal polysomnographic respiratory values in children and adolescents. Chest 2004; 125(3):872–878.

24. Witmans MB, Keens TG, vidson Ward SL, et al Obstructive hypopneas in children and adolescents: normal values. Am J Respir Crit Care Med 2003; 168(12):1540.

25. Marcus C, England S, Annett R, et al. Cardiorespiratory sleep studies in children. Establishment of normative data and polysomnographic predictors of morbidity. American Thoracic Society. Am J Respir Crit Care Med 1999; 160(4):1381–1387.

26. Marcus CL, Chapman D, Davidson Ward S, et al. Clinical practice guideline: diagnosis and management of childhood obstructive sleep apnea syndrome; American Academy of Pediatrics. Pediatrics 2002; 109(4):704–712.

27. Loughlin GM, Brouillete RT, Brooks LJ, et al. Standards and indications for car-diopulmonary sleep studies in children. American Thoracic Society. Am J Respir Crit Care Med 1996; 153(2):866–878.

28. Schechter MS; The Section on Pediatric Pulmonology SoOSAS. Technical report: diagnosis and management of childhood obstructive sleep apnea syndrome. American Academy of Pediatrics. Pediatrics 2002; 109(4):e69.

29. Flemons WW, Buysse D, Redline S, et al. Sleep-related breathing disorders in adults: Recommendations for syndrome definition and measurement techniques in clinical research. Sleep 1999; 22(5):667–689.

30. Cantineau JP, Escourrou P, Sartene R, et al. Accuracy of respiratory inductive plethysmography during wakefulness and sleep in patients with obstructive sleep-apnea. Chest 1992; 102(4):1145–1151.

31. Trang H, Leske V, Gaultier C. Use of nasal cannula for detecting sleep apneas and hypopneas in infants and children. Am J Respir Crit Care Med 2002; 166(4): 464–468.

32. Serebrisky D, Cordero R, Mandeli J, et al. Assessment of inspiratory flow limitation in children with sleep-disordered breathing by a nasal cannula pressure transducer system. Pediatr Pulmonol 2002; 33(5):380–387.

33. Downey R III, Perkin RM, MacQuarrie J. Upper airway resistance syndrome: sick, symptomatic but underrecognized. Sleep 1993; 16(7):620–623.

34. Chervin RD, Ruzicka DL, Wiebelhaus JL, et al. Tolerance of esophageal pressure monitoring during polysomnography in children. Sleep 2003; 26(8):1022–1026.

35. Brouilette R, Hanson D, David R, et al. A diagnostic approach to suspected obstructive sleep apnea in children. J Pediatr 1984; 105(1):10–14.

36. Brietzke SE, Katz ES, Roberson DW. Can history and physical examination reliably diagnose pediatric obstructive sleep apnea/hypopnea syndrome? A systematic review of the literature. Otolaryngol Head Neck Surg 2004; 131(6):827–832.

37. Carroll JL, McColley SA, Marcus CL, et al. Inability of clinical history to distinguish primary snoring from obstructive sleep apnea syndrome in children. Chest 1995; 108(3):610–618.

38. Weatherly RA, Mai EF, Ruzicka DL, et al. Identification and evaluation of obstructive sleep apnea prior to adenotonsillectomy in children: a survey of practice patterns. Sleep Med 2003; 4(4):297–307.

39. Goldstein NA, Pugazhendhi V, Rao SM, et al. Clinical assessment of pediatric obstructive sleep apnea. Pediatrics 2004; 114(1):33–43.

40. Chervin RD, Weatherly RA, Garetz SL, et al. Pediatric sleep questionnaire: prediction of sleep apnea and outcomes. Arch Otolaryngol Head Neck Surg 2007; 133(3): 216–222.

41. Brouillette RT, Morielli A, Leimanis A, et al. Nocturnal pulse oximetry as an abbreviated testing modality for pediatric obstructive sleep apnea. Pediatrics 2000; 105(2):405–412.

42. Brown KA, Laferriere A, Moss IR. Recurrent hypoxemia in young children with obstructive sleep apnea is associated with reduced opioid requirement for analgesia. Anesthesiology 2004; 100(4):806–810.

43. Brown KA, Laferriere A, Lakheeram I, et al. Recurrent hypoxemia in children is associated with increased analgesic sensitivity to opiates. Anesthesiology 2006; 105(4):665–669.

44. Nixon GM, Kermack AS, Davis GM, et al. Planning adenotonsillectomy in children with obstructive sleep apnea: the role of overnight oximetry. Pediatrics 2004; 113 (1 pt 1):e19–e25.

45. Sauerland EK, Harper RM. The human tongue during sleep: electromyographic activity of the genioglossus muscle. Exp Neurol 1976; 51(1):160–170.

46. Remmers JE, Degroot WJ, Sauerland EK, et al. Pathogenesis of upper airway occlusion during sleep. J Appl Physiol 1978; 44(6):931–938.

47. Brouillette RT, Thach BT. A neuromuscular mechanism maintaining extrathoracic airway patency. J Appl Physiol 1979; 46(4):772–779.

48. Brouillette RT, Thach BT. Control of genioglossus muscle inspiratory activity. J Appl Physiol 1980; 49(5):801–808.
49. Marcus CL, McColley SA, Carroll JL, et al. Upper airway collapsibility in children with obstructive sleep apnea syndrome. J Appl Physiol 1994; 77(2):918–924.
50. Isono S, Shimada A, Utsugi M, et al. Comparison of static mechanical properties of the passive pharynx between normal children and children with sleep-disordered breathing. Am J Respir Crit Care Med 1998; 157(4 pt 1):1204–1212.
51. Frank Y, Kravath RE, Pollak CP, et al. Obstructive sleep apnea and its therapy: clinical and polysomnographic manifestations. Pediatrics 1983; 71(5):737–742.
52. Goh DY, Galster P, Marcus CL. Sleep architecture and respiratory disturbances in children with obstructive sleep apnea. Am J Respir Crit Care Med 2000; 162(2 pt 1): 682–686.
53. Morielli A, Ladan S, Ducharme FM, et al. Can sleep and wakefulness be distinguished in children by cardiorespiratory and videotape recordings? Chest 1996; 109(3):680–687.
54. Jeans WD, Fernando DC, Maw AR, et al. A longitudinal study of the growth of the nasopharynx and its contents in normal children. Br J Radiol 1981; 54(638): 117–121.
55. Arens R, McDonough JM, Costarino AT, et al. Magnetic resonance imaging of the upper airway structure of children with obstructive sleep apnea syndrome. Am J Respir Crit Care Med 2001; 164(4):698–703.
56. Arens R, McDonough JM, Corbin AM, et al. Linear dimensions of the upper airway structure during development: assessment by magnetic resonance imaging. Am J Respir Crit Care Med 2002; 165(1):117–122.
57. Arens R, McDonough JM, Corbin AM, et al. Upper airway size analysis by magnetic resonance imaging of children with obstructive sleep apnea syndrome. Am J Respir Crit Care Med 2003; 167(1):65–70.
58. Felman AH, Loughlin GM, Leftridge CA Jr., et al. Upper airway obstruction during sleep in children. AJR Am J Roentgenol 1979; 133(2):213–216.
59. Fernbach SK, Brouillette RT, Riggs TW, et al. Radiologic evaluation of adenoids and tonsils in children with obstructive sleep apnea: plain films and fluoroscopy. Pediatr Radiol 1983; 13(5):258–265.
60. Xu C, Sin S, McDonough JM, et al. Computational fluid dynamics modeling of the upper airway of children with obstructive sleep apnea syndrome in steady flow. J Biomech 2006; 39(11):2043–2054.
61. Donnelly LF, Surdulescu V, Chini BA, et al. Upper airway motion depicted at cine MR imaging performed during sleep: comparison between young Patients with and those without obstructive sleep apnea. Radiology 2003; 227(1):239–245.
62. Shott SR, Donnelly LF. Cine magnetic resonance imaging: evaluation of persistent airway obstruction after tonsil and adenoidectomy in children with Down syndrome. Laryngoscope 2004; 114(10):1724–1729.
63. Marcus CL, Keens TG, Bautista DB, et al. Obstructive sleep apnea in children with Down syndrome. Pediatrics 1991; 88(1):132–139.
64. Donnelly LF, Shott SR, LaRose CR, et al. Causes of persistent obstructive sleep apnea despite previous tonsillectomy and adenoidectomy in children with down syndrome as depicted on static and dynamic cine MRI. AJR Am J Roentgenol 2004; 183(1):175–181.

65. Shott SR, Amin R, Chini B, et al. Obstructive sleep apnea: Should all children with Down syndrome be tested? Arch Otolaryngol Head Neck Surg 2006; 132(4): 432–436.

66. Uong EC, McDonough JM, Tayag-Kier CE, et al. Magnetic resonance imaging of the upper airway in children with Down syndrome. Am J Respir Crit Care Med 2001; 163(3 pt 1):731–736.

67. Lefaivre JF, Cohen SR, Burstein FD, et al. Down syndrome: identification and surgical management of obstructive sleep apnea. Plast Reconstr Surg 1997; 99(3): 629–637.

68. Brouillette RT, Fernbach SK, Hunt CE. Obstructive sleep apnea in infants and children. J Pediatr 1982; 100(1):31–40.

69. Marcus CL, Carroll JL, Koerner CB, et al. Determinants of growth in children with the obstructive sleep apnea syndrome. J Pediatr 1994; 125(4):556–562.

70. Bland RM, Bulgarelli S, Ventham JC, et al. Total energy expenditure in children with obstructive sleep apnoea syndrome. Eur Respir J 2001; 18(1):164–169.

71. Marcus CL. Total energy expenditure in children with obstructive sleep apnoea syndrome. Eur Respir J 2002; 19(6):1215–1216.

72. Bar A, Tarasiuk A, Segev Y, et al. The effect of adenotonsillectomy on serum insulin-like growth factor-I and growth in children with obstructive sleep apnea syndrome. J Pediatr 1999; 135(1):76–80.

73. Selimoglu E, Selimoglu MA, Orbak Z. Does adenotonsillectomy improve growth in children with obstructive adenotonsillar hypertrophy? J Int Med Res 2003; 31 (2):84–87.

74. Nieminen P, Lopponen T, Tolonen U, et al. Growth and biochemical markers of growth in children with snoring and obstructive sleep apnea. Pediatrics 2002; 109 (4):e55.

75. Soultan Z, Wadowski S, Rao M, et al. Effect of treating obstructive sleep apnea by tonsillectomy and/or adenoidectomy on obesity in children. Arch Pediatr Adolesc Med 1999; 153(1):33–37.

76. Nixon GM, Brouillette RT. Sleep and breathing in Prader-Willi syndrome. Pediatr Pulmonol 2002; 34(3):209–217.

77. Nitzan M, Spitzer S, Elian E. Obesity-hypoventilation (Pickwickian) syndrome in a child. Isr J Med Sci 1968; 4(2):264–269.

78. Lugaresi E, Coccagna G, Ceroni GB. Pickwick's syndrome and the primary alveolar hypoventilation syndrome. Acta Neurol Psychiatr Belg 1968; 68(1):15–25.

79. Hirooka M, Inaba Y, Ono T. The Pickwickian syndrome in a child. Tohoku J Exp Med 1969; 98(4):363–372.

80. Bradley TD. Right and left ventricular functional impairment and sleep apnea. Clin Chest Med 1992; 13(3):459–479.

81. Marcus CL, Greene MG, Carroll JL. Blood pressure in children with obstructive sleep apnea. Am J Respir Crit Care Med 1998; 157(4 pt 1):1098–1103.

82. Amin RS, Carroll JL, Jeffries JL, et al. Twenty-four-hour ambulatory blood pressure in children with sleep-disordered breathing. Am J Respir Crit Care Med 2004; 169(8):950–956.

83. Enright PL, Goodwin JL, Sherrill DL, et al. Blood pressure elevation associated with sleep-related breathing disorder in a community sample of white and Hispanic children: the Tucson Children's Assessment of Sleep Apnea study. Arch Pediatr Adolesc Med 2003; 157(9):901–904.

84. Leung LC, Ng DK, Lau MW, et al. Twenty-four-hour ambulatory BP in snoring children with obstructive sleep apnea syndrome. Chest 2006; 130(4):1009–1017.
85. Aljadeff G, Gozal D, Schechtman VL, et al. Heart rate variability in children with obstructive sleep apnea. Sleep 1997; 20(2):151–157.
86. Baharav A, Kotagal S, Rubin BK, et al. Autonomic cardiovascular control in children with obstructive sleep apnea. Clin Auton Res 1999; 9(6):345–351.
87. Ferri R, Curzi-Dascalova L, Del GS, et al. Heart rate variability and apnea during sleep in Down's syndrome. J Sleep Res 1998; 7(4):282–287.
88. Guilleminault C, Connolly S, Winkle R, et al. Cyclical variation of the heart rate in sleep apnoea syndrome. Mechanisms, and usefulness of 24 h electrocardiography as a screening technique. Lancet 1984; 1(8369):126–131.
89. Stradling JR, Thomas G, Warley AR, et al. Effect of adenotonsillectomy on nocturnal hypoxaemia, sleep disturbance, and symptoms in snoring children. Lancet 1990; 335 (8684):249–253.
90. Constantin E, McGregor CD, Cote V, et al. Pulse rate and pulse rate variability decrease after adenotonsillectomy for severe obstructive sleep apnea syndrome. Proc Am Thor Soc 2006; 3:A414.
91. Somers VK, Dyken ME, Clary MP, et al. Sympathetic neural mechanisms in obstructive sleep apnea. J Clin Invest 1995; 96(4):1897–1904.
92. Baruzzi A, Riva R, Cirignotta F, et al. Atrial natriuretic peptide and catecholamines in obstructive sleep apnea syndrome. Sleep 1991; 14(1):83–86.
93. Amin RS, Kimball TR, Kalra M, et al. Left ventricular function in children with sleep-disordered breathing. Am J Cardiol 2005; 95(6):801–804.
94. Amin RS, Kimball TR, Bean JA, et al. Left ventricular hypertrophy and abnormal ventricular geometry in children and adolescents with obstructive sleep apnea. Am J Respir Crit Care Med 2002; 165(10):1395–1399.
95. Shouldice RB, O'Brien LM, O'Brien C, et al. Detection of obstructive sleep apnea in pediatric subjects using surface lead electrocardiogram features. Sleep 2004; 27 (4):784–792.
96. Ebert CS Jr., Drake AF. The impact of sleep-disordered breathing on cognition and behavior in children: a review and meta-synthesis of the literature. Otolaryngol Head Neck Surg 2004; 131(6):814–826.
97. Halbower AC, Mahone EM. Neuropsychological morbidity linked to childhood sleep-disordered breathing. Sleep Med Rev 2006; 10(2):97–107.
98. Weissbluth M, Davis AT, Poncher J, et al. Signs of airway obstruction during sleep and behavioral, developmental, and academic problems. J Dev Behav Pediatr 1983; 4(2):119–121.
99. Ali NJ, Pitson DJ, Stradling JR. Snoring, sleep disturbance, and behaviour in 4-5 year olds. Arch Dis Child 1993; 68(3):360–366.
100. Ali NJ, Pitson D, Stradling JR. Natural history of snoring and related behaviour problems between the ages of 4 and 7 years. Arch Dis Child 1994; 71(1):74–76.
101. Chervin RD, Dillon JE, Bassetti C, et al. Symptoms of sleep disorders, inattention, and hyperactivity in children. Sleep 1997; 20(12):1185–1192.
102. Gozal D, Pope DW Jr. Snoring during early childhood and academic performance at ages thirteen to fourteen years. Pediatrics 2001; 107(6):1394–1399.
103. Ali NJ, Pitson D, Stradling JR. Sleep disordered breathing: effects of adenotonsillectomy on behaviour and psychological functioning. Eur J Pediatr 1996; 155 (1):56–62.

104. Gozal D. Sleep-disordered breathing and school performance in children. Pediatrics 1998; 102(3 pt 1):616–620.

105. Harvey JM, O'Callaghan MJ, Wales PD, et al. Six-month follow-up of children with obstructive sleep apnoea. J Paediatr Child Health 1999; 35(2):136–139.

106. Chervin RD, Ruzicka DL, Giordani BJ, et al. Sleep-disordered breathing, behavior, and cognition in children before and after adenotonsillectomy. Pediatrics 2006; 117 (4):e769–e778.

107. Constantin E, Kermack AS, Creighton D, et al. Adenotonsillectomy improves isSleep, breathing and quality of life, but not behavior. J Pediatr 2007; 150(5): 540–546.

108. Everett AD, Koch WC, Saulsbury FT. Failure to thrive due to obstructive sleep apnea. Clin Pediatr 1987; 26(2):90–92.

109. Mallory GB Jr., Fiser DH, Jackson R. Sleep-associated breathing disorders in morbidly obese children and adolescents. J Pediatr 1989; 115(6):892–897.

110. Marcus CL, Curtis S, Koerner CB, et al. Evaluation of pulmonary function and polysomnography in obese children and adolescents. Pediatr Pulmonol 1996; 21(3): 176–183.

111. Silvestri JM, Weese-Mayer DE, Bass MT, et al. Polysomnography in obese children with a history of sleep-associated breathing disorders. Pediatr Pulmonol 1993; 16(2): 124–129.

112. Redline S, Tishler PV, Schluchter M, et al. Risk factors for sleep-disordered breathing in children. Associations with obesity, race, and respiratory problems. Am J Respir Crit Care Med 1999; 159(5 Pt 1):1527–1532.

113. Tauman R, Gozal D. Obesity and obstructive sleep apnea in children. Paediatr Respir Rev 2006; 7(4):247–259.

114. Kelly A, Marcus CL. Childhood obesity, inflammation, and apnea: what is the future for our children? Am J Respir Crit Care Med 2005; 171(3):202–203.

115. Rosen GM, Muckle RP, Mahowald MW, et al. Postoperative respiratory compromise in children with obstructive sleep apnea syndrome: can it be anticipated? Pediatrics 1994; 93(5):784–788.

116. Spector A, Scheid S, Hassink S, et al. Adenotonsillectomy in the morbidly obese child. Int J Pediatr Otorhinolaryngol 2003; 67(4):359–364.

117. Franco RA Jr., Rosenfeld RM, Rao M. First place–resident clinical science award 1999. Quality of life for children with obstructive sleep apnea. Otolaryngol Head Neck Surg 2000; 123(1 pt 1):9–16.

118. Goldstein NA, Fatima M, Campbell TF, et al. Child behavior and quality of life before and after tonsillectomy and adenoidectomy. Arch Otolaryngol Head Neck Surg 2002; 128(7):770–775.

119. Stewart MG, Glaze DG, Friedman EM, et al. Quality of life and sleep study findings after adenotonsillectomy in children with obstructive sleep apnea. Arch Otolaryngol Head Neck Surg 2005; 131(4):308–314.

120. Rosen CL, Palermo TM, Larkin EK, et al. Health-related quality of life and sleep-disordered breathing in children. Sleep 2002; 25(6):657–666.

121. Schwimmer JB, Burwinkle TM, Varni JW. Health-related quality of life of severely obese children and adolescents. JAMA 2003; 289(14):1813–1819.

122. Mitchell RB, Kelly J, Call E, et al. Quality of life after adenotonsillectomy for obstructive sleep apnea in children. Arch Otolaryngol Head Neck Surg 2004; 130 (2):190–194.

123. Riley DJ, Santiago TV, Edelman NH. Complications of obesity-hypoventilation syndrome in childhood. Am J Dis Child 1976; 130(6):671–674.

124. Suen JS, Arnold JE, Brooks LJ. Adenotonsillectomy for treatment of obstructive sleep apnea in children. Arch Otolaryngol Head Neck Surg 1995; 121(5):525–530.

125. Tauman R, Gulliver TE, Krishna J, et al. Persistence of obstructive sleep apnea syndrome in children after adenotonsillectomy. J Pediatr 2006; 149(6):803–808.

126. Biavati MJ, Manning SC, Phillips DL. Predictive factors for respiratory complications after tonsillectomy and adenoidectomy in children. Arch Otolaryngol Head Neck Surg 1997; 123(5):517–521.

127. Brown KA, Morin I, Hickey C, et al. Urgent adenotonsillectomy: an analysis of risk factors associated with postoperative respiratory morbidity. Anesthesiology 2003; 99(3):586–595.

128. Cote CJ, Sheldon SH. Obstructive sleep apnea and tonsillectomy: do we have a new indication for extended postoperative observation? Can J Anaesth 2004; 51(1): 6–12.

129. Koomson A, Morin I, Brouillette R, et al. Children with severe OSAS who have adenotonsillectomy in the morning are less likely to have postoperative desaturation than those operated in the afternoon. Can J Anaesth 2004; 51(1):62–67.

130. McColley SA, April MM, Carroll JL, et al. Respiratory compromise after adenotonsillectomy in children with obstructive sleep apnea. Arch Otolaryngol Head Neck Surg 1992; 118(9):940–943.

131. Wilson K, Lakheeram I, Morielli A, et al. Can assessment for obstructive sleep apnea help predict postadenotonsillectomy respiratory complications? Anesthesiology 2002; 96(2):313–322.

132. Gregory GA, Kitterman JA, Phibbs RH, et al. Treatment of the idiopathic respiratory-distress syndrome with continuous positive airway pressure. N Engl J Med 1971; 284 (24):1333–1340.

133. Sullivan CE, Issa FG, Berthon-Jones M, et al. Reversal of obstructive sleep apnoea by continuous positive airway pressure applied through the nares. Lancet 1981; 1(8225):862–865.

134. Guilleminault C, Nino-Murcia G, Heldt G, et al. Alternative treatment to tracheostomy in obstructive sleep apnea syndrome: nasal continuous positive airway pressure in young children. Pediatrics 1986; 78(5):797–802.

135. Marcus CL, Ward SL, Mallory GB, et al. Use of nasal continuous positive airway pressure as treatment of childhood obstructive sleep apnea. J Pediatr 1995; 127(1): 88–94.

136. Waters KA, Everett FM, Bruderer JW, et al. Obstructive sleep apnea: the use of nasal CPAP in 80 children. Am J Respir Crit Care Med 1995; 152(2):780–785.

137. Kirk VG, O'Donnell AR. Continuous positive airway pressure for children: a discussion on how to maximize compliance. Sleep Med Rev 2006; 10(2):119–127.

138. Marcus CL, Rosen G, Ward SL, et al. Adherence to and effectiveness of positive airway pressure therapy in children with obstructive sleep apnea. Pediatrics 2006; 117(3):e442–e451.

139. O'Donnell AR, Bjornson CL, Bohn SG, et al. Compliance rates in children using noninvasive continuous positive airway pressure. Sleep 2006; 29(5):651–658.

140. Al-Ghamdi SA, Manoukian JJ, Morielli A, et al. Do systemic corticosteroids effectively treat obstructive sleep apnea secondary to adenotonsillar hypertrophy? Laryngoscope 1997; 107(10):1382–1387.

141. Demain JG, Goetz DW. Pediatric adenoidal hypertrophy and nasal airway obstruction: reduction with aqueous nasal beclomethasone. Pediatrics 1995; 95(3): 355–364.

142. Brouillette RT, Manoukian JJ, Ducharme FM, et al. Efficacy of fluticasone nasal spray for pediatric obstructive sleep apnea. J Pediatr 2001; 138(6):838–844.

143. Alexopoulos EI, Kaditis AG, Kalampouka E, et al. Nasal corticosteroids for children with snoring. Pediatr Pulmonol 2004; 38(2):161–167.

144. Criscuoli G, D'Amora S, Ripa G, et al. Frequency of surgery among children who have adenotonsillar hypertrophy and improve after treatment with nasal beclomethasone. Pediatrics 2003; 111(3):e236–e238.

145. Goldbart AD, Veling MC, Goldman JL, et al. Glucocorticoid receptor subunit expression in adenotonsillar tissue of children with obstructive sleep apnea. Pediatr Res 2005; 57(2):232–236.

146. Goldbart AD, Goldman JL, Veling MC, et al. Leukotriene modifier therapy for mild sleep-disordered breathing in children. Am J Respir Crit Care Med 2005; 172 (3):364–370.

147. Kheirandish L, Goldbart AD, Gozal D. Intranasal steroids and oral leukotriene modifier therapy in residual sleep-disordered breathing after tonsillectomy and adenoidectomy in children. Pediatrics 2006; 117(1):e61–e66.

Index

T - #0025 - 101024 - C4 - 229/152/35 [37] - CB - 9781420060829 - Gloss Lamination